CLEFT PALATE AND CRANIOFACIAL ANOMALIES

Effects on Speech and Resonance

THIRD EDITION

ANN W. KUMMER, PH.D., CCC-SLP, ASHA-F

Senior Director, Division of Speech-Language Pathology
Cincinnati Children's Hospital Medical Center
and
Professor of Clinical Pediatrics and
Professor of Otolaryngology–Head and Neck Surgery
University of Cincinnati Medical Center

with Contributions

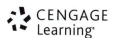

Australia • Brazil • Canada • Mexico • Singapore • Spain • United Kingdom • United States

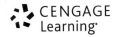
CENGAGE
Learning

**Cleft Palate and Craniofacial Anomalies:
Effects on Speech and Resonance
Third Edition
Ann W. Kummer**

Vice President, Careers & Computing:
  Dave Garza

Director of Learning Solutions: Stephen Helba

Acquisitions Editor: Thomas Stover

Director, Development-Career and Computing:
  Marah Bellegarde

Product Development Manager: Juliet Steiner

Senior Product Manager: Natalie Pashoukos

Editorial Assistant: Cassie Cloutier

Brand Manager: Wendy Mapstone

Market Development Manager:
  Jonathan Sheehan

Senior Production Director: Wendy Troeger

Production Manager: Andrew Crouth

Content Project Manager: Allyson Bozeth

Senior Art Director: David Arsenault

Media Editor: William Overocker

Cover image(s): © istockphoto.com/Anna
  Grabowski; © istockphoto.com/Jeannette
  Meier Kamer

Library of Congress Control Number: 2013934774

ISBN-13: 978-1-133-73236-5

Delmar

Executive Woods

5 Maxwell Drive

Clifton Park, NY 12065

USA

Cengage Learning is a leading provider of customized learning solutions with office locations around the globe, including Singapore, the United Kingdom, Australia, Mexico, Brazil, and Japan. Locate your local office at: **www.cengage.com/global**

Cengage Learning products are represented in Canada by Nelson Education, Ltd.

To learn more about Delmar, visit **www.cengage.com/delmar**

Purchase any of our products at your local college store or at our preferred online store **www.cengagebrain.com**

Notice to the Reader

Printed in the United States of America
2 3 4 5 6 7 18 17 16 15 14

DEDICATION

This book is dedicated to the three people who have influenced me most in my life and have helped me to be the best that I can be. Without their love and support, I would never have had a career and certainly would not have had the opportunity to write this book … now for the third time.

The first dedication is to my father, who was a wonderful, caring, and talented otolaryngologist whom I always admired. Dad, I always wanted to be just like you when I grew up.

The next dedication is to my mother, who is the kindest, most thoughtful, and most caring person that I have ever known. Mom, now that I am grown up, I strive to be more like you.

The final dedication is to my husband, who has supported me, encouraged me, and helped me to focus and succeed in my career. John, you have allowed me to spread my wings and fly. For that I will be eternally grateful!

With all my love, Ann

CONTENTS

PART 3

PART 4

PREFACE

Anticipating the birth of a new baby is usually a very exciting time of life. The expectant couple does many things to prepare for the baby, including setting up a nursery, gathering baby clothes and diapers, and deciding on a name. The parents expect to have a normal baby, with 10 fingers, 10 toes, and an intact face. Usually, they are totally unprepared for the possibility of a different outcome.

Unfortunately, not all babies are born with perfect structures. When a child is born with cleft lip and/or cleft palate or other craniofacial anomalies, this is a true shock, especially because it involves the face. This can be a devastating blow to the family. What was expected to be a very happy and exciting time becomes a very stressful and emotional time for the parents and other family members. It may be impossible for the parents to see past the anomaly in order to really appreciate and bond with their newborn baby.

Cleft lip or palate is the fourth most common birth defect and the first most common facial birth defect. In fact, about 1 in every 600 children born in the United States each year has a cleft of the lip and/or palate. About half of these children have other associated malformations. Cleft palate is a characteristic of well over 400 recognized syndromes.

Although current medical technology is not advanced enough to prevent the occurrence of these birth defects, most of the speech and physical impairments associated with craniofacial anomalies can be improved or even corrected with the help of a team of various professionals. To provide the type of care that these patients require, this group of professionals must be specialists within their field. For true quality care, they must have a thorough understanding of the current methods of evaluation and treatment of these patients.

Considering the prevalence of clefts and craniofacial anomalies in the general population, however, all health care providers should have at least basic knowledge about the management of these patients and appropriate referrals. In particular, speech-language pathologists must be trained in the basic evaluation, treatment, and appropriate referrals of individuals with these anomalies, considering the fact that they often have a significant effect on speech. Certainly, school-based speech-language pathologists are very likely to have children on their caseloads with a history of cleft, craniofacial anomalies, or resonance disorders.

PURPOSE OF THIS BOOK

The purpose of this book is to inform, educate, and excite students and professionals in speech-language pathology and in the medical and dental professions regarding the management of individuals with a history of cleft or craniofacial anomalies. This book is designed to be a textbook for graduate students and also a sourcebook for health care professionals who provide services in this area. My goal in writing this book was to provide readers with a great deal of information, but in a way that is both interesting and easy to read. As an active clinician myself, my intent was to make this book a very practical "how-to" guide, as well as a source of didactic and theoretical information.

My ultimate goal with this book was to improve the knowledge of treating professionals who work with individuals who are affected by a cleft or other craniofacial conditions. It is hoped that with this knowledge, they can positively impact the quality of care provided to this population.

ORGANIZATION

This book was written in a purposeful sequence so that the information from each chapter builds on the information from previous chapters.

Part 1 of this text provides basic information on the normal anatomy of the orofacial structures and the normal physiology of the velopharyngeal valve. Once the normal structures and function are described, information on clefts and craniofacial anomalies is discussed in subsequent chapters. The various causes of these anomalies, including the genetic bases, are reviewed. When the reader has completed the first section, there should be a firm understanding of normal and abnormal facial and velopharyngeal features and the potential causes of abnormalities.

Part 2 of this text includes chapters on the various problems associated with clefts and craniofacial anomalies. In particular, this section covers the effects of these anomalies on feeding, dentition, language, cognition, articulation, resonance, hearing, and psychosocial development. After completing the second section, the reader will have an understanding of the number, types, and complexity of the problems that are secondary to clefts and craniofacial anomalies. It will then be apparent to the reader that there is a need for multidisciplinary management of these patients in an interdisciplinary setting.

Part 3 of this text covers the various diagnostic methods for assessing speech, resonance, and velopharyngeal function. This section includes the perceptual examination of speech and resonance, and the physical examination of the oral cavity and other orofacial structures. There is an overview chapter on instrumentation that is sufficient for graduate students. There are also individual chapters on the various types of instrumental procedures. These chapters are very detailed and are written to provide specific information for practicing clinicians who will be using these procedures.

Part 4 of this book discusses the treatment of speech and resonance disorders secondary to clefts, craniofacial anomalies, and velopharyngeal dysfunction. This section includes surgical management, prosthetic management, and speech therapy.

Part 5 of this book is short but important because it emphasizes the fact that many disciplines are needed to provide care for patients affected by clefts or craniofacial anomalies. The reader will complete this section with an understanding that quality patient care necessitates interdisciplinary interaction and collaboration in the assessment and treatment of these patients.

FEATURES

- **Chapter outlines:** The outlines of each chapter help readers navigate through the content and find information quickly.

- **Illustrations:** This text includes *433 photos* and *94 line drawings* for a total of *527 illustrations*. These illustrations are meant to enhance comprehension of information and concepts discussed in the chapters.

- **Case studies:** Several chapters include patient case studies to illustrate how chapter information applies to real-life situations.

- **For Review and Discussion:** A list of questions and topics for discussion is included at the end of each chapter. The purpose of this section is to help the reader synthesize and apply information presented in the chapter. Professors can also use this section for class discussion, student homework, or for essay exams.

- **Definitions:** Selected *technical and medical terms* are presented in italics and defined at the first occurrence in the book.

- **Glossary:** There is a glossary of terms at the back of the book that defines all the medical and technical terms that were italicized in the individual chapters. The student may find that studying the glossary is helpful for learning much of the information in the book.

- **Appendices:** The appendices contain resource information for parents and guardians, and include a list of publications and parent support groups.

- **Videos:** There are many videos of various speech and resonance disorders and of diagnostic and treatment techniques.

NEW TO THIS EDITION

- **Chapter order:** The order of some of the chapters and sections has been changed for better flow.

- **Chapter outlines:** The outlines of all chapters were simplified and are more consistent between chapters.

- **New chapter:** Because the individual instrumental chapters are very detailed, there is now a new chapter entitled *Overview of Instrumental Procedures*. This chapter is designed for graduate students and other health care providers who need to know what instrumental procedures are available, but do not need the details of how to actually perform these procedures.

- **Speech Notes:** Chapters regarding anomalies and surgeries have boxed sections called *Speech Notes*. These sections highlight how these anomalies or surgeries affect speech and resonance.

- **New figures:** Almost *150 new figures* (photos and line art) were added to this edition.

- **Phonetic symbols:** In this edition, phonetic symbols, rather than letters, are used for speech sounds, as is done in other speech pathology texts. A key to these symbols is included for physicians and other professionals who are not familiar with phonetic symbols.

- **Glossary:** The glossary has been greatly expanded with many more word definitions.

ONLINE RESOURCES

- **Cleft Notes:** The *Cleft Notes* are basic summaries in table format and are provided for each chapter. There are some compare-and-contrast aspects of these tables to help the student assimilate the information. There are two versions of the Cleft Notes—a blank version for students to use when taking notes or studying, and a filled-out version for instructors/professors.

- **Handouts:** There are online handouts on a variety of topics that are covered in this book. These handouts are designed primarily for parents, but can also be helpful to other professionals who are not familiar with the topic area. The handouts are designed so the user can print them directly from the website. These can be printed and distributed as long as the heading, logo, and content are not altered.

- **Videos:** More than 240 patient videos are online and more will be added over time. These videos Illustrate different speech and resonance disorders, evaluation techniques, and treatment techniques. There are also many videos of nasopharyngoscopy, videofluoroscopy, and even nasometry studies. These videos are designed to help the viewer develop diagnostic and treatment skills. Because the videos are carefully edited, this is better than direct observation of a clinic.

- **PowerPoint® Presentations:** There are PowerPoint presentations for each chapter, which include important figures and photos.

- **Exam and Test Yourself Questions:** There are many multiple-choice questions for each chapter. These can be used by the instructor/ professor for exams or can be given to the students to use for studying the material.

- **eBook:** This book is available as both a printed text and an ebook. It is now possible to purchase single chapters of the ebook.

FORMAT NOTES

Service providers must be sensitive to the emotional and psychological needs of the patient. Sensitivity to the feelings of the patient is often overlooked by well-meaning service providers. It is easy to forget that we deal with real people, not just interesting cases. This lack of sensitivity is sometimes reflected in the terminology that is used in the literature and in daily use. I recall listening to a speech given by an adult who was born with a cleft palate. As he described his childhood, he pointed out that being called a "cleft palate child" evoked very negative feelings. Fortunately, this type of phrase is becoming "politically incorrect," just as the term "harelip" has in the past. Using the anomaly as an adjective to describe the individual is certainly insensitive to the feelings of the person who was born with this anomaly. Therefore, it is preferable to use "patient first" terminology as in "child with a cleft."

The reader will note that the word "child" is frequently used throughout the text for the individual with the anomaly. This is because the speech and resonance disorders secondary to cleft lip/palate and craniofacial anomalies are usually addressed during childhood. However, it should be understood that this information also applies to adults with the same anomalies.

ACKNOWLEDGEMENTS

There are so many people for whom I would like to acknowledge for their help with this edition of the text. I am grateful for the work of several outstanding students, including Brooke Goodall, for her help in researching and updating the literature; Brooke Goodall, Vanessa Hardin, and Nicole Brenza, for help in compiling the video case studies; and Jennifer Hanson, for her work in developing the PowerPoint presentations for each chapter.

Many thanks go to the members of our Resonance Specialty Team at Cincinnati Children's, including Molly Hylton Dow, M.A.; Shyla Miller, M.A.; Allison Flynn, M.A.; Janet H. Middendorf, M.A.; and Meg Toner, M.A. They were very helpful in providing feedback, developing the Cleft Notes, and reviewing videos. In particular, I would like to thank Meg Toner for an excellent job in coordinating the Video Case Studies project. I would like to thank Mary Gilene, our division's project manager, for her invaluable help with EndNote, the handouts, PowerPoints, and many other miscellaneous things. I am indebted to my administrative assistants, Colleen Kinnard (who left me to attend graduate school in speech-language pathology) and Debbie Kleemeier. Both of them helped me in many ways, including editing, formatting, and tracking down permissions.

Thanks to Robert McClurkin, Director of Product Management and Marketing at KayPENTAX, for feedback regarding Chapters 14 and 17; to Sid Khosla, M.D., Assistant Professor in the Department of Otolaryngology–Head and Neck Surgery at the University of Cincinnati, for feedback regarding Chapter 7; and to Mackinnon Webster, Vice President, Strategic Partnerships and Program Development at The Smile Train, for feedback regarding Chapter 23. I especially want to thank the reviewers of this text for their time and efforts. Their comments and suggestions were very valuable.

Special thanks go to Janet H. Middendorf, M.A., who is my colleague and friend. She has helped me and covered patients and clinics for me on many occasions so that I could travel or work on this book! Finally, I'd like to thank the members of the Craniofacial Team at Cincinnati Children's Hospital Medical Center (CCHMC) for being such great colleagues, mentors, and friends! I have learned so much from all of them.

Finally, I would like to acknowledge my husband. This book consumed an enormous amount of my personal time and energy. I could not have done it without his support, encouragement, patience, and understanding.

FEEDBACK

I would like to encourage the readers of this text to contact me by e-mail (ann.kummer@cchmc.org) with suggestions or comments about this text. My goal is to constantly improve this text over time.

FINAL WORDS

Speaking for myself and for all the contributors, we are grateful for the opportunity to present this information to you. We are hopeful that you will be educated, enlightened, and inspired to provide superior clinical services for individuals with clefts or other craniofacial conditions.

Ann W. Kummer

REVIEWERS

Nancye C. Roussel, Ph.D., CCC-SLP
Head, Department of Communicative Disorders
University of Louisiana, Lafayette
Lafayette, Louisiana

Monica C. Devers, Ph.D., CCC-SLP
Interim Dean, School of Health and Human Services
St. Cloud State University
St. Cloud, MN

Dianne Altuna, M.S./CCC-SLP
Lecturer II, Department of
Communication Disorders
University of Texas at Dallas
Dallas, Texas

Ann Blanton, Ph.D., CCC-SLP
Assistant Professor
CSU Sacramento
Sacramento, CA

Key to Phonetic Symbols

(includes only those used in this book)

Vowels

Symbol	Examples
/i/	**bee, see**
/æ/	hat, cat
/ɑ/	father, pot
/ɚ/	teach**er,** moth**er**

Consonants

Symbol	Letters	Examples
ʔ	glottal stop	bu**tt**on, mi**tt**en
/ʃ/	sh	**sh**oe
/ʒ/	zh	mea**s**ure
/ʧ/	ch	**ch**air
/dʒ/	j	**j**ump
/θ/	th	**th**in
/ð/	th	**th**en
/ŋ/	ng	si**ng**

ABOUT THE AUTHOR

ANN W. KUMMER, PH.D., CCC-SLP, is Senior Director of the Division of Speech-Language Pathology at Cincinnati Children's Hospital Medical Center and Professor of Clinical Pediatrics, and Professor of Otolaryngology–Head and Neck Surgery at the University of Cincinnati Medical Center.

Under her direction, the Division of Speech-Language Pathology at Cincinnati Children's has grown to be the largest and one of the most respected programs in the country. Dr. Kummer gives frequent lectures on leadership and professional business practices in speech-language pathology. She is also one of the authors of the text *Business Practices: A Guide for Speech-Language Pathologists*, published by the American Speech-Language-Hearing Association (ASHA) in 2004. She was one of the main developers of workflow software that won the 1995 International Beacon Award through IBM/Lotus. (Derivative software is marketed by Chart Links.)

As a clinician and researcher, Dr. Kummer specializes in speech and resonance disorders secondary to cleft palate, craniofacial anomalies, and velopharyngeal dysfunction. She is a long-term member of the Craniofacial Team at Cincinnati Children's and at Shriners Hospitals for Children in Cincinnati. She also provides services through the multidisciplinary VPI Clinic. She has worked with several international volunteer organizations for cleft palate, and is an active member of the American Cleft Palate–Craniofacial Association (ACPA) and the American Speech-Language Hearing Association (ASHA), serving on many committees.

Dr. Kummer has done several hundred lectures and seminars on a national and international level on cleft palate, craniofacial conditions, resonance disorders, and velopharyngeal dysfunction. She is the author of many professional articles, as well as over 20 book chapters in speech pathology and medical texts. In addition to this text, she is the co-author of the Simplified Nasometric Assessment Procedures (SNAP) Test (1996) and the author of the SNAP-R Test (2005) for the Nasometer II (KayPENTAX, Montvale, N.J.). She holds a patent on the Nasoscope device, which is marketed as the Oral & Nasal Listener (Super Duper, Inc.).

Dr. Kummer has received Honors of the Southwestern Ohio Speech-Language and Hearing Association (1995); Honors of the Ohio Speech-Language and Hearing Association (OSLHA) (1997); the Elwood Chaney Outstanding Clinician Award from the Ohio Speech-Language and Hearing Association (OSLHA) (2012); distinguished alumnus award from the Department of Communication Sciences and Disorders of the University of Cincinnati (1999); and the distinguished alumnus award from the College of Allied Health at the University of Cincinnati (2012). She was elected Fellow of the American Speech-Language-Hearing Association (ASHA) in 2002. She was named one of the top 25 most influential therapists in the United States by Therapy Times (2006); and named one of the 10 Most Inspiring Women in Cincinnati (2007).

Dr. Kummer received her bachelor's and master's degrees from Indiana University and her Ph.D. from the University of Cincinnati.

CONTRIBUTORS

David A. Billmire, M.D.[*]
Professor of Clinical Surgery
University of Cincinnati College of Medicine
Director, Plastic Surgery Division
Cincinnati Children's Hospital Medical Center
Address:
Cincinnati Children's Hospital Medical Center
3333 Burnet Avenue
Cincinnati, Ohio 45229-3039

Richard Campbell, D.M.D., M.S.[*]
Assistant Professor of Clinical Pediatrics
University of Cincinnati College of Medicine
Director, Orthodontics
Division of Pediatric Dentistry
Cincinnati Children's Hospital Medical Center
Address:
Cincinnati Children's Hospital Medical Center
3333 Burnet Avenue
Cincinnati, Ohio 45229-3039

Julia Corcoran, M.D.
Associate Professor of Surgery
Feinberg School of Medicine Northwestern University
Attending Surgeon
Ann and Robert H. Lurie Children's Hospital of Chicago
Address:
Division of Pediatric Plastic Surgery
225 E Chicago Avenue, Box 93
Chicago, IL 60611

Deepak Krishnan, D.D.S.[*]
Assistant Professor of Surgery
Residency Program Director
Division of Oral & Maxillofacial Surgery

Address:
University of Cincinnati College of Medicine
231 Albert Sabin Way
Cincinnati, Ohio 45267-0558

Murray Dock, D.D.S., M.S. D.
Associate Professor of Clinical Pediatrics
University of Cincinnati College of Medicine
Division of Pediatric Dentistry
Cincinnati Children's Hospital Medical Center
Address:
Cincinnati Children's Hospital Medical Center
3333 Burnet Avenue
Cincinnati, Ohio 45229-3039

Robert J. Hopkin, M.D.[*]
Associate Professor of Clinical Pediatrics
University of Cincinnati College of Medicine
Division of Human Genetics
Cincinnati Children's Hospital Medical Center
Address:
Cincinnati Children's Hospital Medical Center
3333 Burnet Avenue
Cincinnati, Ohio 45229-3039

Claire K. Miller, Ph.D.
Program Director, Aerodigestive and Sleep Center
Speech Pathologist III
Division of Speech-Language Pathology
Cincinnati Children's Hospital Medical Center
Address:
Cincinnati Children's Hospital Medical Center
3333 Burnet Avenue
Cincinnati, Ohio 45229-3039

Howard M. Saal, M.D.[*]
Professor of Pediatrics
University of Cincinnati College of Medicine
Director, Clinical Genetics
Division of Human Genetics
Cincinnati Children's Hospital Medical Center

Address:
Cincinnati Children's Hospital Medical Center
3333 Burnet Avenue
Cincinnati, Ohio 45229-3039

Janet R. Schultz, Ph.D.[*]
Professor
Psychology Department
Xavier University
Address:
Xavier University
3800 Victory Parkway
Cincinnati, Ohio 45207-6511

J. Paul Willging, M.D.[*]
Professor
Department of Otolaryngology–Head and Neck Surgery
University of Cincinnati College
    of Medicine
Cincinnati Children's Hospital Medical Center
Address:
Cincinnati Children's Hospital Medical Center
3333 Burnet Avenue
Cincinnati, Ohio 45229-3039

David J. Zajac, Ph.D.
Associate Professor
Department of Dental Ecology and the Craniofacial Center
University of North Carolina at Chapel Hill
Address:
Craniofacial Center
CB# 7450
University of North Carolina at Chapel Hill
Chapel Hill, North Carolina 27599

[*]Denotes current members of the team of The Craniofacial Center, Cincinnati Children's Hospital
  Medical Center, Cincinnati, Ohio

NORMAL STRUCTURES, CLEFTS, AND CRANIOFACIAL ANOMALIES

C H A P T E R

1

ANATOMY AND PHYSIOLOGY: FACIAL, ORAL, AND VELOPHARYNGEAL STRUCTURES

CHAPTER OUTLINE

INTRODUCTION

The nasal, oral, and pharyngeal structures are all very important for normal speech and resonance. Unfortunately, these are the structures that are commonly affected by cleft lip and palate and other craniofacial anomalies. Before the speech-language pathologist can fully understand the effects of oral and craniofacial anomalies on speech and resonance, a thorough understanding of normal structure is important. In addition, knowledge about normal function of the oral structures and the velopharyngeal valve is essential before the speech-language pathologist will be able to effectively evaluate abnormal speech and velopharyngeal dysfunction.

This chapter reviews the basic anatomy of the structures of the orofacial and velopharyngeal complex as they relate to speech production. The physiology of the subsystems of speech, including the velopharyngeal mechanism, is also described. For more detailed information on anatomy and physiology of the speech articulators, the interested reader is referred to other sources (Cassell & Elkadi, 1995; Cassell, Moon, & Elkadi, 1990; Dickson, 1972, 1975; Dickson & Dickson, 1972; Dickson, Grant, Sicher, Dubrul, & Paltan, 1974, 1975; Huang, Lee, & Rajendran, 1998; Kuehn, 1979; Maue-Dickson, 1977, 1979; Maue-Dickson & Dickson, 1980; Maue-Dickson, Dickson, & Rood, 1976; Moon & Kuehn, 1996, 1997, 2004; Perry, 2011; Seikel, King, & Drumright, 2005).

EAR

The *external ear* is comprised of the pinna and the external auditory canal. The *pinna* is the delicate cartilaginous framework of the external ear. It functions to direct sound energy into the *external auditory canal*, which is a skin-lined canal leading from the opening of the external ear to the eardrum.

The *middle ear* is a hollow space within the temporal bone. The *mastoid cavity* connects to the middle ear space posteriorly and is comprised of a collection of air cells within the temporal bone. Both the middle ear and mastoid cavities are lined with a *mucous membrane (mucosa)*, which consists of stratified squamous epithelium and lamina propria. (This should not be confused with *mucus*, which is the clear, viscid secretion from the mucous membranes.)

The *tympanic membrane*, also called the *eardrum*, is considered part of the middle ear. The tympanic membrane transmits sound energy through the ossicles to the inner ear. The three tiny bones in the middle ear are called the *ossicles*, and they include the malleus, incus, and stapes. The *malleus* (hammer) is firmly attached to the tympanic membrane. The *incus* (anvil) articulates with both the malleus and the stapes. The *stapes* acts as a piston to create pressure waves within the fluid-filled cochlea, which is part of the inner ear. The tympanic membrane and ossicles act to amplify the sound energy and efficiently introduce this energy into the liquid environment of the cochlea.

The *Eustachian tube* connects the middle ear with the nasopharynx. The end of this tube that terminates in the nasopharynx is closed at rest. During swallowing, the tensor veli palatini muscle contracts to open the Eustachian tube. This provides ventilation for the middle ear and mastoid cavities, and also results in equalization of air pressure between the middle ear and the environment (Cunsolo, Marchioni, Leo, Incorvaia, & Presutti, 2010; Licameli, 2002; Yoshida, Takahashi, Morikawa, & Kobayashi, 2007).

The *inner ear* consists of the cochlea and semicircular canals. The *cochlea* is composed of a bony spiral tube that is shaped like a snail's shell. Within this bony tube are delicate membranes separating the canal into three separate fluid-filled spaces. The *organ of Corti* is the site where mechanical energy introduced into the cochlea is converted into electrical stimulation conducted by the auditory nerves to the auditory cortex, which results in an awareness of sound. Inner and outer *hair cells* (sensory cells with hair-like properties) of the cochlea may be damaged by a variety of mechanisms, leading to sensorineural hearing loss.

A second function of the inner ear is balance. The *semicircular canals* are the loop-shaped tubular parts of the inner ear that provide a sense of spatial orientation. They are oriented in three planes at right angles to one another. The *saccule* and *utricle* are additional sensory organs within the inner ear. Hair cells within these organs have small calcium carbonate granules that respond to gravity, motion, and acceleration.

FACIAL STRUCTURES

Although the facial structures are familiar to all, some aspects of the face are important to point out for a thorough understanding of congenital anomalies and clefting. The normal facial landmarks can be seen on Figure 1–1A and Figure 1–1B. The student is encouraged to identify the same structures on the photo of the normal infant face shown in Figure 1–1B.

Nose and Nasal Cavity

Starting with the nose, the *nasal root* is where the nose begins at the level of the eyes. The *nasal bridge*, also known as the *nasion*, is the bony structure that is located between the eyes and corresponds with the nasofrontal suture. The nostrils are separated by the *columella* (little column), which is the structure that supports the nasal tip and is between the nostrils. The columella is at the anterior end of the nasal septum and consists of epidermis, cartilage, and mucosa. Ideally, the columella is straight and backed by a straight nasal septum. It must also be long enough so that the nasal tip has an appropriate degree of projection.

The nostrils are frequently referred to as *nares*, although an individual nostril is a *naris*. The *ala nasi* (*ala* is Latin for "wing") is the outside curved side of the nostril, which consists of cartilage. The alae are the two curved sides of the nostril. The *alar rim* is the outside curved edge that surrounds the opening to the nostril on either side, and the *alar base* is the area where the ala meets the upper lip. The *nasal sill* is the base of the nostril opening. The *piriform aperture*, which literally means pear-shaped opening, is the opening to the nostril or nasal cavity. The *nasal vestibule* is the most anterior part of the nasal cavity and is enclosed by the cartilages of the nose.

The *nasal septum*, as can be seen in Figure 1–2, is in the midline and separates the nasal cavity into two halves. The *quadrangular cartilage* forms the anterior nasal septum and projects anteriorly to the columella. (The anterior nasal spine of the maxilla forms a base

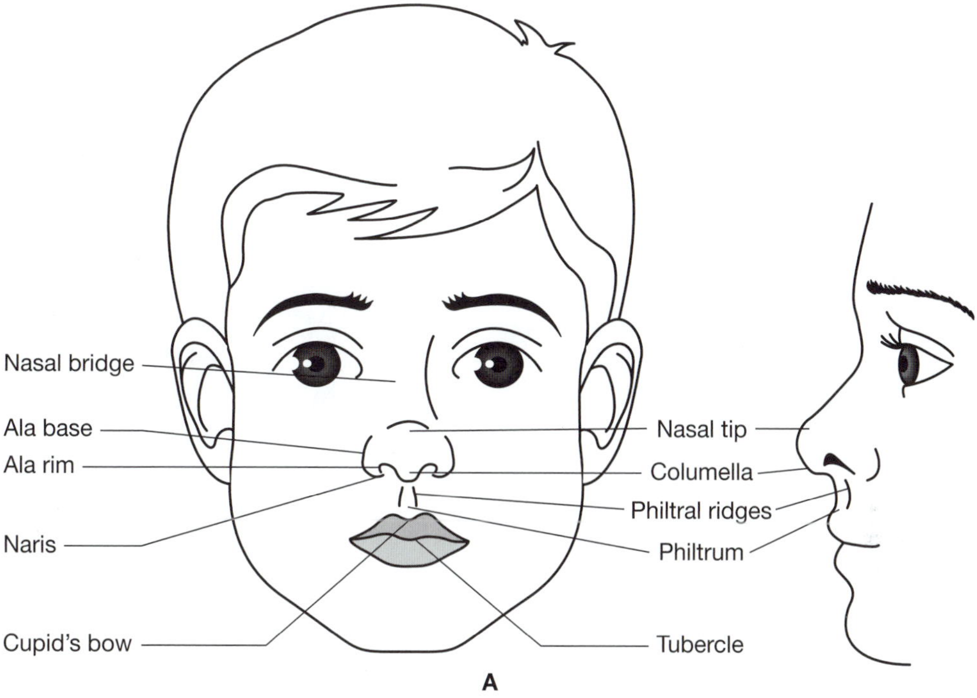

Nasal bridge

Ala base

Ala rim

Naris

Cupid's bow

Nasal tip

Columella

Philtral ridges

Philtrum

Tubercle

A

FIGURE 1–1A   Normal facial landmarks. Note the structures on the diagram.

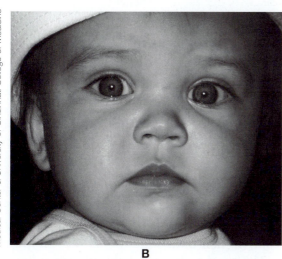

B

FIGURE 1–1B   Normal face. Try to locate the same structures on this infant's face.

for the columella.) The *vomer* is a trapezoidal-shaped bone in the nasal septum. It is positioned perpendicular to the palate and as such, the lower portion of the vomer fits in a groove formed by the median palatine suture line on the nasal aspect of the maxilla. The *perpendicular plate of the ethmoid* projects downward to join the vomer. It is not uncommon for the nasal septum to be less than perfectly straight, particularly in adults. The nasal septum is covered with mucous membrane, which is the lining tissue of the nasal cavity, oral cavity, and the pharynx. The nasal septum and nasal cavity, as well as the oral and pharyngeal cavities, are lined with a mucous membrane.

The *nasal turbinates*, also called *nasal conchae* (*concha*, singular), are paired shelf-like

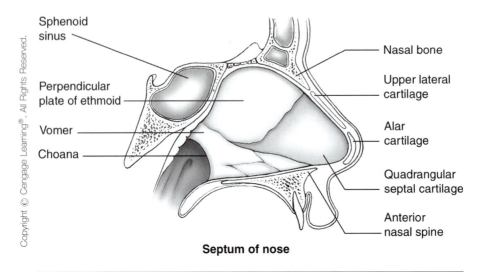

Septum of nose

FIGURE 1–2 The nasal septum and related structures.

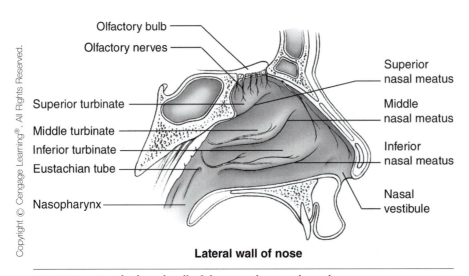

Lateral wall of nose

FIGURE 1–3 The lateral wall of the nose showing the turbinates.

bony structures that are attached to the lateral walls of the nose and protrude into the nasal cavity. They are long, narrow, and curled (Figure 1–3). The curled shape helps to create turbulent airflow (thus their name) within the nose to maximize contact of the inspired air with the nasal mucosa that covers the bones.

The superior and middle turbinates are parts of the ethmoid bone. The inferior turbinates, which are largest, are separate and unique bones of their own.

The nasal turbinates within the nose have three distinct functions. First, the mucous blanket covering the nasal mucosa traps particulate contaminants in order to filter inspired air of gross contaminants. Second, the turbinates warm and humidify the inspired air. This is done as nasal mucosa goes through alternating periods of vascular engorgement and decongestion. These periods alternate between sides every 90 minutes. The period of engorgement of the nasal lining promotes the warming and humidification of the inspired air. The third function of the turbinates is to deflect air superiorly in the nose in order to enhance the sense of smell.

Directly under the turbinates are the superior, middle, and inferior *nasal meatuses* (*meatus*, singular), which are the openings or passageways through which the air flows. At the back of the nasal cavity, on each side of the posterior part of the vomer, is a *choana* (*choanae*, plural), which is a funnel-shaped opening that leads to the nasopharynx.

Finally, the *paranasal sinuses* are air-filled spaces in the bones of the face and skull. These structures are each about the size of a walnut and are shown in Figure 8–5 as they would be seen through computed tomography. There are four pairs of paranasal sinuses: frontal sinuses (in the forehead area), maxillary sinuses (under the cheeks), ethmoid sinuses (between the eyes), and finally, sphenoid sinuses (deep in the skull). These sinuses are connected to the nose by a small opening called an *ostium* (*ostia*, plural).

Upper Lip

The features of the upper lip can be seen in Figure 1–1A. An examination of the upper lip reveals the *philtrum*, which is a long dimple or indentation that courses from the columella down to the upper lip. The philtrum is bordered by the *philtral ridges* on each side. These ridges are actually embryological suture lines that are formed as the segments of the upper lip fuse. The philtrum and philtral ridges course downward from the nose and terminate at the edge of the upper lip.

The top of the upper lip is called the *Cupid's bow* due to its characteristic shape, which includes a rounded configuration with an indentation in the middle. The upper and lower lips are both highlighted by the *white roll*, which is border tissue surrounding the red portion of the lip, called the *vermilion*. On the upper lip, the inferior border of the midsection of the vermilion comes to a point and is somewhat prominent. Therefore, it is referred to as the *labial tubercle*. In its naturally closed position, the upper lip rests over and slightly in front of the lower lip, although the inferior border of the upper lip is inverted.

ORAL STRUCTURES

Oral structures include the tongue, the faucial pillars, and the palate. The palate can be separated into two main parts: the hard palate and the soft palate (Figure 1–4). The *hard palate* is a bony structure that separates the oral cavity from the nasal cavity. The *velum*, frequently referred to as the *soft palate*, is the part of the palate that is muscular and is located in the back of the mouth, just posterior to the hard palate. At the posterior edge of the velum is the pendulous uvula. These structures are discussed in more detail as follows.

Tongue

The tongue resides within the arch of the mandible and fills the oral cavity when the mouth is closed. With the mouth closed, the slight negative pressure within the oral cavity ensures that the tongue adheres to the palate and the tip rests against the alveolar

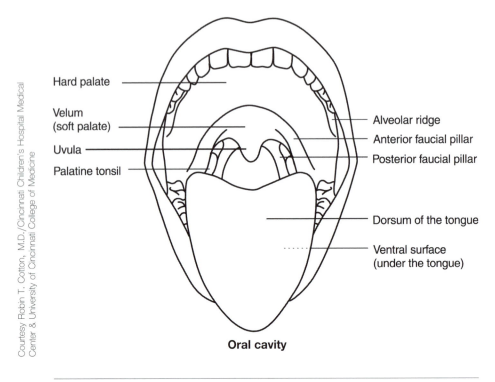

Hard palate

Velum (soft palate)

Uvula

Palatine tonsil

Alveolar ridge

Anterior faucial pillar

Posterior faucial pillar

Dorsum of the tongue

Ventral surface (under the tongue)

Oral cavity

FIGURE 1–4   The structures of the oral cavity.

ridge. The *dorsum* (dorsal surface) is the superior surface of the tongue and the *ventrum* (ventral surface) is the inferior surface of the tongue.

Faucial Pillars

At the back of the oral cavity are bilateral paired (anterior and posterior) curtain-like structures called *faucial pillars* (Figure 1–4). As the velum curves downward toward the tongue on both sides, it forms the anterior faucial pillar. Just behind the anterior pillar is the posterior faucial pillar. These structures contain muscles that assist with velopharyngeal and lingual movement. The *palatine tonsils* (or simply the tonsils) consist of lymphoepithelial tissue and are found between the anterior and posterior

faucial pillars on both sides. Although the tonsils are bilateral, differences in size are common, so it is not unusual for one tonsil to be larger than the other. The *lingual tonsils* are masses of lymphoid tissue that are located at the base of the tongue and extend to the epiglottis (Figure 1–5). The *oropharyngeal isthmus* is the opening from the oral cavity to the pharynx and is bordered superiorly by the velum, laterally by the faucial pillars, and inferiorly by the base of the tongue (see Chapter 8 for more information about tonsils and adenoids).

Hard Palate

The *hard palate* is a bony structure that separates the oral cavity from the nasal cavity. The hard palate forms a rounded dome on the

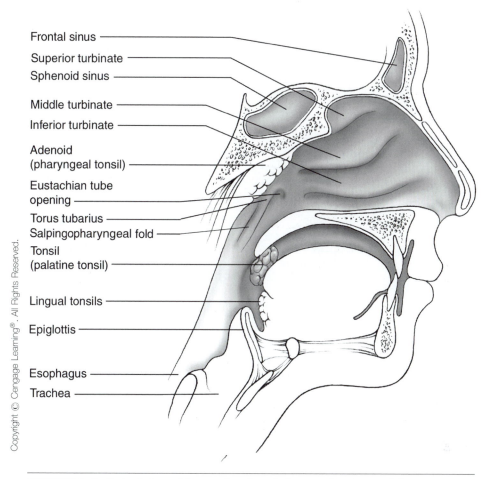

Frontal sinus

Superior turbinate

Sphenoid sinus

Middle turbinate

Inferior turbinate

Adenoid
(pharyngeal tonsil)

Eustachian tube
opening

Torus tubarius

Salpingopharyngeal fold

Tonsil
(palatine tonsil)

Lingual tonsils

Epiglottis

Esophagus

Trachea

FIGURE 1–5   Lateral view of the nasal, oral, and pharyngeal cavities and the structures in these areas.

upper part of the oral cavity, called the *palatal vault*. In addition to serving as the roof of the mouth, it also serves as the floor of the nasal cavity. The outer portion of the hard palate is called the *alveolar ridge, alveolus*, or simply the gum ridge (see Figure 1–4). This ridge forms the base and the bony support for the teeth. The bony frame of the hard palate is covered by a mucoperiosteum. *Mucoperiosteum* consists of a mucous membrane and periosteum. *Periosteum* is a thick, fibrous tissue that covers the surface of bone. The mucosal covering of the hard palate has multiple ridges running transversely, which are called the *rugae*. There is a slight elevation of the mucosa in the middle of the anterior part of the hard palate, called the *incisive papilla*. A narrow seam-like ridge, called the *palatine raphe* (pronounced /ræfeɪ/), forms the midline of the hard palate and runs from the incisive papilla posteriorly over the entire length of the mucosa of the hard palate. At the junction of the hard and soft palate, bilateral midline depressions can often be seen, called the *foveae palati*, which are openings to minor salivary glands.

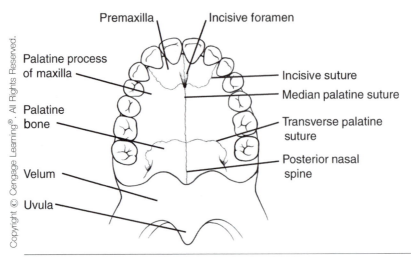

Premaxilla   Incisive foramen

Palatine process
of maxilla

Palatine
bone

Velum

Uvula

Incisive suture

Median palatine suture

Transverse palatine
suture

Posterior nasal
spine

FIGURE 1–6 Bony structures of the hard palate.

The hard palate is made up of fused bony segments that are separated by the incisive foramen and embryological fusion lines (Figure 1–6). By definition, a *foramen* is a hole or opening in a bony structure that allows blood vessels and nerves to pass through to the area on the other side. The *incisive foramen* is located in the alveolar ridge area of the maxillary arch, just behind the central incisors and at the tip of the premaxilla. The *premaxilla* is a triangular-shaped bone bordered on either side by the incisive suture lines. The dental arch of this bony segment contains the central and lateral maxillary incisors.

Behind the incisive suture lines are the paired *palatine processes* of the maxilla, which form the anterior three quarters of the maxilla. These paired bones terminate at the *transverse palatine suture line* (also known as the *palatomaxillary suture line*). Behind the transverse palatine suture line are the paired *horizontal plates* of the palatine bones. These bones form the posterior portion of the hard palate and end with the protrusive posterior nasal spine. The palatine processes of the maxilla and the horizontal plates of the

palatine bones are both paired because they are separated in the midline by the median *palatine suture* (also known as the *intermaxillary suture line*). This midline suture line begins at the incisive foramen and ends at the posterior nasal spine. In some individuals, a *torus palatinus*, or *palatine torus* (Figure 1–7) can be seen as a prominent longitudinal ridge on the oral surface of the hard palate in the area of the median suture line. It can become bigger with age. This finding is a normal variation, rather than an abnormality, and is

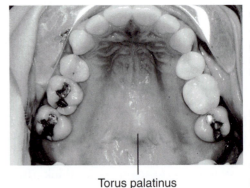

Torus palatinus

FIGURE 1–7 Small torus palatinus.

most commonly seen in Caucasians of northern European descent, Native Americans, or Eskimos. It tends to occur more in females than in males (Garcia-Garcia, Martinez-Gonzalez, Gomez-Font, Soto-Rivadeneira, & Oviedo-Roldan, 2010).

The *sphenoid bone* (an unpaired bone located at the base of the skull), and the *temporal bones* (located at the sides and base of the skull) provide bony attachment for the velopharyngeal musculature. The *pterygoid process* of the sphenoid bone contains the medial pterygoid plate, the lateral pterygoid plate, and the *pterygoid hamulus*, which provides attachments for muscles in the velopharyngeal complex (Figure 1–8).

Velum

The *velum* is attached to the posterior border of the hard palate and is held in place by its internal muscles (Figure 1–4 and Figure 1–6). The velum has an oral surface and a nasal surface. The oral surface of the velum is covered by a mucous membrane that contains fine blood vessels. A thin white line, called the median *palatine raphe*, can be seen coursing down the midline of the velum on the oral surface. The nasal surface of the velum (Figure 1–9) consists anteriorly of pseudostratified, ciliated columnar epithelium, and posteriorly of stratified, squamous epithelium in the area where the velum contacts the posterior pharyngeal wall during closure activities (Ettema & Kuehn, 1994; Kuehn & Kahane, 1990; Moon & Kuehn, 1996, 1997; Serrurier & Badin, 2008).

The anterior portion of the velum has very few muscle fibers. Instead, it consists of the tensor tendon, glandular tissue, *adipose* (fat) tissue, and the *palatine aponeurosis* (also called *velar aponeurosis*) (Figure 1–10). The palatine aponeurosis consists of a sheet of fibrous connective tissue and fibers from the tensor veli palatini tendon. It attaches to the posterior border of the hard palate and courses about

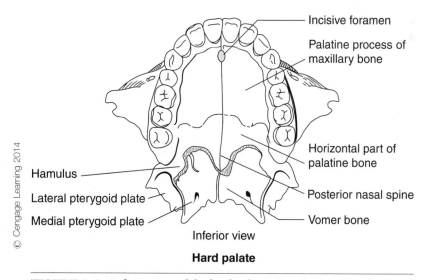

Incisive foramen

Palatine process of maxillary bone

Horizontal part of palatine bone

Posterior nasal spine

Vomer bone

Hamulus

Lateral pterygoid plate

Medial pterygoid plate

Inferior view

Hard palate

© Cengage Learning 2014

FIGURE 1–8 Inferior view of the hard palate. Note the hamulus, the lateral pterygoid plate and the medial pterygoid plate.

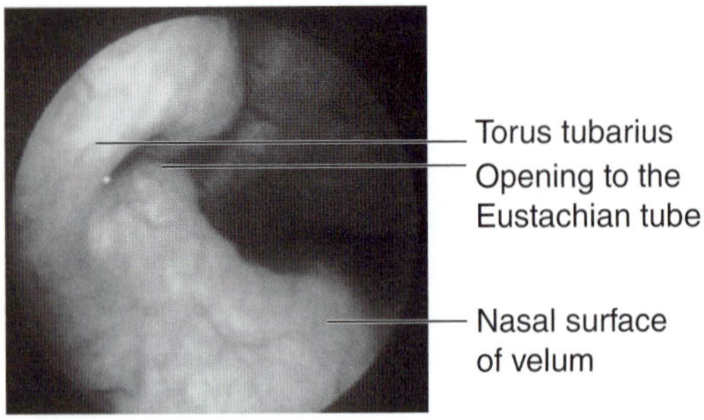

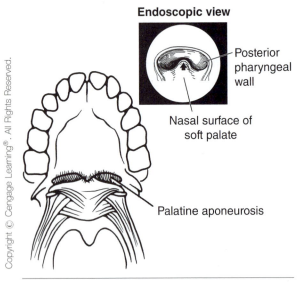

FIGURE 1–9   View of the nasal surface of the velum as seen through nasopharyngoscopy. Note the opening to the Eustachian tube.

1 cm posteriorly through the velum. The palatine aponeurosis provides an anchoring point for the velopharyngeal muscles and adds stiffness to that portion of the velum (Cassell & Elkadi, 1995; Ettema & Kuehn, 1994; (Hwang, Kim, Huan, Han, & Hwang, 2011). The medial portion of the velum contains most of the

Endoscopic view

Posterior pharyngeal wall

Nasal surface of soft palate

Palatine aponeurosis

FIGURE 1–10   Position of the palatine (velar) aponeurosis. This is a sheet of fibrous tissue that is located just below the nasal surface of the velum and consists of periosteum, fibrous connective tissue, and fibers from the tensor veli palatini tendon. It provides an anchoring point for the velopharyngeal muscles and adds stiffness and velopharyngeal flexibility.

muscle fibers, which are described later in this chapter. The posterior portion consists of the same glandular and adipose tissue as can be found in the anterior portion. The velar muscle fibers taper off as they reach the posterior portion of the velum, so few fibers are found in this section.

Uvula

The *uvula* is a teardrop-shaped structure that is typically long and slender (Figure 1–4 and Figure 1–6). It hangs freely from the posterior border of the velum. The uvula consists of mucosa on the surface and connective, glandular, adipose, and vascular tissue underneath. It contains no muscle fibers, however. The uvula does not contribute to velopharyngeal function and actually has no known function. When the velum is short, it may be seen to flip backward during phonation due to the pulling fibers of the musculus uvulae muscle in the velum above.

PHARYNGEAL STRUCTURES

The throat area between the esophagus and the nasal cavity is called the *pharynx*. The adenoids and Eustachian tube are in the upper part of the pharynx. These are discussed in the following sections.

Pharynx

The pharynx is divided into several sections, as can be seen in Figure 1–11. These sections include the *nasopharynx*, which is above the oral cavity and velum and is just posterior to the nasal cavity; the *oropharynx*, which is at the level of the oral cavity or just posterior to the mouth; and the *hypopharynx*, which is below the oral cavity and extends from the epiglottis inferiorly to the esophagus. The back wall of the throat is called the *posterior*

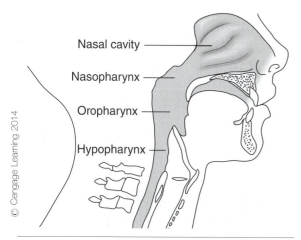

FIGURE 1–11 Sections of the pharynx. The *oropharynx* is at the level of the oral cavity or just posterior to the mouth. The *nasopharynx* is above the oral cavity and velum and is just posterior to the nasal cavity. The *hypopharynx* is below the oral cavity and extends from the epiglottis inferiorly to the esophagus.

pharyngeal wall and the side walls of the throat are called the *lateral pharyngeal walls*. The *adenoids* (also called the *pharyngeal tonsil, adenoid pad*, or just *adenoid*) consist of a singular mass of lymphoid tissue (despite the plural word). Adenoid tissue is found on the posterior pharyngeal wall of the nasopharynx, just behind the velum. Adenoids are usually present in children, but they atrophy with age. Adults have little, if any, adenoid tissue.

Eustachian Tube

The *Eustachian tube* is a membrane-lined tube that connects the middle ear space with the pharynx (Figure 1–5 and Figure 1–9). On each side of the pharynx, the pharyngeal opening of the Eustachian tube is lateral and slightly above the level of the velum during phonation.

The Eustachian tube is closed at rest, which helps prevent the inadvertent contamination of the middle ear by the normal secretions found in the pharynx and back of the nose. During swallowing and yawning, however, the velum raises and the tensor veli palatini muscle contracts to open the proximal end of the tube. This allows middle ear ventilation, which ensures that the pressure inside the ear remains nearly the same as ambient air pressure. In addition, the opening of the tube allows drainage of fluids and debris from the middle ear space.

In the infant or toddler, the Eustachian tube is essentially horizontal, and the pharyngeal opening is small. As the child grows, however, the tube changes to a downward-slanting angle from ear to pharynx, and the opening becomes larger. As a result, the Eustachian tube of an adult is at a 45° angle, and the opening is about the size of the diameter of a pencil. This gradual change in both the angle and width of the tube results in improved ventilation and drainage of the middle ear.

The *torus tubarius* is a ridge that is located posterior to the Eustachian tube opening and is caused by a projection of the cartilaginous portion of the tube. *The salpingopharyngeal folds* originate from the torus tubarius at the opening to the Eustachian tube and then course downward to the lateral pharyngeal wall (see Figure 1–5). These folds consist primarily of glandular and connective tissue (Cunsolo et al., 2010; Dickson, 1975; Lukens, Dimartino, Gunther, & Krombach, 2011).

VELOPHARYNGEAL FUNCTION

Normal velopharyngeal closure is accomplished by the coordinated action of the velum (soft palate), the lateral pharyngeal walls, and the posterior pharyngeal wall (Moon & Kuehn, 1996). These structures function as a valve that serves to close off the nasal cavity from the oral cavity during speech as well as during singing, whistling, blowing,

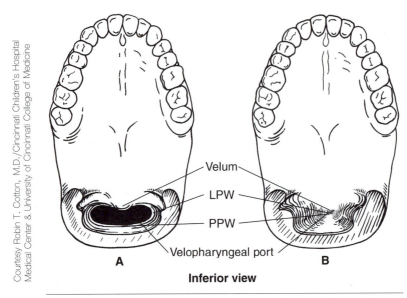

Courtesy Robin T. Cotton, M.D./Cincinnati Children's Hospital Medical Center & University of Cincinnati College of Medicine

Inferior view

FIGURE 1–12 (A and B) An inferior view of the velopharyngeal port. (A) The velopharyngeal port is open for nasal breathing. (B) The velopharyngeal port is closed for speech.

sucking, swallowing, gagging, and vomiting (Nohara et al., 2007). The valve then opens for nasal breathing and production of nasal sounds. As such, the velopharyngeal valve regulates and directs the transmission of sound energy and airflow in the oral and nasal cavities. In looking at the entire velopharyngeal mechanism, it is important to recognize that this is a three-dimensional tube that includes the anterior–posterior dimension, the vertical dimension, and the horizontal dimension. During closure, there must be coordinated movement of all structures in all dimensions so that the velopharyngeal valve can achieve closure like a sphincter. This can be seen in Figure 1–12, which shows an inferior view of the entire sphincter.

Velar Movement

During nasal breathing, the velum drapes down from the hard palate and rests against the base of the tongue (Figure 1–13A). This position contributes to a patent pharynx, which is important for the unobstructed movement of air between the nasal cavity and lungs during normal nasal breathing. During the production of oral speech (and other pneumatic and nonpneumatic activities as noted below), the velum moves in a superior and posterior direction to contact the posterior pharyngeal wall or, in some cases, the lateral pharyngeal walls (Figure 1–13B).

As the velum elevates, it has a type of "knee action" where it bends to provide maximum contact with the posterior pharyngeal wall over a large surface. The point where the velum bends is called the *velar dimple*. This "dimple" is formed by the contraction of the levator muscles where they interdigitate. The velar dimple is usually located at a point that is about 80% of the distance from the hard palate to the end of the velum and can be seen through an intraoral examination. An examination of the nasal surface of the velum through endoscopy would reveal a muscular bulge on the nasal side of the velum

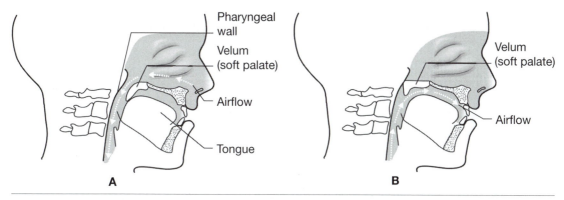

FIGURE 1–13 (A and B)   Lateral view of the velum and posterior pharyngeal wall. (A) The velum rests against the base of the tongue during normal nasal breathing, resulting in a patent airway. (B) The velum elevates during speech and closes against the posterior pharyngeal wall. This allows the air pressure from the lungs and the sound from the larynx to be redirected from a superior direction to an anterior direction to enter the oral cavity for speech.

© Cengage Learning 2014

during phonation. This bulge is called the *velar eminence* and results from the contraction of the musculus uvulae muscles. In fact, it could be said that the musculus uvulae muscles form the "patella" of the levator "knee." The contraction of the musculus uvulae muscles is felt to provide internal stiffness to the velum. In addition, the bulk that this bulge provides in this area helps to achieve velopharyngeal closure in the midline.

As the velum elevates, it also elongates through a process called *velar stretch* (Bzoch, 1968; Mourino & Weinberg, 1975; Pruzansky & Mason, 1962; Simpson & Austin, 1972; Simpson & Chin, 1981; Simpson & Colton, 1980). Because of this stretch factor, the velum is actually longer during function than it is at rest. Therefore, the effective length of the velum is the distance between the posterior border of the hard palate and the point on the posterior pharyngeal wall where there is velar contact during speech. This is measured in a line on the same plane as the hard palate (Satoh, Wada, Tachimura, & Fukuda, 2005). The amount of velar stretch and effective length of the velum varies among individuals and is

dependent on the size and configuration of the pharynx. Simpson and Colton (1980) reported that the amount of velar stretch is highly correlated with the "need ratio," which they defined as the pharyngeal depth divided by the velar length at rest.

When nasal phonemes are produced, the velum is pulled down so that sound energy can enter the nasal cavity. The lowering of the velum is the result of contraction of the palatoglossus muscles and, to a lesser extent, gravity and tissue elasticity (Fritzell, 1979; Kuehn & Azzam, 1978; Moon, Kuehn, & Azzam, 1978; Moon & Kuehn, 1996). Given the speed with which the velum must be lowered for nasal phonemes and then raised for oral phonemes, gravity alone would not be effective (Cheng, Zhao, & Qi, 2006; Lam, Hundert, & Wilkes, 2007).

Lateral Pharyngeal Wall Movement

The lateral pharyngeal walls contribute to velopharyngeal closure by moving medially to close against the velum or, in some cases, to meet in midline behind the velum (Figure 1–14).

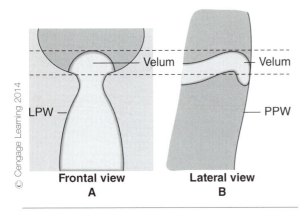

© Cengage Learning 2014

Frontal view
A

Lateral view
B

FIGURE 1–14 (A and B) (A) Frontal view of the lateral pharyngeal walls. The lateral pharyngeal walls move medially to close against the velum on both sides. (B) Lateral view of the velum as it contacts the posterior pharyngeal wall (PPW).

Both lateral pharyngeal walls move during closure, but there is great variation among normal speakers as to the extent of movement (Lam et al., 2007). In addition, there is often asymmetry in movement so that one side may move significantly more than the other side. Although some lateral wall movement can be noted from an intraoral perspective, the point of greatest medial displacement occurs near the level of the hard palate (Iglesias, Kuehn, & Morris, 1980) and velar eminence (Lam et al., 2007; Shprintzen, McCall, Skolnick, & Lencione, 1975). This area is well above the area that can be seen from an intraoral inspection. In fact, at the oral cavity level, the lateral walls may actually appear to bow outward during speech (Lam et al., 2007).

Posterior Pharyngeal Wall Movement

During velar movement, the posterior pharyngeal wall may move forward to assist in achieving contact, although this forward movement may be slight (Iglesias et al., 1980;

Magen, Kang, Tiede, & Whalen, 2003). Some posterior pharyngeal wall movement is noted in most normal speakers, but its contribution to closure seems to be much less than that of the velum and lateral pharyngeal walls. Some normal as well as abnormal speakers have a defined area on the posterior pharyngeal wall that bulges forward during speech. This is called Passavant's ridge and is discussed in the next section.

Passavant's Ridge

Passavant's ridge, first reported by Gustav Passavant in the 1800s, is a shelf-like projection from the posterior pharyngeal wall that occurs inconsistently in some individuals during velopharyngeal activities such as speech, whistling, and blowing (Glaser, Skolnick, McWilliams, & Shprintzen, 1979) (Figure 1–15). Passavant's ridge occurs in both normal and abnormal speakers during active velar and pharyngeal wall movement (Glaser et al., 1979). Passavant's ridge is not a permanent structure. Instead, it is a dynamic structure that occurs during velopharyngeal movement but disappears

Passavant's ridge

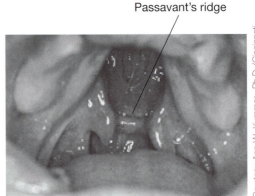

Courtesy Ann W. Kummer, Ph.D./Cincinnati Children's Hospital Medical Center & University of Cincinnati College of Medicine

FIGURE 1–15 Passavant's ridge as noted during phonation. This patient has an open palate due to surgery for maxillary cancer. During phonation, the Passavant's ridge presents as a ridge of muscle on the posterior pharyngeal wall.

during nasal breathing or when velopharyngeal activity ceases (Skolnick & Cohn, 1989). Because Passavant's ridge is a localized projection, it should not be confused with the generalized anterior movement of the posterior pharyngeal wall during speech.

Passavant's ridge is thought to be formed by the contraction of specific fibers of the superior constrictor muscles and possibly of fibers of the palatopharyngeus muscles in the posterior pharynx (Dickson & Dickson, 1972; Finkelstein et al., 1993; Perry, 2011). This forms the muscular ridge, which projects from the posterior pharyngeal wall. Passavant's ridge extends from one lateral pharyngeal wall to the other lateral pharyngeal wall on the opposite side. The vertical location of the ridge is variable among individuals. Although it is across from the free margin of the velum, it is often well below the site of velopharyngeal contact. A study by Glaser and colleagues (1979) of 43 individuals found that the ridge was located opposite the velar eminence in 5% of this group, opposite the vertical portion of the velum in 58%, opposite the uvula in 25%, and below the uvula in 12%. The orientation of the ridge is also variable among individuals. The ridge can be found to point in a superior, anterior, or inferior direction.

Although the location and orientation of the ridge is variable among different speakers, it appears to be in a consistent location for each individual speaker. However, the size of the ridge appears to vary according to the speech sound being produced and the overall degree of velar activity (Skolnick & Cohn, 1989). The size has also been found to be affected by fatigue.

Passavant's ridge is not a prerequisite for normal velopharyngeal function, and it is probably not a compensatory mechanism either. When it is found in individuals with velopharyngeal dysfunction, it does not seem to be correlated with gap size or type of cleft palate.

In addition, the formation of Passavant's ridge does not appear to be associated with the degree of velopharyngeal closure necessary for a specific speech sound. Instead, it has been found to be closely related to the tongue position for vowel production (Honjo, Kojima, & Kumazawa, 1975). When an individual demonstrates Passavant's ridge, it does not occur on all sounds all the time, and when it does occur, it is often delayed, occurring after velopharyngeal closure has been achieved. It is often located well below the level of velar and lateral pharyngeal wall movement. Therefore, the appearance of Passavant's ridge is probably an insignificant finding because it does not indicate an abnormality and it's not relevant when considering appropriate treatment.

Reports of the prevalence of Passavant's ridge in normal speakers range from as little as 9.5% to as high as 80% (Casey & Emrich, 1988; Finkelstein et al., 1991; Skolnick & Cohn, 1989; Skolnick, Shprintzen, McCall, & Rakoff, 1975; Yamawaki, 2003; Yanagisawa & Weaver, 1996). This variation in the reported prevalence may be due to the fact that Passavant's ridge is more prominent, and therefore more easily identified, when the head is hyperextended (Glaser et al., 1979). In a look at the collective results of several studies, Casey and Emrich (1988) found that Passavant's ridge probably occurs in about 23% of individuals with a history of cleft and in 15% of normal speakers.

Muscles of the Velopharyngeal Mechanism

The velopharyngeal sphincter requires the coordinated action of several different muscles, all of which are paired, with one muscle of the pair on each side of the midline (Moon & Kuehn, 1996; Perry, 2011) (Figure 1–16). Many of the muscles in the velopharyngeal complex have their attachments at the medial and lateral pterygoid plates and the pterygoid hamulus of the pterygoid process of the sphenoid bone. Each muscle has been studied extensively and its function defined. However, control of the velopharyngeal valve is very complex, requiring the interaction not only of these muscles but also of the articulators, particularly the tongue. Therefore, much more remains to be learned about the dynamics of the muscles and their interactions during speech (Kao, Soltysik, Hyde, & Gosain, 2008; Perry & Kuehn, 2009; Perry, 2011).

Levator Veli Palatini Muscles

The *levator veli palatini* muscles take up the middle 40% of the entire velum and therefore provide its main muscle mass (Boorman & Sommerlad, 1985; Kuehn & Moon, 2005; Perry, Kuehn, & Sutton, 2011; Nohara,

Tachimura, & Wada, 2006; Shimokawa et al., 2004). The levator muscles are primarily responsible for velar elevation (Smith & Kuehn, 2007). On each side of the nasopharynx, the levator veli palatini muscle originates from the apex of the petrous portion of the temporal bone at the base of the skull. The muscle then courses through an area that is anterior and medial to the carotid canal and inferior to the Eustachian tube (Moon & Kuehn, 1996, 1997). Both muscles enter the velum at a 45° angle and interdigitate (blend together) in the upper surface of the palatine aponeurosis. Contraction of the levator muscles forces the velum to move in a superior and posterior direction (at a 45° angle) in order to close against the posterior pharyngeal wall. Because of the angle of elevation, these muscles are often referred to as the *levator sling* (Mehendale, 2004). The point of

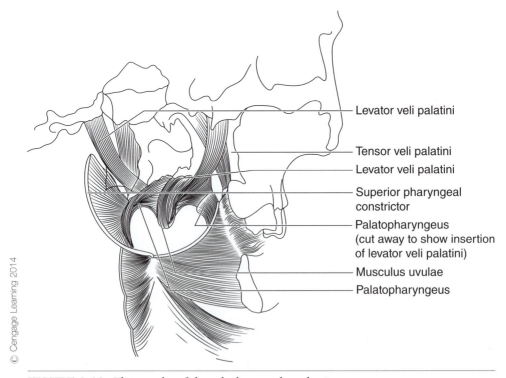

Levator veli palatini

Tensor veli palatini

Levator veli palatini

Superior pharyngeal constrictor

Palatopharyngeus (cut away to show insertion of levator veli palatini)

Musculus uvulae

Palatopharyngeus

© Cengage Learning 2014

FIGURE 1–16   The muscles of the velopharyngeal mechanism.

contraction of the levator muscles, called the *velar dimple*, can be noted on the oral surface of the velum during phonation.

Superior Constrictor Muscles

The upper fibers of the *superior constrictor* (also called *superior pharyngeal constrictor*) muscles are thought to be responsible for the medial displacement (constriction) of the lateral pharyngeal walls to effectively narrow the velopharyngeal port and close against the velum (Iglesias et al., 1980; Shprintzen et al., 1975; Skolnick, McCall, & Barnes, 1973). The paired superior constrictor muscles are located in the upper pharynx and arise from the pterygoid hamulus, pterygomandibular raphe, posterior tongue, posterior mandible, and palatine aponeurosis. They insert posteriorly in the pharyngeal raphe in the midline of the posterior pharyngeal wall.

Palatopharyngeus Muscles

The function of the *palatopharyngeus* muscles is not well understood. The horizontal fibers of these muscles are thought to be associated with the sphincteric action of pulling the lateral pharyngeal walls medially toward the velum (Cassell & Elkadi, 1995; Cheng & Zhang, 2004; Sumida, Yamashita, & Kitamura, 2012). The vertical fibers may assist in the lowering of the velum and could also assist with the elevation of the larynx and the lower portion of the pharynx (Moon & Kuehn, 1996, 1997). Some authors have suggested that this muscle functions as a muscular "hydrostat," which squeezes the posterior aspect of the velum so that it conforms to the shape of the posterior pharyngeal wall, thus resulting in a better velopharyngeal seal (Ettema & Kuehn, 1994; Moon & Kuehn, 1997). The palatopharyngeus muscle originates from the palatine aponeurosis and posterior border of the hard palate and then courses down through the posterior faucial pillars to the pharynx. A few of the vertical fibers of this muscle reach the thyroid cartilage of the larynx.

Palatoglossus Muscles

The *palatoglossus* muscles act antagonistically to the levator veli palatini to depress the velum or elevate the tongue. As such, these muscles are felt to be responsible for the rapid downward movement of the velum for production of nasal consonants in connected speech. On each side, the palatoglossus muscle arises from the palatine aponeurosis of the anterior half of the soft palate and inserts into the posterior lateral aspect of the tongue. It is contained within the anterior faucial pillar and may be subject to possible damage during tonsillectomy.

Salpingopharyngeus Muscles

The *salpingopharyngeus* muscles cannot have a significant role in achieving velopharyngeal closure given its size and location. These muscles arise from the inferior border of the torus tubarius, which is at the upper level of the pharynx. They then course vertically along the lateral pharyngeal wall and under the salpingopharyngeal fold.

Musculus Uvulae Muscles

The *musculus uvulae* muscles contract during phonation and create a bulge on the posterior part of the nasal surface of the velum. It has been postulated that the bulge serves two purposes (Kuehn, Folkins, & Linville, 1988; Moon & Kuehn, 1996, 1997). The first purpose is to provide additional stiffness to the nasal side of the velum during contraction, which prevents velar distortion. The second purpose is to fill in the area of contact between the velum and posterior pharyngeal wall in midline, which helps to assure a firm velopharyngeal seal

(Huang, Lee, & Rajendran, 1997; Kuehn et al., 1988).

It has also been suggested that the musculus uvulae may have an extensor effect on the nasal aspect of the velum, displacing it toward the posterior pharyngeal wall (Huang et al., 1997). The paired musculus uvulae muscles overlie the levator sling in the midline of the posterior velum and originate from the area of the palatine aponeurosis. They are the only intrinsic muscles of the velum and, as such, they are contained solely within the velum and do not extend beyond its borders (Moon & Kuehn, 1996; Kuehn & Moon, 2005). They are positioned side by side and extend to the free edge of the soft palate, superficial to the levator veli palatini. It should be noted that the name of this muscle is somewhat misleading in that it does not exist within the uvula. In fact, the uvula contains very few muscle fibers and does not contribute to velopharyngeal closure (Ettema & Kuehn, 1994; Kuehn & Kahane, 1990; Moon & Kuehn, 1996, 1997).

Tensor Veli Palatini Muscles

The *tensor veli palatini* muscles are responsible for opening the Eustachian tubes in order to enhance middle ear aeration and drainage, as noted above (Ghadiali, Swarts, & Doyle, 2003). Although these muscles are the main contributors to the palatine aponeurosis, the tensor is not positioned in a way to either raise or lower the velum. Therefore, these muscles probably contribute little, if anything, to velopharyngeal closure. The tensor veli palatini muscle on each side originates from the membranous portion of the Eustachian tube cartilage and the scaphoid fossa spine of the sphenoid bone (Barsoumian, Kuehn, Moon, & Canady, 1998). Additional slips arise from the lateral aspect of the medial pterygoid plate and the spine of the sphenoid. The tensor veli palatini muscle then courses vertically down

from the skull base to pass around the pterygoid hamulus. This redirects the muscle tendon 90° medially, where it contributes to the palatine aponeurosis in the superior and anterior region of the velum.

It is important to stress that the muscles of the velopharyngeal mechanism do not work in isolation. In fact, each motor movement is probably the result of the synergistic activities of several muscles. For example, the position and force of closure of the velopharyngeal valve varies with different activities, as will be discussed later. These variations are probably due to variations in the relative contribution of the levator veli palatini, palatoglossus, and palatopharyngeus muscles (Moon, Smith, Folkins, Lemke, & Gartlan, 1994). The complexity of the interaction of the muscles of the velopharyngeal mechanism has been studied, but further research is needed before this interaction is fully understood.

Velopharyngeal Motor and Sensory Innervation

The motor and sensory innervation of the velopharyngeal mechanism arises from the cranial nerves in the medulla. The following section describes the specific innervation for motor movement and sensation.

Motor innervation for the muscles that contribute to velopharyngeal closure comes from the pharyngeal plexus (Figure 1–17). The *pharyngeal plexus* is a network of nerves that lies along the posterior wall of the pharynx and consists of the pharyngeal branches of the glossopharyngeal nerve (CN IX) and the vagus nerve (CN X). Innervation of the velar muscles with these nerves occurs through the brainstem nucleus ambiguus and retrofacialis (Cassell & Elkadi, 1995; Kennedy & Kuehn, 1989; Moon & Kuehn, 1996). The palatoglossus muscle has also been found to receive

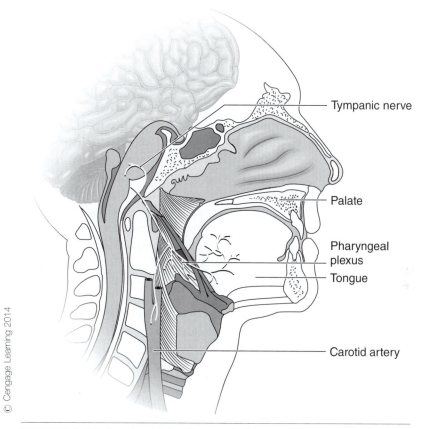

Tympanic nerve

Palate

Pharyngeal plexus

Tongue

Carotid artery

© Cengage Learning 2014

FIGURE 1–17   Position of the pharyngeal plexus.

innervation from the hypoglossal nerve (CN XII) (Cassell & Elkadi, 1995). The tensor veli palatini, which does not contribute to velopharyngeal closure, receives motor innervation from the mandibular division of the trigeminal nerve (CN V).

Sensory innervation of both the hard and soft palate is believed to derive from the greater and lesser palatine nerves, which arise from the maxillary division of the trigeminal nerve (CN V). The faucial and pharyngeal regions of the oral cavity are innervated by the glossopharyngeal nerve (CN IX). The facial nerve (CN VII) and vagus nerve (CN X) might also contribute to sensory innervation (Perry, 2011). Although the peripheral distribution of

sensory fibers may travel along different cranial nerve routes, they all appear to terminate in the spinal nucleus of the trigeminal nerve (Cassell & Elkadi, 1995). It has been reported that the cutaneous sensory nerve endings are more prolific in the anterior portion of the oral cavity but diminish in quantity as they course toward the posterior regions of the mouth (Cassell & Elkadi, 1995).

VARIATIONS IN VELOPHARYNGEAL CLOSURE

Velopharyngeal closure between individuals, and even within an individual, is not always the same. Each individual has a certain basic pattern of closure that is dependent on the relative contributions of the muscles within the component structures. Despite this basic pattern, the height, strength, and timing of closure vary with the type of activity. For example, closure is much higher and firmer with nonpneumatic activities (i.e., vomiting) when compared to speech. More subtle variations in closure are found during speech production, based on the type of phoneme produced, the phonemic context, and the rate of speech.

Patterns of Velopharyngeal Closure

The relative contribution of the velopharyngeal structures to closure varies among both normal and abnormal speakers. In fact, distinct patterns of velopharyngeal closure can be identified, based on the extent of movement of the soft palate and pharyngeal walls (Croft, Shprintzen, & Rakoff, 1981; Finkelstein, Talmi, Nachmani, Hauben, & Zohar, 1992; Igawa, Nishizawa, Sugihara, & Inuyama, 1998; Perry, 2011; Shprintzen, Rakoff, Skolnick, & Lavorato, 1977; Siegel-Sadewitz & Shprintzen, 1982; Skolnick & Cohn, 1989; Skolnick et al., 1973; Witzel & Posnick, 1989). These basic patterns of closure can be seen in Figure 1–18.

The *coronal pattern* of closure is the most common and is accomplished by the posterior movement of the soft palate closing against a broad area of the posterior pharyngeal wall. There may also be anterior movement of the posterior pharyngeal wall. With this closure pattern, there is minimal contribution of the lateral pharyngeal walls. Witzel and Posnick (1989) studied 246 individuals who underwent nasopharyngoscopy for evaluation of velopharyngeal function. Nasopharyngoscopy is an endoscopic procedure in which a flexible

fiberoptic scope is inserted through the nose until it reaches the nasopharynx, allowing visual observation and analysis of the velopharyngeal mechanism (see Chapter 17 for more information). In this study, they found that 68% of their patients demonstrated a coronal pattern of closure.

The next most common pattern of closure is the *circular pattern*. This pattern occurs when the soft palate moves posteriorly, the posterior pharyngeal wall moves anteriorly, and the lateral pharyngeal walls move medially. In this case, all the velopharyngeal structures contribute to closure, and the closure pattern resembles a true sphincter. Witzel and Posnick (1989) found this pattern in 23% of the individuals in their study. Another 5% had a circular pattern with Passavant's ridge. Although Passavant's ridge seems to be most common in individuals with a circular pattern of closure, it is also found with the other patterns of velopharyngeal closure (Skolnick & Cohn, 1989).

The least common pattern of closure is the *sagittal pattern*. This was found in only 4% of the patients in the Witzel and Posnick study (1989). With this pattern, the lateral pharyngeal walls move medially to meet in midline behind the velum, and there is minimal posterior displacement of the soft palate to effect closure. Of note is the fact that the prevalence of the different patterns of closure is similar in frequency in both normal speakers and those with velopharyngeal dysfunction (Croft et al., 1981).

To try to explain the differences in movement patterns, Finkelstein and colleagues studied 42 consecutive individuals who were undergoing uvulopalatopharyngoplasty (UPPP), which is the partial excision of the velum and uvula to resolve sleep apnea. The velopharyngeal valve was studied through an oral examination and also through an endoscopic examination. They found that individuals with a deep oropharynx tended to show a

Lateral view of VP closure

**Patterns of VP closure
as viewed through nasopharyngoscopy**

Coronal

Sagittal

Circular

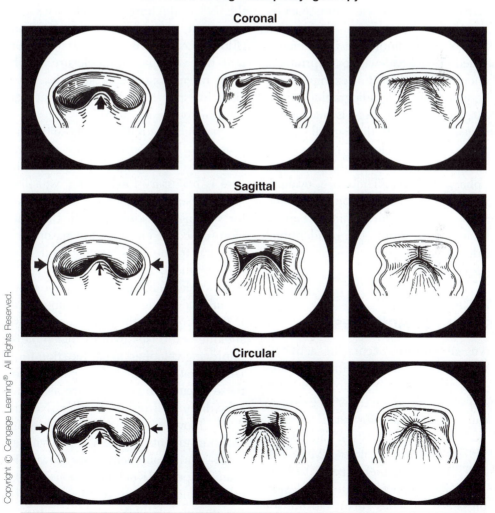

FIGURE 1–18   Patterns of velopharyngeal closure as viewed from above.

sagittal or circular pattern of closure, whereas individuals with a flat oropharynx showed a coronal pattern of closure. These researchers concluded that there must be minor differences in muscular orientation among individuals to account for the different pharyngeal configurations at rest and during speech (Finkelstein et al., 1992, 1993).

The variations in the basic patterns of closure among individuals are important to recognize and understand. This is particularly true in the evaluation process, because the basic pattern of closure may have an impact on the diagnosis of velopharyngeal dysfunction and the type of intervention that is ultimately recommended (Siegel-Sadewitz & Shprintzen, 1982; Skolnick et al., 1973). For example, on a lateral videofluoroscopy (a radiographic procedure), it may appear as if there is inadequate velopharyngeal closure with the sagittal pattern of closure, even when closure is complete, because the velum does not close against the posterior pharyngeal wall. Therefore, evaluating all of the velopharyngeal structures and their contribution to closure is important so that the basic closure pattern can be identified and considered when making treatment recommendations.

Pneumatic versus Nonpneumatic Activities

Velopharyngeal closure occurs in activities other than speech. If these activities are categorized into pneumatic and nonpneumatic functions, a characteristic and distinct closure pattern can be identified for each category (Flowers & Morris, 1973; Matsuya, Yamaoka, & Miyasaki, 1979; Shprintzen, Lencione, McCall, & Skolnick, 1974). In fact, there seems to be a separate neurological mechanism for closure during nonspeech activities versus closure for speech.

Nonpneumatic activities include swallowing, gagging, and vomiting. With these activities, the velum is raised very high in the pharynx and the lateral pharyngeal walls close tightly along their entire length. Closure appears to be almost exaggerated and is very firm, as viewed through videofluoroscopy. This type of closure is necessary because the purpose of closure in these cases is to allow substances to pass through the oral cavity while preventing nasal regurgitation. In swallowing, velopharyngeal closure is further assisted by the back of the tongue, which raises against the velum, thus pushing the velum up and back (Flowers & Morris, 1973). It is important to note that velopharyngeal closure may be complete for nonpneumatic activities but insufficient for speech or other pneumatic activities (Shprintzen et al., 1975).

Pneumatic activities are those that utilize air pressure (both positive and negative) as a result of velopharyngeal closure. Positive pressure is necessary for blowing, whistling, singing, and speech. Negative pressure is needed for sucking and kissing. With these activities, closure occurs lower in the nasopharynx and appears to be less exaggerated than with nonpneumatic activities.

It would be tempting to assume that closure for all pneumatic activities is about the same. If that were true, then the use of blowing and sucking exercises would be beneficial in improving velopharyngeal function for speech. Unfortunately, the closure patterns for all of these pneumatic activities are also physiologically different from each other (Nohara et al., 2007). Blowing, for example, requires generalized movements of the velopharyngeal structures—and levator activity for blowing is higher than for speech (Kuehn & Moon, 1994). On the other hand, speech requires precise, rapid movements of these structures; the point of contact even varies during speech, as is discussed in the next section. When comparing velopharyngeal closure during singing and speech, the velopharyngeal port is closed longer and tighter in singing than in speech, particularly on the higher pitches (Austin, 1997).

Timing of Closure

Voice onset and velopharyngeal closure must be closely coordinated during speech. Velar movement for oral sounds must begin prior to the onset of phonation so that the velopharyngeal valve is completely closed when phonation begins. If complete closure is not achieved before activation of the sound source, then speech may be *hypernasal* (characterized by too much sound in the nasal cavity during speech production) (Ha, Sim, Zhi, & Kuehn, 2004).

The timing of closure for an oral sound has been found to be somewhat dependent on the type of phoneme. Kent and Moll (1969) found evidence to suggest that the velar elevating gesture for a stop begins earlier and is executed more rapidly when the stop is voiceless rather than voiced. The production of nasal consonants during an utterance has an additional effect on velopharyngeal function and timing. The velum remains elevated, and closure is maintained throughout the utterance as long as oral consonants or vowels are being produced. As a nasal consonant (/m/, /n/, /ŋ/) is produced, the velum lowers quickly and the pharyngeal walls move away from midline, thus opening the velopharyngeal valve to allow for nasal resonance. Speech segments with many oral-nasal combinations make the temporal requirements for velar movement more challenging. This can be a problem if there is tenuous velopharyngeal closure (Jones, 2006). In addition, vowels that precede or follow the nasal consonant will be slightly affected by the anticipatory lowering of the velum just before the nasal consonant and

by the slight delay in raising the velum just after the nasal consonant (Bunnell, 2005). Therefore, the timing of closure requires constant fine adjustments throughout an utterance, depending on the phonemic needs. Missed timing may have implications for the perception of resonance or nasality.

Height of Closure

Even as velopharyngeal closure is maintained throughout oral speech, there are slight variations in contact due to the type of phoneme being produced and its phonemic environment (Flowers & Morris, 1973; Moll, 1962; Moon & Kuehn, 1997; Shprintzen et al., 1975; Simpson & Chin, 1981).

The height of velar closure is affected by the movement and height of the tongue during articulation of the sound and also by the phoneme's requirements for intraoral air pressure (Tom, Titze, Hoffman, & Story, 2001). In general, velar heights are slightly greater for consonants than for vowels. High-pressure consonants (plosives, fricatives, and affricates), especially those that are voiceless, have the greatest heights when compared to other consonants. High vowels have a higher velar height than low vowels (Moll, 1962; Moon & Kuehn, 1997), possibly due to the elevation of the back of the tongue during the production of these sounds.

Firmness of Closure

The same factors that increase the height of velar contact during speech also increase the firmness of closure. Therefore, velopharyngeal closure force is greater on consonants than on vowels, and it is greatest on high-pressure consonants, particularly fricatives (Kuehn & Moon, 1998). High vowels are associated with a greater degree of closure force than low vowels (Kuehn & Moon, 1998; Moll, 1962; Moon, Kuehn, & Huisman, 1994). Moll (1962) has shown that vowels adjacent to a nasal consonant, particularly when preceding the consonant, have less closure force than those adjacent to oral consonants. A decline in overall closure force occurs with fatigue (Kuehn & Moon, 2000). Considering all of these factors, changes in velar position are the result of the interaction of a number of variables, including vowel height and the type of consonant (Seaver & Kuehn, 1980). Therefore, velar position must be changed and coordinated with each syllable production (Karnell, Linville, & Edwards, 1988).

Rate and Fatigue

Rapid speech can affect the efficiency of velar movement, thus compromising velopharyngeal closure. It has been shown that when speech rate increases, the height of closure decreases and is less firm (Moll & Shriner, 1967), presumably due to the difficulty in achieving appropriate height and contact with the rapid rate. Therefore, as speech rate increases, it can become more hypernasal.

Muscular fatigue can also affect the height and firmness of closure. Even normal speakers become "nasal" when they are tired. Young children are often described as "whiny" at the end of the day, especially when they are tired. The term "whiny" actually describes an increase in hypernasality due to velar fatigue. Even blowing for an extended period of time, as when playing a wind instrument, can result in velar fatigue (Tachimura, Nohara, Satoh, & Wada, 2004).

Changes with Growth and Age

The maturational changes in the craniofacial skeleton result in changes in the relationships of the pharyngeal structures and the size of the cavities of the vocal tract (pharyngeal, oral, and nasal). The differences in the vocal tract anatomy among an infant, a child, and an adult are significant and account for the differences in the quality of the "voice" at different stages of development.

Although the cranium approaches adult size relatively early in childhood, the facial bones continue to grow into adolescence or early adulthood. The growth of the mandible and maxillary bones is somewhat affected by the development of dentition. As these structures grow and mature, they move down and forward relative to the cranium. Both the maxilla and mandible are similar in size in males and females until around 14 years of age. After that age, these facial bones continue to grow in males until around age 18, whereas there is very little additional growth in females (Tineshev, 2010; Ursi, Trotman, McNamara, & Behrents, 1993). Despite the changes in the size of the mandible and maxilla over time, there are relatively minor changes in shape, even during the various occlusal stages (Kent & Vorperian, 1995).

The size of the pharynx changes greatly during maturation. The newborn pharynx is estimated to be approximately 4 cm long. In fact, the velum and epiglottis are in close proximity, resulting in a very short pharynx (which partly accounts for the infant's high-pitched voice). In contrast, the adult pharynx is approximately 20 cm long. It has been shown that with age and height, there is a linear increase in the length of the pharynx for both boys and girls (Rommel et al., 2003; Stellzig-Eisenhauer, 2001).

In addition to the increase in length, there is an increase of approximately 80% in the volume of the nasopharynx from infancy to adulthood (Bergland, 1963). Because there is more vertical than horizontal growth, there is very little change in the anterior–posterior dimension of the nasopharynx (Bergland, 1963; Kent & Vorperian, 1995; Tourne, 1991). However, there is significant change in the angle of the posterior pharyngeal wall and its relationship to the velum. In a newborn, the oropharynx curves slightly to form the naso-pharynx. At around age 5, the posterior pha-ryngeal wall of the nasopharynx and oropharynx meet at an oblique angle. Because of the position of the pharyngeal wall, velo-pharyngeal closure in children typically occurs with the back of the velum (under the bend) against the pharyngeal wall (and most likely against the adenoid tissue). By puberty, how-ever, the inclination of the nasopharynx changes so that the posterior pharyngeal wall meets the velum at almost a right angle (Kent, 1976; Kent & Vorperian, 1995). As a result, velopharyngeal closure in adults tends to be with the top of the velum against the pharyn-geal wall that is slightly above it. Fortunately, the angle of the pharyngeal wall changes at the same time as the downward and slightly forward growth of the maxilla and thus the velum. In addition, the velum increases in both length and thickness at this stage. Therefore, despite these changes in structure and velo-pharyngeal relationships, the competency of velopharyngeal closure is maintained.

Another factor that changes the relative dimensions of the pharyngeal space and can introduce some instability in velopharyngeal function is the presence and size of the adenoid tissue. The adenoid pad is positioned on the posterior pharyngeal wall in the area of velopharyngeal closure. In young children, the adenoid pad can be prominent in size and in many cases, it actually assists with closure. As a result, young children actually have veloadenoi-dal (rather than velopharyngeal) closure (Croft, Shprintzen, & Ruben, 1981; Kent & Vorperian,

1995; Maryn, Van Lierde, De Bodt, & Van Cauwenberge, 2004; Skolnick et al., 1975).

A gradual process of involution and atrophy of the adenoid tissue begins before puberty, but a more sudden involution may occur with puberty. However, the velopharyngeal mecha-nism is usually able to adapt to the anatomic changes that occur with adenoid atrophy in such a way that velopharyngeal function is maintained. In addition, there may be an increase in velopharyngeal movement follow-ing adenoid involution—so that a more mature pattern of velopharyngeal closure is adopted (Kent & Vorperian, 1995). However, in indi-viduals with a history of cleft palate or tenuous velopharyngeal closure, these compensations may not be possible. As a result, the changes that occur in the adenoid pad as the individual moves through puberty may result in the onset of velopharyngeal insufficiency that requires surgical intervention (Mason & Warren, 1980; Siegel-Sadewitz & Shprintzen, 1986; Van Demark & Morris, 1983; Abdel-Aziz, Dewidar, El-Hoshy, & Aziz, 2009). Finally, the effect of aging on velopharyngeal function has been studied. Hoit and colleagues (1994) found no differences in nasal airflow in ages up to 80 years, suggesting that velopharyngeal func-tion does not deteriorate with age.

PHYSIOLOGICAL SUBSYSTEMS FOR SPEECH: PUTTING IT ALL TOGETHER

Speech is the result of the coordination of several physiological subsystems, including respiration, phonation, resonance, and articu-lation. The velopharyngeal valve must function in coordination with the other subsystems of speech for speech to be produced normally and with good intelligibility. To understand the importance of these subsystems and the need for coordination, it may be helpful to review how sound is produced.

Every instrument that is capable of producing sound needs at least three components: (1) a vibrating mechanism to produce sound, (2) a stimulating force that can set the vibration in motion, and (3) a resonating mechanism to damp or amplify the sound. In human speech, the vocal folds are the vibrating mechanism, the force of breath pressure is the stimulating force, and the cavities of the vocal tract provide the resonating mechanism for sound energy (Baken, 1987; Sataloff, Heman-Ackah, & Hawkshaw, 2007).

During speech, all movements must be done quickly and with accuracy. In addition, the action of every muscle is influenced by the actions of other muscles in the system; the movements of each structure are influenced by movements of other structures; and every phoneme is influenced by other phonemes around it (Kollia, Gracco, & Harris, 1995). Because of this, there must be good coordination of all aspects of the physiological subsystems.

It is almost as if each subsystem is a player on a "team." Each player must be able to execute its role and also learn how to work with the other players. If it is a good player, the other team players will be more effective as well. If it is a poor player, however, this will make the job of the other team players much more difficult, and they will function less effectively. Overall, the complexity of speech production cannot be overstated. The following is a discussion of the role of each subsystem on the "team."

Respiration

Respiration is essential for life support, but it is also essential for speech. The air from the lungs is what provides the initiating force for phonation and the air pressure for articulation. During quiet breathing, the inspiratory and expiratory phases are relatively long and usually about equal in duration. During speech, however, inspiration occurs very quickly. Subglottic air pressure is then maintained under the vocal folds during the entire phrase or sentence. The expiratory phase is relatively long and varies, depending on the length of the produced utterance. Both the inspiratory and expiratory phases must be controlled by the speaker during speech production.

Phonation

Phonation is the sound that is generated by the vocal folds as they begin to vibrate. This sound, called voice, is used for the production of all vowel sounds and about half of the consonant sounds. Some consonants are voiceless, however. Therefore, the vocal folds must vibrate for voiced sounds, stop vibrating abruptly for voiceless sounds, and then vibrate again for the next vowel or voiced consonant (Bailly, Henrich, & Pelorson, 2010; Kent & Moll, 1969; Takemoto, Mokhtari, & Kitamura, 2010; Tsai, Chen, Shau, & Hsiao, 2009). In the simple two-syllable phrase "a cup," the vocal folds vibrate on the vowel, stop on the /k/, vibrate on the vowel, and stop again on the /p/. This requires a great deal of neuromotor coordination and control.

Phonation is initiated when the vocal folds close and air from the lungs creates subglottic pressure. This air pressure forces the bottom of the vocal folds open and then continues to move upward to open the top of the vocal folds. The low pressure created behind the fast-moving air column causes the bottom of the folds to close, followed by the top folds. This is called the *Bernoulli Effect*. The closure of the vocal folds cuts off the air column and releases a pulse of air. This completes one vibratory cycle. The cycles repeat for vocal fold vibration, resulting in a type of buzzing sound (which is later modified by resonance). During phonation, there is continuous adduction (or closing) of the vocal folds as they vibrate for voiced phonemes and periodic abduction (or opening) of the vocal folds as voiceless sounds are produced. Air pressure must be maintained throughout the utterance so that it can continue to provide the force for phonation.

Prosody

Prosody refers to the stress, intonation, and rhythm of speech. In connected speech, articulation is influenced by the stress of individual phonemes and the intonation of the utterance. *Stress* is related to increased laryngeal and subglottic pressure during the production of a syllable. Stressed syllables are higher in pitch and intensity, longer in duration, and produced with greater articulatory precision as compared with unstressed syllables. *Rhythm* refers to the alteration of stressed and unstressed syllables and the relative timing of each. *Intonation* refers to the frequent changes in pitch throughout an utterance, as controlled by subtle changes in vocal fold length and mass. These changes influence the rate of vibration of the vocal folds and the tension of the muscles of the larynx. Although there are changes in pitch throughout connected speech, the pitch of the voice tends to drop to a lower frequency at the end of each statement and rise to a higher frequency at the end of a question. Both stress and intonation are used for emphasis and also to help to convey meaning. For example, the words "desert" and "dessert" have different meanings that are conveyed through differences in the place of stress. When the sentence "Well, that's just fine" is uttered as if it has an exclamation point, it has a different meaning than when it is spoken as if it has a period at the end. The differences in meaning are conveyed by differences in the stress and intonation.

Resonance and Velopharyngeal Function

Once phonation has begun, air pressure from the lungs and sound energy from the vocal folds travel in a superior direction in the vocal tract. The sound energy vibrates throughout the cavities of the supraglottic tract, beginning with the pharyngeal cavity and then including the oral cavity and/or nasal cavity. The resultant shaping of the sound energy adds the resonant quality to speech.

Several factors can affect the resonance and the overall acoustic product of the voice. These factors include the size and shape of the cavities of the vocal tract. This effect can be compared to what happens when you blow across the lip of a bottle. When the bottle is mostly full, the resonating space is small, and the resulting sound is high in pitch. When the bottle is almost empty and therefore leaves a larger resonating cavity, the sound is deeper in pitch. Variation in the size and shape of the resonating cavities among individuals is often determined by age and gender. For example, infants have very small resonating cavities; thus, the vocal quality is very high in pitch. Women and children usually have a shorter vocal tract than men; therefore, they have higher formant frequencies in their vocal product. An additional consideration is the wall thickness of the cavities. A thick pharyngeal wall can absorb sound, whereas a thinner wall can reflect sound. The changes in vibration that result from all of these factors produce the resonance and give the perception of timbre or vocal quality (Sataloff, 1992).

The velopharyngeal valve is very important for normal speech and resonance because it is responsible for regulating and directing the transmission of sound energy and airflow into the appropriate cavities (nasal or oral) during speech. During the production of oral speech sounds (all sounds with the exception of /m/, /n/, and /ŋ/), the velopharyngeal valve closes, thus blocking off the nasal cavity from the oral cavity. This allows the sound energy and air pressure to be directed anteriorly into the oral cavity. During the production of nasal sounds, the velopharyngeal valve opens, which allows the nasal cavity to be *coupled* (sharing acoustic energy) with the oral and pharyngeal cavities.

Articulation

The sound that results from phonation and resonance is further altered for individual speech sounds by the articulators. The oral *articulators* include the lips, the jaws (including the teeth), and the tongue. (The velum is also an articulator for speech.) The oral articulators alter the acoustic product for different speech sounds in two ways. First, they can vary the size and shape of the oral cavity through movement and articulatory placement. In addition, the articulators can modify the manner in which the sound, and particularly the airstream, is released.

Both vowels and voiced oral consonants require oral resonance for production, and many consonants also require oral air pressure. For the production of vowels, the tongue and jaws modify the size and shape of the oral cavity, but there is little constriction of the sound energy or air pressure. The differentiation of vowel sounds is determined by tongue height (high, mid, or low), tongue position (front, central, back), and lip rounding (present or absent).

On the other hand, consonants are produced by partial or complete obstruction of the oral cavity, which results in a buildup of air pressure in the oral cavity. Intraoral air pressure provides the force for the production of all pressure-sensitive consonants (plosives, fricatives, and affricates). *Plosive phonemes* (/p/, /b/, /t/, /d/, /k/, /g/) are produced with a buildup of intraoral pressure and then a sudden release. *Fricative phonemes* (/f/, /v/, /s/, /z/, /ʃ/, /ʒ/, /h/) require a gradual release of air pressure through a small or restricted opening. *Affricate phonemes* (/ʧ/, /ʤ/) are a combination of plosive and fricative phonemes (/ʧ/ = /t/ + /ʃ/ and /ʤ/ = /d/ + /ʒ/). As such, affricate sounds require a buildup of intraoral air pressure and then release through a narrow opening. Consonants are differentiated not only by the manner of production (plosives, fricatives, affricates, liquids, and glides) but also by the place of production (bilabial, labiodental, lingual-alveolar, palatal, velar, and glottal) and voicing (voiced or voiceless).

Subsystems as "Team Players"

It can be said that during speech production, each subsystem is like a member of a team. For the team to reach its goal of normal speech production, each subsystem must work smoothly and efficiently with the others.

Just as on a team, if one subsystem is a poor player, it can affect the function of other team members (subsystems) and ultimately affect the team goal. For example, velopharyngeal dysfunction can affect respiration, phonation, and articulation. It can cause an alteration of respiration during speech because the loss of air through the nose causes the individual to take more frequent breaths to replenish the airflow. Phonation may be altered if the individual compensates for inadequate oral airflow for voiceless sounds by substituting phonated sounds (e.g., n/s). On the other hand, the individual may use a breathy voice to mask the sound of hypernasality. The loss of oral airflow due to velopharyngeal dysfunction can affect articulation of pressure-sensitive consonants, causing the individual to produce sounds in the pharynx rather than the oral cavity. Overall, it is important to understand that the subsystems are interrelated and dependent on each other to reach the goal of normal speech production.

SUMMARY

The anatomy of the face, oral cavity, and velopharyngeal valve is well documented and is easy to describe and to understand. On the other hand, the physiology of the velopharyngeal mechanism, particularly as it relates to speech, is very complex and not well understood. There is still much to be learned regarding the roles of the various muscles, the interaction of velopharyngeal function with articulation, and the neuromotor controls required for coordination of velopharyngeal function with the other subsystems of speech. A thorough understanding of the anatomy and physiology of the vocal tract is particularly important in the management of speech and resonance disorders.

FOR REVIEW AND DISCUSSION

1. Why is it important to understand normal structure when working with individuals with a history of cleft lip and palate?

2. What are the facial landmarks and structures that may be relevant to the study of cleft lip?

3. Describe the internal nasal structures and the various functions of the nasal turbinates.

4. List the oral structures that can be seen when looking in the mouth.

5. List the suture lines of the hard palate. Why do you think they are called "suture" lines? Explain how they are formed.

6. Describe the movement of the velopharyngeal structures and the role of the velopharyngeal muscles in closing and opening the velopharyngeal valve.

7. What are the physiological subsystems of speech, and how do they interact with each other for normal speech? Describe how a problem with one subsystem may affect other subsystems.

8. What are the types of velopharyngeal closure patterns among normal and abnormal speakers? Why do you think it is important to understand the basic patterns of speech when evaluating abnormal speakers?

9. Discuss the effects of type of activity, type of phoneme, rate of speech, and fatigue on velopharyngeal closure. Given the known effect of these factors on velopharyngeal closure, how would this affect the way you evaluate velopharyngeal function for speech?

10. How does velopharyngeal closure change with growth and adenoid involution? How could these changes potentially affect speech?

REFERENCES

Abdel-Aziz, M., Dewidar, H., El-Hoshy, H., & Aziz, A. A. (2009). Treatment of persistent post-adenoidectomy velopharyngeal insufficiency by sphincter pharyngoplasty. *International Journal of Pediatric Otorhinolaryngology*, 73(10), 1329–1333.

Austin, S. F. (1997). Movement of the velum during speech and singing in classically trained singers. *Journal of Voice*, 11(2), 212–221.

Bailly, L., Henrich, N., & Pelorson, X. (2010). Vocal fold and ventricular fold vibration in period-doubling phonation: Physiological description and aerodynamic modeling. *Journal of the Acoustic Society of America*, 127(5), 3212–3222.

Baken, R. J. (1987). *Clinical measurement of speech and voice*. Boston: College-Hill Press.

Barsoumian, R., Kuehn, D. P., Moon, J. B., & Canady, J. W. (1998). An anatomie study of the tensor veli palatini and dilatator tubae muscles in relation to the Eustachian tube and velar function. *The Cleft Palate–Craniofacial Journal*, 35(2), 101–110.

Bergland, O. (1963). The bony nasopharynx. *Acta Odontologica Scandinavia*, 21(Suppl. 35), 1–137.

Boorman, J. C., & Sommerlad, B. C. (1985). Levator palati and palatal dimples: Their anatomy, relationship, and clinical significance. *British Journal of Plastic Surgery*, 38(3), 326–332.

Bunnell, H. T. (2005). The acoustic phonetics of nasality: A practical guide to acoustic analysis. *Perspectives on Speech Science and Orofacial Disorders*, 15(2), 3–10.

Bzoch, K. F. (1968). Variations in velopharyngeal valving: The factor of vowel changes. *Cleft Palate Journal*, 5, 211–218.

Casey, D. M., & Emrich, L. J. (1988). Passavant's ridge in patients with soft palatectomy. *Cleft Palate Journal*, 25(1), 72–77.

Cassell, M. D., & Elkadi, H. (1995). Anatomy and physiology of the palate and velopharyngeal structures. In R. J. Shprintzen & J. Bardach (Eds.), *Cleft palate speech management: A multidisciplinary approach* (pp. 45–62). St. Louis, MO: Mosby.

Cassell, M. D., Moon, J. B., & Elkadi, H. (1990). Anatomy and physiology of the velopharynx. In J. Bardach & H. L. Morris (Eds.), *Multidisciplinary management of cleft lip and palate*. Philadelphia: Saunders.

Cheng, N. X., & Zhang, K. Q. (2004). The applied anatomic study of palatopharyngeus muscle. *Chinese Journal of Plastic Surgery*, 20(5), 384–387.

Cheng, N., Zhao, M., & Qi, K. (2006). Lateral radiographic comparison for velar movement between palatoplasty with velopharyngeal muscular reconstruction and modified Von Langenbeck's procedure. *Zhongguo Xiu Fu Chong Jian Wai Ke Za Zhi*, 20(5), 515–518.

Croft, C. B., Shprintzen, R. J., & Rakoff, S. J. (1981). Patterns of velopharyngeal valving in normal and cleft palate subjects: A multiview videofluoroscopic and nasendoscopic study. *Laryngoscope*, 91(2), 265–271.

Croft, C. B., Shprintzen, R. J., & Ruben, R. J. (1981). Hypernasal speech following adenotonsillectomy. *Otolaryngology—Head & Neck Surgery*, 89(2), 179–188.

Cunsolo, E., Marchioni, D., Leo, G., Incorvaia, C., & Presutti, L. (2010). Functional anatomy of the Eustachian tube. *International Journal of Immunopathology and Pharmacology*, 23(Suppl. 1), 4–7.

Dickson, D. R. (1972). Normal and cleft palate anatomy. *Cleft Palate Journal, 9,* 280–93.

Dickson, D. R. (1975). Anatomy of the normal velopharyngeal mechanism. *Clinics in Plastic Surgery, 2*(2), 235–248.

Dickson, D. R., & Dickson, W. M. (1972). Velopharyngeal anatomy. *Journal of Speech and Hearing Research, 15*(2), 372–381.

Dickson, D. R., Grant, J. C., Sicher, H., Dubrul, E. L., & Paltan, J. (1974). Status of research in cleft palate anatomy and physiology, Part 1. *Cleft Palate Journal, 11,* 471–492.

Dickson, D. R., Grant, J. C., Sicher, H., Dubrul, E. L., & Paltan, J. (1975). Status of research in cleft lip and palate: Anatomy and physiology, Part 2. *Cleft Palate Journal, 12*(1), 131–156.

Ettema, S. L., & Kuehn, D. P. (1994). A quantitative histologic study of the normal human adult soft palate. *Journal of Speech and Hearing Research, 37,* 303–313.

Finkelstein, Y., Lerner, M. A., Ophir, D., Nachmani, A., Hauben, D. J., & Zohar, Y. (1993). Nasopharyngeal profile and velopharyngeal valve mechanism. *Plastic and Reconstructive Surgery, 92*(4), 603–614.

Finkelstein, Y., Talmi, Y. P., Kravitz, K., Bar-Ziv, J., Nachmani, A., Hauben, D. J., & Zohar, Y. (1991). Study of the normal and insufficient velopharyngeal valve by the "Forced Sucking Test." *Laryngoscope, 101* (11), 1203–1212.

Finkelstein, Y., Talmi, Y. P., Nachmani, A., Hauben, D. J., & Zohar, Y. (1992). On the variability of velopharyngeal valve anatomy and function: A combined peroral and nasendoscopic study. *Plastic & Reconstructive Surgery, 89*(4), 631–639.

Flowers, C. R., & Morris, H. L. (1973). Oral pharyngeal movements during swallowing and speech. *Cleft Palate Journal, 10,* 181–191.

Fritzell, B. (1979). Electromyography in the study of the velopharyngeal function—A review. *Folia Phoniatrica, 31*(2), 93–102.

Garcia-Garcia, A. S., Martinez-Gonzalez, J. M., Gomez-Font, R., Soto-Rivadeneira, A., & Oviedo-Roldan, L. (2010). Current status of the torus palatinus and torus mandibularis. *Medicina Oral Patología Oral y Cirugía Bucal, 15*(2), e353–360.

Ghadiali, S. N., Swarts, J. D., & Doyle, W. J. (2003). Effect of tensor veli palatini muscle paralysis on Eustachian tube mechanics. *The Annals of Otology, Rhinology, and Laryngology, 112*(8), 704–711.

Glaser, E. R., Skolnick, M. L., McWilliams, B. J., & Shprintzen, R. J. (1979). The dynamics of Passavant's ridge in subjects with and without velopharyngeal insufficiency—A multi-view videofluoroscopic study. *Cleft Palate Journal, 16*(1), 24–33.

Ha, S., Sim, H., Zhi, M., & Kuehn, D. P. (2004). An acoustic study of the temporal characteristics of nasalization in children with and without cleft palate. *The Cleft Palate–Craniofacial Journal, 41*(5), 535–543.

Hoit, J. D., Watson, P. J., Hixon, K. E., McMahon, P., & Johnson, C. L. (1994). Age and velopharyngeal function during speech production. *Journal of Speech and Hearing Research, 37*(2), 295–302.

Honjo, L., Kojima, M., & Kumazawa, T. (1975). Role of Passavant's ridge in cleft palate speech. *Archives of Otorhinolaryngology, 211*(3), 203–208.

Huang, M. H., Lee, S. T., & Rajendran, K. (1997). Structure of the musculus uvulae: Functional and surgical implications of an anatomic study. *The Cleft Palate–Craniofacial Journal, 34*(6), 466–474.

Huang, M. H., Lee, S. T., & Rajendran, K. (1998). Anatomic basis of cleft palate and velopharyngeal surgery: Implications from a fresh cadaveric study. *Plastic & Reconstructive Surgery, 101*(3), 613–27; Discussion 628–629.

Hwang, K., Kim, D. J., Huan, F., Han, S. H., & Hwang, S. W. (2011). Width of the levator aponeurosis is broader than the tarsal plate. *Journal of Craniofacial Surgery, 22* (3), 1061–1063.

Igawa, H. H., Nishizawa, N., Sugihara, T., & Inuyama, Y. (1998). A fiberscopic analysis of velopharyngeal movement before and after primary palatoplasty in cleft palate infants. *Plastic & Reconstructive Surgery, 102*(3), 668–674.

Iglesias, A., Kuehn, D. P., & Morris, H. L. (1980). Simultaneous assessment of pharyngeal wall and velar displacement of selected speech sounds. *Journal of Speech and Hearing Research, 23*, 429–446.

Jones. (1989). From page 1–6.

Jones, D. L. (2006). Patterns of oral-nasal balance in normal speakers with and without cleft palate. *Folia Phoniatrica et Logopaedica, 58*(6), 383–391.

Kao, D. S., Soltysik, D. A., Hyde, J. S., & Gosain, A. K. (2008). Magnetic resonance imaging as an aid in the dynamic assessment of the velopharyngeal mechanism in children. *Plastic and Reconstructive Surgery, 122*(2), 572–577.

Karnell, M. P., Linville, R. N., & Edwards, B. A. (1988). Variations in velar position over time: A nasal videoendoscopic study. *Journal of Speech and Hearing Research, 31*(3), 417–424.

Kennedy, J. G., & Kuehn, D. P. (1989). Neuroanatomy of speech. In D. P. Kuehn, M. L. Lemme, & J. M. Baumgartner (Eds.), *Neural bases of speech, hearing, and language* (pp. 111–145). Boston: College-Hill Press.

Kent, R. D. (1976). Anatomical and neuromuscular maturation of the speech mechanism: Evidence from acoustic studies. *Journal of Speech and Hearing Research, 19*(3), 421–447.

Kent, R. D., & Moll, K. L. (1969). Vocal-tract characteristics of the stop cognates. *Journal of the Acoustical Society of America, 46* (6), 1549–1555.

Kent, R. D., & Vorperian, H. K. (1995). Development of the craniofacial-oral-laryngeal anatomy: A review. *Journal of Medical Speech-Language Pathology, 3*(3), 145–190.

Kollia, H. B., Gracco, V. L., & Harris, K. S. (1995). Articulatory organization of mandibular, labial, and velar movements during speech. *The Journal of the Acoustical Society of America, 98*(3), 1313–1324.

Kuehn, D. P. (1979). Velopharyngeal anatomy and physiology. *Ear, Nose & Throat Journal, 58*(7), 316–321.

Kuehn, D. P., & Azzam, N. A. (1978). Anatomical characteristics of palatoglossus and the anterior faucial pillar. *Cleft Palate Journal, 15*, 349–359.

Kuehn, D. P., Folkins, J. W., & Linville, R. N. (1988). An electromyographic study of the musculus uvulae. *Cleft Palate Journal, 25* (4), 348–355.

Kuehn, D. P., & Kahane, J. C. (1990). Histologic study of the normal human adult soft palate. *Cleft Palate Journal, 27*, 26–34.

Kuehn, D. P., & Moon, J. B. (1994). Levator veli palatini muscle activity in relation to intraoral air pressure variation. *Journal of Speech & Hearing Research, 37*(6), 1260–1270.

Kuehn, D. P., & Moon, J. B. (1998). Velopharyngeal closure force and levator veli palatini activation levels in varying phonetic contexts. *Journal of Speech, Language & Hearing Research, 41*(1), 51–62.

Kuehn, D. P., & Moon, J. B. (2000). Induced fatigue effects on velopharyngeal closure force. *Journal of Speech, Language & Hearing Research, 43*(2), 486–500.

Kuehn, D. P., & Moon, J. B. (2005). Histologic study of intravelar structures in normal human adult specimens. *The Cleft Palate– Craniofacial Journal, 42*(5), 481–489.

Lam, E., Hundert, S., & Wilkes, G. H. (2007). Lateral pharyngeal wall and velar movement and tailoring velopharyngeal surgery: Determinants of velopharyngeal incompetence resolution in patients with cleft palate. *Plastic and Reconstructive Surgery, 120*(2), 495–505; discussion 506–507.

Licameli, G. R. (2002). The eustachian tube. Update on anatomy, development, and function. *Otolaryngologic Clinics of North America, 35*(4), 803–809.

Lukens, A., Dimartino, E., Gunther, R. W., & Krombach, G. A. (2011). Functional MR imaging of the Eustachian tube in patients with clinically proven dysfunction: Correlation with lesions detected on MR images. *European Radiology.*

Magen, H. S., Kang, A. M., Tiede, M. K., & Whalen, D. H. (2003). Posterior pharyngeal wall position in the production of speech. *Journal of Speech, Language & Hearing Research, 46*(1), 241–251.

Maryn, Y., Van Lierde, K., De Bodt, M., & Van Cauwenberge, P. (2004). The effects of adenoidectomy and tonsillectomy on speech and nasal resonance. *Folia Phoniatric Logopedia, 56*(3), 182–191.

Mason, R. M., & Warren, D. W. (1980). Adenoid involution and developing hypernasality in cleft palate. *Journal of Speech & Hearing Disorders, 45*(4), 469–480.

Matsuya, T., Yamaoka, M., & Miyasaki, T. (1979). A fiberoscopic study of velopharyngeal closure in patients with operated cleft palates. *Plastic & Reconstructive Surgery, 63*(4), 497–500.

Maue-Dickson, W. (1977). Cleft lip and palate research: An updated state of the art. Section II. Anatomy and physiology. *Cleft Palate Journal, 14*(4), 270–287.

Maue-Dickson, W. (1979). The craniofacial complex in cleft lip and palate: An update review of anatomy and function. *Cleft Palate Journal, 16*(3), 291–317.

Maue-Dickson, W., & Dickson, D. R. (1980). Anatomy and physiology related to cleft palate: Current research and clinical implications. *Plastic & Reconstructive Surgery, 65*(1), 83–90.

Maue-Dickson, W., Dickson, D. R., & Rood, S. R. (1976). Anatomy of the Eustachian tube and related structures in age-matched human fetuses with and without cleft palate. *Transactions of the American Academy of Ophthalmology and Otolaryngology, 82*(2), 159–164.

Mehendale, F. V. (2004). Surgical anatomy of the levator veli palatini: A previously undescribed tendonous insertion of the anterolateral fibers. *Plastic and reconstructive surgery, 114*(2), 307–315.

Moll, K. (1962). Velopharyngeal closure on vowels. *Journal of Speech and Hearing Research, 5,* 30–37.

Moll, K. L., & Shriner, T. H. (1967). Preliminary investigation of a new concept of velar activity during speech. *Cleft Palate Journal, 4,* 58.

Moon, J. B., & Kuehn, D. P. (1996). Anatomy and physiology of normal and disordered velopharyngeal function for speech. *National Center for Voice and Speech, 9* (April), 143–158.

Moon, J. B., & Kuehn, D. P. (1997). Anatomy and physiology of normal and disordered velopharyngeal function for speech. In K. R. Bzoch (Ed.), *Communicative disorders related to cleft lip and palate* (4th ed., pp. 45–47). Austin, TX: Pro-Ed.

Moon, J. B., & Kuehn, D. P. (2004). Anatomy and physiology of normal and disordered velopharyngeal function for speech. In K. R. Bzoch (Ed.), *Communicative disorders related to cleft lip and palate* (5th ed.), Austin, TX: Pro-Ed.

Moon, J., Kuehn, D. P., & Huisman, J. (1994). Measurement of velopharyngeal closure force during vowel production. *The Cleft Palate–Craniofacial Journal*, *31*, 356–363.

Moon, J., Smith, A., Folkins, J., Lemke, J., & Gartlan, M. (1994). Coordination of velopharyngeal muscle activity during positioning of the soft palate. *The Cleft Palate–Craniofacial Journal*, *31*, 45–55.

Mourino, A. P., & Weinberg, B. (1975). A cephalometric study of velar stretch in 8- and 10-year-old children. *Cleft Palate Journal*, *12*, 417–435.

Nohara, K., Kotani, Y., Ojima, M., Sasao, Y., Tachimura, T., & Sakai, T. (2007). Power spectra analysis of levator veli palatini muscle electromyogram during velopharyngeal closure for swallowing, speech, and blowing. *Dysphagia*, *2*, 135–139.

Nohara, K., Tachimura, T., & Wada, T. (2006). Levator veli palatini muscle fatigue during phonation in speakers with cleft palate with borderline velopharyngeal incompetence. *The Cleft Palate–Craniofacial Journal*, *43*, 103–107.

Perry, J. L. (2011). Anatomy and physiology of the velopharyngeal mechanism. *Seminars in Speech and Language*, *32*(2), 83–92.

Perry, J. L., & Kuehn, D. P. (2009). Magnetic resonance imaging and computer reconstruction of the velopharyngeal mechanism. *Journal of Craniofacial Surgery*, *20* (Suppl. 2), 1739–1746.

Perry, J. L., Kuehn, D. P., & Sutton, B. P. (2011). Morphology of the Levator Veli Palatini Muscle Using Magnetic Resonance Imaging. *Cleft Palate and Craniofacial Journal*, October 24, 2011. Epub ahead of print.

Pruzansky, S., & Mason, R. (1962). The "stretch factor" in soft palate function. *Journal of Dental Research*, *48*, 972.

Rommel, N., Bellon, E., Hermans, R., Smet, M., De Meyer, A. M., Feenstra, L., Dejaeger, E., Veereman-Wauters, G. (2003). Development of the orohypopharyngeal cavity in normal infants and young children. *The Cleft Palate–Craniofacial Journal*, *40*(6), 606–611.

Sataloff, R. T. (1992, December). The human voice. *Scientific American*, 108–115.

Sataloff, R. T., Heman-Ackah, Y. D., Hawkshaw, M. J. (2007). Clinical anatomy and physiology of the voice. *Otolaryngologic clinics of North America*, *40*(5), 909–929.

Satoh, K., Wada, T., Tachimura, T., & Fukuda, J. (2005). Velar ascent and morphological factors affecting velopharyngeal function in patients with cleft palate and noncleft controls: A cephalometric study. *International Journal of Oral and Maxillofacial Surgery*, *34*(2), 122–126.

Seaver, E. J., & Kuehn, D. P. (1980). A cineradiographic and electromyographic investigation of velar positioning in nonnasal speech. *Cleft Palate Journal*, *17*(3), 216–226.

Seikel, J. A., King, D. W., Drumright, D. G. (2005). Anatomy & physiology for speech, language, and hearing (3rd ed.). Clifton Park, NY: Thomson Delmar Learning.

Serrurier, A., & Badin, P. (2008). A three-dimensional articulatory model of the velum and nasopharyngeal wall based on MRI and CT data. *Journal of the Acoustic Society of America, 123*(4), 2335–2355.

Shimokawa, T., Yi, S. Q., Izumi, A., Ru, F., Akita, K., Sato, T., & Tanaka, S. (2004). An anatomical study of the levator veli palatini and superior constrictor with special reference to their nerve supply. *Surgical and Radiological Anatomy, 26*(2), 100–105.

Shprintzen, R. J., Lencione, R. M., McCall, G. N., & Skolnick, M. L. (1974). A three-dimensional cinefluoroscopic analysis of velopharyngeal closure during speech and nonspeech activities in normals. *Cleft Palate Journal, 11*, 412–428.

Shprintzen, R. J., McCall, G. N., Skolnick, M. L., & Lencione, R. M. (1975). Selective movement of the lateral aspects of the pharyngeal walls during velopharyngeal closure for speech, blowing, and whistling in normals. *Cleft Palate Journal, 12*(1), 51–58.

Shprintzen, R. J., Rakoff, S. J., Skolnick, M. L., & Lavorato, A. S. (1977). Incongruous movements of the velum and lateral pharyngeal walls. *Cleft Palate Journal, 14*(2), 148–157.

Siegel-Sadewitz, V. L., & Shprintzen, R. J. (1982). Nasopharyngoscopy of the normal velopharyngeal sphincter: An experiment of biofeedback. *Cleft Palate Journal, 19*(3), 194–200.

Siegel-Sadewitz, V. L., & Shprintzen, R. J. (1986). Changes in velopharyngeal valving with age. *International Journal of Pediatric Otorhinolaryngology, 11*(2), 171–182.

Simpson, R. K., & Austin, A. A. (1972). A cephalometric investigation of velar stretch. *Cleft Palate Journal, 9*, 341–351.

Simpson, R. K., & Chin, L. (1981). Velar stretch as a function of task. *Cleft Palate Journal, 18*(1), 1–9.

Simpson, R. K., & Colton, J. (1980). A cephalometric study of velar stretch in adolescent subjects. *Cleft Palate Journal, 17*(1), 40–47.

Skolnick, M. L., & Cohn, E. R. (1989). *Videofluoroscopic studies of speech in patients with cleft palate.* New York: Springer-Verlag.

Skolnick, M. L., McCall, G., & Barnes, M. (1973). The sphincteric mechanism of velopharyngeal closure. *Cleft Palate Journal, 10*, 286–305.

Skolnick, M. L., Shprintzen, R. J., McCall, G. N., & Rakoff, S. (1975). Patterns of velopharyngeal closure in subjects with repaired cleft palate and normal speech: A multi-view videofluoroscopic analysis. *Cleft Palate Journal, 12*, 369–376.

Smith, B. E., & Kuehn, D. P. (2007). Speech evaluation of velopharyngeal dysfunction. *The Journal of Craniofacial Surgery, 18*(2), 251–261.

Stellzig-Eisenhauer, A. (2001). The influence of cephalometric parameters on resonance of speech in cleft lip and palate patients. An interdisciplinary study. *Journal of Orofacial Orthopedics, 62*(3), 202–223.

Sumida, K., Yamashita, K., & Kitamura, S. (2012). Gross anatomical study of the human palatopharyngeus muscle throughout its entire course from origin to insertion. *Clinical Anatomy, 25*(3), 314–323.

Tachimura, T., Nohara, K., Satoh, K., & Wada, T. (2004). Evaluation of fatigability of the levator veli palatini muscle during continuous blowing using power spectra analysis. *The Cleft Palate–Craniofacial Journal, 41*(3), 320–326.

Takemoto, H., Mokhtari, P., & Kitamura, T. (2010). Acoustic analysis of the vocal tract during vowel production by finite-difference time-domain method. *Journal of the Acoustic Society of America, 128*(6), 3724–3738.

Tineshev, S. A. (2010). Age dynamics and secular changes of indices characterizing the neurocranium and facial cranium in ethnic Bulgarian 7-17-year-old children from the region of the Eastern Rhodopes. *Folia Med (Plovdiv), 52*(4), 32–38.

Tom, K., Titze, I. R., Hoffman, E. A., & Story, B. H. (2001). Three-dimensional vocal tract imaging and formant structure: Varying vocal register, pitch, and loudness. *Journal of the Acoustical Society of America, 109*(2), 742–747.

Tourne, L. P. (1991). Growth of the pharynx and its physiologic implications. *American Journal of Orthodontics and Dentofacial Orthopediatrics, 99*(2), 129–139.

Tsai, C. G., Chen, J. H., Shau, Y. W., & Hsiao, T. Y. (2009). Dynamic B-mode ultrasound imaging of vocal fold vibration during phonation. *Ultrasound in Medicine & Biology, 35*(11), 1812–1818.

Ursi, W. J., Trotman, C. A., McNamara, J. A., Jr., & Behrents, R. G. (1993). Sexual dimorphism in normal craniofacial growth. *Angle Orthodontist, 63*(1), 47–56.

Van Demark, D. R., & Morris, H. L. (1983). Stability of velopharyngeal competency. *Cleft Palate Journal, 20*(1), 18–22.

Witzel, M. A., & Posnick, J. C. (1989). Patterns and location of velopharyngeal valving problems: Atypical findings on video naso-pharyngoscopy. *Cleft Palate Journal, 26*(1), 63–67.

Yamawaki, Y. (2003). Forward movement of posterior pharyngeal wall on phonation. *American Journal of Otolaryngology, 24*(6), 400–404.

Yanagisawa, E., & Weaver, E. M. (1996). Passavant's ridge: Is it a functional structure? *Ear Nose Throat Journal, 75*(12), 766–767.

Yoshida, H., Takahashi, H., Morikawa, M., & Kobayashi, T. (2007). Anatomy of the bony portion of the eustachian tube in tubal stenosis: Multiplanar reconstruction approach. *Annals of Otology, Rhinology and Laryngology, 116*(9), 681–686.

C H A P T E R

2

CLEFTS OF THE LIP AND PALATE

CHAPTER OUTLINE

INTRODUCTION

Cleft lip and palate is the fourth most common birth defect and the most common congenital defect of the face. A cleft of the lip affects facial aesthetics, whereas a cleft of the palate can affect feeding, middle ear function, and speech. Clefts vary in type and severity, but typically follow the path of normal embryological suture lines.

This chapter begins with a general description of a cleft and its associated malformations. It then goes on to describe the embryological development of the lip and palate, and the various types of clefts that can occur when there is a disruption in this development. Particular emphasis is placed on submucous cleft palate because this anomaly can cause significant problems with speech and resonance, but is not always easy to identify. The effect of the cleft on the anatomy of the lip, palate, and adjacent structures is described. Potential functional problems secondary to the cleft are also noted.

WHAT IS A CLEFT

A *cleft* is an abnormal opening or a fissure in an anatomical structure that is normally closed. A cleft lip is the result of failure of parts of the lip to come together early in the life of a fetus. Cleft palate occurs when the sections of the roof of the mouth do not fuse normally during fetal development, leaving an opening between the oral cavity and the nasal cavity. Clefts can vary in length and in width, depending on the degree of fusion of the individual parts. It is important to note that when there is a cleft lip and/or palate, the structures are all present but have not fused together normally. However, the structures may be *hypoplastic*, where tissues (i.e., bone, muscles, and nerves) are underdeveloped in their formation.

A cleft of the lip and/or palate is a *congenital* condition (present at birth due to either an inherited condition or something that occurred during the pregnancy). Because a cleft is due to a disruption in embryological development, clefts typically follow the normal embryological fusion lines. The interference in embryological development of the midface and oral cavity can also be associated with malformations of the nose, eyes, and other facial structures as well (Mossey, Little, Munger, Dixon & Shaw, 2009; Yu, Serrano, Miguel, Ruest, & Svoboda, 2009). When other congenital anomalies occur along with the cleft lip and palate, they usually have a genetic etiology and are part of a "multiple malformation" syndrome (Jones, 1988; Sekhon, Ethunandan, Markus, Gopalkrishnan, & Rao, 2010).

A cleft lip presents with more serious cosmetic concerns than a cleft palate, but a cleft palate presents with more serious functional problems, particularly with speech and hearing. Individuals born with both cleft lip and cleft palate are at risk for problems with aesthetics, feeding, speech, resonance, and hearing. Although there are many commonalities in the appearance of the basic clefting conditions, clefts also give rise to unique anatomical and functional deviations. These deviations are due to variations in etiology and differences in the forms of treatment that the patient has undergone. Therefore, the severity in aesthetics and function ranges from barely noticeable to severely affected and malformed.

EMBRYOLOGICAL DEVELOPMENT

A basic knowledge of embryological development and the sequence of lip and palate formation helps the clinician to understand why clefts occur as they do. This knowledge also relates to how clefts are described and classified.

Embryological development of the face and palate is dependent on the formation of neural crest cells in the embryo. These cells migrate at different rates to form the structures of the skull and face. If migration of the neural crest cells fails to take place or if the migration is delayed, this can affect the formation of facial structures and can cause clefts or other craniofacial anomalies.

Embryological development of the lip and alveolus begins at around 6 to 7 weeks of gestation and starts at the incisive foramen. Figure 2–1 shows the direction of embryological closure of the sutures lines. Fusion begins at the incisive foramen and then proceeds in an anterior direction to form the alveolus through the fusion of the bilateral incisive suture lines. Closure then proceeds to form the base of the anterior nose and finally the upper lip. The median and two lateral lip segments are then fused, forming the philtrum and philtral lines. This completes the formation of the upper lip.

Embryological development of the palate starts at around 8 to 9 weeks of gestation. Prior to palate formation, the tongue is in a high and posterior position, in the area of the posterior nasal cavity. The palatal shelves are vertical and positioned on each side of the tongue.

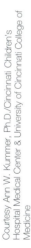
Courtesy Ann W. Kummer, Ph.D./Cincinnati Children's Hospital Medical Center & University of Cincinnati College of Medicine

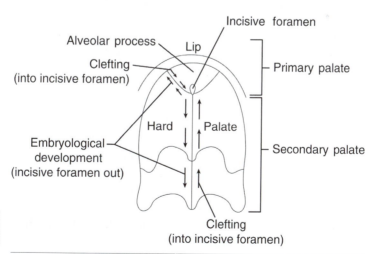

FIGURE 2–1 Embryological development and patterns of clefting. Embryological development proceeds from the incisive foramen out to the periphery. Clefting patterns begin at the periphery and follow the lines of normal embryological fusion towards the incisive foramen to the point of that disruption. The classification of clefts as affecting either the primary palate or the secondary palate is based on embryological development, with the incisive foramen as the dividing point between the two.

Around the seventh or eighth week of gestation, the tongue begins to gradually drop down. When this occurs, the palatal shelves move slowly from a vertical to a horizontal position. They then begin to fuse, first with the premaxilla at the incisive foramen and then with each other. As can be noted in Figure 2–1, the process of fusion begins at the incisive foramen and then proceeds between the palatal shelves, moving in a posterior direction along the median palatine suture line. This completes the formation of the hard palate. The vomer, forming a portion of the nasal septum, moves downward. It fuses with the superior surface of the hard palate, thus completing the separation of the nasal cavity. Once the hard palate is formed, the velum is fused in midline, forming the median raphe. Lastly, the uvula is formed. It can be theorized that fusion of the oral surface of the velum slightly precedes fusion of the nasal surface, which would explain the occasional occurrence of an occult submucous cleft (on the nasal surface only). Fusion of the hard palate and velum is usually complete by 12 weeks of gestation.

CAUSES OF CLEFTS

Because embryological fusion goes from the incisive foramen out (forward for the alveolus and lip and backward for the hard palate and velum), anything that disrupts that process will cause a cleft from that point all the way to the periphery (lip or uvula). Therefore, as can be seen in Figure 2–1, clefting patterns begin at the periphery and follow the lines of normal embryological fusion toward the incisive foramen to the point of that disruption. A "complete" cleft is one that follows the embryological

fusion line(s) all the way through to the incisive foramen.

Clefts can occur due to disruptions or delays in cell migration or palatal shelf movement. There are several basic causes of clefts and related craniofacial anomalies, including chromosomal disorders and genetic disorders, which are both *endogenous* (internal) factors. Recently, older parental age has also been linked with an increased risk for both cleft lip and cleft palate (Bille et al., 2005; Martelli et al., 2010). Clefts can also be caused by environmental teratogens or by mechanical factors in utero. These are both considered *exogenous* (external) factors.

Environmental *teratogens* are substances that can cause congenital malformations. Teratogens that have been associated with cleft lip and/or palate include cigarette smoke (Honein, Paulozzi, & Watkins, 2001; Reiter et al., 2012); certain drugs, such as phenytoin (Dilantin), valium, and corticosteroids (Edwards et al., 2003); and lead pollution (Vinceti et al., 2001). Certain viruses, including rubella and even influenza (Metneki, Puho, & Czeizel, 2005), have been found to be risk factors for the pathogenesis of clefts. Even maternal nutritional deficiencies have been implicated in causing malformations. Lack of maternal vitamin B-6 has been associated with clefting (Munger et al., 2004). In the past, folic acid deficiency was thought to be a cause of orofacial clefts because it is important for embryonic and fetal development of the neural tube. However, recent studies have found that folic acid fortification during pregnancy has not reduced the prevalence of clefting in large populations (Bille, Knudsen, & Christensen, 2005; Castilla, Orioli, Lopez-Camelo, Dutra Mda, & Nazer-Herrera, 2003; Hashmi, Waller, Langlois, Canfield, & Hecht, 2005; Munger et al., 2004; Ray, Meier, Vermeulen, Wyatt, &

Cole, 2003). Although the evidence linking low levels of folic acid to clefting is presently equivocal, there is strong evidence for the role of folic acid in the prevention of neural tube defects (Simmons, Mosley, Fulton-Bond, & Hobbs, 2004). Finally, maternal obesity has been found to cause an increased risk for orofacial clefts (Moore, Singer, Bradlee, Rothman, & Milunsky, 2000).

Mechanical interference can also affect embryonic development and cause clefts. For example, one of the causes of Pierre Robin sequence with cleft palate is mechanical interference due to crowding in utero. In this case, the crowding may cause the head to be pushed down, thus restricting the forward and downward growth of the mandible. Because the position of the tongue is determined by the position of the mandible, this leaves the tongue up high, causing interference with palate formation. The result is typically a wide, bell-shaped cleft palate (as opposed to a V-shaped cleft that occurs due to other causes of disruption).

Although various causes of clefts have been identified, the etiology of clefting in a single individual is complex and may involve a combination of factors. Several genes can contribute to clefting. These genes may lead to a genetic predisposition for a cleft, but may not cause expression of the cleft unless combined with certain environmental factors. In fact, in most cases the cause of the cleft is not due to just one factor, but instead is due to the interaction of several factors. This is called *multifactorial inheritance*.

CLASSIFICATION OF CLEFTS

Because there are different types of clefts with different combinations, the naming and classification of clefts can be a challenge. Although several classification systems have been proposed over the years, the system that has gained the most universal acceptance is the one proposed by Kernahan and Stark (1958). Kernahan and Stark recommended that clefts be classified based on embryological development, with two basic categories: clefts of the primary palate and clefts of the secondary palate, with the incisive foramen as the dividing point between the two. This division can be viewed schematically on the right side of Figure 2–1.

The *primary palate* includes the structures that are anterior to the incisive foramen. These are the structures that fuse around 7 weeks of gestation and include the alveolus and also the lip (even though the terminology is primary "palate"). The *secondary palate* includes the structures that are posterior to the incisive foramen. These are the structures that fuse around 9 weeks of gestation and include the hard palate (excluding the alveolus) and the velum. Clefts can be of the primary palate, secondary palate, or both.

Although this basic classification system is used most commonly by professionals, a modification of the Kernahan and Stark classification system was later proposed by Kernahan (1971). Because clefts vary in severity, this system is more detailed. It uses a "striped-Y" figure as a means of identifying the extent of the cleft classification, as noted in Figure 2–2. The upper arms of the Y represent the primary palate, and the base of the Y represents the secondary palate. The Y form is divided into sections that are numbered. The upper stems of the Y are divided into three segments, with the right side numbered as 1, 2, and 3 and the left side numbered as 4, 5, and 6. The most anterior segment represents the lip; the middle segment represents the alveolus; and the

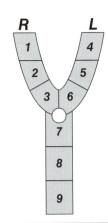

FIGURE 2–2 The Kernahan striped Y for cleft classification. The upper arms of the Y represent the primary palate and the base represents the secondary palate. The most anterior segment represents the lip, the middle segment represents the alveolus, and the posterior segment represents the area between the alveolus and the incisive foramen. The secondary palate (hard and soft palate) is also divided into sections to represent the areas of the velum and hard palate. The segments affected by the cleft are darkened on the diagram so that a visual representation can be made of the type and extent of the cleft. If there is a submucous cleft, the affected segments are marked with crosshatch marks.

posterior segment represents the area between the alveolus and the incisive foramen. The secondary palate (hard and soft palate) is also divided into three sections, and these are numbered as 7, 8, and 9. When the segments affected by the cleft are darkened on the diagram, a visual representation can be made of the type and extent of the cleft. If there is a submucous cleft, the affected segments are marked with crosshatch marks. Using this figure, the extent of a cleft can be described or illustrated.

CLEFTS OF THE PRIMARY PALATE

As noted above, the primary palate includes structures anterior to the incisive foramen.

Therefore, clefts of the primary palate include the lip, and often include the alveolus.

Types and Severity

There are various types of clefts of the primary palate and various degrees of severity, as can be seen in Figure 2–3. A cleft of the primary palate can be "complete," which means that it extends through the entire lip, nostril sill, and alveolus to the incisive foramen. When the term "complete cleft lip" is used, it often refers to a complete cleft of the primary palate. If the cleft does not extend to the incisive foramen, it is considered "incomplete." An incomplete cleft lip can be as minor as a small, subcutaneous notch in the vermilion, or it may involve the entire lip and part of the alveolus.

In addition to incomplete or complete, a cleft of the primary palate can be unilateral

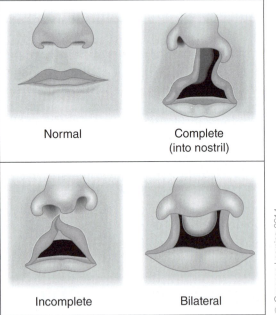

FIGURE 2–3 A normal lip and basic types of cleft lip. On the drawings of clefts, note the short columella and the distortion of the ala on the affected side.

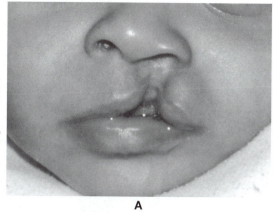

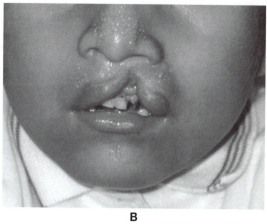

A

B

FIGURE 2–4 (A and B)   Patients with a unilateral incomplete cleft of the primary palate (lip and alveolus).

(on the right or the left side) or bilateral (on both sides). If the cleft is unilateral, it most often occurs on the left side (Jensen, Kreiborg, Dahl, & Fogh-Andersen, 1988; Kim & Baek, 2006; McWilliams, Morris, & Shelton, 1990). Figure 2–4 (A and B) illustrates examples of a unilateral incomplete cleft of the lip and alveolus. Figure 2–5 (A–D) shows examples of a unilateral complete cleft of the primary palate (lip and alveolus). Figure 2–6 (A–D) shows examples of bilateral incomplete cleft of the lip. Finally, Figure 2–7 (A–C) shows infants with bilateral complete cleft of the primary palate.

A bilateral cleft of the lip results in the complete separation of the tissue that would normally form the philtrum. The philtral tissue segment that is isolated due to the bilateral cleft is called the *prolabium*. When a bilateral cleft courses through the lip and also through both incisive suture lines in the alveolus to the incisive foramen, it separates the triangle-shaped premaxilla bone. Therefore, when there is a complete bilateral cleft of the lip and alveolus, both the prolabium and the premaxilla are separated. In many cases, these structures are positioned in an extremely

anterior position at birth so that they appear to extend from the tip of the nose. In Figure 2–7, the prolabium appears as tissue that is attached to the tip of the nose and the premaxilla is isolated and in an anterior position.

By examining an unrepaired cleft lip closely, one can see that all the structures are present, including the philtral dimple and both of the philtral ridges. The cleft passes just to the lateral side of the philtral ridge. On the cleft side, the lip is short and the Cupid's bow is twisted up into the cleft. Although cleft lip can occur in isolation, it is more often found to be associated with a cleft palate.

In rare cases, a *form fruste* (or *microform cleft*) may occur (Figure 2–8). A form fruste is a partial or arrested form of a cleft lip. In Figure 2–8 (A and B), the overlying skin is intact, but the underlying muscle, nasal cartilage, and oral sphincter function usually are significantly affected. Whether the cleft is complete or incomplete, if it extends through the nostril sill, it will cause distortion of the nose. Another infrequent finding with regard to the cleft lip is a *Simonart's band* (Figure 2–9), which is a strand of soft tissue in the area of the cleft. A Simonart's band is due

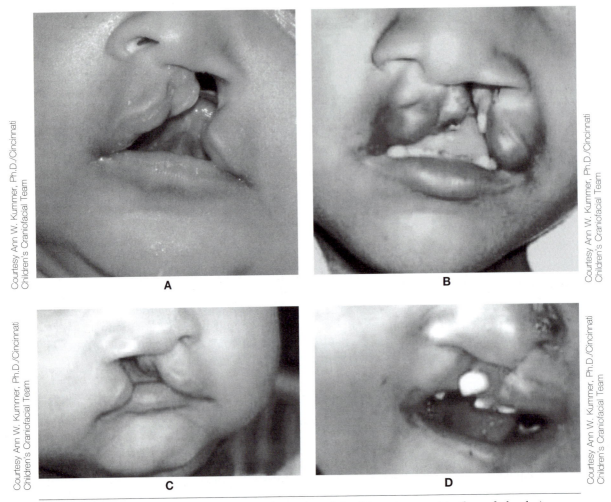

FIGURE 2–5 (A–D)   Patients with a unilateral complete cleft of the primary palate (lip and alveolus).

to partial, yet incomplete, embryonic fusion of the upper lip; it has no particular clinical significance, and the treatment is the same as in a complete cleft lip.

Effects on Structure and Function

Because a complete cleft of the lip and alveolus courses through the nostril sill, the nose can be adversely affected. The nose may appear to be very wide and flattened due to the separation

of the *orbicularis oris muscle*, which is the muscle that encircles the mouth and functions by closing the lips. This muscle is not only divided but also misaligned and curves upward along the edges of the vermilion. The wide space within the cleft can further distort the nose by spreading the nasal ala. In fact, the wider the cleft, the more distorted the nasal features will be.

The formation of the columella may also be adversely affected by a cleft lip, causing it to be abnormally short. If the cleft is unilateral,

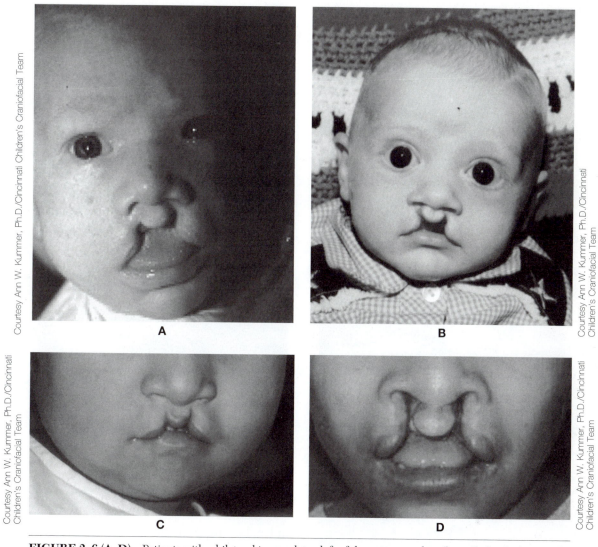

Courtesy Ann W. Kummer, Ph.D./Cincinnati Children's Craniofacial Team

Courtesy Ann W. Kummer, Ph.D./Cincinnati Children's Craniofacial Team

Courtesy Ann W. Kummer, Ph.D./Cincinnati Children's Craniofacial Team

Courtesy Ann W. Kummer, Ph.D./Cincinnati Children's Craniofacial Team

A   **B**

C   **D**

FIGURE 2–6 (A–D)   Patients with a bilateral incomplete cleft of the primary palate (lip and alveolus). Note the distortion of the nose.

the columella will be short on the cleft side and positioned obliquely, with its base deviated toward the noncleft side. When the cleft is bilateral and complete, the columella may be so short that it is virtually nonexistent, giving the appearance that the prolabium and pre-maxilla are attached to the tip of the nose. In less common cases, as in the case of a forme fruste, the lip is essentially intact, but there still may be evidence of the nasal deformity and the muscle discontinuity that are typically found with cleft lip.

Clefts of the primary (and secondary) palate often result in nasal cavity deformities that tend to reduce its size. The nasal cavity is smaller in individuals with unilateral cleft lip

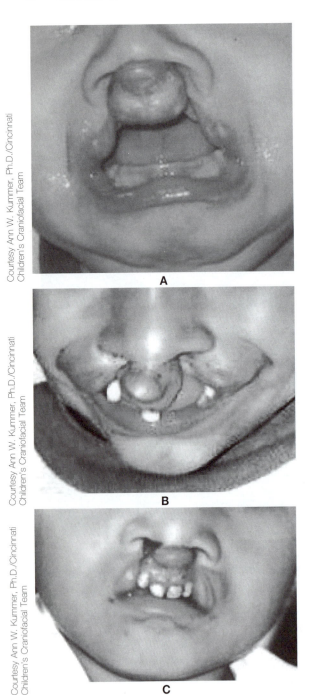

FIGURE 2–7 (A–C)   Patients with a bilateral complete cleft lip.

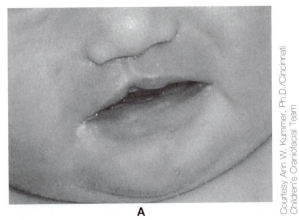

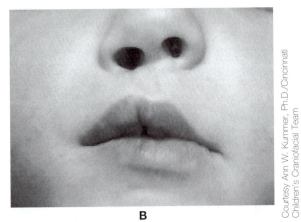

FIGURE 2–8 (A and B)   Patients with a forme fruste (or microform cleft). This is a partially arrested form of cleft lip.

and palate than in those with bilateral clefts. Although the nasal cavity continues to grow with age, it remains about 30% smaller than normal due to the inherent dysplasia of the tissues and possibly due to the restrictive effects of surgical correction (Drake, Davis, & Warren, 1993; Reiser, Andlin-Sobocki, Mani, & Holmstrom, 2011).

Finally, a cleft of the primary palate may result in dental and occlusal abnormalities, and also small oral cavity size. Dental interference of tongue tip movement or crowding in the

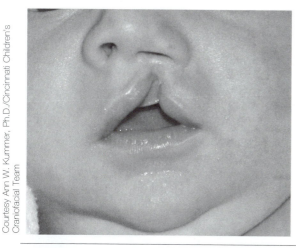

FIGURE 2–9 Patient with a Simonart's band, which is a strand of soft tissue in the area of the cleft due to partial, yet incomplete embryonic fusion of the upper lip.

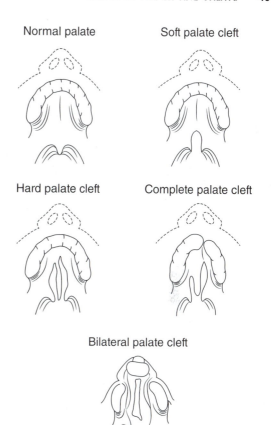

Normal palate   Soft palate cleft

Hard palate cleft   Complete palate cleft

Bilateral palate cleft

FIGURE 2–10 A normal palate and various types of cleft palate.

anterior portion of the oral cavity can cause specific articulation errors on anterior speech sounds, and the small cavity size can affect resonance.

CLEFTS OF THE SECONDARY PALATE

As previously discussed, the secondary palate includes structures posterior to the incisive foramen. Therefore, clefts of the secondary palate include the uvula and usually the velum, and often include the hard palate.

Types and Severity

As with cleft lip, a cleft palate can be either incomplete or complete and can occur with various degrees of severity, as shown in Figure 2–10. An incomplete cleft palate may be as slight as a line in the midline of the uvula or a bifid uvula. A more severe incomplete cleft palate may extend into the velum or into part of the hard palate. A complete cleft of the secondary palate goes through the uvula and the velum, and then follows the median palatine suture line through the hard palate all the way to the incisive foramen. The vomer bone, which forms the bottom part of the nasal septum, is usually attached to the larger of the two palatal segments in a unilateral cleft, and is not attached to either segment in a bilateral cleft. A cleft palate can occur with or without a cleft lip. Isolated cleft palate (with no involvement of the lip) is more frequently associated with a syndrome, and thus with other anomalies. Figures 2–11A and 2–11B show two patients, each with a repaired unilateral cleft

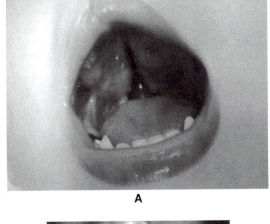

A

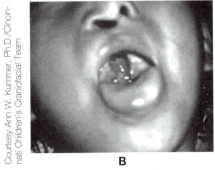

B

FIGURE 2–11 (A and B) (A) Unrepaired complete cleft palate (hard palate and velum). The right unilateral cleft lip has been repaired. (B) Wide unrepaired cleft palate (hard palate and velum).

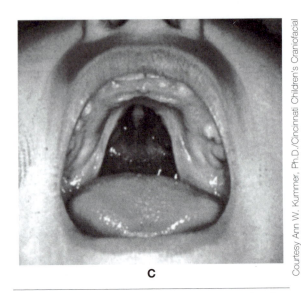

C

FIGURE 2–11C (C) A wide, bell–shaped cleft palate with no cleft lip is characteristic of Pierre Robin sequence.

lip and an unrepaired complete cleft palate. Figure 2–11C shows a child with a wide unrepaired cleft palate with no involvement of the primary palate. A wide, bell-shaped cleft palate with no cleft lip is characteristic of Pierre Robin sequence. Figures 2–12A and 2–12B show examples of a bilateral complete cleft lip and palate. The prolabium and premaxilla are isolated and in an anterior position. The vomer portion of the nasal septum can be viewed through the cleft of the palate.

Some patients will demonstrate a *palatal fistula* or hole in the palate after the palate is repaired. This should not be confused with an unrepaired incomplete cleft. This type of fistula is actually due to a partial *dehiscence* (or breakdown) of the cleft repair. The fistula can be located anywhere in the hard palate or velum but will always be located along the embryological or surgical suture lines (Figure 2–13). In addition, patients who have had a cleft of the primary palate may have a residual *nasolabial fistula*, located in the alveolus just under the upper lip. This fistula is often left deliberately by the surgeon during the initial repair in order to allow for unrestricted maxillary growth for a period of time. It is later closed by an alveolar bone graft when the permanent teeth begin to erupt. For more information about fistulas, see Chapter 7 and Chapter 8.

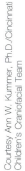

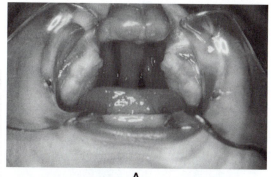

A

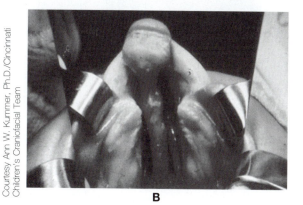

B

FIGURE 2–12 (A and B) Patients with a bilateral complete cleft of the lip and palate (primary and secondary palate). Note the prolabium, premaxilla, and the nasal septum.

Effects on Structure and Function

With cleft palate there are additional abnormalities of the anatomy other than the obvious. If the cleft goes entirely through the velum, the velar aponeurosis is conspicuously absent (Dickson, 1972; Koch, Grzonka, & Koch, 1998; Rittler et al., 2011), and the orientation of the levator veli palatini, palatopharyngeus, and musculus uvulae muscles is necessarily altered. In the case of the levator veli palatini muscles, the muscle origins (from the temporal bones of the base of the skull) are normal. However, the muscle insertions, which should

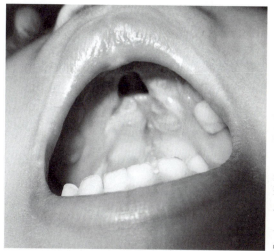

FIGURE 2–13 Palatal fistula. A palatal fistula is a hole in the palate that occurs due to a partial dehiscence (or breakdown) of the cleft repair. The fistula can be located anywhere in the hard palate or velum, but will always be located along the embryological or surgical suture lines.

interdigitate (interlock like fingers) in the midline of the velum, are necessarily abnormal due to the open cleft. Instead of a midline insertion, the levator muscle on each side inserts onto the posterior border of the cleft hard palate, thus rendering these muscles essentially nonfunctional (Dickson, 1972; Dickson, Grant, Sicher, Dubrul, & Paltan, 1974, 1975; Kriens, 1975; Maue-Dickson, 1979; Maue-Dickson & Dickson, 1980; Mehendale, 2004). Even fibers of the palatopharyngeus muscle insert abnormally into the hard palate. As a result, rather than being amuscular, the anterior one-third of the velum contains the muscle fibers of both the levator veli palatini and the palatopharyngeus muscles (Dickson, 1972). With cleft palate, the musculus uvula muscles, which are intrinsic muscles that sit side by side in the midline of the velum, are typically hypoplastic. This abnormal configuration of muscles with cleft palate has been referred to as the *cleft muscle of Veau*. Figure 2–14A shows the orientation of the

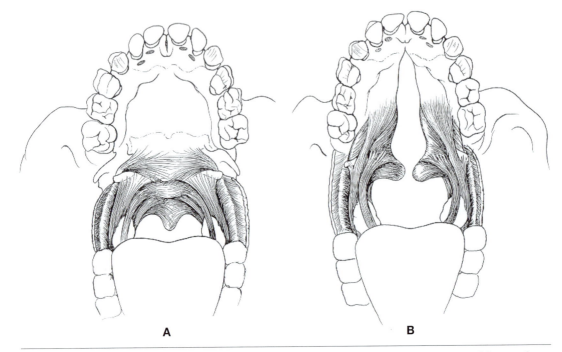

A   **B**

FIGURE 2–14 (A and B)   (A) Illustration of normal velar musculature. Note the orientation of the muscles in midline. (B) Abnormal muscle orientation due to a cleft palate. As a result of the cleft, the anterior one–third of the velum contains the muscle fibers of the levator veli palatini and the palatopharyngeus muscles. Instead of inserting into the midline of the velum, these muscles are inserted into the posterior border of the hard palate. This abnormal orientation is called the *cleft muscle of Veau*.

Courtesy Robin T. Cotton, M.D./Cincinnati Children's Hospital Medical Center & University of Cincinnati College of Medicine

velar muscles in a normal palate and velum. Figure 2–14B shows the abnormal orientation of the muscles when there is a cleft.

One goal of cleft palate surgery is to correct the orientation of the muscles in order to achieve normal function. Despite surgical attempts to normalize the muscle orientation, individuals with a repaired cleft of the velum have great variability in the insertion point of the muscles and in the muscle mass (Hassan & Askar, 2007; Moon & Kuehn, 1997). Therefore, the function of the muscles following surgery can be difficult to predict. In addition, the velum may be abnormally short or thin due to the absent aponeurosis and hypoplasia of the levator veli palatini and musculus uvulae muscles (Dickson, 1972). It has been estimated that

about 20% to 30% of individuals with a history of cleft palate are likely to have velopharyngeal insufficiency (Bardach, 1995) due to either a short velum or a poor velar movement as a result of abnormal muscles. (Velopharyngeal insufficiency causes defective speech and resonance. See Chapter 7 for more information.)

Individuals with a history of cleft palate are at high risk for early feeding problems and nasal regurgitation (see Chapter 5). They are also at high risk for otitis media and associated conductive hearing loss (see Chapter 8). This is due to malfunction of the Eustachian tube (Sheer, Swarts, & Ghadiali, 2010), which connects the middle ear to the posterior pharynx. The Eustachian tube is normally closed in its resting position. In response to changes in external air pressure, the individual usually swallows (or yawns) to relieve the pressure in the ears. The act of swallowing or yawning causes the tensor veli palatini muscle to contract to open the pharyngeal end of the tube. As the Eustachian tube opens, it allows fluids to drain from the middle ear into the pharynx. It also results in the equalization of air pressure between the middle ear and the environment. If the tensor veli palatini muscle does not function normally, as is common when there is a history of cleft palate, this results in poor ventilation of the middle ear. This can lead to bacterial infection, inflammation, and the accumulation of fluids. The buildup of fluids impairs the conduction of sound through the ossicles, resulting in a conductive hearing loss. If this fluid buildup and inflammation become chronic, permanent damage to the middle ear, to the surrounding structures, and to hearing can result.

As noted previously, the nasal cavity space can be compromised by developmental defects secondary to cleft lip and palate. Cleft palate alone can include abnormalities of both the cartilaginous and bony septum, causing a nasal septal deviation that can alter nasal cavity size (Sandham & Murray, 1993). The nasopharyngeal anatomy also appears to be altered in individuals with a history of cleft palate (Fukushiro and Trindade, 2005; Satoh, Wada, Tachimura, & Fukuda, 2005; Smahel, Kasalova, & Skvarilova, 1991; Smahel & Mullerova, 1992). These differences included a reduction of the nasopharyngeal airway due to a decrease in depth of the nasopharyngeal bony framework and the posterior displacement of the maxilla. The findings of reduced nasal cavity size and reduced nasopharyngeal depth can explain the high incidence of both upper airway obstruction and mouth breathing in the cleft palate population (Liu, Warren, Drake, & Davis, 1992; Rosé, Thissen, Otten, & Jonas, 2003; Warren & Drake, 1993; Warren, Hairfield, & Dalston, 1990, 1991). This

is a particular concern when the cleft palate is due to Pierre Robin sequence because of the posterior position of the tongue. Therefore, a first treatment priority for these patients is to ensure adequate breathing. (See Chapter 3 for more information about Pierre Robin sequence.)

SUBMUCOUS CLEFT PALATE

A *submucous cleft palate* is a congenital defect that affects the underlying structure of the palate, whereas the oral surface mucosa is intact. The exact pathogenesis of submucous cleft is not clearly understood, but it is probably related to delayed embryological development of the nasal surface of the palate when compared to the oral surface. A submucous cleft can range in severity from a dysplastic or slightly bifid uvula to a cleft under the oral mucosa that courses through the muscles of velum and bone of the hard palate all the way to the area of the incisive foramen. Submucous cleft is usually more apparent on the nasal surface of the velum, as observed through nasopharyngoscopy. It often causes the musculus uvulae muscles to be dysplastic and may also cause abnormal insertion of the levator veli palatini muscle into the border of the hard palate. Like an open cleft palate, a submucous cleft often occurs as part of a generalized syndrome of multiple malformations (Reiter, Haase, & Brosch, 2010).

Types and Severity

Submucous clefts can vary in type, from one that is obvious on the oral side of the velum to one that is only apparent by viewing the nasal side of the velum through endoscopy. They can also range in severity from a dysplastic or slightly bifid uvula to a cleft under the oral mucosa that courses all the way to the area of the incisive foramen.

Overt Submucous Cleft

An *overt submucous cleft palate* is one that can be seen on the oral surface and therefore, can be identified through an intraoral examination alone. The diagnosis is made by observation of one or more of the classic stigmata, which include a bifid or hypoplastic uvula, a zona pellucida, or a notch in the posterior border of the hard palate.

Abnormalities of the uvula vary in appearance. In some cases, the uvula is clearly bifid, with two distinct pendulous structures (Figure 2–15A) instead of a single pedicle. In other cases, a bifurcation is not easily appreciated. The uvula may even appear as one structure, but with a line down the middle (Figure 2–15B) or may appear to be *hypoplastic* (small and underdeveloped) (Figure 2–15C). A bifid or

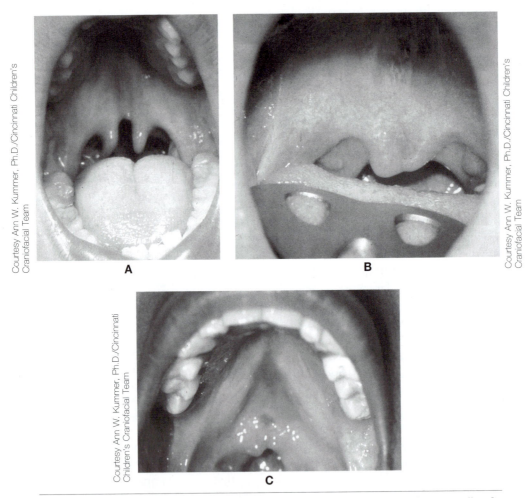

Courtesy Ann W. Kummer, Ph.D./Cincinnati Children's Craniofacial Team

A

B

C

FIGURE 2–15 (A–E)   (A) Submucous cleft palate with bifid uvula and zona pellucida. (B) Submucous cleft that is more subtle, but still very noticeable. Note the hypoplastic uvula with a faint line in the middle, and the zona pellucida. (C) Submucous cleft with obvious diastasis of the velar musculature. Note how the muscles insert into the hard palate, resulting in an inverted "V" shape. *(continues)*

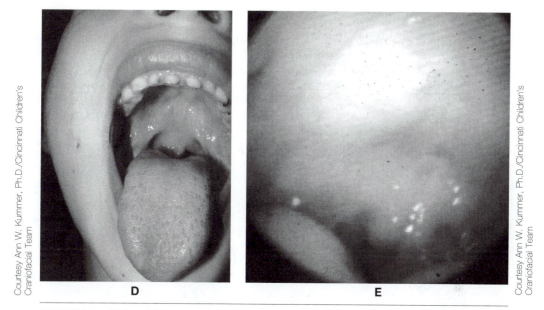

Courtesy Ann W. Kummer, Ph.D./Cincinnati Children's Craniofacial Team

Courtesy Ann W. Kummer, Ph.D./Cincinnati Children's Craniofacial Team

FIGURE 2–15 (A–E) (*Continued*) (D) Submucous cleft that is noted only during phonation. Note the subtle inverted "V" during velar elevation, indicating an abnormality in the insertion of the levator veli palatini muscle. (E) Submucous cleft that is characterized by a hypoplastic uvula with a thin line in the middle.

hypoplastic uvula can be an isolated anomaly with no submucous cleft of the velum and normal speech. This makes sense when one remembers that embryological development of the palate starts at the incisive foramen and finishes with the uvula. However, the observation of a bifid or hypoplastic uvula suggests that embryological development was disrupted at some point during secondary palate formation. Therefore, when it is noted, it is important to rule out an associated submucous cleft that extends into the velum (and even into the hard palate). A submucous cleft of the velum can result in velopharyngeal insufficiency with hypernasal speech (Reiter, Brosch, Wefel, Schlomer, & Haase, 2011; Shprintzen, Schwartz, Daniller, & Hoch, 1985).

In addition to a bifid uvula, an inspection of the velum may reveal a *zona pellucida* (Figures 2–15A and B). This is a bluish area in the middle of the velum and is the result of

thin mucosa with a lack of the normal underlying muscle mass. The velum may also appear to be in the shape of an inverted "V" at rest, but especially with phonation (Figure 2–15D). This shape is due to the *diastasis* (separation) of the paired levator veli palatini muscle, with abnormal insertion of these muscles into the posterior border of the hard palate rather than into the midline of the velum. With phonation, this abnormal muscle insertion makes the velum appear to "tent up" toward the hard palate. The submucous cleft can extend into the hard palate, all the way to the incisive foramen. When this is the case, the V-shaped abnormality can be viewed underneath the surface of the mucoperiosteum. Sometimes, the defect is not as obvious and may just look like a minor defect in the velum (Figure 2–15E).

A third indication of a submucous cleft is a notch in the midline of the posterior border of the hard palate. This can be found through palpation of bony edge of the palate. (For information on palpation of the palate, see Chapter 12, "Orofacial Examination.") A notch in the hard palate may be present, even when an intraoral examination shows an apparently intact uvula and velum (Malata, Cooter, & Batchelor, 1993; Shprintzen et al., 1985). This is due to the fact that part of the submucous cleft may be occult (hidden from view). Figure 2–16 shows various degrees of

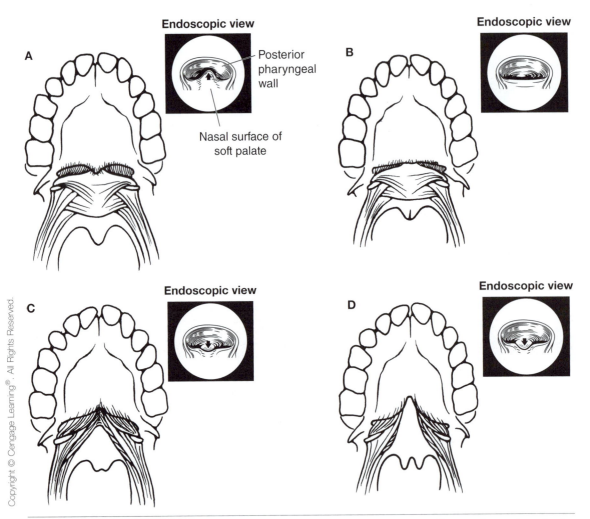

FIGURE 2–16 (A–D) Degrees of severity of a submucous cleft palate and the effect on the uvula and velar musculature. The endoscopic view of the nasal surface of the velum can be seen in the circles. (A) A normal velum and uvula with normal velar musculature. (B) A bifid uvula but normal velum with no involvement of the velar musculature. This type of submucous cleft is unlikely to affect velopharyngeal function. (C) A bifid uvula and submucous cleft that extends through the velum to the hard palate. This type of submucous cleft affects the muscle orientation of the velum and could affect velopharyngeal function and thus speech. (D) A bifid uvula and submucous cleft that extends through the velum and partially through the hard palate. This type of submucous cleft affects the velar musculature and has the potential to affect speech.

severity of a submucous cleft and the effect of the defect on the musculature.

Occult Submucous Cleft

An *occult submucous cleft* is a defect in the velum that is not apparent on the oral surface (Abdel-Aziz, Dewidar, El-Hoshy, & Aziz, 2009). In fact, it can only be appreciated by viewing the nasal surface of the velum through nasopharyngoscopy. Because the word "occult" means "hidden" or "not revealed," this malformation is aptly named. The occult submucous cleft is not embryologically or genetically different from other variations of the submucous cleft. Instead, the occult submucous cleft represents a point on the continuum of severity of submucous cleft and cleft palate.

The diagnosis of occult submucous cleft is only pursued if the patient has velopharyngeal insufficiency of unknown etiology, as there is no obvious physical abnormality of the velum. McWilliams et al. (1990) used the term *congenital palatal insufficiency (CPI)* to describe characteristics of velopharyngeal insufficiency with no history of cleft palate and no apparent evidence of submucous cleft or other known etiology. It is possible that individuals previously identified with CPI actually had an occult submucous cleft. With the help of nasopharyngoscopy, which is an endoscopic procedure, it is now possible to identify the velar abnormalities that commonly occur on the nasal surface only and could not be viewed through videofluoroscopy.

Figure 2–17 is an endoscopic view of the velum showing the nasal surface. On the posterior edge of the velum, there is a small indentation, and on the nasal surface there is a depression rather than a rounded bulky mass of the musculus uvulae muscles. These characteristics, and the absence of an abnormality

on the oral surface, are typical of an occult submucous cleft. In patients with velopharyngeal insufficiency of unknown etiology, surgeons have reported finding abnormalities on the nasal surface of the velum as the velum is dissected for a pharyngeal flap for correction. In a study of 52 patients without overt cleft palate who were undergoing pharyngeal flap surgery, Trier (1983) found that 48 patients (92%) demonstrated abnormal anatomy of the velum, which explained the velopharyngeal insufficiency.

Individuals with an occult submucous cleft have some of the same abnormalities as those with an overt submucous cleft. The musculus uvulae muscles are either absent or deficient (Croft, Shprintzen, Daniller, & Lewin, 1978; Finkelstein, Hauben, Talmi, Nachmani, & Zohar, 1992), and there is abnormal insertion of the levator muscles into the hard palate. In the case of occult submucous cleft, this can

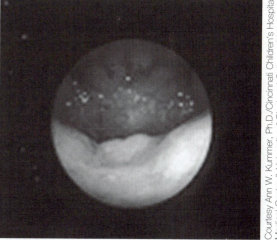

Courtesy Ann W. Kummer, Ph.D./Cincinnati Children's Hospital Medical Center & University of Cincinnati College of Medicine

FIGURE 2–17 An endoscopic view of the velum showing the nasal surface. It can be seen that the edge of the velum has a depression rather than a rounded muscle mass of the musculus uvulae muscles. This depression is an indication of a submucous cleft.

often be seen through nasopharyngoscopy as a V-shaped midline defect with a flattening or depression in the area of the velar eminence.

Effects on Structure and Function

The effect of a submucous cleft on structure and function depends greatly on the type and extent of the defect, as it does with an overt cleft. Abnormalities in the morphology of the velum can particularly affect velopharyngeal function and therefore speech. These abnormalities can also cause nasal regurgitation with swallowing, especially during the first year of life. With submucous cleft palate, there is an increased risk for middle ear disease with conductive hearing loss due to abnormalities of the tensor veli palatini muscle, which can cause Eustachian tube malfunction (Garcia Velasco, Ysunza, Hernandez, & Marquez, 1988; Saad, 1980; Schwartz, Hayden, Rodriquez, Shprintzen, & Cassidy, 1985; Sheahan, Miller, Earley, Sheahan, & Blayney, 2004).

Although individuals with a submucous cleft are at risk for dysfunction of the velopharyngeal valve, many people with this abnormality have normal speech, normal middle ear function, and no history of nasal regurgitation with swallowing. McWilliams (1991) studied a group of 130 patients with submucous cleft and found that 44% remained asymptomatic into adulthood. Therefore, the mere presence of a submucous cleft should not be a concern if there is normal speech. It is important, however, that the individual and the family be counseled regarding this abnormality, for several reasons. The family should be informed that a full adenoidectomy with a submucous cleft is usually contraindicated due to the risk that this will cause velopharyngeal insufficiency (Saunders, Hartley, Sell, &

Sommerlad, 2004). In addition, the family should be counseled regarding the genetic risk for additional offspring with submucous cleft, cleft palate, or associated syndromes.

Treatment of Submucous Cleft

The literature and most professionals do not support the prophylactic surgical correction of the physical stigmata of submucous cleft palate, because many individuals with a submucous cleft have normal speech, swallowing, and middle ear function. Instead, surgical correction is indicated only if there is evidence of velopharyngeal insufficiency that is affecting speech (Abdel-Aziz et al., 2009; Chen, Wu, & Noordhoff, 1994; Garcia Velasco et al., 1988; Gosain, Conley, Marks, Larson, 1996). It is therefore important to wait until speech has fully developed before considering surgical correction so that speech and velopharyngeal function can be adequately evaluated. For optimal speech results, however, it is best to surgically correct the defect as soon as a velopharyngeal insufficiency is diagnosed (Reiter et al., 2011).

When surgical correction is necessary and the child is still very young, a palatoplasty is often done initially to improve the orientation of the muscles for better function. If this is not effective, if the individual is older, or if there is significant velopharyngeal insufficiency, a pharyngeal flap or sphincter pharyngoplasty is done, either alone or in combination with a palatoplasty (Carlisle, Sykes, & Singhal, 2011).

FACIAL CLEFTS

Most clefts follow the embryological suture lines of the lip and palate. However, other types of clefts can occur due to failure of neural crest cell migration, which results in the lack of fusion of the facial processes, including the branchial arches. In addition, *amniotic bands* (loose strands of tissue that have ruptured from the amnion) are thought to be responsible for certain types of facial clefts (Hukki et al., 2004; Rintala, Leisti, Liesmaa, & Ranta, 1980). Facial clefts are usually very severe and are accompanied by many other anomalies.

Types and Severity

One type of facial cleft is the oblique cleft, which can be unilateral (Figure 2–18A) or bilateral (Figure 2–18B). This is an extremely disfiguring congenital anomaly of the face that affects the skeletal and soft tissue structures (Kuriyama, Udagawa, Yoshimoto, Ichinose, & Suzuki, 2008). An oblique cleft begins at the mouth and then courses laterally, horizontally, and upward so that it may affect the facial bones, nasal structures, orbits, and even the ears.

Another type of facial cleft is the midline (median) cleft (Figure 2–19, A–E). This type of cleft can be very mild so that there is only a notch in the midline of the vermilion or a slight cleft of the upper lip (Figure 2–19A). However, midline clefts are often associated with a spectrum of other midline anomalies, such as bifid nose (Miller, Grinberg, & Wang, 1999; Patel & Tantri, 2010), frontonasal *dysplasia* (abnormal tissue development) (Hodgkins et al., 1998), and *hypertelorism*, which is wide spacing between the eyes (Figure 2–19, B–E). Midline clefts can also affect brain development, causing cranial base anomalies, an *encephalocele* (which is a congenital gap in the skull, with herniation of brain tissue into the nose or palate), or an absent *corpus callosum* (nerve fibers that allow communication between the cerebral hemispheres). In severe cases, a midline cleft may be associated with *holoprosencephaly*, which is failure of the forebrain to divide into two hemispheres (Figure 2–19F).

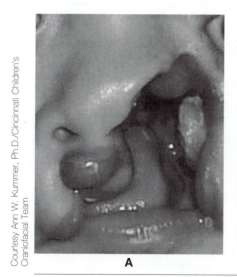
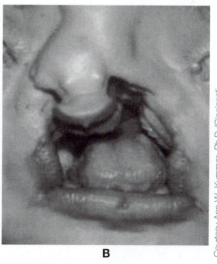

Courtesy Ann W. Kummer, Ph.D./Cincinnati Children's Craniofacial Team

Courtesy Ann W. Kummer, Ph.D./Cincinnati Children's Craniofacial Team

A   **B**

FIGURE 2–18 (A and B) Oblique facial clefts. (A) Left unilateral facial cleft affecting the nose and orbit. (B) Bilateral facial clefts.

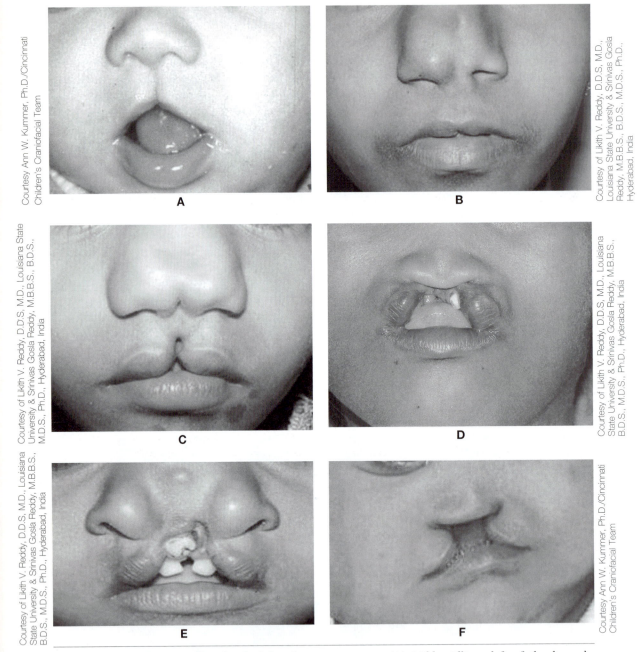

FIGURE 2–19 (A–F) Midline facial clefts of varying severity. (A) Mild midline cleft of the lip only. (B–E) Midline facial clefts that affect the nose. F. Midline facial cleft with holoprosencephaly, a condition in which there is failure of the forebrain to divide into the two hemispheres.

Effects on Structure and Function

Facial clefts are often severe and may be accompanied by other significant craniofacial anomalies or other medical conditions. Related anomalies may involve malformations of the ears, eyes, nose, facial bones, jaws, or skull. As a general rule, whenever there are abnormalities on the outside of the head (face and/or skull), there are often corresponding abnormalities on the inside of the head. Whenever there are abnormalities on the inside of the head (face and/or skull), there are often corresponding functional abnormalities. For example, the observation of external ear malformations would suggest the possibility of internal ear anomalies of the ossicles and perhaps even of the cochlea. The internal anomalies would lead to the functional problems of hearing loss. In another example, the observation of *hypertelorism* (wide-spaced eyes) and abnormal skull shape may suggest internal brain anomalies that could result in functional problems with cognition and language. Outside anomalies typically affect appearance and aesthetics. Inside anomalies typically affect function (i.e., cognition, language, speech, resonance, hearing, feeding, and swallowing).

PREVALENCE OF CLEFTS

Because the cause of clefts is a combination of both genetic and environmental factors, estimates of the prevalence of clefts necessarily vary from one population to another. In addition, prevalence figures are harder to obtain for submucous cleft, which may occur without obvious symptoms. However, the following information provides a general estimate of prevalence of clefts and how this prevalence tends to vary with different populations.

Prevalence of Cleft Lip and Palate

Cleft lip and palate is the fourth most common birth defect and the most common congenital defect of the face. The prevalence of clefts is usually quoted as one in every 600 live births in the United States (Cleft Palate Foundation, 2011), although this varies with racial background. (This estimate does not include the prevalence of bifid uvula, submucous cleft palate, or noncleft velopharyngeal insufficiency.) Once a couple has a child with a cleft, their risk of having another child with a cleft is 2–5%. Note that in epidemiology, the term *incidence* refers to the number of new cases of a disease or disorder in a given population, such as the number of persons becoming ill with a certain disease. On the other hand, the term *prevalence* refers to a measure of existing cases of a disorder in a given population. Therefore, prevalence refers to the number of cases of clefts in the general population.

About 10–15% of individuals with cleft lip (with or without cleft palate) have a related syndrome. In contrast, 40–50% of individuals with cleft palate only have a related syndrome (Cleft Palate Foundation, 2011). In fact, there are about 400 recognized syndromes that include cleft lip and/or cleft palate as one of its features. When cleft palate occurs as part of a syndrome, there are usually other associated craniofacial malformations as well as other malformations and medical conditions (Beriaghi et al., 2009; Jones, 1988; Rollnick & Pruzansky, 1981; Shprintzen et al., 1985). In addition to cleft lip and palate, these other types of congenital craniofacial anomalies can also affect communication development and communication skills.

The prevalence of clefts varies significantly depending on racial background. The prevalence is highest in Native Americans (1 in 300), then Asians (1 in 500), and then Caucasians (1 in 800). The prevalence of clefts is lowest for those of African descent (1 in 2000) (Gorlin, Cohen, & Hennekam, 2001).

There is evidence to show that there are differences between males and females in the types of clefts typically presented. Cleft lip, with or without cleft palate, occurs about twice as often in males than in females and is usually more severe in males. On the other hand, cleft palate occurs about twice as frequently in females as in males (Jensen et al., 1988; Maresova, Veleminska, & Mullerova, 2004). Although the reason for these differences between genders is not clearly understood, it has been speculated that it could be related to differences in the timing of the development of the lip and palate in the embryo. Burdi and Silvey (1969) found that, in the male human embryo, the horizontal positioning and subsequent closure of the secondary palate occurs earlier than in the female embryo. Because the palatal shelves are open longer in the female, there is a greater period of time during which there is susceptibility to environmental teratogens.

Prevalence of Submucous Cleft

Several studies have reported the prevalence of bifid uvula in a primarily Caucasian population to be between 0.2% and 2.0% (Bagatin, 1985; Gorlin, Cervenka, & Pruzansky, 1971; Meskin, Gorlin, & Isaacson, 1964; Saad, 1980; Wharton & Mowrer, 1992). One study compared the occurrence of bifid uvula in four races (Shapiro, Meskin, Cervenka, & Pruzansky, 1971). They reported bifid uvula to be prevalent in 10.25% of Native American Chippewa, 9.96% of Japanese, 1.44% of whites, and 0.27% of blacks. It is interesting that this relative frequency by race is similar to the relative frequency of cleft lip and palate. Although these studies reported the preva-

lence of bifid uvula, it is important to note that children with bifid uvula often have the additional characteristics of submucous cleft palate, including velopharyngeal insufficiency and hypernasal speech (Rivron, 1989).

Several studies have attempted to determine the prevalence of submucous cleft in the general population (Bagatin, 1985; Gosain, Conley, Santoro, & Denny, 1999). Gosain and colleagues (1996) summarized the results of several studies in the literature and stated that prevalence of the classic stigmata of submucous cleft palate among the general population is between 0.02% and 0.08%.

Although a submucous cleft may be noticed at birth or soon after, especially if there are early feeding problems, an occult submucous cleft is usually not discovered until the child begins to speak and has evidence of hypernasality. In some cases, the defect is not noted for years or is never discovered, especially if it is asymptomatic and not causing any problems with speech. Therefore, the prevalence of occult submucous cleft is not known.

The prevalence of submucous cleft palate in individuals with clefts of the primary palate has been found to be significantly greater than the prevalence of submucous cleft palate found in the general population (Gosain et al., 1999; Kono, Young, & Holtmann, 1981). Because of this increased risk, it is important for individuals with cleft lip to be thoroughly examined for submucous cleft. Early detection of submucous cleft associated with cleft lip is important for the prevention of middle ear problems and for the proper management of velopharyngeal insufficiency, if it occurs.

Individuals with submucous cleft palate are at high risk for velopharyngeal insufficiency resulting in hypernasality. Studies have shown that overall, one-fourth to one-half of individuals with submucous cleft will have associated velopharyngeal dysfunction (Bagatin, 1985;

Garcia Velasco et al., 1988; Kono et al., 1981; Sullivan, Vasudavan, Marrinan, & Mulliken, 2011). On the other hand, it is important to recognize that most individuals with a submucous cleft will have normal speech (Park et al., 2000).

Prevalence of Facial Clefts

Fortunately, facial clefts are very rare. The exact prevalence of facial clefts is unknown, and estimates vary greatly because of the rarity of their occurrence and the lack of standard methods of data collection (Cooper, Ratay, & Marazita, 2006; Darzi & Chowdri, 1993).

SUMMARY

Cleft lip and palate is a common birth defect that presents in a variety of ways. There are different types of clefts, such as clefts of the primary palate and clefts of the secondary palate. There are also different degrees of severity, from a bifid uvula to complete cleft palate, or a notch in the lip to a bilateral complete cleft of the lip and alveolus. A submucous cleft is a type of cleft that is not readily apparent because it affects the underlying structures of the velum while leaving the oral surface intact. When a cleft occurs, it is the result of a disruption in embryological development. Many craniofacial syndromes include cleft palate as part of the phenotype.

As will be noted in subsequent chapters, cleft lip and cleft palate can affect the development of communication skills in a variety of ways. Therefore, health care providers, particularly members of a cleft palate or craniofacial team, need to be aware of this so that appropriate intervention can be initiated.

FOR REVIEW AND DISCUSSION

1. Beginning with the incisive foramen, describe the process and direction of embryological development of the lip and palate.

2. What are possible causes of clefts? Given these causes, what do you think could be done to reduce the risk of clefting in a population?

3. What is meant by the terms "primary palate" and "secondary palate"? What structures are included? How does this classification system relate to embryological development?

4. List different types of clefts of the primary palate. What are the potential functional problems with regard to these clefts? What professional disciplines may be involved in treatment?

5. List different types of clefts of the secondary palate. What are the potential functional problems with regard to these clefts? What professional disciplines may be involved in treatment?

6. Describe the possible characteristics of a submucous cleft palate. Why is this type of cleft often undetected at birth? Discuss the occurrence of submucous cleft as it relates to embryological development.

7. What structures may be involved in a facial cleft? In addition to the obvious aesthetic concerns, what are some reasons that these types of clefts are of particular concern?

References

Abdel-Aziz, M., Dewidar, H., El-Hoshy, H., & Aziz, A. A. (2009). Treatment of persistent post-adenoidectomy velopharyngeal insufficiency by sphincter pharyngoplasty. *International Journal of Pediatric Otorhinolaryngology, 73*(10), 1329–1333.

Bagatin, M. (1985). Submucous cleft palate. *Journal of Maxillofacial Surgery, 13*(1), 37–38.

Bardach, J. (1995). Secondary surgery for velopharyngeal insufficiency. In R. J. Shprintzen & J. Bardach (Eds.), *Cleft palate speech management: A multidisciplinary approach* (pp. 277–294). St. Louis, MO: Mosby.

Beriaghi, S., Meyers, S. L., Jensen, S. A., Kaimal, S., Chan, C. M., & Schaefer, G. B. (2009). Cleft lip and palate: Association with other congenital malformations. *The Journal of Clinical Pediatric Dentistry, 33*(3), 207–210.

Bille, C., Knudsen, L. B., & Christensen, K. (2005). Changing lifestyles and oral clefts occurrence in Denmark. *The Cleft Palate–Craniofacial Journal, 42*(3), 255–259.

Bille, C., Skytthe, A., Vach, W., Knudsen, L. B., Nybo Andersen, A. M., Murray, J. C., & Christensen, K. (2005). Parents age and the risk of oral clefts. *Epidemiology, 16*(3), 311–316.

Burdi, A. R., & Silvey, R. G. (1969). Sexual differences in closure of the human palatal shelves. *Cleft Palate Journal, 6*, 1–7.

Carlisle, M. P., Sykes, K. J., & Singhal, V. K. (2011). Outcomes of sphincter pharyngoplasty and palatal lengthening for velopharyngeal insufficiency: A 10-year experience. *Archives of Otolaryngology Head and Neck Surgery, 137*(8), 763–766.

Castilla, E. E., Orioli, I. M., Lopez-Camelo, J. S., Dutra Mda, G., & Nazer-Herrera, J. (2003). Preliminary data on changes in neural tube defect prevalence rates after folic acid fortification in South America. *American Journal of Medical Genetics Part A, 123*(2), 123–128.

Chen, K. T., Wu, J., & Noordhoff, S. M. (1994). Submucous cleft palate. *Chang Keng I Hsueh: Chang Gung Medical Journal, 17*(2), 131–137.

Cleft Palate Foundation. (2011). Available at http://www.cleft.com.

Cooper, M. E., Ratay, J. S., & Marazita, M. L. (2006). Asian oral-facial cleft birth prevalence. *The Cleft Palate–Craniofacial Journal, 43*(5), 580–589.

Croft, C. B., Shprintzen, R. J., Daniller, A. L, & Lewin, M. L. (1978). The occult submucous cleft palate and the musculus uvulae. *Cleft Palate Journal, 15*, 150–154.

Darzi, M. A., & Chowdri, N. A. (1993). Oblique facial clefts: A report of Tessier numbers 3, 4, 5, and 9 clefts. *The Cleft Palate–Craniofacial Journal, 30*(4), 414–415.

Dickson, D. R. (1972). Normal and cleft palate anatomy. *Cleft Palate Journal, 9*, 280–93.

Dickson, D. R., Grant, J. C., Sicher, H., Dubrul, E. L., & Paltan, J. (1974). Status of research in cleft palate anatomy and physiology, Part 1. *Cleft Palate Journal, 11*, 471–492.

Dickson, D. R., Grant, J. C., Sicher, H., Dubrul, E. L., & Paltan, J. (1975). Status of research in cleft lip and palate: Anatomy and physiology, Part 2. *Cleft Palate Journal, 12*, 131–156.

Drake, A. F., Davis, J. U., & Warren, D. W. (1993). Nasal airway size in cleft and noncleft children. *Laryngoscope, 103*(8), 915–917.

Edwards, M. J., Agho, K., Attia, J., Diaz, P., Hayes, T., et al. (2003). Case-control study of cleft lip or palate after maternal use of topical corticosteroids during pregnancy. *American Journal of Medical Genetics Part A, 120*(4), 459–463.

Finkelstein, Y., Hauben, D. J., Talmi, Y. P., Nachmani, A., & Zohar, Y. (1992). Occult and overt submucous cleft palate: From peroral examination to nasendoscopy and back again. *International Journal of Pediatric Otorhinolaryngology, 23*(1), 25–34.

Fukushiro, A. P., & Trindade, I. E. (2005). Nasal airway dimensions of adults with cleft lip and palate: Differences among cleft types. *Cleft Palate Journal, 42*(4), 396–402.

Garcia Velasco, M., Ysunza, A., Hernandez, X., & Marquez, C. (1988). Diagnosis and treatment of submucous cleft palate: A review of 108 cases. *Cleft Palate Journal, 25*(2), 171–173.

Gorlin, R. J., Cervenka, J., & Pruzansky, S. (1971). Facial clefting and its syndromes. *Birth Defects Original Article Series, 7*(7), 3–49.

Gorlin, R., Cohen, M. J., & Hennekam, R. C. M. (2001). *Syndromes of the head and neck* (4th ed.). New York: Oxford University Press.

Gosain, A. K., Conley, S. F., Marks, S., & Larson, D. L. (1996). Submucous cleft palate: Diagnostic methods and outcomes of surgical treatment. *Plastic & Reconstructive Surgery, 97*(7), 1497–1509.

Gosain, A. K., Conley, S. F., Santoro, T. D., & Denny, A. D. (1999). A prospective evaluation of the prevalence of submucous cleft palate in patients with isolated cleft lip versus controls. *Plastic & Reconstructive Surgery, 103*(7), 1857–1863.

Hashmi, S. S., Waller, D. K., Langlois, P., Canfield, M., & Hecht, J. T. (2005). Prevalence of nonsyndromic oral clefts in Texas: 1995–1999. *American Journal of Medical Genetics Part A, 134*(4), 368–372.

Hassan, M. E., & Askar, S. (2007). Does palatal muscle reconstruction affect the functional outcome of cleft palate surgery? *Plastic and Reconstructive Surgery, 119*(6), 1859–1865.

Hodgkins, P., Lees, M., Lawson, J., Reardon, W., Leitch, J., Thorogood, P., et al. (1998). Optie disc anomalies and frontonasal dysplasia. *British Journal of Ophthalmology, 82*(3), 290–293.

Honein, M. A., Paulozzi, L. J., & Watkins, M. L. (2001). Maternal smoking and birth defects: Validity of birth certificate data for effect estimation. *Public Health Reports, 116*(4), 327–335.

Hukki, J., Balan, P., Ceponiene, R., Kantola-Sorsa, E., Saarinen, P., & Wikstrom, H. (2004). A case study of amnion rupture sequence with acalvaria, blindness, and clefting: Clinical and psychological profiles. *Journal of Craniofacial Surgery, 15*(2), 185–191.

Jensen, B. L., Kreiborg, S., Dahl, E., & Fogh-Andersen, P. (1988). Cleft lip and palate in Denmark, 1976–1981: Epidemiology, variability, and early somatic development. *Cleft Palate Journal, 25*(3), 258–269.

Jones, M. C. (1988). Etiology of facial clefts: Prospective evaluation of 428 patients. *Cleft Palate Journal, 25*(1), 16–20.

Kernahan, D. A. (1971). The striped Y-A symbolic classification for cleft lip and palate. *Plastic & Reconstructive Surgery, 47*(5), 469–470.

Kernahan, D. A., & Stark, R. B. (1958). A new classification for cleft lip and cleft palate. *Plastic & Reconstructive Surgery, 22*, 435.

Kim, N. Y., & Baek, S. H. (2006). Cleft sidedness and congenitally missing or malformed permanent maxillary lateral incisors in Korean patients with unilateral cleft lip and alveolus or unilateral cleft lip and palate.

American Journal of Orthodontics and Dentofacial Orthopedics, 130(6), 752–758.

Koch, K. H., Grzonka, M. A., & Koch, J. (1998). Pathology of the palatal aponeurosis in cleft palate. *The Cleft Palate–Craniofacial Journal, 35*(6), 530–534.

Kono, D., Young, L., & Holtmann, B. (1981). The association of submucous cleft palate and clefting of the primary palate. *Cleft Palate Journal, 18*(3), 207–209.

Kriens, O. (1975). Anatomy of the velopharyngeal area in cleft palate. *Clinical Plastic Surgery, 2*(2), 261–288.

Kuriyama, M., Udagawa, A., Yoshimoto, S., Ichinose, M., & Suzuki, H. (2008). Tessier number 7 cleft with oblique clefts of bilateral soft palates and rare symmetric structure of zygomatic arch. *Journal of Plastic, Reconstructive & Aesthetic Surgery, 61*(4), 447–450.

Liu, H., Warren, D. W., Drake, A. F., & Davis, J. U. (1992). Is nasal airway size a marker for susceptibility toward clefting? *The Cleft Palate–Craniofacial Journal, 29*(4), 336–339.

Malata, C. M., Cooter, R. D., & Batchelor, A. G. (1993). Submucous cleft palate with a discontinuous bony deformity. *The Cleft Palate–Craniofacial Journal, 30*(6), 590–592.

Maresova, K., Veleminska, J., & Mullerova, Z. (2004). The development of intracranial relations in patients with complete unilateral cleft lip and palate in relation to surgery method and gender aspect. *Acta Chirurgiae Plasticae, 46*(3), 89–94.

Martelli, D. R., Cruz, K. W., Barros, L. M., Silveira, M. F., Swerts, M. S., & Martelli Jr., H. (2010). Maternal and paternal age, birth order and interpregnancy interval evaluation for cleft lip-palate. *Brazilian Journal of Otorhinolaryngology, 76* (1), 107–112.

Maue-Dickson, W. (1979). The craniofacial complex in cleft lip and palate: An update review of anatomy and function. *Cleft Palate Journal, 16*(3), 291–317.

Maue-Dickson, W., & Dickson, D. R. (1980). Anatomy and physiology related to cleft palate: Current research and clinical implications. *Plastic & Reconstructive Surgery, 65*(1), 83–90.

McWilliams, B. J. (1991). Submucous clefts of the palate: How likely are they to be symptomatic? *The Cleft Palate–Craniofacial Journal, 28*(3), 247–249; Discussion 250–251.

McWilliams, B. J., Morris, H. L., & Shelton, R. L. (1990). *Cleft palate speech*. Philadelphia: B. C. Decker.

Mehendale, F. V. (2004). Surgical anatomy of the levator veli palatini: A previously undescribed tendinous insertion of the anterolateral fibers. *Plastic & Reconstructive Surgery, 114*(2), 307–315.

Meskin, L., Gorlin, R., & Isaacson, R. (1964). Abnormal morphology of the soft palate: The prevalence of a cleft uvula. *Cleft Palate Journal, 3*, 342–346.

Metneki, J., Puho, E., & Czeizel, A. E. (2005). Maternal diseases and isolated orofacial clefts in Hungary. *Birth Defects Research, 73*(9), 617–623.

Miller, P. J., Grinberg, D., & Wang, T. D. (1999). Midline cleft. Treatment of the bifid nose. *Archives of Facial Plastic Surgery, 1*(3), 200–203.

Moon, J. B., & Kuehn, D. P. (1997). Anatomy and physiology of normal and disordered velopharyngeal function for speech. K. R. Bzoch (Ed.), *Communicative disorders related to cleft lip and palate*. Austin, TX: Pro-Ed.

Moore, L. L., Singer, M. R., Bradlee, M. L., Rothman, K. J., & Milunsky, A. (2000). A prospective study of the risk of congenital defects associated with maternal obesity and diabetes mellitus. *Epidemiology, 11*(6), 689–694.

Mossey, P. A., Little, J., Munger, R. G., Dixon, M. J., & Shaw, W. C. (2009). Cleft lip and palate. *Lancet, 374*(9703), 1773–1785.

Munger, R. G., Sauberlich, H. E., Corcoran, C., Nepomuceno, B., Daack-Hirsch, S., et al. (2004). Maternal vitamin B-6 and folate status and risk of oral cleft birth defects in the Philippines. *Birth Defects Research, 70* (7), 464–471.

Park, S., Saso, Y., Ito, O., Tokioka, K., Kato, K., et al. (2000). A retrospective study of speech development in patients with submucous cleft palate treated by four operations. *Scandinavian Journal of Plastic and Reconstructive Surgery and Hand Surgery, 34*(2), 131–136.

Patel, N. P., & Tantri, M. D. (2010). Median cleft of the upper lip: A rare case. *The Cleft Palate–Craniofacial Journal, 47*(6), 642–644.

Ray, J. G., Meier, C., Vermeulen, M. J., Wyatt, P. R., & Cole, D. E. (2003). Association between folic acid food fortification and congenital orofacial clefts. *Journal of Pediatrics, 143*(6), 805–807.

Reiser, E., Andlin-Sobocki, A., Mani, M., & Holmstrom, M. (2011). Initial size of cleft does not correlate with size and function of nasal airway in adults with unilateral cleft lip and palate. *Journal of Plastic Surgery and Hand Surgery, 45*(3), 129–135.

Reiter, R., Haase, S., & Brosch, S. (2010). Submucous *The Cleft Palate*–an often late diagnosed malformation. *Laryngo- Rhino-Otologie, 89*(1), 29–33.

Reiter, R., Brosch, S., Ludeke, M., Fischbein, E., Haase, S., Pickhard, A., & Maier, C. (2012). Genetic and environmental risk factors for submucous cleft palate. *European Journal of Oral Sciences, 120*(2), 97–103.

Reiter, R., Brosch, S., Wefel, H., Schlomer, G., & Haase, S. (2011). The submucous cleft palate: Diagnosis and therapy. *International Journal of Pediatric Otorhinolaryngology, 75*(1), 85–88.

Rintala, A., Leisti, J., Liesmaa, M., & Ranta, R. (1980). Oblique facial clefts: Case report. *Scandinavian Journal of Plastic & Reconstructive Surgery, 14*(3), 291–297.

Rittler, M., Cosentino, V., Lopez-Camelo, J. S., Murray, J. C., Wehby, G., et al. (2011). Associated anomalies among infants with oral clefts at birth and during a 1-year follow-up. *American Journal of Medical Genetics A, 155A*(7), 1588–1596.

Rivron, R. P. (1989). Bifid uvula: Prevalence and association in otitis media with effusion in children admitted for routine otolaryngological operations. *Journal of Laryngology and Otology, 103*(3), 249–252.

Rollnick, B. R., & Pruzansky, S. (1981). Genetic services at a center for craniofacial anomalies. *Cleft Palate Journal, 18*(4), 304–313.

Rosé, E., Thissen, U., Otten, J. E., & Jonas, I. (2003). Cephalometric assessment of the posterior airway space in patients with cleft palate after palatoplasty. *The Cleft Palate–Craniofacial Journal, 40*(5), 498–503.

Saad, E. F. (1980). The underdeveloped palate in ear, nose, and throat practice. *Laryngoscope, 90*(8, Pt. 1), 1371–1377.

Sandham, A., & Murray, J. A. (1993). Nasal septal deformity in unilateral cleft lip and palate. *The Cleft Palate–Craniofacial Journal, 30*(2), 222–226.

Satoh, K., Wada, T., Tachimura, T., & Fukuda, J. (2005). Velar ascent and morphological factors affecting velopharyngeal function in patients with cleft palate and noncleft controls: A cephalometric study. *International Journal of Oral and Maxillofacial Surgery, 34*(2), 122–126.

Saunders, N. C., Hartley, B. E., Sell, D., & Sommerlad, B. (2004). Velopharyngeal insufficiency following adenoidectomy.

Clinical Otolaryngology and Allied Sciences, 29(6), 686–688.

Schwartz, R. H., Hayden, G. F., Rodriquez, W. J., Shprintzen, R. J., & Cassidy, J. W. (1985). The bifid uvula: Is it a marker for an otitis prone child? *Laryngoscope, 95*(9, Pt. 1), 1100–1102.

Sekhon, P., Ethunandan, M., Markus, A., Gopalkrishnan, K., & Rao, B. (2010). Congenital anomalies associated with cleft lip and palate—an analysis of 1632 consecutive patients. *The Cleft Palate–Craniofacial Journal, 48*(4), 371–378.

Shapiro, B. L., Meskin, L. H., Cervenka, J., & Pruzansky, S. (1971). Cleft uvula: A microform of facial clefts and its genetic basis. *Birth Defects Original Article Series, 7*(7), 80–82.

Sheahan, P., Miller, L, Earley, M. J., Sheahan, J. N., & Blayney, A. W. (2004). Middle ear disease in children with congenital velopharyngeal insufficiency. *The Cleft Palate–Craniofacial Journal, 41*(4), 364–367.

Sheer, F. J., Swarts, J. D., & Ghadiali, S. N. (2010). Finite element analysis of Eustachian tube function in cleft palate infants based on histological reconstructions. *The Cleft Palate–Craniofacial Journal, 147*(6), 600–610.

Shprintzen, R. J., Schwartz, R. H., Daniller, A., & Hoch, L. (1985). Morphologic significance of bifid uvula. *Pediatrics, 75*(3), 553–561.

Simmons, C. J., Mosley, B. S., Fulton-Bond, C. A., & Hobbs, C. A. (2004). Birth defects in Arkansas: Is folic acid fortification making a difference? *Birth Defects Research, 70*(9), 559–564.

Smahel, Z., Kasalova, P., & Skvarilova, B. (1991). Morphometric nasopharyngeal characteristics in facial clefts. *Journal of Craniofacial Genetics and Developmental Biology, 11*(1), 24–32.

Smahel, Z., & Mullerova, I. (1992). Nasopharyngeal characteristics in children with cleft lip and palate. *The Cleft Palate–Craniofacial Journal, 29*(3), 282–286.

Sullivan, S. R., Vasudavan, S., Marrinan, E. M., & Mulliken, J. B. (2011). Submucous cleft palate and velopharyngeal insufficiency: Comparison of speech outcomes using three operative techniques by one surgeon. *The Cleft Palate–Craniofacial Journal, 48*(5), 561–570.

Trier, W. C. (1983). Velopharyngeal incompetency in the absence of overt cleft palate: Anatomic and surgical considerations. *Cleft Palate Journal, 20*(3), 209–217.

Vinceti, M., Rovesti, S., Bergomi, M., Calzolari, E., Candela, S., et al. (2001). Risk of birth defects in a population exposed to environmental lead pollution. *Science of the Total Environment, 278*(1–3), 23–30.

Warren, D. W., & Drake, A. F. (1993). Cleft nose. Form and function. *Clinics in Plastic Surgery, 20*(4), 769–779.

Warren, D. W., Hairfield, W. M., & Dalston, E. T. (1990). The relationship between nasal airway size and nasaloral breathing in cleft lip and palate. *Cleft Palate Journal, 27*(1), 46–51; Discussion 51–52.

Warren, D. W., Hairfield, W. M., & Dalston, E. T. (1991). Nasal airway impairment: The oral response in cleft palate patients. *American Journal of Orthodontics & Dentofacial Orthopedics, 99*(4), 346–353.

Wharton, P., & Mowrer, D. E. (1992). Prevalence of cleft uvula among school children in kindergarten through grade five. *The Cleft Palate–Craniofacial Journal, 29*(1), 10–12; Discussion 13–14.

Yu, W., Serrano, M., Miguel, S. S., Ruest, L. B., & Svoboda, K. K. (2009). Cleft lip and palate genetics and application in early embryological development. *Indian Journal of Plastic Surgery, 42*, 35–50.

CHAPTER

3

THE GENETICS EVALUATION AND COMMON CRANIOFACIAL SYNDROMES

HOWARD M. SAAL, M.D.

CHAPTER OUTLINE

INTRODUCTION

Congenital anomalies occur in 3% to 5% of all live births. They are among the most common causes of hospitalization in childhood. There are numerous causes of congenital anomalies, with contributions from both genetic and environmental factors.

Cleft lip and palate and other craniofacial anomalies make up a significant percentage of congenital anomalies. The reported prevalence of cleft lip, with or without cleft palate, ranges from about 0.2 to 2.3 per 1000 births, whereas the reported prevalence of cleft palate only ranges from 0.1 to 1.1 per 1000 births (Gorlin, Cohen, & Hennekam, 2001; Mitchell, 2009; Mossey & Little, 2002; Rahimov, Jugessur, & Murray, 2012). The variability of the prevalence estimates reflects differences by racial background and environmental teratogens, and in the inclusion criteria of the studies (e.g., live births only or including fetal deaths) (Mitchell, 2009). Other craniofacial anomalies frequently encountered are craniosynostosis, hemifacial microsomia, submucous cleft palate, and velopharyngeal insufficiency. Because there is usually a significant genetic component to the pathogenesis of most craniofacial disorders, it is important for each child born with these conditions to have a complete genetic evaluation and follow-up evaluations as the child grows and develops.

The purpose of this chapter is to first describe the components of the genetics evaluation and the information that is important to obtain in order to arrive at a genetics diagnosis. The reader will then learn about the types and causes of dysmorphology. This chapter includes a description of the genetics of clefting and the incidence of clefts. Finally, common craniofacial syndromes will be described.

THE GENETICS EVALUATION

The purpose of the genetics evaluation is as follows: (1) to make a diagnosis; (2) to determine the natural history of a condition, which will assist with anticipatory management for medical and developmental issues; (3) to determine recurrence risks for the parents and other close family members, which may include information regarding availability of prenatal diagnosis for future pregnancies; and (4) to provide genetic psychosocial counseling and family support, which is often the most important function of the genetics evaluation. It is clear that the genetics evaluation is an important component of the early management of the child born with a craniofacial disorder, and the findings can significantly influence long-term medical and educational management and ultimate outcomes.

The genetics evaluation is somewhat different from the standard medical evaluation because greater emphasis is placed on the pregnancy and on family history (Abuelo, 2002; Jones & Jones, 2009; McDonald-McGinn, Driscoll, & Matthews, 2009). Additionally, most cases of craniofacial disorders are treated as chronic conditions with a need for long-term, integrated management.

Prenatal History

The prenatal history is an essential component of the genetics evaluation. It is particularly important to determine whether the fetus had any exposure to teratogens. A *teratogen* is a chemical or physical agent that can interfere with the normal embryological processes. Teratogens can include drugs, radiation, viruses, or any other outside agent that can result in abnormal fetal development. Therefore, information regarding maternal exposure (e.g., medications or radiation) and maternal illnesses (e.g., infections or diabetes) during pregnancy can be helpful in determining a diagnosis.

Several common medications can act as teratogens and cause orofacial and other disorders if taken during pregnancy. These include anticonvulsants, corticosteroids, and benzodiazepines (for anxiety or insomnia) (Mitchell, 2009). Some of these medications are still prescribed to pregnant women, such as anticonvulsants, because it is assumed that their benefit in controlling seizures outweighs the risks for fetal anomalies. Alcohol and smoking are other significant teratogens. In addition to causing developmental disabilities and growth delays, their use has been associated with cleft lip, cleft palate, and Pierre Robin sequence.

Medical History

The medical history of the newborn with a craniofacial disorder is usually straightforward and uncomplicated. Any and all perinatal complications should be noted, especially if there are any respiratory problems, seizures, heart defects, or congenital anomalies. Knowledge of birth weight, length, and head circumference can give valuable clues to diagnosis, because many syndromes are associated with low birth weight or small head size. Other disorders, such as Beckwith-Wiedemann syndrome, are associated with large body size for gestational age. The infant who is abnormally small or large for gestational age often has other underlying medical issues that require greater attention. Although any congenital anomaly can give a clue to the diagnosis, specific birth defects are most often associated with genetic conditions, including structural heart anomalies, seizures, eye anomalies, and genital anomalies.

For the older child, it is important to determine whether he or she has been previously diagnosed with a syndrome, disorder, or condition. Previous medical examination results can be particularly valuable, including those from an ophthalmologic or neurologic evaluation. A history of major illnesses, hospitalizations, and surgeries is important to obtain. Finally, a list of current and even past medications can be helpful.

Developmental History

The developmental history is important and should include comprehensive information about early developmental milestones, especially those regarding gross motor and language development. A history of early developmental interventions, especially those related to speech and physical therapy, should be determined. School performance information should be obtained, including the history of special therapies, the need for special education, and the results of any developmental or intelligence testing. It should also be noted which grades were repeated, if any, and for what reasons, including school absences for illnesses or medical interventions, specific learning disorders, and issues with behavior and socialization.

Feeding History

Early feeding problems are common in infants with cleft palate due to a difficulty with achieving suction and also difficulty with compression of the nipple against the palate due to the cleft. These problems are usually resolved quickly with simple feeding modifications. Other anatomic disorders related to feeding difficulty include tongue-based airway obstruction, which occurs with Pierre Robin sequence, choanal atresia or stenosis, and submucous cleft palate.

If the infant has persistent feeding problems beyond the first week of life, this may suggest an underlying neurological condition, which can be important to know when determining a genetics diagnosis. Multiple neurological disorders can be associated with feeding disorders, including chromosome anomalies, other genetic disorders associated with poor tone, congenital myotonic dystrophy, spinal muscular atrophy, and congenital brain anomalies. If no etiology for a feeding disorder can be identified, further evaluation with a feeding specialist or a feeding team may be beneficial.

The evaluation of the older child should include a history of feeding difficulties and feeding modifications. It is also important to determine whether any current feeding issues exist and how they are being managed.

Family History

What really distinguishes the genetics evaluation from a standard medical evaluation is the

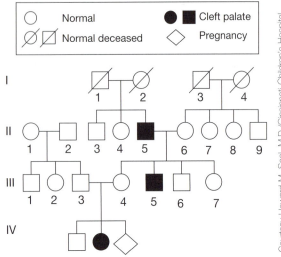

FIGURE 3–1   A pedigree, which is a pictorial representation of family members and their line of descent.

comprehensiveness of the family history. A *pedigree* is developed, which is a pictorial representation of family members and their line of descent (Figure 3–1). This can be used by the geneticist to analyze inheritance, particularly for certain traits or anomalies. It is important to extend the pedigree to four generations, if enough information is available. It can be valuable to identify whether any of the parents are related in any way (called *consanguinity*) because this can give insight into rare autosomal recessive disorders. The presence of multifactorial disorders, such as cleft lip or cleft palate, may be seen in other first- and second-degree relatives and may alter the genetic counseling regarding recurrence risks.

Any and all medical problems in relatives are noted, with special attention to infertility or miscarriages, birth defects (e.g., cleft lip, cleft palate, congenital heart defects, etc.), major medical disorders or illnesses, and early deaths. Developmental disabilities in the family are also important to note.

Physical Examination

The physical examination of the child with a craniofacial disorder is straightforward. As with any examination, attention is given to the growth parameters (weight, height or length, and head circumference). *Microcephaly*, which is a small head size, is important to note as it can indicate poor brain growth or development. Children with microcephaly often have underlying genetic conditions and are at greater risk for developmental disabilities. Poor weight gain may indicate poor feeding or possibly a genetic condition associated with small stature, such as a chromosome disorder.

In addition to the standard physical examination, the clinical geneticist is trained to perform a dysmorphology examination. In this part of the examination, the physician examines the child for abnormal features that may not be familial, but are specific to the child and can be indicative of a specific disorder or syndrome. This may include measurements of the eyes, ears, mouth, nose, and numerous other structures. It is helpful to identify specific *dermatoglyphics*, which are creases on the hands or changes in the fingerprints that can give clues to early developmental problems. The neurologic examination is especially helpful because this can give insight regarding the child's muscle tone, level of function, and degree of social interaction.

Photographs are taken of the patient at each visit. It is often helpful to look at earlier photographs that the parents bring to the visit, as well as photographs of other family members. It is also helpful to examine the parents and siblings for features similar to those of the patient.

Laboratory and Imaging Studies

After the history is reviewed and the examination is completed, it is necessary to determine whether laboratory studies are needed. Children with chromosome disorders usually have multiple dysmorphic features and anomalies, although there are some conditions in which there may be only a few specific clinical features. Chromosome studies can help to confirm a clinical suspicion based on the presenting features, by identifying known common and even rare syndromes.

If a specific chromosome anomaly is suspected (e.g., trisomy 13; Down syndrome which is also known as trisomy 21; or Turner syndrome), then specific testing with chromosome analysis is done. If velocardiofacial syndrome (deletion 22q11 syndrome) is suspected, then a fluorescence in situ hybridization (FISH) study is performed to confirm the deletion on chromosome 22q11.2 (Bartsch et al., 2003; Oh, Workman, & Wong, 2007).

Many children with chromosome disorders have rare deletions and duplications. When a chromosome disorder is suspected because of multiple congenital anomalies and/or the presence of developmental delays or intellectual disabilities, the most useful diagnostic test is a microarray analysis. This is a DNA-based study that can identify most chromosome anomalies, including submicroscopic duplications and deletions (Manning & Hudgins, 2010).

In addition to the laboratory studies, it is often helpful to obtain X-rays to determine bone maturation or to identify specific skeletal syndromes. An MRI scan of the brain can help identify structural anomalies in children with serious developmental disorders, microcephaly, or neurological disorders.

Finally, referral to other physicians may be necessary as part of a complete genetics assessment. An ophthalmology examination should be done for all children with cleft palate only, because *myopia* (nearsightedness) is a clue to the diagnosis of Stickler syndrome and may be severe enough to cause retinal detachment. Children with suspected heart defects, such as those with velocardiofacial syndrome, should have an echocardiogram. If a heart anomaly is found, the child should be evaluated by a cardiologist.

Genetic Counseling

After all the above are completed, the family is seen for genetic counseling. This is usually the longest part of the genetics evaluation because the family is counseled regarding the issues of heredity and development. Part of the process involves discussion of natural history of the suspected condition and planning for medical interventions. Families often have questions regarding cause of the condition and the recurrence risks for themselves, their child, and for other family members. For many genetic disorders, recurrence risks are known and can be shared with the family. There is ongoing research to determine the relative recurrence risk of cleft lip and palate on the basis of not only genetic background but also various environmental influences (e.g., smoking, alcohol use, and dietary factors, etc.). This will be useful in genetic counseling in the future, and possibly for the development of future preventive measures (Kohli & Kohli, 2012).

In addition to discussing recurrence risks, it is also important to identify the prenatal testing for the condition and reproductive options. Amniocentesis can be performed for prenatal identification of chromosome anomalies and specific known genetic disorders, using molecular analysis. For some birth defects, such as cleft lip with or without cleft palate, fetal ultrasound studies are the only test available for prenatal diagnosis. Unfortunately, prenatal therapy for most birth defects is not available.

Because many genetic disorders have associated developmental disabilities, referrals for developmental testing, including a speech and language evaluation, are often indicated. It is also important to plan for school interventions, with referrals to school system or community agencies for special services as necessary.

Psychosocial Counseling

Last, the genetics evaluation should include both recognition of the difficulty of having a child with a birth defect and offers of psychosocial support for the family. It is essential to identify community and national resources for the family, such as local, state, and national support groups and meetings. Specific websites can be shared with the family members to help them find educational and support resources.

DYSMORPHOLOGY

Dysmorphology is the study of abnormal shape or form. Any clinical abnormalities that are of significant medical or cosmetic consequence, especially those requiring medical intervention, are considered major anomalies. On the other hand, those abnormal features that have clinical diagnostic implications but are of minimal medical or cosmetic significance and require no intervention are considered minor anomalies. Minor anomalies occur in less than 5% of the population. The diagnosis of many genetic and craniofacial disorders depends upon the identification of specific dysmorphic features—both major and minor anomalies.

It is important to understand the underlying pathogenesis of congenital anomalies. *Morphogenesis* is the process of embryonic tissue formation. *Dysmorphogenesis* describes errors in this process. These errors result in *dysmorphic* (abnormally formed) features. Factors that can cause these abnormalities can be related to external nongenetic forces, usually attributable to abnormal fetal environment or disruption of normal development, or they may be due to intrinsic genetic or developmental abnormalities.

MALFORMATIONS AND DEFORMATIONS

Most craniofacial anomalies are malformations. A *malformation* is a morphologic anomaly that results from an intrinsically abnormal developmental process and is due to a genetic etiology (Jones, 2006). Cleft lip and many cases of cleft palate are examples of malformations. Mental retardation may also be considered a malformation if it results from a genetic etiology or from a brain malformation. Genetic factors can cause a *dysplasia*, which refers to an abnormal organization of cells into tissues, which leads to the malformation. The *craniosynostoses* are the commonly encountered dysplasias. These usually represent the abnormal development of the cranial skeleton, with other skeletal structures or tissues often being affected as well.

Some birth defects may arise as a result of abnormal mechanical forces on an otherwise normal structure. An anomaly that is caused by physical forces in the fetal environment is called a *deformation* or *deformity* (Jones, 2006c). Deformations usually result in the abnormal shape or form of a completely formed organ or structure. Classic examples of fetal deformations include clubfoot and *plagiocephaly* (abnormal skull shape).

Deformations occur when external forces disrupt the development of an intrinsically normal structure. A *disruption* causes a morphologic defect due to an extrinsic breakdown or interference with a normal developmental process. Because teratogens interfere with the normal embryological processes, they are often implicated in disruptions. Examples of teratogens that cause birth defects include alcohol, anticonvulsants (such as hydantoin, valproic acid, and carbamazepine), and vitamin A analogs (such as retinoic acid), which can cause ear anomalies, hearing loss, brain anomalies, and congenital heart defects.

Physical disruption of normal development can also occur. For example, *amniotic bands* occur when the *amnion*, the membrane surrounding the embryo and fetus, ruptures, leaving strands of tissue floating in the amniotic cavity. These strands can attach to limbs, the head, or other body parts and act as tourniquets, cutting off blood supply to developing structures. This results in amputates of limbs and digits, cleft lip, and other oral and facial deformities (Figure 3–2, A–B). Even some

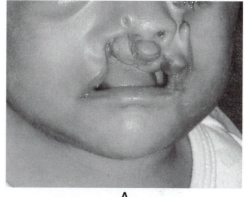

Courtesy Howard M. Saal, M.D./Cincinnati Children's Hospital Medical Center & University of Cincinnati College of Medicine

A

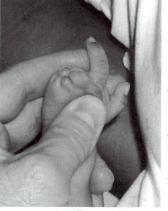

Courtesy Howard M. Saal, M.D./Cincinnati Children's Hospital Medical Center & University of Cincinnati College of Medicine

B

FIGURE 3–2 (A and B) Amniotic band deformities. (A) Facial cleft and deformity due to amniotic bands. (B) Finger amputations due to amniotic bands.

maternal illnesses can result in disruptions, such as maternal diabetes, which can cause vertebral, heart, and even brain anomalies.

Syndromes and Associations

A *syndrome* is a pattern of multiple anomalies that are pathogenically related, and therefore have a common known or suspected cause. Because craniofacial syndromes affect the facial features, they can cause affected individuals to look alike, even when there is no family relationship. An example of this is Down syndrome. Many children with craniofacial conditions have underlying syndromes as the cause of the specific craniofacial anomaly. Recognizing a specific syndrome is important for medical management and is a focus of genetic counseling.

An *association* is a nonrandom occurrence of a pattern of multiple anomalies in two or more individuals that are not a known syndrome or sequence. In an association, the pathogenesis is not known, and therefore a genetic etiology cannot be discerned. An association is a diagnosis of exclusion; in other words, a genetic, developmental, or teratogenic etiology must first be excluded before making the diagnosis of an association. Because no genetic etiology can be discerned, the recurrence risks for associations are no greater than the risks for the general population. One example of an association is VATER (vertebral, anal, tracheoesophageal, and renal) association. In VATER association, one can see vertebral anomalies; anorectal anomalies (imperforate anus); tracheoesophageal fistula; and renal, radial, and other limb anomalies. In VATER association, the etiology is not known and there appears to be no increased recurrence risk than that in the general population.

Pierre Robin Sequence

In contrast to a syndrome or association, a *sequence* describes a series of anomalies that result from a single initiating event, anomaly, or mechanical factor. The best-known and perhaps the best understood example is Pierre Robin sequence (Figure 3–3). In this sequence, the initiating event is *micrognathia* (small mandible), with the secondary consequence of *glossoptosis* (posterior placement of the tongue) and obstruction of the upper airway. This is often accompanied by a wide, bell-shaped cleft palate if the posterior position of the tongue interferes with normal palate closure. Pierre Robin sequence can occur in isolation due to mechanical forces in utero, but it is often

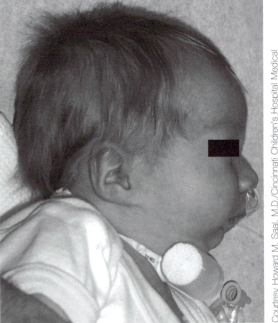

Courtesy Howard M. Saal, M.D./Cincinnati Children's Hospital Medical Center & University of Cincinnati College of Medicine

FIGURE 3–3   Pierre Robin sequence with the characteristic micrognathia (small mandible).

associated with a syndrome (e.g., Stickler syndrome, Treacher Collins syndrome, velocardiofacial syndrome, and fetal alcohol syndrome). Recurrence risks are related to the underlying cause of the micrognathia.

After birth, the upper airway may be obstructed due to the glossoptosis. This can be serious enough to cause life-threatening respiratory distress. There are many approaches to airway management for affected infants, and the treatment must be individualized for each child. The first approach is to keep the infant in a prone position. Gravity then causes the tongue to fall forward, relieving the glossoptosis for some infants. Sometimes it is necessary to use a *nasopharyngeal airway tube*, which goes through the nose and the pharynx below the region of tongue obstruction. This tube may be needed until 3 or 4 months of age. Some infants do not respond adequately to such conservative treatments and therefore require a *tracheostomy*, which is surgical placement of a tube directly in the trachea in order to bypass the area of upper airway obstruction. Usually the tracheostomy remains in place until after the palate is repaired, or until about14 months. Unfortunately, the presence of the tracheostomy prevents or interferes with vocalizations, often leading to further speech issues in addition to those related to the cleft palate.

A newer procedure to manage patients with Pierre Robin sequence and tongue-based obstructive apnea is mandibular distraction (Fritz & Sidman, 2004; Hong, McNeil, Kearns, & Magit, 2012; Sidman, Sampson, & Templeton, 2001). With this procedure, an *osteotomy* (fracture or cut) is created on both sides of the mandible, and the two segments of the mandible are separated. They are pulled apart gradually (over several days or weeks) until there is adequate lengthening of the mandible to relieve the obstruction due to glossoptosis. This procedure can be done in early infancy and usually

results in normal respiration and feeding. (See Chapter 19 for more information.)

Most infants with Pierre Robin sequence also have early feeding problems. Some of these infants respond to short periods of feeding with a *nasogastric tube* (NG-tube), which is placed through the nose into the stomach. In more severe cases, a *gastrostomy tube* (G-tube) is needed. A G-tube is placed directly into the stomach for feeding.

GENETICS OF CLEFTS

As has been noted, cleft lip (CL), with or without cleft palate (CL ± P), is a very common birth defect. Boys are affected more frequently than girls, by a ratio of 3:2 (Wyszynski, Beaty, & Maestri, 1996). A left-sided cleft lip is more common than a right-sided cleft, and both occur more frequently than bilateral CL ± P.

Genetics of Nonsyndromic Cleft Lip (± Cleft Palate)

Although most cases of CL ± P are isolated—that is, there are no associated syndromes or other birth defects—there still is a substantial underlying genetic pathogenesis. This is supported by the fact that the recurrence risk for CL ± P is elevated for affected individuals, their parents, and even their siblings. For the child with CL ± P and his or her parents, the recurrence risk with each future pregnancy is in the range of 3%–5%—in other words, a 30- to 45-fold increase over baseline risk. After a second child is born with CL ± P, the recurrence risk rises to 10%–15%, consistent with an increased genetic contribution. With the birth of a third first-degree relative that is affected, the recurrence risk increases to 25%–50%, consistent with autosomal dominant or recessive inheritance. The recurrence risk is also influenced by the severity of the CL ± P. For a child born with bilateral cleft lip and cleft palate, the recurrence risk is 5.6% for a bilateral cleft lip and palate, 4.1% for a unilateral cleft lip and cleft palate, and 2.6% for a unilateral cleft lip without cleft palate (Fraser, 1970).

In some families, there are multiple individuals affected with CL ± P. This can represent a more significant underlying genetic influence or predisposition. In these families, the inheritance may appear to be autosomal dominant. In particular, Van der Woude syndrome has been identified with autosomal-dominant inheritance of clefts. In addition to having cleft lip and/or cleft palate, most individuals with this syndrome also have bilateral pits in the lower lip. Because this is an autosomal dominant syndrome, the recurrence risk with Van der Woude syndrome is 50% rather than the typical 3% to 5% when there is a nonsyndromic cleft.

There are significant racial differences in the incidence of CL ± P. For those of African descent, the risk is only 1 in 2000, for Caucasian populations the incidence is 1 in 800, and for Asians it is 1 in 500. The incidence of CL ± P appears to be highest in Native Americans, with 1 in 300 being affected. Even with these data, recurrence risks are similar among all racial and ethnic groups (Gorlin et al., 2001; Wyszynski et al., 1996).

A great deal of research is underway to find the genes that cause or predispose to isolated (nonsyndromic) CL ± P. Specific genes that are active during early craniofacial development have been implicated in the etiology of CL ± P, including transforming growth factor-alpha retinoic acid receptor; transforming growth factor beta; MSX1 (Lidral et al., 1998); and IRF6, the gene (Rahimov et al., 2012; Zucchero et al., 2004). To date, 17 genes have been associated with nonsyndromic orofacial cleft.

If the prevalence of CL ± P were determined on the basis of inheritance of a single gene, one would expect recurrence risks of 25% or 50%, as would be seen in autosomal recessive or autosomal dominant inheritance, respectively. However, other genes that are inherited from both parents modify the effects of this predisposing gene. In addition, environmental factors also influence whether the child is actually born with an orofacial cleft. These environmental factors may include maternal smoking, alcohol intake, metabolic changes, or nutritional deficiencies. Even fetal positioning, blood flow, and placental factors can affect whether a cleft actually occurs.

Genetics of Syndromic Cleft Lip (± Cleft Palate)

Although most cases of CL ± P are isolated birth defects, some are caused by underlying genetic syndromes or are part of a multiple congenital anomaly disorder. Gorlin and colleagues (2001) has estimated that there are over 400 distinct syndromes associated with facial clefts. Some of the syndromes associates with CL ± P are noted in Table 3–1.

TABLE 3–1 Syndromes Associated with Cleft Lip (±Cleft Palate)

Amniotic bands

CHARGE syndrome

Diabetic embryopathy

Fetal alcohol syndrome

Hemifacial microsomia

Opitz syndrome

Orofaciodigital syndrome Type I (OFD I)

Popliteal pterygium syndrome

Trisomy 13

Van der Woude syndrome

Wolf-Hirschhorn syndrome

Some patients have CL ± P with multiple anomalies in what appears to be an underlying syndrome, although a diagnosis cannot be made because the pattern of anomalies is not one that has been previously described. Approximately 40% to 50% of patients seen by a geneticist have syndromes that are either rare or possibly unique. These patients are diagnosed as having *provisionally unique syndromes* until other patients with the same syndromic pattern are identified and reported.

Genetics of Cleft Palate Only (CPO)

In contrast to CL ± P, cleft palate only (CPO) is much more likely to be associated with an underlying syndrome or other congenital anomalies. CP is a component of numerous syndromes (Table 3–2). The London Dysmorphology Database lists 485 syndromes, excluding chromosome disorders, in which cleft palate may be a feature (Baraitser & Winter, 1991; Fryns & de Ravel, 2002). A prospective analysis at the Craniofacial Center at Cincinnati Children's Hospital showed that approximately 55% of all cases of CP were syndromic or associated with additional anomalies (Stanier & Moore, 2004).

TABLE 3–2 Syndromes Primarily Associated with Cleft Palate

CHARGE syndrome

Fetal alcohol syndrome

Fetal hydantoin syndrome

Hemifacial microsomia

Kabuki syndrome

Stickler syndrome

Van der Woude syndrome

Velocardiofacial syndrome

© Cengage Learning 2014

CLEFT AND CRANIOFACIAL SYNDROMES

Syndromes are diagnosed based on the pattern of major and minor malformations (Jones & Jones, 2009). Table 3–3 shows cleft and craniofacial syndromes and their typical features and concerns. In addition, some of the more common are discussed below.

Beckwith-Wiedemann Syndrome

Beckwith-Wiedemann syndrome (Figure 3–4) is a genetic disorder that results in prenatal and postnatal overgrowth. Children with Beckwith-Wiedemann syndrome are usually born large for gestational age (often more than 10 pounds at birth). Some are born with an umbilical hernia or even an *omphalocele*, where part of the intestine is outside of the abdomen in the region of the umbilical cord. There is a risk for severe neonatal *hypoglycemia* (low blood sugar), which can result in seizures and can even be life threatening.

Patients with Beckwith-Wiedemann syndrome often have accelerated growth during early childhood, which can result in *hemihypertrophy*, where one side of the body grows faster and larger than the other side, leading to asymmetry. A major feature of this syndrome is *macroglossia* (very large tongue). The large tongue can cause Pierre Robin sequence with cleft palate (Dios, Posse, Sanroman, & Garcia, 2000; Laroche, Testelin, & Devauchelle, 2005).

Children with Beckwith-Wiedemann syndrome have a significant risk of developing a *Wilms tumor* (a malignant tumor of the kidney), a *hepatoblastoma* (a malignant tumor of the liver), or other malignant tumors in the abdomen. The risk for developing such tumors is between 5% and 8%, with most cases occurring before 8 years. For this reason, a

TABLE 3–3 Craniofacial Conditions: Syndromes, Associations, and Sequences

Amniotic Bands

Etiology	Caused by restricted development of parts of the fetus due to constriction of amniotic bands.
Inheritance	Sporadic
Phenotypic Features	**Clefts:** Bands can affect development of the lip or palate if they are in the mouth. **Craniofacial features:** Facial deformities if the bands restrict the face. **Other:** Clubfoot deformity; limb, hand and finger anomalies or amputations.
Functional Concerns	Communication disorders related to cleft palate.

Apert Syndrome (aka: Acrocephalosyndactly Type I)

Etiology	Mutation of a gene on the long arm of chromosome 10 (10q25.3-q26). **FGFR2 (10q26)** Causes premature closure of the coronal sutures so that the skull grows laterally, but not anteriorly.
Inheritance	Autosomal dominant: 50% recurrence risk
Phenotypic Features	**Clefts:** Cleft palate occurs infrequently. **Craniofacial features:** Similar to Crouzon syndrome, including a prominent forehead with a flat occiput, exophthalmos, hypertelorism, antimongoloid slant, strabismus and midface hypoplasia/retrusion, Class III malocclusion, low set ears; upper airway obstruction. **Other:** Syndactyly of fingers and toes; developmental disabilities.
Communication Concerns	Communication disorders related to upper airway obstruction; mental retardation; cleft palate, and Class III malocclusion.

Beckwith-Wiedemann Syndrome

Etiology	Some are due to mutations in the short arm of chromosome 11 (11p15).
Inheritance	Sporadic
Phenotypic Features	**Craniofacial features:** Hypertrophic facial features; macroglossia. **Other:** Large at birth, neonatal hypoglycemia; organ macromegaly; hemihypertrophy; umbilical hernia; omphalocele; abnormalities of kidneys, pancreas and adrenal cortex; at risk for Wilms tumor, hepatablastoma and malignant tumors of the abdomen. Macroglossia can cause feeding issues; upper airway obstruction and sleep apnea; and dental malocclusion and ultimately, prognathia.
Communication Concerns	Communication disorders related to macroglossia and dental malocclusion.

CHARGE Association

Etiology	Sporadic. Due to mutations on the CHD7 gene (located on Chromosome 8) Due to mutations on chromosomes 7 and 8
Inheritance	Autosomal dominant (most cases new mutation)
Phenotypic Features	**Clefts:** Robin sequence, cleft lip and palate **Primary features:** **C**oloboma **H**eart disease **A**tresia of the choanae **R**etarded growth and development

(continues)

TABLE 3–3 (continued)

	Genital anomalies, cryptorchidism, micropenis, hypogonadism, delayed puberty Ear anomalies, hearing loss and deafness **Other:** micrognathia; brain and cranial nerve anomalies; abnormal or absent pituitary gland; and developmental disability
Communication Concerns	Communication disorders related to hearing loss, cleft palate, and the presence of neurological dysfunction.

Crouzon Syndrome

Etiology	Mutation along the long arm of chromosome 10 (10q25.3-q26). **FGFR2 (10q26)** Causes premature closure of the coronal sutures so that the skull grows laterally, but not anteriorly.
Inheritance	Autosomal dominant: 50% recurrence risk
Phenotypic Features	**Clefts:** Cleft palate and submucous cleft palate is occasionally seen in these patients. **Craniofacial features:** Features similar to Apert syndrome, including a broad forehead, flat occiput, exophthalmos, hypertelorism, antimongoloid slant, strabismus and midface hypoplasia/retrusion, Class III malocclusion; low set ears. **Other:** Can have hydrocephalus or agenesis of the corpus callosum; occasional developmental disabilities.
Communication Concerns	Communication disorders related to developmental disabilities or brain anomalies (if present), cleft palate, Class III malocclusion, and upper airway obstruction.

Down Syndrome (aka: Trisomy 21 Syndrome)

Etiology	Extra copy of chromosome 21
Inheritance	Sporadic
Phenotypic Features	**Clefts:** Clefts are not part of this syndrome. **Craniofacial features:** Upward slanting of the palpebral fissures with epicanthal folds on the inner corner of the eyes; micrognathia; macroglossia and/or protruding tongue; broad face; short neck; low set ears. **Other:** Short limbs resulting in short stature; a crease across one or both palms; hypotonia; congenital heart defects; gastroesophageal reflux; breathing issues and obstructive sleep apnea; mild to moderate mental retardation.
Communication Concerns	Communication disorders related to developmental disability and large or hypotonic tongue.

Ectrodactyly-Ectodermal Dysplasia-Cleft Syndrome (EEC Syndrome)

Etiology	Genetic defect on the long arm of chromosome 7 (7q11.2-q21.3)
Inheritance	Autosomal dominant: 50% recurrence risk
Phenotypic Features	**Clefts:** Cleft lip and cleft palate are common **Craniofacial features:** Partial anodontia or microdontia; maxillary and malar hypoplasia; photophobia; defects of the lacrimal duct system; ossicular anomalies. **Other:** Ectrodactyly (deficiency or absence of one or more central digits of the hand or foot), sometimes referred to as a "lobster-claw" deformity; ectodermal dysplasia (dry skin and mucosa, dry, sparse hair); absent sweat glands.
Communication Concerns	Voice issues, particularly breathiness, due to lack of vocal fold hydration. Communication disorders related to the cleft and conductive hearing loss.

(continues)

TABLE 3–3 (continued)

Fetal Alcohol Syndrome (FAS)

Etiology	Teratogenic (Usually 4-6 alcoholic drinks per day)
Inheritance	Teratogenic
Phenotypic Features	**Clefts:** Pierre Robin sequence and cleft palate, and cleft lip. **Craniofacial features:** Short palpebral fissures; short nose, flat philtrum and thin upper lip; microcephaly. **Other:** Small size at birth; heart defects, including ventricular septal defect (VSD), atrial septal defect (ASD); mental retardation (average intelligence is about 65); severe behavior problems, hyperactivity, poor judgment, difficulty interpreting social cues, behavioral problems.
Communication Concerns	Communication disorders related to the mental retardation and neurological dysfunction.

Fetal Hydantoin Syndrome (aka: Fetal Dilantin Syndrome)

Etiology	**Teratogenic due to use of Dilantin for seizures during pregnancy.**
Inheritance	**Teratogenic**
Phenotypic Features	**Clefts: Clefts are not part of this syndrome.** **Craniofacial features: Microcephaly; minor dysmorphic craniofacial features** **Other: Intrauterine growth restriction; limb defects; hypoplastic nails; developmental delay or mental retardation.**
Communication Concerns	**Communication disorders related to developmental delay or mental retardation.**

Hemifacial Microsomia (HFM) (aka: Oculo-Auriculo-Vertebral (OAV) Dysplasia, Facio-Auriculo-Vertebral Spectrum (FAV) or Goldenhar Syndrome)

Etiology	Sporadic
Recurrence Risk	Autosomal dominant: 50% recurrence risk
Phenotypic Features	**Clefts:** Cleft lip and/or palate in about 15% of cases **Craniofacial features:** Facial asymmetry due to unilateral hypoplasia of the face, malar, maxillary, and/or mandibular processes; cleft-like extension of corner of mouth; ear anomalies, including microtia or anotia and preauricular tags or pits; eye anomalies including colobomas of upper eyelid, epibulbar lipodermoids, microphthalmia; dysplasia or aplasia of temporomandibular joint, affecting the opening of the mouth and excursion of mandible. **Other:** Cervical vertebral anomalies **Note:** Hemifacial microsomia is usually unilateral but can be bilateral, although more severe on one side.
Communication Concerns	Communication disorders related to velopharyngeal insufficiency or incompetence, hearing loss, or asymmetric oral structures.

Moebius Syndrome

Etiology	Absence or under development of abducent nerve (CN VI) and facial nerve (CN VII)
Inheritance	2 to 20 cases per million births

(continues)

TABLE 3–3 (continued)

Phenotypic Features	**Clefts:** Clefts are not part of this syndrome. **Craniofacial features:** Abnormalities in movement of cheeks, lips, and eyes, resulting in a flat, "mask-type" facies; strabismus; occasional hearing loss if cranial VIII is affected; occasional breathing and/or in swallowing problems. **Other:** Limb abnormalities, including clubbed feet, missing digits; chest wall abnormalities.
Communication Concerns	Communication disorders related to the inability to produce bilabial and sometimes labio-dental sounds for speech; inability to smile, move the eyes or mouth, or show facial expression; and possible hearing problems.

Opitz G Syndrome (aka: BBB syndrome, Opitz-Frias Syndrome, Hypertelorism-Hypospadias Syndrome)

Etiology	One form is caused by a mutation in the MID1 gene on the X chromosome. Another form is caused by a mutation in an unidentified gene on chromosome 22.
Inheritance	If X-linked: Recessive inheritance If related to chromosome 22, autosomal dominant: 50% recurrence risk
Phenotypic Features	**Clefts:** Laryngeal cleft, cleft lip, cleft palate **Craniofacial features:** Hypertelorism; flat nasal bridge; thin upper lip; and low set ears. **Other:** Hypospadias; cryptorchidism; imperforate anus, heart defects; inguinal hernias; absent corpus callosum; learning disabilities and mental retardation.
Communication Concerns	Communication disorders related to long-term tracheostomy management; cleft palate; learning disabilities and mental retardation.

Orofaciodigital Syndrome Type I (OFD I)

Etiology	X-linked
Inheritance	Dominant in females; usually lethal in males
Phenotypic Features	**Clefts:** cleft lip, cleft palate, midline cleft lip **Craniofacial features:** Hypertelorism; lobulated tongue; multiple hyperplastic oral frenula; notching in alveolar ridge; broad nose; hydrocephalus, absence of corpus callosum. **Other:** Syndactyly or clinodactyly; dry skin and dry, sparse hair; missing teeth; renal cysts; mental retardation or developmental disabilities.
Communication Concerns	Communication disorders related to the cleft, mental retardation or developmental disabilities. The lobulated tongue does not usually affect speech.

Pfeiffer Syndrome

Etiology	Mutation in the fibroblast growth factor receptor (FGFR genes) on the short arm of chromosome 8 (8p11.2-p12). Causes premature closure of the coronal sutures.
Inheritance	Autosomal dominant: 50% recurrence risk
Phenotypic Features	**Clefts:** Cleft palate is rare. **Craniofacial features:** Coronal craniosynostosis, midface hypoplasia, shallow orbits with exophthalmos, hypertelorism; tracheal anomalies and upper airway stenosis; hearing loss **Other:** Broad thumbs and great toes. **Note:** Type I is most common; Type 2 and Type 3 have the same clinical features, but are more severe. The craniosynostosis involves multiple sutures, giving the skull a cloverleaf appearance. Death in early childhood is common.
Communication Concerns	Communication disorders related to the mental retardation or hearing loss.

(continues)

TABLE 3–3 (continued)

Pierre Robin Sequence

Etiology	Micrognathia that may be due to crowding in utero, or may be genetic as part of a syndrome (e.g., Stickler's syndrome or velocardiofacial syndrome). Micrognathia interferes with the downward progression of the tongue and the closure of the velum.
Inheritance	Depends on if it is due to genetic factors or mechanical factors in utero.
Phenotypic Features	**Clefts:** Usually a wide bell-shaped cleft palate. **Craniofacial features:** Micrognathia; glossoptosis; airway and feeding issues, particularly at birth. **Other:** None
Communication Concerns	Communication disorders related to the cleft and airway obstruction.

Popliteal Pterygium Syndrome

Etiology	Mutations of the interferon regulatory factor *IRF6* gene on the long arm of chromosome 1 (1q32.3-q41).
Inheritance	Autosomal dominant
Phenotypic Features	**Clefts:** Usually includes cleft lip and cleft palate **Craniofacial features:** Lip pits near the center of the lower lip; tissue connecting the eyelids or jaws; missing teeth. **Other:** Webs of skin behind the knee; abnormal genitals, including cryptorchidism; learning disabilities or mild cognitive problems
Communication Concerns	Communication disorders related to jaw restriction, learning disabilities or cognitive problems.

Stickler Syndrome

Etiology	Mutations on the short arm of chromosome 6 (6p21).
Recurrence Risk	Autosomal dominant: 50% recurrence risk
Phenotypic Features	**Clefts:** Pierre Robin sequence with characteristic bell-shaped cleft palate. **Craniofacial features:** Pierre Robin sequence with the characteristics of micrognathia, glossoptosis and wide bell-shaped cleft palate; a wide, flat face with midface hypoplasia; epicanthal folds; sensorineural hearing loss, high myopia and risk for retinal detachments. **Other:** Early onset of osteoarthritis and other joint disorders.
Communication Concerns	Communication disorders related to cleft palate and hearing loss.

Saethre-Chotzen Syndrome (aka: Acrocephalosyndactyly Type 3 or Chotzen syndrome)

Etiology	Complete or partial deletion of the TWIST gene. Causes premature closure of the coronal sutures so that the skull grows laterally, but not anteriorly. Most common craniosynostosis syndrome-but may not have craniosynostosis.
Inheritance	Autosomal dominant: 50% recurrence risk
Phenotypic Features	**Clefts:** Cleft palate or submucous cleft palate **Craniofacial features:** Coronal synostosis; ptosis of the eyelids; midface hypoplasia; external ear anomalies; **Other:** Mental retardation occurs infrequently.
Communication Concerns	Communication disorders related to cleft palate or mental retardation if present.

(continues)

TABLE 3–3 (continued)

Treacher Collins Syndrome

Etiology	Mutations on the long arm of chromosome 5 (5q32-q33.3)
Inheritance	Autosomal dominant: 50%-variable expressivity
Phenotypic Features	**Clefts:** Clefts occur infrequently, despite Pierre Robin sequence with pronounced micrognathia. **Craniofacial features:** Downward slanting of the palpebral fissures; colobomas of the lower eyelids; microtia or middle ear anomalies; hypoplastic zygomatic arches and malar hypoplasia; and macrostomia or microstomia; micrognathia; glossoptosis
Communication Concerns	Communication disorders related to conductive hearing loss and micrognathia

Trisomy 21 Syndrome

Etiology	Duplication of chromosome 21
Inheritance	Chromosomal, usually sporadic
Phenotypic Features	**Clefts:** Cleft lip and palate. May have a midline cleft. **Craniofacial Features:** Severe eye defects; midline facial deformities. **Other:** Severe brain anomalies including holoprosencephaly; congenital heart defects; polydactyly; spina bifida; severe to profound mental retardation.
Communication Concerns	Most infants die before their first birthday.

Van der Woude Syndrome

Etiology	Mutation of interferon regulatory growth factor 6 (IRF6) gene on the long arm of chromosome (11q.32-41).
Inheritance	Autosomal dominant: 50% recurrence risk
Phenotypic Features	**Clefts:** Cleft lip and palate **Craniofacial features:** Bilateral lip pits on the lower lip; missing teeth.
Communication Concerns	Communication disorders related to the cleft.

Velocardiofacial Syndrome (VCFS) (aka: DiGeorge syndrome or 22q11.2 Syndrome)

Etiology	Second most common genetic syndrome, following Down syndrome (Trisomy 21) as most common
Inheritance	Chromosomal, Autosomal dominant: 50%
Phenotypic Features	**Primary Features:** • **Velo:** velopharyngeal dysfunction causing hypernasality, usually secondary an occult submucous cleft or pharyngeal hypotonia. • **Cardio:** minor cardiac and vascular anomalies including ventriculoseptal deviation (VSD); atrial septal defect (ASD); patent ductus arteriosis (PDA); pulmonary stenosis; tetralogy of Fallot; right-sided aortic arch; medially displaced internal carotid arteries; and tortuosity of the retinal arteries. Parents often report a history of heart murmur at birth. • **Facial:** microcephaly, long face with vertical maxillary excess; micrognathia (small jaw) or retruded mandible, often with a Class II malocclusion; nasal anomalies including wide nasal bridge, narrow alar base and bulbous nasal tip; narrow palpebral fissures (slit-like eyes); malar flatness; thin upper lip; minor auricular anomalies; abundant scalp hair and others. • **Other:** Long slender digits; hyperextensibility of the joints; short stature, usually below the 10%ile in weight and height; Pierre Robin sequence (cleft palate, micrognathia,

(continues)

TABLE 3–3 (continued)

glossoptosis with airway obstruction); umbilical and inguinal hernias; laryngeal web; gross and fine motor delays; various brain anomalies; social disinhibition; risk of onset of psychosis in adolescence; learning disabilities and concrete thinking; mild to moderate mental retardation.

Communication Concerns	Communication disorders related to velopharyngeal insufficiency; pharyngeal hypotonia; verbal apraxia; conductive and/or sensorineural hearing loss; laryngeal anomalies and developmental disabilities.

Wolf-Hirschhorn syndrome

Etiology	Deletion or missing portion of short arm of chromosome 4
Inheritance	Usually sporadic, Autosomal dominant: 50%
Phenotypic Features	**Clefts:** Cleft Palate is common **Craniofacial features:** Distinctive facial appearance which is likened to a Greek helmet; hypertelorism; coloboma of the iris; prominent nasal bridge; microcephaly; micrognathia; short philtrum; dysplastic ears and periauricular tag; occasional hearing loss **Other:** Congenital heart defects; small stature and poor growth; renal anomalies; hypotonia; developmental disabilities or severe to profound mental retardation.
Communication Concerns	Communication disorders related to developmental disabilities and mental retardation; and hearing loss if present.

© Cengage Learing 2014

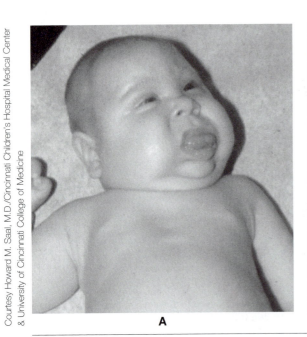
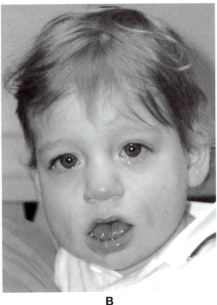

Courtesy Howard M. Saal, M.D./Cincinnati Children's Hospital Medical Center & University of Cincinnati College of Medicine

A

B

FIGURE 3–4 (A and B) Beckwith-Wiedemann syndrome with macroglossia. (A) A newborn with the severe macroglossia, which can cause respiratory problems and feeding difficulties for newborns. (B) Child with macroglossia and open mouth posture. This causes speech problems.

child with Beckwith-Wiedemann syndrome should receive a renal and abdominal ultrasound examination at least every 4 months.

Development in Beckwith-Wiedemann syndrome is usually normal, although there is a risk for developmental delay if neonatal hypoglycemia is prolonged. The large tongue may contribute to abnormal cranial and dental growth, including *prognathism* (a large mandible). The large tongue often causes obstructive breathing; eating problems; and, of course, speech problems. Resonance can be affected not only by cleft palate but also by the size of the tongue, which can block the transmission of acoustic energy in the oral cavity. For these reasons, some children with Beckwith-Wiedemann syndrome require surgical reduction of the tongue (Shuman, Beckwith, Smith, & Weksberg, 2010).

CHARGE Syndrome

CHARGE syndrome (Figure 3–5) is an acronym for **c**oloboma, **h**eart defect, choanal **a**tresia, **r**etarded growth and/or development, **g**enitourinary anomalies, and **e**ar anomalies and/or deafness (Hsueh, Yang, Lu, & Hsu, 2004). A diagnosis of CHARGE syndrome requires at least four of the six clinical features, and one of the features must be the presence of *choanal atresia* (a blockage at the back of the nasal passage) or *colobomas* (congenital defects of the eye, including a notch in the lower eyelid or defects of the iris or retina).

The colobomas of CHARGE syndrome usually affect the retina, causing significant visual impairment (McMain et al., 2008; Plomp et al., 1998). The heart defects are often very serious and life threatening. Genitourinary anomalies are usually related to *micropenis*

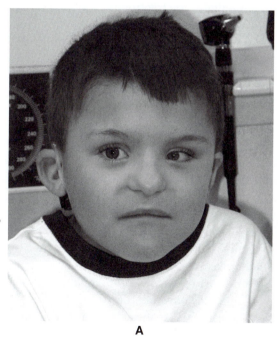
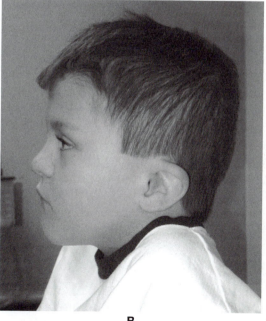

Courtesy Howard M. Saal, M.D./Cincinnati Children's Hospital Medical Center & University of Cincinnati College of Medicine

A   **B**

FIGURE 3–5 (A and B) CHARGE syndrome. (A) There is a defect in the left eye and a hearing aid on the child's right. (B) Note the mild ear anomaly.

(small penis) or *cryptorchidism* (undescended testicles) in males. These may be related to pituitary abnormalities that may also be manifested in adolescence as delayed or absent puberty or amenorrhea. External ear anomalies, hearing loss, and deafness are very common as well. Brain anomalies are often found, and there may be abnormalities or absence of the pituitary gland, which affects growth and genitourinary development. Although some individuals with CHARGE syndrome have normal intelligence, mental retardation is seen in most patients and is often severe to profound. Cleft lip and/or cleft palate occurs in many patients with CHARGE association (Jongmans et al., 2006). Speech and language disorders related to clefts are often complicated by the coexistence of mental retardation and deafness.

Down Syndrome

Down syndrome is the most common chromosome disorder, with an incidence of 1/700 live births. It is associated with intellectual disability, hypotonia, short stature, increased risk for hypothyroidism, leukemia, middle ear disease, and celiac disease. Approximately 50% of individuals with Down syndrome are born with a congenital heart defect. Cleft lip and/or cleft palate occurs infrequently in Down syndrome. However, affected individuals have speech and language disorders due to poor oral-motor function, conductive hearing loss, and intellectual impairment (Bull, 2011).

Fetal Alcohol Syndrome (FAS)

Fetal alcohol syndrome is caused by exposure to significant amounts of alcohol during gestation, particularly during the first trimester. Although the precise amount of alcohol intake necessary to cause fetal alcohol syndrome remains unknown, it is generally accepted that women who consume two alcoholic drinks daily during pregnancy are at risk for delivering babies with small birth size. The intake of more drinks per day can cause other serious clinical issues (Jones, 2006; Jones & Smith, 1973).

The classic signs of fetal alcohol syndrome include low birth weight, microcephaly, dysmorphic facial features with narrow *palpebral fissures* (eye slits), thin upper lip, short nose, flat philtrum, and occasionally cleft lip and/or cleft palate. Congenital heart defects are common, particularly *ventricular septal defect* (VSD) (discontinuity of tissue that separates the lower chambers of the heart). Developmental delays and intellectual disabilities are almost universal. The average intelligence quotient in this population has been estimated to be 63 (Jones, 2006). In addition, older children with fetal alcohol syndrome often have severe behavior problems including hyperactivity, distractibility, poor judgment, and difficulty interpreting social cues (Jones, 2006; Nash, Sheard, Rovet, & Koren, 2008; Streissguth et al., 1991).

Hemifacial Microsomia

Hemifacial microsomia (Figure 3–6) is a condition with numerous names, including oculo-auriculo-vertebral (OAV) or facio-auriculo-vertebral (FAV) spectrum, and even Goldenhar syndrome if there are *epibulbar lipodermoids* (fatty cysts) on the *sclerae* (white portion) of the eyeball. This is a relatively common multiple anomaly disorder with a birth incidence of 1 in 3000 to 5000 live births (Jones, 2006). Most cases are sporadic, although some familial cases have been reported.

The primary feature of hemifacial microsomia is hypoplasia of the maxilla, mandible, and ear on the affected side(s). Hemifacial microsomia is usually unilateral (hence the

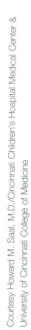

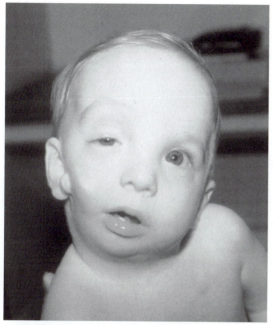

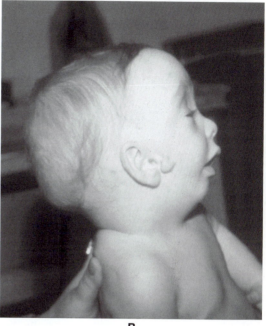

A **B**

FIGURE 3–6 (A and B) (A) A boy with hemifacial microsomia. He has severe facial asymmetry exacerbated by cervical spine abnormalities and fusion. (B) The lateral view shows severe dysplasia of the right ear and an ear tag.

name), although about 30% of the cases have bilateral involvement (Gorlin et al., 2001). The right side tends to be affected more often than the left, and boys are affected more frequently than girls (Jones, 2006).

The hypoplasia of hemifacial microsomia may affect the temporomandibular joint, limiting the extent of mouth opening. An intraoral evaluation may reveal an occlusal cant and unilateral velar paresis. Cleft lip and/or cleft palate are seen in about 15% of affected patients. There can also be weakness of the facial nerve (Cranial Nerve VII) on the affected side. Ear involvement ranges from mild aplasia to *anotia* (absence of the external auditory canal). Anomalies of the eyes can occur, including colobomas of the upper eyelid or retina and *microphthalmia* (small eyes).

Brain anomalies can be seen in this population, including hydrocephalus, *encephaloceles* (protrusions of the brain through openings in the skull), and absence of the corpus callosum. Vertebral anomalies are found in about 15% of cases and usually involve the cervical vertebrae. Serious heart defects and kidney abnormalities can occur, leading to significant morbidity (Strömland et al., 2007).

Although most patients with hemifacial microsomia have normal intelligence, learning disabilities and mental retardation may occur if there are anomalies of the brain. Speech disorders are common due to dental malocclusion, limited mouth opening, cleft palate, and velar paralysis or paresis.

Kabuki Syndrome

Kabuki syndrome (Figure 3–7), also called Kabuki makeup syndrome after the dramatic appearance of the Kabuki actors, is a

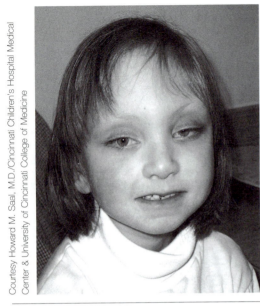

Courtesy Howard M. Saal, M.D./Cincinnati Children's Hospital Medical Center & University of Cincinnati College of Medicine

FIGURE 3–7 Kabuki syndrome. Note the wide palpebral fissures (eye openings) with eversion (turning out) of the lateral portion of the lower lid, external ear anomalies, arched eyebrows, and a broad nasal tip.

distinctive genetic condition. Facial features include wide palpebral fissures with eversion (turning out) of the lateral portion of the lower lid, external ear anomalies, arched eyebrows, and a broad nasal tip. Other anomalies can include cleft palate and submucous cleft palate, vertebral anomalies, congenital heart defects, and low muscle tone (Hannibal et al., 2011). Speech and language is usually affected by mild to moderate intellectual impairment and cleft palate, if present.

Neurofibromatosis Type 1

Neurofibromatosis type 1 (Figure 3–8) is one of the most common autosomal dominant genetic disorders, with a prevalence of approximately 1/3000 individuals (Friedman, Birch & Greene, 1993). The diagnosis of neurofibromatosis type 1 is usually made by clinical evaluation and the presence of two or more

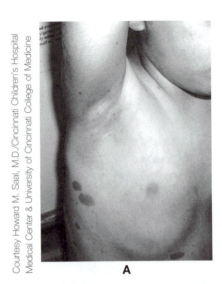

Courtesy Howard M. Saal, M.D./Cincinnati Children's Hospital Medical Center & University of Cincinnati College of Medicine

A

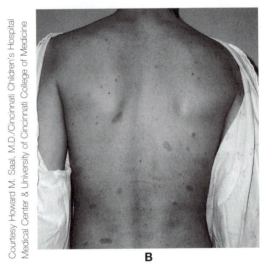

Courtesy Howard M. Saal, M.D./Cincinnati Children's Hospital Medical Center & University of Cincinnati College of Medicine

B

FIGURE 3–8 (A and B) Neurofibromatosis 1. Note the café au lait spots on the skin.

clinical features out of seven. The seven features are (1) six or more *café au lait macules* (pigmented spots the color of "coffee with milk") >5 mm in prepubertal individuals or >15 mm post-puberty; (2) two or more neurofibromas or a single plexiform neurofibroma (usually larger and spongy in texture); (3) freckling in the axillae or the inguinal region; (4) an optic pathway tumor (diagnosed with magnetic resonance imaging [MRI]); (5) two or more Lisch nodules (small hamartomas or benign tumors) of the iris; (6) osseous lesions of the sphenoid wing of the cranium or long bone bowing (usually of the tibia); (7) a first-degree relative with neurofibromatosis type 1 diagnosed with the above criteria (Viskochil, 2002).

Although patients with neurofibromatosis type 1 rarely have craniofacial anomalies, a significant number of individuals with this disorder have velopharyngeal dysfunction, causing resonance disorders (Zhang et al., 2012). Neurofibromatosis type 1 is the second most common syndrome associated with velopharyngeal dysfunction in the VPI Clinic at Cincinnati Children's Hospital Medical Center. In addition, these children often have delays in speech sound and language develop-

ment (Thompson, Viskochil, Stevenson, & Chapman, 2010).

Opitz G Syndrome

Opitz G syndrome (Figure 3–9) is a condition that has many names, including hypertelorism-hypospadias syndrome, Opitz BBB syndrome, and Opitz-Frias syndrome. The typical manifestations of Opitz G syndrome are hypertelorism and *hypospadias* in affected males (where the orifice of the penis is proximal to its normal location). Other features that may be seen include imperforate anus, cryptorchidism, congenital heart defects, inguinal hernias, mental retardation, and learning disabilities.

One characteristic that can be very serious is a laryngeal cleft. This abnormality in the development of the larynx can lead to swallowing disorders, aspiration pneumonia, and speech

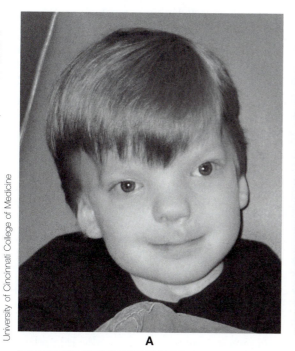
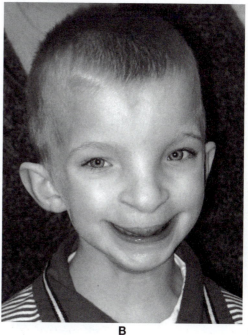

Courtesy Howard M. Saal, M.D./Cincinnati Children's Hospital Medical Center & University of Cincinnati College of Medicine

Courtesy Howard M. Saal, M.D./Cincinnati Children's Hospital Medical Center & University of Cincinnati College of Medicine

A　　　**B**

FIGURE 3–9 (A and B) Opitz syndrome. In both cases, note the hypertelorism (wide-spaced eyes) and evidence of a cleft lip.

problems. Many patients require long-term tracheostomy management as a result. CL + P is frequently seen in this population. In fact, Opitz G syndrome is the second most common identifiable cause of syndromic CL + P at the Craniofacial Center at Cincinnati Children's Hospital Medical Center.

Orofaciodigital Syndrome Type I (OFD I)

Orofaciodigital syndrome type I (OFD I) (Figure 3–10) is an X-linked dominant condition. Therefore, affected females can have affected daughters, but it is usually lethal in males (Goodship, Platt, Smith, & Burn, 1991; Prattichizzo et al., 2008). Infants born with this condition often have a midline cleft lip with multiple oral *frenulae* (oral tissue webs), cleft palate, and tongue abnormalities that include lobulations and notching. There is often hypertelorism, with a broad nose and hair that is coarse and sparse. There may be abnormal or missing teeth with decreased enamel. Digital anomalies include *brachydactyly* (short fingers), variable degrees of *syndactyly* (fusion or webbing of the digits), or *clinodactyly* (curved or bent digits). Renal anomalies may be seen, including the presence of renal cysts. Brain

anomalies have been reported, including hydrocephalus and absence of the corpus callosum.

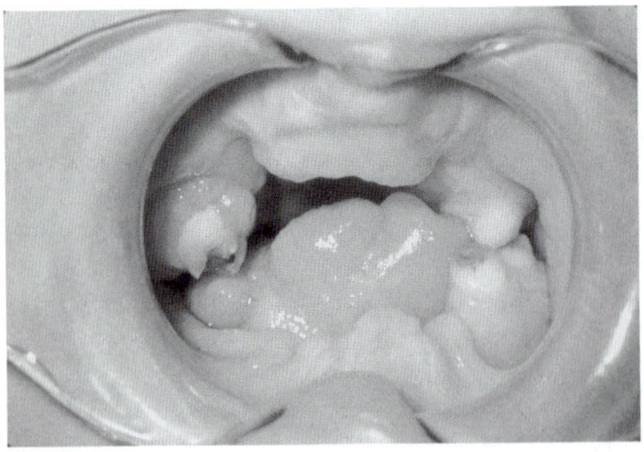

Developmental disabilities are common in this population, especially in the presence of brain anomalies (Jones, 2006). Speech and language difficulties are generally related to the cleft palate and developmental disabilities.

Stickler Syndrome

Stickler syndrome (Figure 3–11) is the most common cause of Pierre Robin sequence and among the most common syndromic causes of cleft palate. It is an autosomal dominant disorder with *variable expressivity*, so individuals with this condition may have just a few or all of the clinical features associated with this syndrome.

In addition to the Pierre Robin sequence, there are characteristic facial features of Stickler syndrome that include micrognathia in infancy, a flat facial profile, *epicanthal folds* (folds of skin over the medial portion of the openings of the eyes or palpebral fissures), a small nose, flat nasal bridge, and midface hypoplasia. In addition, Stickler syndrome is characterized by high *myopia* (severe nearsightedness), which is usually progressive. There is also a high risk for retinal detachments, so these patients must be followed closely by an ophthalmologist. Most individuals with Stickler's syndrome have a high frequency hearing loss, which may be complicated by the conductive hearing loss secondary to middle ear effusion due to the cleft palate (Antunes, Alonso, & Paula, 2012; Nowak, 1998). Therefore, they should be followed with serial audiograms. Finally, there is a risk for early onset osteoarthritis.

Development is usually normal with Stickler syndrome and affected individuals are not at risk for learning disabilities. Speech and language problems are usually related to the cleft palate, hearing loss, and in some instances, problems related to tracheostomy.

Courtesy Howard M. Saal, M.D./Cincinnati Children's Hospital Medical Center & University of Cincinnati College of Medicine

FIGURE 3–10 Orofaciodigital syndrome type 1. Note the lobulations and fissures of the tongue.

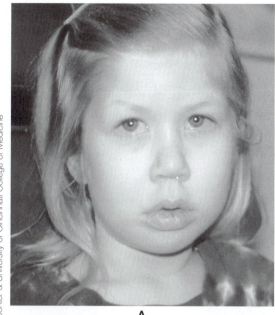

A

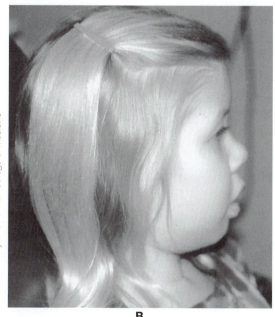

B

Courtesy Howard M. Saal, M.D./Cincinnati Children's Hospital Medical Center & University of Cincinnati College of Medicine

FIGURE 3–11 (A and B) Stickler syndrome. (A) This girl has the characteristic features of a flat facial profile, small nose, and flat nasal bridge. (B) Note the micrognathia. She was also born with Pierre Robin sequence due to the micrognathia, which is typical of this syndrome.

Treacher Collins Syndrome

Treacher Collins syndrome (Figure 3–12) is also called mandibulofacial dysostosis. It is an autosomal dominant condition with variable expressivity, which makes it difficult to predict the outcome of offspring of affected individuals.

The classic features of Treacher Collins syndrome include downward-slanting palpebral fissures, colobomas of the lower eyelids, micrognathia, hypoplasia of the maxilla and zygomatic arches, *macrostomia* (a large mouth), *microtia* (small or dysplastic ear), and atresia of the external auditory canal (Martelli-Junior et al., 2009; Posnick & Ruiz, 2000). Conductive hearing loss is common due to middle ear anomalies. Treacher Collins syndrome usually includes Pierre Robin sequence, although most individuals with this condition do not have clefts, despite pronounced micrognathia.

Intelligence is usually normal in this population. Speech disorders are common due to the hearing loss and micrognathia. The speech disorders are exacerbated when cleft palate or airway obstruction is also present.

Trisomy 13

Trisomy 13 (Figure 3–13) is a disorder where the baby is born with an extra copy of chromosome 13. The incidence of this disorder is about 1 in 5000 live births (Jones, 2006).

Trisomy 13 is associated with multiple serious life-endangering birth defects, including severe brain anomalies, congenital heart defects, *polydactyly* (extra fingers and/or toes), spina bifida, and severe eye defects. Unilateral or bilateral CL ± P is seen in 60% to 80% of cases (Jones, 2006). Many infants with trisomy 13 have a midline cleft lip and midline facial deformities. This usually denotes *holoprosencephaly*, which is the failure of the brain to

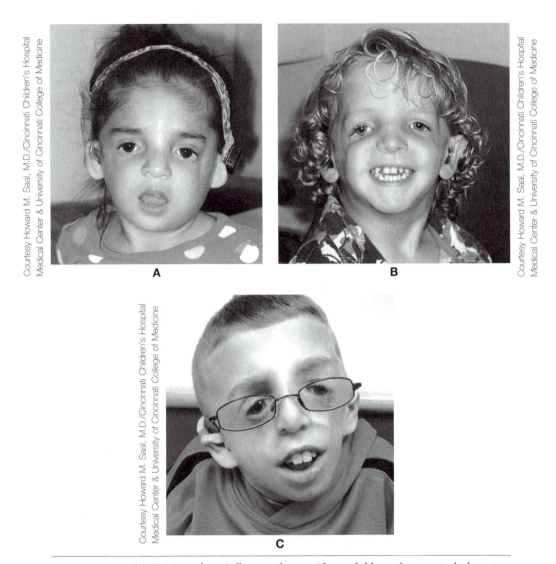

FIGURE 3–12 (A–C)   Treacher Collins syndrome. These children show typical characteristics, including micrognathia, severe hypoplasia of the zygomatic arches, down-slanting palpebral fissures, and secondary low-set ears. Hearing loss is common. You will note that all three children are wearing a hearing aid.

divide into the two hemispheres. Over 90% of affected children die before their first birthday, usually from a central nervous system or cardiac event. Therefore, patients with trisomy 13 are rarely seen in a craniofacial center.

Children who do survive for several years are usually severely to profoundly intellectually disabled and require a great deal of care. They tend to have severe feeding difficulties that require *nasogastric feeding* (feeding through a tube that is placed through the nose to the stomach). Because most children with trisomy 13 do not survive beyond 1 year of age, a gastrostomy is rarely performed to assist with feeding.

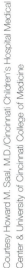

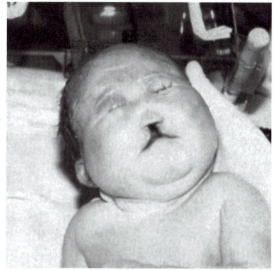

FIGURE 3–13 A newborn female with trisomy 13 and holoprosencephaly. Note the midline cleft lip and cleft palate.

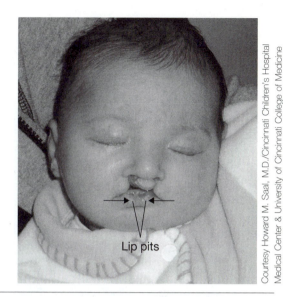

FIGURE 3–14 Van der Woude syndrome. This infant has a bilateral cleft lip and cleft palate. The bilateral lip pits (that show with mild swelling) on the lower lip are a diagnostic feature of this syndrome.

Van der Woude Syndrome

Van der Woude syndrome (Figure 3–14) is characterized by bilateral lip pits on the lower lip (Jones, 2006). Other features described in Van der Woude syndrome include cleft lip and/or cleft palate and missing teeth. Development is usually normal, and speech problems are usually related to the cleft palate. Van der Woude syndrome may be responsible for up to 3% of cases with cleft lip (Murray et al., 1990; Malik et al., 2010).

Velocardiofacial Syndrome (22q11.2 Deletion Syndrome)

Velocardiofacial (VCFS) (Figure 3–15), also known as 22q11.2 deletion syndrome, conotruncal face syndrome, and DiGeorge syndrome, is the most common syndrome associated with velopharyngeal dysfunction. The prevalence is estimated at approximately 1 in 2000 to 1 in 4000 live births (Kobrynski &

Sullivan, 2007; Shprintzen, 2000). More than 180 different associated features have been reported with VCFS. The most common features are velopharyngeal dysfunction, congenital heart defects, and dysmorphic facial features (Goldmuntz, 2005; Shprintzen, 1994, 2000; Vantrappen et al., 1999).

At the Velopharyngeal Insufficiency Clinic at Cincinnati Children's Hospital, velocardiofacial syndrome is diagnosed in about 20% of individuals with velopharyngeal dysfunction in the absence of overt cleft palate, although some of these patients have submucous cleft palate. VCFS is also the third most common cause of cleft palate. The cleft palate is often associated with Pierre Robin sequence, and therefore these infants must be monitored for the respiratory and feeding complications.

Approximately 75% of children with VCFS followed in the Division of Human Genetics at Cincinnati Children's Hospital Medical Center

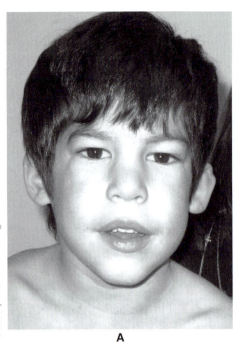

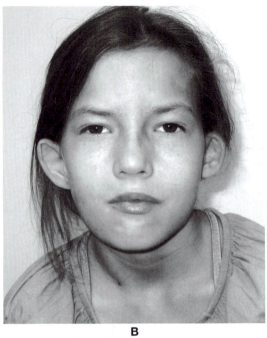

A

B

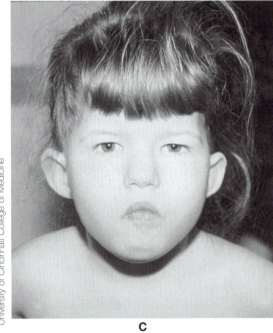

C

FIGURE 3–15 (A–C) Velocardiofacial syndrome. In all three examples, note the long, narrow face; broad nasal tip; narrow palpebral fissures (eye openings); and ear anomalies.

are born with congenital heart defects. Cardiac defects of the aorta, the ventricular septum (the tissue which separates the two lower chambers of the heart), the pulmonary artery, and the pulmonary valve are common. These particular abnormalities of the heart and related blood vessels are called *conotruncal defects* because of their location and development. In the population of children born with conotruncal heart defects, 10% to 15% have velocardiofacial syndrome. Therefore, any child with a cleft palate or velopharyngeal insufficiency and a congenital heart defect should be evaluated for VCFS (Goldmuntz, 2005; Marino, Digilio, Toscano, Giannotti, & Dallapiccola, 1999; Ryan et al., 1997).

In addition to the cardiac anomalies, vascular anomalies are common with VCFS. This includes tortuosity and medial displacement of the carotid arteries (Even-Or, Wohlgelernter, & Gross, 2005; Johnson, Gentry, Rice, & Mount, 2010; Ross, Witzel, Armstrong, & Thomson, 1996; Witt, Miller, Marsh, Muntz, & Grames, 1998). The pulsation of the carotid arteries can often be viewed on the pharyngeal wall through nasopharyngoscopy. Knowledge of the possible displacement of the carotid arteries in the posterior pharyngeal wall is important for the surgeon to placement of a pharyngeal flap.

The facial characteristics associated with velocardiofacial syndrome include microcephaly, narrow palpebral fissures, a wide nasal root, a bulbous nose, vertical maxillary excess, a thin upper lip, a long face, micrognathia, and minor auricular anomalies (Dyce et al., 2002). Additional physical features include short stature, usually below the 10th percentile, and long, tapered fingers.

Individuals with VCFS can have a myriad of medical problems, including kidney or urinary tract anomalies, obesity, and failure to thrive in infancy (Ryan et al., 1997). A subgroup of

patients have DiGeorge sequence, which also includes hypoplasia or absence of the thymus (the organ in the chest that is the source of T-lymphocytes) or parathyroid glands (that make a hormone to regulate calcium levels in the blood) (Fomin et al., 2010; Stevens, Carey, & Shigeoka, 1990). There can be seizures from hypocalcemia or serious infections from abnormal T-lymphocyte function (Chao, Chao, Hwang, & Chung, 2009; Ryan et al., 1997; Tsai, Lian, & Chen, 2009). Other common medical problems include chronic middle ear effusion, presumably due to tensor veli palatini dysfunction, and airway problems caused by a narrow airway, laryngotracheal anomalies, or a laryngeal web (Dyce, 2002).

Infants with velocardiofacial syndrome often have characteristics of hypotonia or oral apraxia. Many of these children have problems with sucking because of structural anomalies of the palate and/or poor oral-motor skills. Speech sound disorders are common and are caused by a combination of velopharyngeal insufficiency or incompetence, and oral-motor dysfunction. If a pharyngoplasty is needed for velopharyngeal dysfunction, the prognosis for total correction is somewhat guarded due to the pharyngeal hypotonia and oral-motor problems.

Learning disabilities, reading difficulty, difficulty with abstraction, and overall cognitive problems are common with velocardiofacial syndrome (Antshel, Conchelos, Lanzetta, Fremont, & Kates, 2005; Jacobson et al., 2010; Kok & Solman, 1995). Intelligence tends to be in the low to normal range (Golding-Kushner, Weller, & Shprintzen, 1985). Educational goals must therefore focus on the development of language and communication skills.

Individuals with velocardiofacial syndrome often have behavior or socialization difficulties (Swillen et al., 1997). In addition, psychiatric problems are seen in many of affected individuals, with an increased incidence of schizophrenia and schizo-affective disorder that manifest around the second decade (Heineman-de Boer, Van Haelst, Cordia-de Haan, & Beemer, 1999; Karayiorgou et al., 1995). There is also an increased incidence of depression and bipolar disorder.

Velocardiofacial syndrome is caused by a gene deletion on the long arm (q arm) of chromosome 22, in the area of band 11 (thus 22q11.2 deletion syndrome). This can be diagnosed with a *fluorescent in situ hybridization* (FISH) test or a microarray analysis.

Although most individuals with velocardiofacial syndrome demonstrate this deletion, approximately 10% of patients with velocardiofacial syndrome do not have a demonstrable deletion on chromosome 22. It is assumed that these individuals have a mutation or genetic rearrangement of the critical region on chromosome 22 that cannot yet be detected by current diagnostic tests. Most identified cases represent new deletions with no prior family history, but 10–20% of cases have a parent with features of the syndrome.

Wolf-Hirschhorn Syndrome (4p-syndrome)

Wolf-Hirschhorn syndrome is a rare chromosome disorder that is caused by a deletion or missing portion of the short arm of chromosome 4 (hence 4p- syndrome). Affected patients have a distinctive facial appearance, likened to a Greek helmet because of the presence of *hypertelorism* (wide-spaced eyes) and a prominent nasal bridge. A cleft lip and/or palate is a common feature. Most patients are very small, grow poorly, and have microcephaly. They may have heart defects, and seizures are very common. Developmental disabilities are universal in this disorder. Most patients have severe to profound mental

retardation and significant communication disorders (Jones, 2006).

GENETICS OF CRANIOSYNOSTOSIS

Craniosynostosis is the premature fusion of one or more cranial sutures, which causes the skull to grow abnormally, resulting in a misshaped head. The distortion of the skull depends on the sutures that are involved. If the sagittal suture is involved, the lateral growth of the skull will be prevented. Therefore, the growth occurs in an anterior–posterior (AP) direction, resulting in frontal bossing and *scaphacephaly*, where the skull is oblong from front to back. On the other hand, if the coronal suture is involved, the skull cannot expand in the AP direction, causing *brachycephaly*, which is a short skull. When multiple sutures are involved, there may be asymmetry of the skull, called *plagiocephaly*. *Dolichocephaly* is the long, narrow skull that is often seen with prematurity and typically resolves on its own.

Although not as common as cleft lip and/or cleft palate, craniosynostosis occurs in about 1 in 2000 to 1 in 2500 live births (Hunter & Rudd, 1976, 1977). Most cases are isolated, limited to the fusion of a single cranial suture, and have no associated malformations. These cases are usually without a genetic etiology. Children with isolated craniosynostosis have an excellent prognosis for normal health, growth, and neurodevelopment.

When craniosynostosis involves more than one suture or when there are other congenital anomalies, it is likely that there is a genetic etiology. Over 100 syndromes include craniosynostosis as a feature (Cohen, 1991; Gorlin et al., 2001; Rice, 2008). See Table 3–3 for a list of some of the common craniosynostosis syndromes. Most craniosynostosis syndromes are inherited in an autosomal dominant manner. Recently, the genes that cause the common craniosynostosis syndromes have been identified (Robin, 1999; Wilkie, 1997).

The prognosis for children who have a craniosynostosis syndrome is more guarded than with isolated craniosynostosis and it depends upon the specific syndrome diagnosed. If brain development is impaired by the cranium or there is an increase in intracranial pressure (ICP), mental retardation can result. Craniotomy and skull reshaping procedures are often required, both for normal brain development and function, and also to improve the aesthetics.

CRANIOSYNOSTOSIS SYNDROMES

Apert Syndrome

Apert syndrome (Figure 3–16) includes midface hypoplasia and shallow orbits, resulting in *exophthalmos* (protrusion of the eyeballs). There is also hypertelorism, strabismus, and a beaked-shape nose (Cohen & Kreiborg, 1992; Jones, 2006). There can be a cleft palate or a very narrow palate, causing dental crowding (Hohoff, Joos, Meyer, Ehmer, & Stamm, 2007). Narrowing of the upper nasal and pharyngeal airway or choanal stenosis are common and result in significant upper airway obstruction and hyponasality. Finally, individuals with Apert syndrome have syndactyly of the fingers and toes. The webbing may be of soft tissue, but it can also include the bone.

Although normal intelligence is found in some patients, most patients with Apert syndrome have some degree of developmental disability, including mild to moderate retardation.

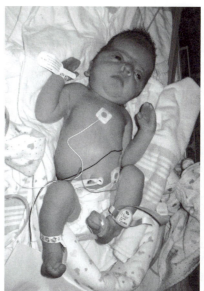

FIGURE 3–16 Apert syndrome. In addition to her craniosynostosis, this girl has syndactyly (webbing) of the fingers and toes of all four extremities.

Communication disorders are common, including articulation disorders due to the small oral cavity and narrow palate, and hyponasality secondary to upper airway obstruction.

Crouzon Syndrome

Crouzon syndrome (Figure 3–17) is the most common craniosynostosis syndrome and is caused by premature closure of the coronal sutures. This creates facial features that are similar to those in Apert syndrome, including midface hypoplasia, shallow orbits, exophthalmos, hypertelorism, and strabismus. Cleft palate and submucous cleft palate occur, but infrequently (Jones, 2006; Robin, 1999).

In contrast to Apert syndrome, there are no digital anomalies with Crouzon syndrome. Developmental disabilities can occur if there is hydrocephalus or agenesis of the corpus callosum. However, children with Crouzon syndrome usually exhibit normal development.

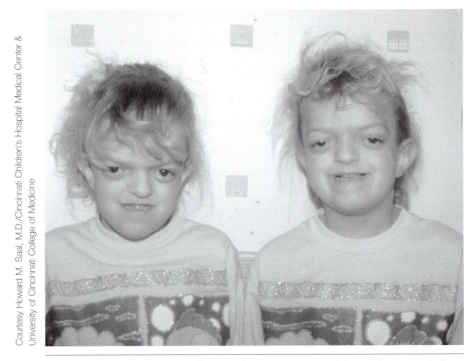

Courtesy Howard M. Saal, M.D./Cincinnati Children's Hospital Medical Center & University of Cincinnati College of Medicine

FIGURE 3–17 Crouzon syndrome. These monozygotic (identical) twin girls have typical features, including shallow orbits with prominent eyes.

Pfeiffer Syndrome

Pfeiffer syndrome (Figure 3–18) is genetically *heterogeneous* (caused by different genes). In most patients with classic Pfeiffer syndrome, the craniofacial features are similar to those seen in Crouzon syndrome, including coronal craniosynostosis, midface hypoplasia, shallow orbits with exophthalmos, and hypertelorism (Plomp et al., 1998). However, Pfeiffer syndrome type 1 also includes broad thumbs and great toes with variable degrees of syndactyly. Hearing loss and cleft palate are occasionally seen. Intelligence is usually normal.

Pfeiffer syndromes type 2 and type 3 are more serious, with limb contractures, airway obstruction, and occasional gastrointestinal disorders. Pfeiffer syndrome type 2 involves multiple sutures, resulting in a "cloverleaf skull" and severe midface hypoplasia and exophthalmos. Pfeiffer syndrome type 3 is usually associated with tracheal anomalies and upper airway stenosis (Stone, Trevenen, Mitchell, & Rudd, 1990). Mental retardation, often severe, is seen in almost all children with Pfeiffer syndrome type 2 and type 3. Death in early childhood is common, especially in Pfeiffer syndrome type 2, which is more likely to be associated with cloverleaf skull and more serious upper airway obstruction.

Saethre-Chotzen Syndrome

Saethre-Chotzen syndrome (Figure 3–19) is known to cause variable degrees of craniosynostosis, especially coronal synostosis. Facial features can be variable, but often include *ptosis* (drooping of the eyelids); midface

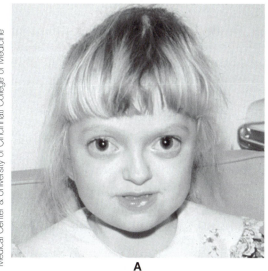
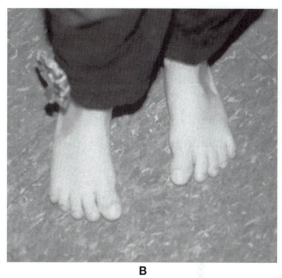

Courtesy Howard M. Saal, M.D./Cincinnati Children's Hospital Medical Center & University of Cincinnati College of Medicine

Courtesy Howard M. Saal, M.D./Cincinnati Children's Hospital Medical Center & University of Cincinnati College of Medicine

A **B**

FIGURE 3–18 (A and B) Pfeiffer syndrome. (A) This girl has shallow orbits similar to those seen in Crouzon syndrome. (B) She also has broad, deviated great toes.

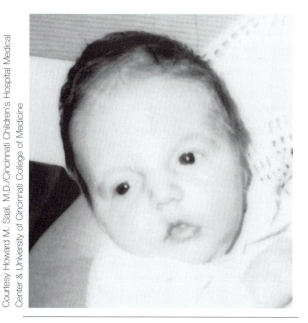

Courtesy Howard M. Saal, M.D./Cincinnati Children's Hospital Medical Center & University of Cincinnati College of Medicine

FIGURE 3–19 Saethre-Chotzen syndrome. This boy has a depressed nasal bridge and down-slanting palpebral fissures.

hypoplasia; a crumpled appearance to the top of the external ear; and mild digit anomalies (e.g., syndactyly or brachydactyly).

Some individuals have broad thumbs and/or great toes with medial deviation of the great toes. A small number of individuals will have cleft palate or submucous cleft palate (Stoler, Rogers, & Mulliken, 2009).

Intelligence in Saethre-Chotzen syndrome is usually normal, although there is an increased risk for developmental disabilities, including mental retardation. Most patients do not have significant speech or language difficulties unless they have cleft palate or mental retardation.

SUMMARY

Patients who present with craniofacial anomalies should be seen for a complete genetics evaluation. This is important so that an appropriate diagnosis can be made and recurrence risks can be determined. Identification of a genetic syndrome is also important because it allows the physician to counsel the family regarding the natural course of the disorder and the potential medical, developmental, and communication problems that are typically associated with the syndrome. Armed with this knowledge, the family, in collaboration with the medical professionals from the craniofacial team, can plan appropriate medical, surgical, therapeutic, and educational interventions in order to achieve the best possible outcome for the child.

FOR REVIEW AND DISCUSSION

1. Why is a genetics evaluation recommended for children born with cleft lip and palate? Why is it particularly important for children born with cleft palate only (without cleft lip)?

2. What is the purpose of the genetics evaluation, and how can the results affect the management of the child?

3. Describe the components of a genetics evaluation and why each component is important.

4. What is the difference between a deformation and malformation? What are the differences among a syndrome, sequence, and association? Describe the series of events that result in Pierre Robin sequence.

5. What is the approximate prevalence of cleft lip and palate? How does it vary with racial groups?

6. What syndromes are particularly associated with cleft lip?

7. What does the presence of bilateral lip pits indicate, and why is it important to identify the lip pits?

8. Describe some syndromes that are associated with cleft palate.

9. What is the difference between Pierre Robin sequence and Stickler syndrome? Which is more serious and why?

10. What are the characteristics of velocardiofacial syndrome? Why do you think identification of this syndrome often occurs in the school years rather than in infancy?

11. What is craniosynostosis, and what are some syndromes that include this as a characteristic? What are potential functional problems with craniosynostosis syndromes?

REFERENCES

Abuelo, D. (2002). Genetic evaluation and counseling for craniofacial anomalies. *Medicine & Health Rhode Island, 85*(12), 373–378.

Antshel, K. M., Conchelos, J., Lanzetta, G., Fremont, W., & Kates, W. R. (2005). Behavior and corpus callosum morphology relationships in velocardiofacial syndrome (22q11.2 deletion syndrome). *Psychiatry Research, 138*(3), 235–245.

Antunes, R. B., Alonso, N., & Paula, R. G. (2012). Importance of early diagnosis of Stickler syndrome in newborns. *Journal of Plastic Reconstructive and Aesthetic Surgery, 65*(8), 1029–1034.

Baraitser, M., & Winter, R. (1991). Update on the London Dysmorphology Database. *The Cleft Palate–Craniofacial Journal, 28*(3), 318.

Bartsch, O., Nemeckova, M., Kocarek, E., Wagner, A., Puchmajerova, A., Poppe, M., Ounap, K., et al. (2003). DiGeorge/velocardiofacial syndrome: FISH studies of chromosomes 22q11 and 10p14, and clinical reports on the proximal 22q11 deletion. *American Journal of Medical Genetics A, 117A*(1), 1–5.

Bull, M. J., & Committee on Genetics. (2011). Health supervision for children with Down syndrome. *Pediatrics, 128*(2), 393–496.

Chao, P. H., Chao, M. C., Hwang, K. P., & Chung, M. Y. (2009). Hypocalcemia impacts heart failure control in DiGeorge 2 syndrome. *Acta Paediatrica, 98*(1), 195–198.

Cohen, M. M., Jr. (1991). Etiopathogenesis of craniosynostosis. *Neurosurgery Clinics of North America, 2*(3), 507–513.

Cohen, M. M., Jr., & Kreiborg, S. (1992). Upper and lower airway compromise in the Apert syndrome. *American Journal of Medical Genetics, 44*(1), 90–93.

Dios, P. D., Posse, J. L., Sanroman, J. F., & Garcia, E. V. (2000). Treatment of macroglossia in a child with Beckwith-Wiedemann syndrome. *Journal of Oral and Maxillofacial Surgery, 58*(9), 1058–1061.

Dyce, O., McDonald-McGinn, D., Kirschner, R. E., Zackai, E., Young, K., & Jacobs, I. N. (2002). Otolaryngologic manifestations of the 22q11.l deletion syndrome. *Archives of Otolaryngology-Head & Neck Surgery, 128*(12), 1408–1412.

Even-Or, E., Wohlgelernter, J., & Gross, M. (2005). Medial displacement of the internal carotid arteries in velocardiofacial syndrome. *Israel Medical Association Journal, 7*(11), 749–750.

Fomin, A. B., Pastorino, A. C., Kim, C. A., Pereira, C. A., Carneiro-Sampaio, M., et al. (2010). DiGeorge Syndrome: A not so rare disease. *Clinics, 65*(9), 865–869.

Fraser, F. C. (1970). The genetics of cleft lip and cleft palate. *American Journal of Human Genetics, 22*(3), 336–352.

Friedman, J. M., Birch, P., & Greene, C. (1993). National Neurofibromatosis Foundation International Database. *American Journal of Medical Genetics, 45*(1), 88–91.

Fritz, M. A., & Sidman, J. D. (2004). Distraction osteogenesis of the mandible. *Current Opinion in Otolaryngology & Head & Neck Surgery, 12*(6), 513–518.

Fryns, J. P., & de Ravel, T. J. (2002). London Dysmorphology Database, London Neurogenetics Database and Dysmorphology Photo Library on CD-ROM [Version 3] 2001R. M. Winter, M. Baraitser, Oxford University Press, ISBN 019851-780, pound sterling 1595. *Human Genetics Journal, 111*(1), 113.

Golding-Kushner, K. J., Weller, G., & Shprintzen, R. J. (1985). Velocardiofacial syndrome: Language and psychological profiles. *Journal of Craniofacial Genetics & Developmental Biology, 5*(3), 259–266.

Goldmuntz, E. (2005). DiGeorge syndrome: New insights. *Clinics in Perinatology, 32*(4), 963–978.

Goodship, J., Platt, J., Smith, R., & Burn, J. (1991). A male with type I orofaciodigital syndrome. *Journal of Medical Genetics, 28*(10), 691–694.

Gorlin, R., Cohen, M. J., & Hennekam, R. C. M. (2001). *Syndromes of the head and neck* (4th ed.). New York: Oxford University Press.

Hannibal, M. C., Buckingham, K. J., Ng, S. B., Ming, J. E., Beck, A. E., McMillin, M. J., Gildersleeve, H. R., et al. (2011). Spectrum of MLL2 (ALR) mutations in 110 cases of

Kabuki syndrome. *American Journal of Medical Genetics A*, 155A(7), 1511–1516.

Heineman-de Boer, J. A., Van Haelst, M. J., Cordia-de Haan, M., & Beemer, F. A. (1999). Behavior problems and personality aspects of 40 children with velocardiofacial syndrome. *Genetic Counseling*, 10(1), 89–93.

Hohoff, A., Joos, U., Meyer, U., Ehmer, U., & Stamm, T. (2007). The spectrum of Apert syndrome: Phenotype, particularities in orthodontic treatment, and characteristics of orthognathic surgery. *Head & Face Medicine*, 3, 10.

Hong, P., McNeil, M., Kearns, D. B., & Magit, A. E. (2012). Mandibular distraction osteogenesis in children with Pierre Robin sequence: Impact on health-related quality of life. *International Journal of Pediatric Otorhinolaryngology*, 76(8), 1159–1163.

Hsueh, K. F., Yang, C. S., Lu, J. H., & Hsu, W. M. (2004). Clinical characteristics of CHARGE syndrome. *Journal of Chinese Medical Association*, 67(10), 542–546.

Hunter, A. G., & Rudd, N. L. (1976). Craniosynostosis. I. Sagittal synostosis: Its genetics and associated clinical findings in 214 patients who lacked involvement of the coronal suture(s). *Teratology*, 14(2), 185–193.

Hunter, A. G., & Rudd, N. L. (1977). Craniosynostosis. II. Coronal synostosis: Its familial characteristics and associated clinical findings in 109 patients lacking bilateral polysyndactyly or syndactyly. *Teratology*, 15(3), 301–309.

Jacobson, C., Shearer, J., Habel, A., Kane, F., Tsakanikos, E., & Kravariti, E. (2010). Core neuropsychological characteristics of children and adolescents with 22q11.2 deletion. *Journal of Intellectual Disability Research*, 54(8), 701–713.

Johnson, M. D., Gentry, L. R., Rice, G. M., Mount, D. L. (2010). A case of congenitally absent left internal carotid artery: Vascular malformations in 22q11.2 deletion syndrome. *The Cleft Palate–Craniofacial Journal*, 47(3), 314–317.

Jones, K. L. (2006). *Smith's recognizable patterns of human malformation* (6th ed.). Philadelphia: Elsevier.

Jones, K. L., & Smith, D. W. (1973). Recognition of the fetal alcohol syndrome in early infancy. *Lancet*, 2(7836), 999–1001.

Jones, M. C., & Jones, K. L. (2009). Syndromes of orofacial clefting. In J. E. Lossee & R. E. Kirschner (Eds.), *Comprehensive Cleft Care* (pp. 107–127). New York: McGraw-Hill.

Jongmans, M. C., Admiraal, R. J., van der Donk, K. P., Vissers, L. E., Baas, A. F., Kapusta, L., van Hagen, J. M., et al. (2006). CHARGE syndrome: The phenotypic spectrum of mutations in the CHD7 gene. *Journal of Medical Genetics*, 43(4), 306–314.

Karayiorgou, M., Morris, M. A., Morrow, B., Shprintzen, R. J., Goldberg, R., Borrow, J., Gos, A., et al. (1995). Schizophrenia susceptibility associated with interstitial deletions of chromosome 22qll. *Proceedings of the National Academy of Sciences of the United States of America*, 92(17), 7612–7616.

Kohli, S. S., & Kohli, V. S. (2012). A comprehensive review of the genetic basis of cleft lip and palate. *Journal of Oral and Maxillofacial Pathology*, 16(1), 64–72.

Kok, L. L., & Solman, R. T. (1995). Velocardiofacial syndrome: Learning difficulties and intervention. *Journal of Medical Genetics*, 32(8), 612–618.

Laroche, C., Testelin, S., & Devauchelle, B. (2005). Cleft palate and Beckwith-Wiedemann syndrome. *The Cleft Palate–Craniofacial Journal*, 42(2), 212–217.

Lidral, A. C., Romitti, P. A., Basart, A. M., Doetschman, T., Leysens, N. J., Daack-Hirsch, S., Semina, E. V., et al. (1998). Association of MSX1 and TGFB3 with nonsyndromic clefting in humans. *American Journal of Human Genetics*, 63(2), 557–568.

Malik, S., Kakar, N., Hasnain, S., Ahmad, J., Wilcox, E. R., & Naz, S. (2010). Epidemiology of Van der Woude syndrome from mutational analyses in affected patients from Pakistan. *Clinical Genetics*, 78(3), 247–256.

Manning, M., & Hudgins, L. (2010). Array-based technology and recommendations for utilization in medical genetics practice for detection of chromosomal abnormalities. *Genetics in Medicine*, 12(11), 742–745.

Marino, B., Digilio, M. C., Toscano, A., Giannotti, A., & Dallapiccola, B. (1999). Congenital heart defects in patients with DiGeorge/velocardiofacial syndrome and del22qll. *Genetic Counseling*, 10(1), 25–33.

Martelli-Junior, H., Coletta, R. D., Miranda, R. T., Barros, L. M., Swerts, M. S., & Bonan, P. R. (2009). Orofacial features of Treacher Collins syndrome. *Medicina Oral Patologia Oral y Cirugia Bucal*, 14(7), E344–348.

McDonald-McGinn, D. M., Driscoll, D. A., & Matthews, M. (2009). Prenatal and genetic counseling. In J. E. Lossee & R. E. Kirschner (Eds.), *Comprehensive Cleft Care* (pp. 71–82). New York: McGraw-Hill.

McMain, K., Blake, K., Smith, I., Johnson, J., Wood, E., Tremblay, F., & Robitaille, J. (2008). Ocular features of CHARGE syndrome. *Journal of the American Association for Pediatric Ophthalmology and Strabismus*, 12(5), 460–465.

Mitchell, L. E. (2009). Epidemiology of cleft lip and palate. In J. E. Lossee & R. E. Kirschner (Eds.), *Comprehensive Cleft Care* (pp. 35–42). New York: McGraw-Hill.

Mossey, P. A., & Little, J. (2002). Epidemiology of oral clefts: An international perspective. In D. F. Wyszynski (Ed.), *Cleft Lip and Palate. From Origin to Treatment* (pp. 127–144). New York: Oxford University Press.

Murray, J. C., Nishimura, D. Y., Buetow, K. H., Ardinger, H. H., Spence, M. A., Sparkes, R. S., Falk, R. E., Falk, P. M., Gardner, R. J., Harkness, E. M., et al. (1990). Linkage of an autosomal dominant clefting syndrome (Van der Woude) to loci on chromosome Iq. *American Journal of Human Genetics*, 46(3), 486–491.

Nash, K., Sheard, E., Rovet, J., & Koren, G. (2008). Understanding fetal alcohol spectrum disorders (FASDs): Toward identification of a behavioral phenotype. *The Scientific World Journal*, 8, 873–882.

Nowak, C. B. (1998). Genetics and hearing loss: A review of Stickler syndrome. *Journal of Communication Disorders*, 31(5), 437–454.

Oh, A. K., Workman, L. A., & Wong, G. B. (2007). Clinical correlation of chromosome 22q11.2 fluorescent in situ hybridization analysis and velocardiofacial syndrome. *The Cleft Palate–Craniofacial Journal*, 44(1), 62–66.

Plomp, A. S., Hamel, B. C., Cobben, J. M., Verloes, A., Offermans, J. P., Lajeunie, E., Fryns, J. P., et al. (1998). Pfeiffer syndrome type 2: Further delineation and review of the literature. *American Journal of Medical Genetics*, 75(3), 245–251.

Posnick, J. C., & Ruiz, R. L. (2000). Treacher Collins syndrome: Current evaluation, treatment, and future directions. *The Cleft Palate–Craniofacial Journal*, 37(5), 434.

Prattichizzo, C., Macca, M., Novelli, V., Giorgio, G., Barra, A., & Franco, B. (2008). Mutational spectrum of the oral-facial-digital type 1 syndrome, a study on a large collection of patients. *Human Mutation*, 29(10), 1237–1246.

Rahimov, F., Jugessur, A., & Murray, J. C. (2012). Genetics of nonsyndromic orofacial clefts. *The Cleft Palate–Craniofacial Journal*, 49(1), 73–91.

Rice, D. P. (2008). Clinical features of syndromic craniosynostosis. *Frontiers of Oral Biology*, 12, 91–106.

Robin, N. H. (1999). Molecular genetic advances in understanding craniosynostosis. *Plastic and Reconstructive Surgery*, 103 (3), 1060–1070.

Ross, D. A., Witzel, M. A., Armstrong, D. C., & Thomson, H. G. (1996). Is pharyngoplasty a risk in velocardiofacial syndrome? An assessment of medially displaced carotid arteries. *Plastic and Reconstructive Surgery*, 98(7), 1182–1190.

Ryan, A. K., Goodship, J. A., Wilson, D. L., Philip, N., Levy, A., Seidel, H., & Schuffenhauer, S., et al. (1997). Spectrum of clinical features associated with interstitial chromosome 22q11 deletions: A European collaborative study. *Journal of Medical Genetics*, 34(10), 798–804.

Shuman, C., Beckwith, J. B., Smith, A. C., & Weksberg, R. (2000). Beckwith-Wiedemann Syndrome. In R. A. Pagon, T. D. Bird, C. R. Dolan, et al. (Eds.). GeneReviews™ Seattle (WA): University of Washington, Seattle.

Sidman, J. D., Sampson, D., & Templeton, B. (2001). Distraction osteogenesis of the mandible for airway obstruction in children. *Laryngoscope*, 111(7), 1137–1146.

Shprintzen, R. J. (1994). Velocardiofacial syndrome and DiGeorge sequence. *Journal of Medical Genetics*, 31(5), 423–424.

Shprintzen, R. J. (2000). Velocardiofacial syndrome. *Otolaryngologic Clinics of North America*, 33(6), 1217–1240.

Stanier, P., & Moore, G. E. (2004). Genetics of cleft lip and palate: Syndromic genes contribute to the incidence of non-syndromic clefts. *Human Molecular Genetics*, 13(Spec. No. 1), R73–81.

Stevens, C. A., Carey, J. C., & Shigeoka, A. O. (1990). DiGeorge anomaly and velocardiofacial syndrome. *Pediatrics*, 85(4), 526–530.

Stoler, J. M., Rogers, G. F., & Mulliken, J. B. (2009). The frequency of palatal anomalies in Saethre-Chotzen syndrome. *The Cleft Palate–Craniofacial Journal*, 46(3), 280–284.

Stone, P., Trevenen, C. L., Mitchell, L., & Rudd, N. (1990). Congenital tracheal stenosis in Pfeiffer syndrome. *Clinical Genetics*, 38(2), 145–148.

Streissguth, A. P., Aase, J. M., Clarren, S. K., Randels, S. P., LaDue, R. A., & Smith, D. F. (1991). Fetal alcohol syndrome in adolescents and adults. *Journal of the American Medical Association*, 265(15), 1961–1967.

Strömland, K., Miller, M., Sjögreen, L., Johansson, M., Joelsson, B. M., Billstedt, E., Gillberg, C., et al. (2007). Oculo-auriculo-vertebral spectrum: Associated anomalies, functional deficits and possible developmental risk factors. *American Journal of Medical Genetics A*, 143A(12), 1317–1325.

Swillen, A., Devriendt, K., Legius, E., Eyskens, B., Dumoulin, M., et al. (1997). Intelligence and psychosocial adjustment in velocardiofacial syndrome: A study of 37 children and adolescents with VCFS. *Journal of Medical Genetics*, 34(6), 453–458.

Thompson, H. L., Viskochil, D. H., Stevenson, D. A., & Chapman, K. L. (2010). Speech-language characteristics of children with neurofibromatosis type 1. *American Journal of Medical Genetics A*, 152A(2), 284–290.

Tsai, P. L., Lian, L. M., & Chen, W. H. (2009). Hypocalcemic seizure mistaken for idiopathic epilepsy in two cases of DiGeorge syndrome (chromosome 22q11 deletion syndrome). *Acta Neurology Taiwan, 18*(4), 272–275.

Vantrappen, G., Devriendt, K., Swillen, A., Rommel, N., Vogels, A., Eyskens, B., Gewillig, M., et al. (1999). Presenting symptoms and clinical features in 130 patients with the velocardiofacial syndrome. *Genetic Counseling, 10*(1), 3–9.

Viskochil, D. (2002). Genetics of neurofibromatosis 1 and the NF1 gene. *Journal of Child Neurology, 17*(8), 562–570; Discussion 562–570.

Wilkie, A. O. (1997). Craniosynostosis: Genes and mechanisms. *Human Molecular Genetics, 6*(10), 1647–1656.

Witt, P. D., Miller, D. C., Marsh, J. L., Muntz, H. R., & Grames, L. M. (1998). Limited value of preoperative cervical vascular imaging in patients with velocardiofacial syndrome. *Plastic and Reconstructive Surgery, 101*(5), 1184–1195; Discussion 1196–1189.

Wyszynski, D. F., Beaty, T. H., & Maestri, N. E. (1996). Genetics of nonsyndromic oral clefts revisited. *The Cleft Palate–Craniofacial Journal, 33*(5), 406–417.

Zhang, I., Husein, M., Dworschak-Stokan, A., Jung, J., Matic, D. B., et al. (2012). Neurofibromatosis and velopharyngeal insufficiency: Is there an association? *Journal of Otolaryngology-head & Neck Surgery, 41*(1), 58–64.

Zucchero, T. M., Cooper, M. E., Maher, B. S., Daack-Hirsch, S., Nepomuceno, B., et al. (2004). Interferon regulatory factor 6 (IRF6) gene variants and the risk of isolated cleft lip or palate. *New England Journal of Medicine, 351*(8), 769–780.

CHAPTER

4

GENETICS AND PATTERNS OF INHERITANCE

ROBERT J. HOPKIN, M.D.

CHAPTER OUTLINE

INTRODUCTION

Craniofacial anomalies, like many other conditions, tend to recur in families. The risk for recurrence, however, is variable, depending on interactions of multiple environmental and genetic factors. The purpose of this chapter is to briefly review the modes of inheritance that may influence the occurrence of craniofacial anomalies. The first part of the chapter reviews DNA, genes, chromosomes, and the cell cycle. (See Table 4–1 for a diagram of a cell's genetic material.) The second part of the chapter discusses the principles of Mendelian inheritance, including autosomal recessive, autosomal dominant, and X-linked patterns. The last portion of the chapter focuses on complex, or non-Mendelian, inheritance. Particular attention is placed on multifactorial inheritance, the pattern associated with most cases of cleft palate—or cleft lip with or without cleft palate.

CELL ANATOMY

All living things contain cells they are a fundamental building block of life. Although each tissue contains cells that are differentiated to perform specific specialized functions, all cells have certain traits in common (Figure 4–1). A cell is a ball of protoplasm coated in a membrane. Each cell contains *organelles*, which perform specific functions (i.e., metabolizing energy, building complex molecules such as proteins, and breaking down waste products). The genetic material (instructions for cell and tissue functions) is contained in the *nucleus*, which is separated from the rest of the cell by a lipid membrane with specialized proteins. These proteins regulate transport of chemicals into and out of the nucleus. Within the nucleus is another structure called the *nucleolus*, in which genes are actively transcribed. The nucleus communicates directly with the endoplasmic reticulum, which is a complex system of membranes that control transport of proteins and lipids throughout the cell. The rough endoplasmic reticulum is associated with smaller organelles called ribosomes that put proteins together.

Other important organelles include mitochondria, where energy metabolism takes place; golgi apparatus, where specialized complex molecules are formed; lysosomes, where complex molecules are broken down; and cytoskeleton, which provides structural support for the cell.

DEOXYRIBONUCLEIC ACID (DNA) AND GENES

For centuries, scientists wondered how the information needed to organize and direct the development of an organism was transmitted from a single cell to a mature individual with complex organs and tissues. This process became more apparent with the discovery of DNA within genes.

Deoxyribonucleic Acid (DNA)

In 1869, Friedrich Miescher discovered a substance in cell nuclei that he called "nuclein." The name was eventually changed to deoxyribonucleic acid or DNA. In 1944, Avery, Macleod, and McCarthy demonstrated

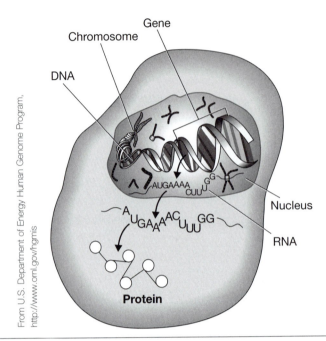

FIGURE 4–1   Diagram of a cell demonstrating that genetic material in the form of DNA is organized into chromosomes. Each chromosome contains thousands of genes. A gene is transcribed into RNA. The messenger RNA is transported outside the nucleus and translated into an amino acid sequence. The amino acid 'polypeptide' is then modified into a functional protein. This sequence of events occurs for the vast majority of genes. Changes in the DNA sequence of a gene are called mutations. Mutations can change the structure of the protein and interfere with its normal function.

that *deoxyribonucleic acid,* or *DNA,* is the substance that carries hereditary information in bacteria and that all genes carry discrete segments of DNA (McKusick, 1997).

DNA is a nucleic acid made up of building blocks called *nucleotides.* Nucleotides consist of a 5-carbon sugar (deoxyribose) chemically bonded to a phosphate group and a nitrogenous base. The nitrogenous bases can be divided into two groups: *purines* (adenine and guanine) and *pyrimidines* (thymine and cytosine). The nucleotides are linked together through the phosphate groups at the fifth and third carbons of the sugar to form long unbranching *polymers,* which are large molecules (macromolecules) composed of repeating structural units. These are arranged in an antiparallel (going in opposite directions) *dou-*

ble helix (coiled ladder) such that the nitrogenous bases are paired according to specific rules. A purine is always paired with a pyrimidine. In fact adenine (A) is always paired with thymine (T), and guanine (G) is always paired with cytosine (C). For example, if one strand contains the sequence 5'GGATTCG3', the complementary sequence would be 3'CCTAAGC5'. The numbers 5' and 3' indicate the direction of the strand. The strands are held together by hydrogen bonds between A-T pairs and C-G pairs (Strachan & Read, 1996).

Replication

Replication is the process of making two identical DNA molecules from one. The complementary nature of the double helix allows

DNA to serve as a template for its own replication. The two double strands separate and another newly synthesized strand is added to each original, making two complete double strands. This process is complex, but it must take place quickly to allow for rapid cell division and growth. In humans, over 3.5×10^4 nucleotides must be precisely matched for each cell division. The process starts at several sites along a DNA molecule simultaneously. When DNA is replicated, a replication bubble forms as the double helix is unwound and the complementary strands are separated. Nucleotides are then added sequentially to each single strand, forming new complementary strands. The final result is two identical double helix molecules of DNA (Strachan & Read, 1996).

The process of replicating DNA is very carefully controlled to prevent errors. In addition, there are proofreading and repair mechanisms to preserve the exact sequence of nucleotides (Strachan & Read, 1996). Fortunately, errors are rare; however, they do occur. When a change in the sequence of a molecule of DNA occurs, it is referred to as a *mutation*. The mutation can be as small as a substitution of a single base pair or as large as the deletion of an entire chromosome. Mutations may have important consequences for the cell and for the individual.

Genes

A *gene* is a submicroscopic functional unit of heredity consisting of a discrete segment of a DNA strand within a chromosome. A *chromosome* is a single, linear double strand of DNA with associated proteins. These proteins function to organize and compact the DNA and/or function in regulating gene activity. Thousands of genes are found in each chromosome. The order of the nucleotides in the DNA of an individual gene determines the information

coded by that gene. Each gene consists of a promoter region that functions as the starting point for the gene's activity and serves as an on–off switch, a coding region that contains the information needed to make the amino acid polymer (called a polypeptide) that will eventually become a functional protein, and regulatory elements that determine how much of that protein will be made. The coding portion of all genes is interrupted by segments of noncoding DNA called *introns*. The segments that code for amino acids are called *exons* (referring to expressed segments). The exons and introns are essential for normal gene function.

Even small changes in the coding region of a gene may lead to changes in function through several mechanisms. Mutations may disrupt gene function, leading to early termination of translation and often to an unstable or nonfunctional product. Deletions and insertions of one or more nucleotides can disrupt gene function by changing, adding, or deleting important amino acids. These changes in the DNA can result in various diseases or malformations.

Changes in DNA can also affect the regulation of gene expression. Both over- and underexpression of genes can result in a disease or malformation. For example, mutations in the MSX2 gene that lead to increased function in the protein result in craniosynostosis. On the other hand, loss of function for the same gene leads to delayed closure of cranial sutures and persistence of fontanels into adulthood (Wilkie et al., 2000).

In spite of the highly regulated process of DNA replication and repair, no two individuals share the exact same DNA sequence, with the exception of identical twins. In fact, much of the DNA in humans is variable. This normal variability among individuals is called *polymorphism*. Polymorphisms are very common (seen in virtually all genes) and contribute to the uniqueness of each individual. Mutations lead to new variations in the DNA. New variants that do not contribute to disease or that improve function may become more common over time, whereas changes that lead to disease tend to remain rare or be eliminated (Cummings, 1997).

Ribonucleic Acid (RNA)

DNA is found primarily in the nucleus of the cells. However, the processes controlled by the genes take place in the cytoplasm of the cell, which is outside the nucleus. The genetic information therefore must be transported from the nucleus to the cytoplasm. This is done through the RNA.

Ribonucleic acid (RNA) is similar to DNA in that it is a linear polymer composed of a 5-carbon sugar (ribose is the sugar in RNA rather than deoxyribose that is in DNA) bound to a phosphate group and a nitrogenous base. The nitrogenous bases differ slightly from those in DNA in that RNA contains the pyrimidine uracil in place of thymine. RNA is a single-stranded molecule rather than a double-stranded helix that characterizes DNA. The RNA is created as a single complementary strand of a DNA template through a process called *transcription*.

Amino acids are the building blocks of proteins. A sequence of amino acids is called a *polypeptide*. The RNA is read in the cytoplasm and determines which amino acids will be incorporated into the polypeptide. Each amino acid is specified by a group of three nucleotides called a codon. Most amino acids can be coded by more than one codon. Thus, some changes in the nucleotide sequence may not result in changes in the protein. These changes are called conservative mutations (Cummings, 1997).

The portions of a gene that determine the amino acid sequence for a polypeptide are referred to as the *coding region*. The coding region is divided into exon segments, separated by introns. The introns are removed, or "spliced out," from the RNA following transcription. The exons are then spliced together to form a continuous RNA coding sequence. It is critical that the process of removing introns and splicing the remaining RNA segments together starts and stops at the correct point. An error of one nucleotide can result in an RNA transcript that codes for a nonfunctional protein.

RNA that has had the introns removed is called *messenger RNA*, or *mRNA*. mRNA is transported from the nucleus to the cytoplasm to function as a template for protein synthesis. In the cytoplasm of the cell, organelles called *ribosomes* attach to the mRNA and translate the nucleotides into the specified amino acid sequence, forming a polypeptide. The polypeptides are then processed to form the functional proteins (Mange & Mange, 1999).

The flow of genetic information, therefore, proceeds from DNA through transcription, to RNA. RNA is then translated into an amino acid sequence, forming a protein. In addition, it has recently been discovered that transporting genetic information to the cytoplasm of the cell for translation is only one of the functions of RNA. Several genes have been discovered that produce RNA transcripts, but no protein. Some of these have been shown to specifically regulate other genes. In fact, functional RNA is now thought to play an important role in regulating gene expression (Kim & Nam, 2006).

CHROMOSOMES

As noted previously, chromosomes are linear double strands of DNA with associated proteins that function to organize and compact the DNA in a cell. In most human cells, the DNA is organized into 46 chromosomes. This can be seen in a *karyotype*, which is a visual profile of an individual's chromosomes. Chromosomal analysis is done by drawing blood, growing the cells in a culture, and then analyzing the white blood cells. A karyotype is made by photographing the chromosomes and then arranging the chromosomes in pairs for display and assessment. A karyotype of normal human chromosomes can be seen in Figure 4–2.

Together the chromosomes contain a complete set of genetic instructions for cell replication and differentiation. This complete set of instructions for a particular organism or species is called the *genome* (Cummings, 1997).

Each chromosome has a narrowed region called a *centromere*. The centromere is critical for normal cell division; however, the location of the centromere is quite variable. In some cases, it is in the middle of the chromosome, dividing it into approximately equal halves. Chromosomes with a centrally located centromere are referred to as *metacentric*. The

centromere may also be off center, leading to a short p arm. The "p" may be thought of as *petit*, which is the French word for "small." The long arm is referred to as the q arm. The "q" is simply the letter after "p." Chromosomes with this structure are referred to as *submetacentric*. Finally, the centromere may be very close to one end of the chromosome. These chromosomes are *acrocentric*. The location of the centromere and the length of the chromosome give each chromosome a characteristic shape, which allows them to be distinguished from one another. Traditionally, chromosomes are labeled according to length, with the longest being number 1.

Each of 22 chromosomes has two copies, one from each parent. These chromosomes are called *autosomes*. The chromosomes in the 23rd pair are referred to as the *sex chromosomes* (X and Y) because of their role in gender determination. If a person inherits two X chromosomes (one from each parent), that

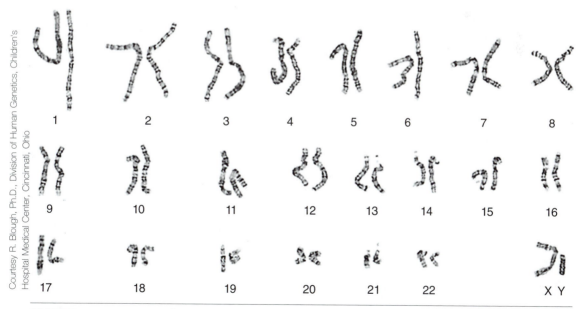

Courtesy R. Blough, Ph.D., Division of Human Genetics, Children's Hospital Medical Center, Cincinnati, Ohio

1 2 3 4 5 6 7 8

9 10 11 12 13 14 15 16

17 18 19 20 21 22 X Y

FIGURE 4–2 Karyotype of normal human chromosomes. It is traditional to align chromosomes so that the 'p' arm is on top.

person will be female. If an X (from the mother) and a Y (from the father) are inherited, the person will be male. The normal chromosomal makeup is written as 46,XX for a female or 46, XY for a male (Keagle & Brown, 1999).

Chromosomes can be specially stained to reveal a pattern of light- and dark-colored bands. This allows specific segments of the chromosome to be identified. Specific chromosomal locations are referred to by the chromosome number, followed by "p" or "q" to indicate the arm, and finally the band number, which indicates its location relative to the centromere and the other bands on that arm of the chromosome. This system is used to describe the rough location of genes in gene mapping studies. For example, a gene may be mapped to lp36. This means that the gene is found on the short arm of chromosome 1 in the band labeled 36. Figure 4–3 shows an *ideogram* (a schematic drawing of the banding pattern of a chromosome) for chromosome 1. The bands can be further subdivided in some cases, allowing for more specific localization to be described. Even with the best current-staining techniques, it is not possible to identify individual genes on a chromosome. The smallest bands that can be distinguished still contain multiple genes (Mange & Mange, 1999).

Cell Cycle

Cells in the body alternate between states of active division and states of nondivision. When a cell is in the process of preparing for and undergoing cell division, the sequence of events is called the *cell cycle*. The frequency of the cell cycle depends on the type of cell and the rate of growth of the organism at the time. The steps in each cycle are very similar for all types of *somatic cells*, which include all cells in the body with the exception of those for reproduction.

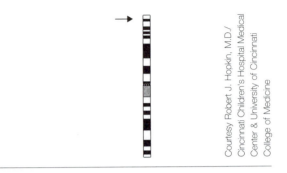

FIGURE 4–3 Ideogram (schematic drawing of the banding pattern) of chromosome 1: Note the light and dark bands. Each chromosome has a unique but consistent banding pattern that allows it to be distinguished from other chromosomes. The arrow indicates band lp36.

Cell division can be divided into two major processes: *mitosis*, which is the process of separating duplicated chromosomes and reconstitution of two cell nuclei, and *cytokinesis*, which is the separation of the cell cytoplasm to form two distinct cells with separate cell membranes. During mitosis, a complete identical set of chromosomes is distributed to each daughter cell. It is critical for the process to be accurate and precise in order for the cells to function normally. The chromosomes contain the genes and therefore the instructions that govern cell function. If errors (mutations) occur in either the separation of the chromosomes or the process of DNA replication, they often have serious consequences for the cell. The process of division takes about 1 hour. The time between cell divisions is called *interphase*. Cells spend much more time in interphase than in active division.

Mitosis takes place in the somatic cells and results in daughter cells that have the same number of chromosomes (46) as the parent cell. In contrast, *meiosis* occurs only in the production of *gametes*, which are sperm from the testes and ova (eggs) from the ovaries. This process results in 23 chromosomes for sperm cells and ova cells, rather than 46. When sperm and the ova combine to form a zygote, the organism will have 46 chromosomes. (If sperm and eggs each contained 46 chromosomes at conception, the new combined cell would contain double that number, or 92 chromosomes. This number would double with each generation!) During meiosis, cells undergo one round of DNA replication but two rounds of cell division. This produces four cells, each with a single copy of each chromosome (Griffiths, Miller, Suzuki, Lewontin, & Gelbart, 1996).

In men, meiosis occurs continuously following puberty and produces four sperm cells per original cell. This results in the availability of large numbers of mature sperm on a continual basis. In women, meiosis starts in fetal life but then arrests until puberty. Following puberty, one *oocyte* (a female gamete) per menstrual cycle completes meiosis. Errors in meiosis may have serious consequences because they result in abnormalities in every cell in a developing organism (Keagle & Brown, 1999).

Chromosomal Abnormalities

Chromosomal mutations may include changes in the number of copies of an individual chromosome. Loss of one copy of a chromosome results in *monosomy*, which is the presence of a single copy of a chromosome. The gain of one extra copy of a chromosome for a total of three chromosomes results in *trisomy*. Figure 4–4 shows a karyotype of trisomy 13. Most monosomies and trisomies end in early miscarriage.

The only monosomy that commonly results in the birth of living infants is monosomy X. This results in Turner syndrome. Turner syndrome is characterized by short stature, webbed neck, and lack of sexual maturation.

The presence of the Y chromosome with no X results in early miscarriage.

Survival is possible for several trisomies, including trisomy for 13, 18, 21, or X. Individuals born with an extra copy of X (47, XXX, or 47, XXY) may be relatively healthy and difficult to distinguish from the general population. The presence of an extra copy of the Y chromosome is also compatible with healthy survival. However, individuals with more than one extra copy of a sex chromosome will generally have medical and developmental problems. Trisomy 13 and 18 may result in live-born infants; however, these infants typically have multiple severe birth defects and rarely survive more than a few weeks. Trisomy 13 is frequently associated with cleft lip and palate and other craniofacial malformations. Trisomy 18 can lead to Pierre Robin sequence and cleft palate, in addition to many other malformations. Those with trisomy 21 have Down syndrome, which is associated with mental retardation, congenital heart disease, low muscle tone, and distinct facial features. Trisomies for other chromosomes result in early miscarriage.

Trisomies and monosomies result from a failure in meiosis. The abnormal number of chromosomes results from *nondisjunction*, which is the failure of one or more chromosomes to separate in cell division. Nondisjunction can be seen in both sperm and egg development. The cause of nondisjunction is not known, but the risk for nondisjunction and related chromosomal abnormalities increases with advancing maternal age. For example, the risk for trisomy 21 (which causes Down syndrome) in a pregnancy to a 20-year-old woman is approximately 1:2000. The risk for a pregnancy to a 45-year-old woman is approximately 1:20. The risk for nondisjunction rises slowly with age at first but increases more rapidly after age 35. For this reason, pregnant

Courtesy R. Blough, Ph.D., Division of Human Genetics, Children's Hospital Medical Center, Cincinnati, Ohio

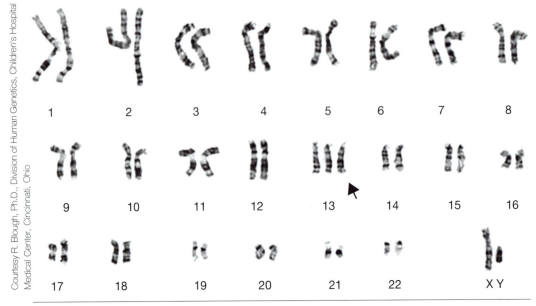

FIGURE 4–4 Karyotype of human chromosomes demonstrating trisomy 13.

women over age 35 are offered chromosomal analysis through amniocentesis. The risk for nondisjunction in men remains relatively stable with advancing age (Randolph, 1999).

Mosaicism is the presence of cells with two or more different genetic contents in a single individual. This may be caused by nondisjunction in mitosis. Because errors in mitosis affect only the daughter cells descended from the cell in which the error occurred, in many cases the abnormal cells may simply be eliminated or the functions of the cell may not be seriously impaired. However, if nondisjunction occurs in mitosis early in embryonic development, it may result in serious malformations. The effect of the abnormal cells depends on the ratio of normal versus abnormal cells and the distribution of the each cell type (Mange & Mange, 1999).

Chromosomal abnormalities, other than the gain or loss of an entire chromosome, can also occur. These include deletions, duplications, inversions, and translocations.

When part of a chromosome becomes separated and lost, this is called a *deletion*. Deletions have been reported for all chromosomes. The location of the deletion is designated by the chromosome number, a "p" (for the short arm) or "q" (for the long arm), and the number of the band where the break occurred. For example, a deletion of the short arm of chromosome 4 with a break point in band 16 in a female could be written 46,XXdel (4)(pl6). Figure 4–5 shows ideograms of a normal and a deleted chromosome 4. This deletion would result in Wolf-Hirschhorn syndrome (see Chapter 3). Deletions are often accompanied by multiple malformations, including facial clefts or other craniofacial malformations. However, unlike the example above, many deletions do not result in recognizable genetic syndromes.

Pure *duplications* of part of a chromosome are rare. Like deletions, chromosomal duplications are usually associated with multiple malformations and developmental handicaps. The pattern of malformations and severity of developmental disability depend on the size and location of the duplication. Even when the size and location are known, it can be difficult to predict what malformations will result and the long-term outcome for an individual patient. Combinations of deletion and duplication frequently result from unbalanced translocations (Kaiser-Rogers & Rao, 1999).

Translocations are the result of a transfer of genetic material between two or more chromosomes. *Inversions* occur when a portion of a chromosome is turned 180° from its usual orientation. Translocations and inversions may not be associated with any abnormalities in the individual because the total amount of genetic material may be unchanged. A problem occurs only if the break points are located in areas that disrupt a gene or genes. Translocations and inversions that do not result in the gain or loss of DNA have approximately a 10% risk for associated malformations or developmental disabilities. This is not surprising, as only approximately 10% of our DNA is in genes. The DNA that is not in genes also has important functions. It contains regulatory information that helps control gene expression and regulates the interactions between genes. Translocations and inversions may, however, increase the risk for infertility or birth defects

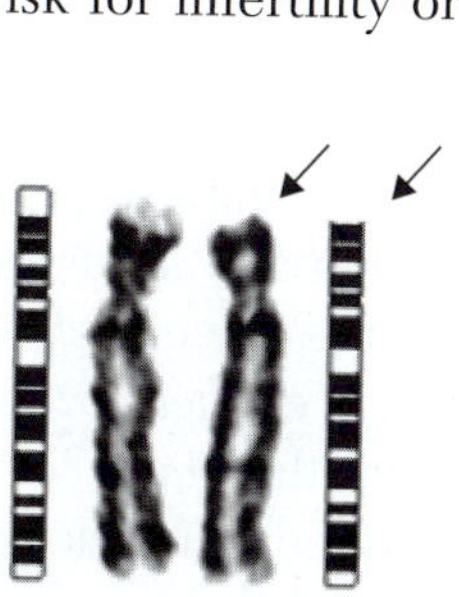

in the children of an asymptomatic individual who carries the chromosomal rearrangement.

Chromosomal abnormalities, as discussed above, involve multiple genes and large amounts of DNA. Therefore, they are relatively easy to detect. All of these types of chromosomal abnormalities can be associated with cleft lip, cleft palate, or other craniofacial malformations. It is important to identify people with chromosomal abnormalities because their needs and associated risks may be different from those of patients with isolated craniofacial malformations or single gene disorders. Fortunately, chromosomal abnormalities account for only a small portion of birth defects and genetic diseases. Smaller mutations involving only single genes are collectively more common, even though the individual disorders are often rare.

Chromosome Analysis

In order to discover abnormalities in the chromosomes, they must be visualized. The chromosomes are condensed enough to be easily viewed under a microscope, but only during certain stages of the cell cycle. Fortunately, by stimulating white blood cells to divide simultaneously, large numbers of cells can be expected to reach the same stage of the cell cycle at about the same time. This greatly improves the efficiency of chromosomal analysis. There are also chemicals that lead to an arrest of cell division at certain stages of the cell cycle. Thus, the cell cycle can be controlled to maximize the number of cells appropriate for analysis (Keagle & Gersen, 1999).

Some chromosomal abnormalities involve only very short segments that are too small to be seen using routine chromosomal analysis. With special techniques, such as *fluorescence in situ hybridization*, or FISH, some submicroscopic segments of DNA can be identified by a

Courtesy R. Blough, Ph.D., Division of Human Genetics, Children's Hospital Medical Center, Cincinnati, Ohio

FIGURE 4–5 Normal and deleted human chromosome 4 with ideograms. The arrows indicate the deleted segment at 4p16. This deletion is associated with Wolf-Hirschhorn syndrome.

cytogenetic laboratory. (*Cytogenetics*, which literally means "cell genetics," is the branch of genetics that is concerned with the structure and function of the chromosomes within the cell.) This procedure involves the use of a nucleic acid probe labeled with a fluorescent dye that localizes a specified DNA segment. For example, the deletion of chromosome 22qll.2, associated with velocardiofacial syndrome (see Chapter 4), is usually not visible on chromosomal analysis, but is seen using FISH in the majority of cases. Syndromes caused by deletions large enough to contain several genes, but too small to be seen on routine cytogenetic analysis, are referred to as *contiguous gene syndromes*. In most, if not all, cases, the problems associated with the syndrome are caused by the loss of function of several important contiguous genes (Kaiser-Rogers & Rao, 1999).

See Table 4–1 for a list of some microdeletion contiguous gene syndromes.

Until recently, it has only been possible to look for submicroscopic deletions by ordering site-specific testing for specific changes that were suspected based on the pattern of malformations. In other words, someone had to recognize the condition first and then look for the genetic abnormality. New technology using SNPs (single nucleotide polymorphisms) and CGH (comparative genomic hybridization) microarray analysis allows assessment of thousands of loci simultaneously (Le Caignec et al., 2005; Schoumans et al., 2005; Ting et al., 2006). This has greatly increased the ability to detect small cytogenetic rearrangements that lead to malformation syndromes. In addition, because of the number of individual probes, this technology allows a much more precise assessment of the size of any deletion or duplication identified. Using microarray technology, it is now possible to determine exactly which genes are deleted or duplicated, even when deletions or duplications are too small to be detected with standard chromosomal analysis. Microarray analysis has therefore become a very important tool for the initial evaluation of suspected genetic disease.

MENDELIAN INHERITANCE

The common patterns of inheritance and the rules that govern them were first outlined by Mendel in 1866 in his studies on peas (McKusick, 1997). Therefore, these patterns are known as Mendelian inheritance and include autosomal recessive, autosomal dominant, and X-linked patterns. These patterns depend on whether the individual is *homozygous* (has two of the same *alleles* or copies of a gene for a trait), or *heterozygous* (has two different alleles of the gene).

Mendel described four rules of inheritance. He discovered the following:

1. Genes come in pairs, one from each parent.

TABLE 4–1   Examples of Microdeletion Contiguous Gene Syndromes

Velocardiofacial syndrome	del 22qll.2
Wolf-Hirschhorn syndrome	del 4pl6.3
Cri du chat syndrome	del 5pl5
Prader-Willi syndrome	del 15qllql3
Miller-Dieker syndrome	del 17pl3.3
Langer-Giedion syndrome	del 8q24
Smith-Magenis syndrome	del 17pll.2
Kallmann syndrome	del Xp22.3
X-linked ichthyosis	del Xp22.3
Jacobsen syndrome	del llq24.1
Williams syndrome	del 7qll.23

2. A pair of genes can have different *alleles* (copies), which are variations of a gene. Some of these are dominant and will exert their effects over the effects of the other allele. Other alleles are recessive and will be manifest only when the genes are similar or the same alleles.

3. At meiosis, alleles segregate from each other; each gamete carries only one allele of the pair.

4. The segregation of alleles for one trait is independent of the segregation of alleles from other genes for other traits.

These principles have remained valid (with only a few modifications) since they were first described.

Pedigrees

In determining a pattern of inheritance for a condition in a family, it is helpful to have a systematic way of collecting and recording the family history. A system has been developed, called a *pedigree*, which is a pictorial representation of family members and their line of descent. This system is used to record the inheritance of traits or anomalies affecting several members of a family. It allows the important findings to be recorded in a short period of time. Most families can be easily described for three to four generations on a single page. In addition, with minimal training and a little practice, pedigrees can be simply and quickly drawn by hand during the course of a brief interview (Mange & Mange, 1999). Three sample pedigrees are illustrated in Figure 4–6.

Autosomal Recessive Inheritance

All people carry genes with mutations that are capable of causing disease. Fortunately, we inherit two copies of each gene, one from each parent, and in many cases one copy that functions normally is sufficient. Individuals who have one abnormal copy of a gene and are without detectable abnormalities are referred to as *carriers*. They are heterozygous, having two different alleles of a gene—one normal and one abnormal.

In *autosomal recessive* conditions, traits of the typical *phenotype* (group of typical characteristics associated with a genetic condition) manifest only when mutations are present in both copies of a gene. Therefore, they only occur with the individual who is homozygous for the genes of that condition.

When two heterozygous carriers of an autosomal recessive condition mate, each parent has an equal probability of passing on either the normal or the abnormal allele to their offspring. Therefore, the risk that the child would receive an abnormal copy of the gene from each parent and be affected with the condition is 25% for each pregnancy. In addition, there is a 50% risk that the child will receive a single copy of the mutation and become a carrier, and a 25% risk that the child will receive a normal copy of the sequence of genes from both parents and be a noncarrier. If two individuals with the same autosomal recessive condition have children together, all of their children will be affected because both parents have only abnormal alleles to pass on (Mueller & Cook, 1997). In all autosomal recessive conditions, males and females are affected in equal numbers.

There are approximately 30,000 different genes in each cell, and on average each person carries six to seven potentially disease-causing mutations. Therefore, the chance that both members of a couple will carry mutations in the same gene is very small. The probability of two people carrying abnormalities in the same genes is greatly increased if they are related,

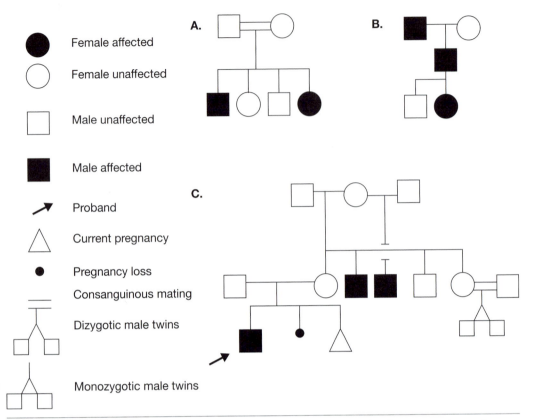

FIGURE 4–6 (A) Symbols used in pedigree construction with three sample pedigrees. (A) demonstrates probable autosomal recessive inheritance. Note recurrence in siblings with unaffected parents and consanguinity. Multifactorial inheritance cannot be ruled out based on the information given. (B) demonstrates autosomal dominant inheritance. Note father-to-son transmission and recurrence in several generations. (C) demonstrates X-linked recessive inheritance. Note occurrence of multiple males born to unaffected female relatives over multiple generations. In drawing a pedigree, horizontal lines connecting two individuals indicate mating between them. Children are indicated by vertical lines with squares or circles to indicate the sex of the child. If more than one child is born to a couple, a horizontal line intersects the vertical line to allow each child to be appropriately recorded. If a parent has children with more than one partner additional lines can be drawn as seen in the first generation of family C. Divorce or separation can be indicated by as hash mark and space in the line connecting two individuals (not shown). If more than one trait is being recorded in a family, the affected individuals can be indicated by shading only one quadrant, for example the upper left for trait 1, the lower left for trait 2, and so on. If still more traits are recorded, different colors or patterns of shading can be added.

because relatives share genetic material. Thus, *consanguinity*, which is mating between related individuals, leads to increased risk that both the members of the couple carry the same disease-causing mutations of the same genes. The closer the relationship, the more genetic material the two individuals have in common and therefore the greater the risk. This is one explanation for the high incidence of genetic disorders in isolated or inbred populations. Although the parents of individuals affected by an autosomal recessive condition are often not affected because they are merely carriers, recurrence of the condition with additional offspring is common.

Occasionally, two people with the same autosomal recessive trait have a child who is unaffected. An example of this would be autosomal recessive hearing loss. This can be explained by *heterogeneity*, which occurs when a specific phenotype can be caused by mutations of different genes (Mueller & Cook, 1997).

See Table 4–2 for a list of some autosomal recessive conditions that can be associated with cleft lip or cleft palate.

Recurrence in more than one generation is uncommon because carrier frequency is low for most autosomal recessive conditions. For example, cystic fibrosis is one of the most common autosomal recessive disorders, affecting 1:2500 live births among populations of Northern European descent. The carrier frequency in that population is 1:25. That means a carrier would have a 24/25 probability of reproducing with a noncarrier in a population with random choice of partners. However, in some populations, a relatively small number of original ancestors has led to a high frequency of carriers for certain disorders. This is known as a *founder effect*. When this occurs, it is often possible to trace family lines to a single common ancestor who brought a trait into a population. More frequently, a founder effect is implied by a high frequency of a few mutations in a large population. For example, three mutations account for 98% of Tay-Sachs disease in the Ashkenazi Jewish population (Rutledge & Percy, 1997).

Genetic testing for carrier status can help couples in making reproductive decisions if they are from a high-risk population or if there is a family history of the disorder that indicates a high probability that one or both partners may be carriers for that condition. Testing is currently available for some of the more common autosomal recessive diseases, such as cystic fibrosis, sickle cell anemia, and Tay-Sachs disease. Prenatal testing for some autosomal recessive conditions is also available to distinguish affected individuals from carriers.

Autosomal Dominant Inheritance

In autosomal dominant conditions, traits of the typical phenotype manifest when mutations are present in either of the two copies of a gene. Therefore, both homozygous and heterozygous individuals will have features of the condition. As a result, pedigrees from families with autosomal dominant conditions demonstrate different findings than are seen with autosomal recessive inheritance.

When two individuals with a dominant condition mate, there is a 75% chance that they will pass the condition to their offspring, because each parent is probably heterozygous (25% of offspring will inherit disease-causing mutations from each parent, 50% will inherit a single mutation, and 25% will not inherit a mutation). When one individual has a dominant condition and an unaffected partner mate,

TABLE 4–2 Examples of Autosomal Recessive Craniofacial Syndromes

Smith-Lemli-Opitz syndrome

Meckel-Gruber syndrome

Baller-Gerold syndrome

Oral-facial-digital syndrome type II

Insley-Astley syndrome

Dubowitz syndrome

Roberts syndrome

Toriello-Carey syndrome

Varadi-Papp syndrome

there is a 50% risk with each pregnancy of passing the condition to their offspring (who will be heterozygotes). As with autosomal recessive conditions, the number of affected males and females with autosomal dominant conditions is approximately equal.

Homozygotes (persons with two abnormal alleles) for autosomal dominant disorders often have a more severe phenotype than heterozygotes. For example, achondroplasia is the most common form of short-limbed dwarfism. Homozygous offspring of parents with achondroplasia have a severe phenotype, with a small chest and pulmonary hypoplasia that is incompatible with survival beyond the first few days of life (Winter & Baraitser, 1996).

Autosomal dominant pedigrees often show that at least one parent is affected. If neither parent has the condition, the affected individual is presumed to carry a new mutation that is causing the condition. For some autosomal dominant conditions, the new mutation rate is high and may account for a large percentage of affected individuals, as in Pfieffer syndrome (Winter & Baraitser, 1996).

Many autosomal dominant conditions have *variable expressivity* (variation in the phenotype associated with a single condition). This may cause affected individuals to be missed if the phenotype is not appropriately defined. For example, in Van der Woude syndrome, affected members of the same family may have lip pits, cleft lip, cleft palate, or a combination of these. Obviously, an individual with isolated lip pits could be missed if only individuals with cleft lip are identified when a family history is obtained. Most, if not all, autosomal dominant conditions demonstrate some degree of variable expressivity (Mueller & Cook, 1997).

Incomplete penetrance is the lack of a recognizable phenotype in an individual who carries a mutation that may cause an autosomal dominant trait or condition. At times, it may be difficult to distinguish between minimal expression caused by variable expressivity and true incomplete penetrance. Some families have members who have no abnormal findings (nonpenetrance) but have transmitted the trait to their children. Other individuals may have only one feature of a condition (variable expressivity) but may transmit the complete condition to their children. The factors that determine the penetrance and expressivity for a given trait are not well understood, but they include different mutations in the same gene, modification of genes that interact with the gene that causes the disorder, environmental influences, and random variation (Mueller & Cook, 1997; Murray, 1995).

Many genes have more than one function and may therefore be associated with multiple seemingly unrelated abnormalities. For example, neurofibromatosis type 1 is associated with growth of large nerve sheath tumors, called *neurofibromas*; pigmentary abnormalities of the skin; bony dysplasias; and learning disabilities. This *pleiotropy* (the phenomenon where a single mutant gene can affect multiple, unrelated systems) can contribute to the variability in genetic syndromes, because each function of a gene can have either variable expression or nonpenetrance (Mueller & Cook, 1997).

For examples of autosomal dominant craniofacial syndromes, see Table 4–3.

X-Linked and Y-Linked Inheritance

X-linked inheritance refers to conditions caused by mutations in genes on the X chromosome. X-linked inheritance is unique because males inherit only one allel of the X chromosome, whereas females inherit two copies.

TABLE 4–3 Examples of Autosomal Dominant Craniofacial Syndromes
Apert syndrome
Branchio-oto-renal syndrome
Crouzon syndrome
Distichiasis-lymphedema syndrome
Ectrodactyly ectodermal dysplasia clefting syndrome
Opitz Frias syndrome
Stickler syndrome
Treacher-Collins syndrome
Van der Woude syndrome
Waardenburg syndrome

© Cengage Learing 2014

TABLE 4–4 Examples of X-Linked Recessive Craniofacial Syndromes
Chitayat syndrome
X-linked cleft palate
Oro-facial-digital syndrome type VIII
VATER with hydrocephaly
Lenz microphthalmia
Lowe syndrome
Oto-palato-digital syndrome type II
Simpson-Golabi-Behmel syndrome
SCARF syndrome
Say-Meyer syndrome

© Cengage Learing 2014

There are many X-linked recessive conditions that affect males almost exclusively. A female is likely to have no more than mild effects, if there are any effects at all. Carrier females transmit the defective genes to 50% of their sons, who will be affected, and 50% of their daughters, who will be carriers. Affected males pass the mutation to 100% of their daughters. There is no father-to-son transmission because fathers do not give an X chromosome to their sons (Mueller & Cook, 1997).

See Table 4–4 for examples of X-linked recessive disorders.

X-linked dominant inheritance is rare, with only a few disorders known. With X-linked dominant disorders, all daughters of affected males inherit the disorder. Sons of affected males never inherit the disorder because they receive the Y chromosome from the father. Affected females can transmit the disorder to offspring of both sexes. There is an excess of affected females in pedigrees for X-linked dominant disorders. Many X-linked dominant disorders are lethal to affected males.

See Table 4–5 for a list of X-linked dominant disorders.

TABLE 4–5 Examples of X-Linked Dominant Syndromes
Goltz syndrome
Conradi chondrodysplasia punctate
Oral-facial-digital syndrome type I
Melnick-Needles ostoedysplasty
Aicardi syndrome
Incontinentia pigmenti
X-linked hypophosphataemic rickets
Rett syndrome

© Cengage Learing 2014

There are a number of X-linked conditions that cannot be clearly categorized as either X-linked recessive or X-linked dominant. They often have effects on females who are heterozygous, but they may affect males more severely. This group of disorders is often lumped with X-linked recessive disorders in the medical literature but should more appropriately be referred to simply as X-linked. Some examples of this pattern include Aarskog syndrome, Opitz BBBG syndrome, Alport syndrome, Coffin-Lowry syndrome, fragile X syndrome, and Fabry disease. This group of disorders is characterized by variable expressivity and high levels of nonpenetrance in females, but with complete penetrance and more uniform expression in males.

Of course Y-linked disorders only affect males. Because there are relatively few genes on the Y chromosome and the only major Y-linked traits are for male gender and sperm production, the transmission of other types of traits from a father to his son is considered diagnostic of autosomal dominant inheritance.

NON-MENDELIAN INHERITANCE

Many disorders that tend to recur in families do not follow the basic rules of Mendelian inheritance. The remainder of this chapter reviews some of the mechanisms involved in the inheritance of these disorders.

Multifactorial Inheritance

Some human disorders result from an interaction of multiple genes with environmental influences. This is called *multifactorial inheritance*. Environmental factors known to increase risks for birth defects are called *teratogens* (Murray, 1995). Common examples of teratogens include ethanol, cigarette smoke, anti-epileptic medications, maternal diabetes, and congenital infections. Most, if not all, teratogens exert their effects by interfering with the regulation of gene expression.

Inherited traits and inherited abnormalities associated with multifactorial inheritance can be divided into two categories: continuous variation and threshold.

Some inherited traits that exhibit continuous variation include height, weight, intelligence, and blood pressure. These traits are not easily distinguished from normal variation because the boundary between normal and abnormal is arbitrary, and there will be large numbers of people in the borderline area. In many cases, "abnormal" is defined as greater than two standard deviations from the mean. Although this can be used to define abnormality, it may or may not be significant to the affected individual.

Threshold abnormalities involve a trait that is either present or absent; therefore, the abnormality is usually not difficult to identify. These abnormalities include cleft lip/palate, pyloric stenosis, and neural tube defects. With a threshold disorder, as the number of risk factors for the trait increases, the additive risk may cross a boundary or threshold, resulting in expression of the trait.

In the case of cleft lip with or without cleft palate, a few of the possible risk factors that contribute to the total risk have been identified. Recent evidence has led to the estimate that variations in 4 to 12 genes contribute most of the genetic risk for cleft lip, with or without cleft palate. Candidate genes include TGFA, RARA, BCL3, and END1 (Lidral & Moreno, 2005). Some environmental influences that affect risk for cleft lip have also been identified. Maternal smoking, for example, raises the risk for cleft lip (Shaw et al., 1996); whereas maternal supplementation of folic acid may decrease recurrence risk (Jia et al., 2011; Tolarova & Harris, 1995). The interaction between genes and environmental factors may be additive in multifactorial disorders. For example, the risk attributed to a rare polymorphism of the TGFA gene is small (one- to twofold). The risk associated with maternal smoking is also small (1.5- to twofold). One study found that when both heavy maternal smoking and the high-risk allele of TGFA were present, the risk jumped to three- to elevenfold compared to the control group risk (Shaw et al., 1996).

The risk for recurrence of a multifactorial trait in family members can be estimated by doing population studies. This is done by gathering empirical data and looking at variables that may correlate with risk for the condition in question. In the case of cleft lip only, a few of the possible risk factors that contribute to the total risk have been identified. For example, cleft lip is more common in boys than girls. It is therefore predicted by the multifactorial model that if a woman has cleft lip, the recurrence risk in the family will be higher than the risk if a man has cleft lip, and that the brothers of an affected individual will be at higher risk than sisters. Both of these predictions have been studied, but the results have been inconsistent. If both parents have cleft lip, the recurrence risk should be still higher because risk factors could be inherited from each parent. In fact, the greater the number of affected relatives, the higher the predicted risk. This prediction has been verified in cleft lip and cleft palate families.

The estimated recurrence risk for future children in a family with one individual with cleft palate is 3% to 5%. If there are two affected first-degree relatives, the risk goes up to approximately 9% to 15%, depending on which family members have cleft lip (Curtis, Fraser, & Warburton, 1961; Wyszynski, Zeiger, Tilli, Bailey-Wilson, & Beaty, 1998). The reason for the range depends on the gender of the person(s) affected and how closely related the affected individuals are to the pregnancy. For example, if a family has an affected mother and an affected female child, the recurrence risk will be greater than an affected father who has a brother with cleft lip. There are two reasons for this difference. First, the incidence of cleft lip is lower in females than males, so affected female relatives probably have more risk factors than would be seen in an affected male relative. The other issue is how closely related the affected relatives are to the pregnancy at risk. In the case of an affected parent and child for a subsequent pregnancy, both affected individuals are first-degree relatives not only to each other but also to the pregnancy in question. In the scenario with the affected father and his affected brother, the individuals are first-degree relatives, but the pregnancy is not as closely related to both, and therefore the child is less likely to inherit all of the potential risk factors.

The severity of the defect is also predicted to impact the recurrence risk. For example, one would predict that the recurrence risk in a family with a child who has a bilateral cleft lip would be higher than if the child had a unilateral cleft, because the bilateral cleft is a more severe defect. Most studies have supported this prediction. The presence of cleft palate with cleft lip, on the other hand, has not been found to correlate well with recurrence risk in spite of being clinically more difficult to manage (Crawford & Sofaer, 1987; Grosen et al., 2010).

The risk for multifactorial disorders is increased in close relatives because they tend to share similar genetic backgrounds and similar environmental risk factors. However, recurrences of multifactorial disorders do not follow a predictable pattern and are usually lower than the 25% or 50% that is predicted for Mendelian disorders. For example, the recurrence risk for first-degree relatives of a person with a cleft lip is in the range of 3% to 5%, and even lower for more distant relatives. Of course, the recurrence risk for multifactorial disorders is greater in consanguineous matings and inbred populations, as it is for Mendelian-inherited disorders, because of the amount of shared genetic material. In addition, isolated populations often have the same environmental exposures.

There are several variations of the multifactorial model. These include the *oligogenic model*. According to this model, a trait may be determined by the interaction of multiple genes, with little environmental influence. Usually, a small number of genes contribute most of the risk. For example, one model of risk for cleft palate estimates that six major genes contribute most of the risk for non-syndromic cleft palate (Fitzpatrick & Farrall, 1993). The major gene model assumes that abnormalities in one of several genes known to influence risk for a trait contribute most of the risk, but that the remaining risk is defined by environmental factors. This model has been suggested for isolated cleft lip recurrence risk estimation (Farrall & Holder, 1992). Multifactorial inheritance is very difficult to study because it is complicated by heterogeneity, small effects of each risk factor, incomplete penetrance, and complex interactions. On the other hand, some of the most common human diseases demonstrate multifactorial inheritance.

See Table 4–6 for examples of human diseases demonstrating multifactorial inheritance.

Recent advances in informatics and genetics have greatly increased the ability to study the additive effects of multiple genetic factors or of interacting factors related to specific birth defects. This area of study, referred to as *genomics*, began with the Human Genome Project. Genomics differs from traditional genetics, which focuses on the specific effects of a single gene. Instead, genomics focuses on the interacting effects of multiple genes and may include various environmental as well as genetic influences. Therefore, this is likely to be a powerful tool for elucidating the etiology of multifactorial disorders. For example, unlike a specific gene in the microdeletion that is known to cause the heart disease in Williams syndrome, a specific gene has not been identified that explains the developmental abnormalities in velocardiofacial syndrome. Through genomics, there is now evidence that the interactions between several of the deleted genes contribute additively to explain these developmental disabilities. Therefore, loss of any one gene may not cause any recognized problems, but loss of several causes a recognizable pattern of abnormality (Vitelli & Baldini, 2003). Genomics is also allowing analysis of very large amounts of data in a short period of time. For example, it is now possible to sequence the entire genome of an individual and compare the genetic makeup of a child to both parents. This has already contributed to identifying genes for multiple very rare disorders that have Mendelian inheritance and is expected to help elucidate the cause of multifactorial disorders as well. It is now possible to identify genetic causes for some disorders with as few as one to three affected individuals.

TABLE 4–6 Examples of Multifactorial Traits

Cleft lip with or without cleft palate

Cleft palate

Velopharyngeal insufficiency (VPI)

Diabetes mellitus

Alzheimer disease

Alcoholism

Athrosclerotic heart disease

Mental retardation

Colon cancer

Bipolar disease

Anticipation

Some inherited disorders show a tendency to have more severe manifestations or an earlier age of onset with succeeding generations. This phenomenon is known as *anticipation*. For many years, anticipation was assumed to be due to sampling errors or ascertainment bias. However, studies have proven that there is a genetic basis for anticipation in some diseases.

All disorders with proven anticipation have a common mechanism. They are all caused by large expansions of nucleotide repeats. The most common repeats occur with the nucleotides of CAG. As the number of repeats expands, it becomes unstable so that in the next generation there is a tendency for the number of repeats to be greater. This, in turn, leads to an earlier age of onset and a more severe phenotype. Disorders caused by CAG repeats include Huntington's disease, spinocerebellar ataxias, and other adult-onset neurodegenerative disorders. A second group of diseases is caused by unstable expansion of untranslated triplet repeats. Fragile X syndrome, the most common inherited form of mental retardation, is caused by a large expansion of an untranslated CGG repeat.

Imprinting

Historically, it was assumed that the two complementary copies of the same gene have equivalent function. However, some genes function differently, depending on whether they were inherited maternally or paternally. This phenomenon is called *imprinting* (Butler, 2002; Tilghman, 1999). If a gene is maternally imprinted, the allele inherited from the mother is not expressed. The opposite is true for genes that are paternally imprinted. This has been demonstrated in a small number of disorders, including Beckwith-Weidemann syndrome, Prader-Willi syndrome, Angelman syndrome, and Russell-Silver syndrome. It appears that imprinting is important in growth control and brain development (Butler, 2002). It may also play an important role in carcinogenesis (Tilghman, 1999).

SUMMARY

The principles of inheritance and genetics that are covered in this chapter are fundamental to the understanding of most human malformations. Accurate counseling for parents and other family members concerning long-term prognosis and recurrence risks depends on correct diagnosis and identification of the appropriate patterns of inheritance. In addition, an understanding of the basis of malformation syndromes is important for appropriate management of the patient. For example, the needs of a child with cleft lip caused by an unbalanced chromosomal translocation are likely to differ from those of a child with cleft lip due to multifactorial inheritance. As new insights are discovered into the causes of genetic disease and birth defects, it will become increasingly important to understand these principles and apply them to improved treatment for each affected patient or family.

FOR REVIEW AND DISCUSSION

1. Describe the "anatomy" of a chromosome and all of its contents.

2. Define DNA and RNA, and list their contents. What are their similarities and differences?

3. How many chromosomes are in human cells? Describe how the 23rd pair of chromosomes determines gender.

4. What is meant by *monosomy* and *trisomy*? What common syndrome is due to trisomy 21?

5. Which is likely to cause more abnormalities—a chromosomal defect or single gene defect? Why do you think that is the case?

6. Cleft palate is often described as the result of multifactorial inheritance. Explain what that means and what the factors might be that can cause cleft palate.

7. What is X-linked inheritance? Is it more serious in boys or girls? Why?

8. What can a pedigree tell you, and why should it be done for individuals with a craniofacial anomaly?

9. What is a phenotype? How does it relate to variable expressivity? Why is it important to know about variable expressivity when evaluating a genetic syndrome in a family?

REFERENCES

Butler, M. G. (2002). Imprinting disorders: Non-Mendelian mechanisms affecting growth. *Journal of Pediatric Endocrinology, 15*(Suppl. 5), 1279–1288.

Crawford, M., & Sofaer, J. (1987). Cleft lip with or without cleft palate: Identification of sporadic cases with a high level of genetic predisposition. *Journal of Medical Genetics, 24,* 163–169.

Cummings, M. (1997). *Human heredity* (4th ed.). Eagan, MD: West/Wadsworth.

Curtis, E., Fraser, F., & Warburton, D. (1961). Congenital cleft lip and palate. *American Journal of Diseases in Childhood, 102,* 853–857.

Farrall, M., & Holder, S. (1992). Familial recurrence-pattern analysis of cleft lip with or without cleft palate. *American Journal of Human Genetics, 50,* 270–277.

Fitzpatrick, D., & Farrall, M. (1993). An estimation of the number of susceptibility loci for isolated cleft palate. *Journal of Craniofacial Genetics and Developmental Biology, 13,* 230–235.

Griffiths, A., Miller, J., Suzuki, D., Lewontin, R., & Gelbart, W. (1996). *An introduction to genetic analysis* (6th ed.). New York: W. H. Freeman and Company.

Grosen, D., Chevrier, C., Skytthe, A., Bille, C., Molsted, K., et al. (2010). A cohort study of recurrence patterns among more than 54,000 relatives or oral cleft cases in Denmark: support for the multifactorial threshold model of inheritance. *Journal of Medical Genetics, 47*(3), 162–168.

Jia, Z. L., Shi, B., Chen, C. H., Shi, J. Y., Wu, J., et al. (2011). Maternal malnutrition, environmental exposure during pregnancy and the risk of non-syndromic orofacial clefts. *Oral Disorders, 17*(6), 584–589.

Kaiser-Rogers, K., & Rao, K. (1999). Structural chromosomal rearrangements. In S. Gersen & M. Keagle (Eds.), *The principles of clinical cytogenetics* (pp. 191–228). Totowa, NJ: Humana Press.

Keagle, M., & Brown, J. (1999). DNA, chromosomes, and cell division. In S. Gersen & M. Keagle (Eds.), *The principles of clinical cytogenetics* (pp. 11–30). Totowa, NJ: Humana Press.

Keagle, M., & Gersen, S. (1999). Basic laboratory procedures. In M. Keagle & S. Gersen (Eds.), *The principles of clinical cytogenetics* (pp. 71–90). Totowa, NJ: Humana Press.

Kim, N. V., & Nam, J. W., (2006). Genomics of microRNA. *Trends in Genetics, 22*(3), 165–173.

Le Caignec, C., Boceno, M., Saugier-Veber, P., Jacquemont, S., Joubert, M., David, A., et al. (2005). Detection of genomic imbalances by array-based comparative genomic hybridization in fetuses with multiple malformations. *Journal of Medical Genetics, 42,* 121–128.

Lidral, A. C., & Moreno L. M. (2005). Progress toward discerning the genetics of cleft lip. *Current Opinion in Pediatrics, 17,* 731–739.

Mange, E., & Mange, A. (1999). *Basic human genetics* (2nd ed.). Sunderland, MA: Sinauer Associates.

McKusick, V. (1997). History of medical genetics. In D. Rimoin, J. Connor & R. Pyeritz (Eds.), *Emery and Rimoin's principles and practice of medical genetics* (3rd ed., *vol. 1,* pp. 1–30). New York: Churchill Livingstone.

Mueller, R., & Cook, J. (1997). Mendelian inheritance. In D. Rimoin, J. Connor & R. Pyeritz (Eds.), *Emery and Rimoin's principles and practice of medical genetics* (3rd ed., vol. *1,* pp. 87–102). New York: Churchill Livingstone.

Murray, J. C. (1995). Face facts: Genes, environment, and clefts. *American Journal of Human Genetics,* 57(2), 227–232.

Randolph, L. (1999). Prenatal cytogenetics. In S. Gersen & M. Keagle (Eds.), *The principles of clinical cytogenetics* (pp. 259–316). Totowa, NJ: Humana Press.

Rutledge, S., & Percy, A. (1997). Gangliosidoses and related lipid storage diseases. In D. Rimoin, J. Connor & R. Pyeritz (Eds.), *Emery and Rimoin's principles and practice of medical genetics* (3rd ed., *vol. 2,* pp. 2105–2130). New York: Churchill Livingstone.

Schoumans, J., Ruivenkamp, C., Holmberg, E., Kyllerman, M., Anderlid, B. M., et al. (2005). Detection of chromosomal imbalances in children with idiopathic mental retardation by array-based comparative genomic hybridization (array-CGH). *Journal of Medical Genetics, 42,* 699–705.

Shaw, G., Wasserman, G., Lammer, E., O'Malley, C., Murray, J., et al. (1996). Orofacial clefts, parental cigarette smoking, and transforming growth factor-alpha gene variants. *American Journal of Human Genetics, 58,* 551–561.

Strachan, T., & Read, A. (1996). *Human molecular genetics.* New York: Wiley-Liss.

Tilghman, S. M. (1999). The sins of the fathers and mothers: Genomic imprinting in mammalian development. *Cell, 96*(2), 185–193.

Ting, J. C., Ye, Y., Thomas, G. H., Ruczinski, L., & Pevsner, J. (2006). Analysis and visualization of chromosomal abnormalities in SNP data with SNPscan. *Bioinformatics, 7*(1), 25.

Tolarova, M., & Harris, J. (1995). Reduced recurrence of orofacial clefts after periconceptional supplementation with high-dose folic acid and multivitamins. *Teratology, 51,* 71–78.

Vitelli, F., & Baldini, A. (2003). Generating and modifying DiGeorge syndrome-like phenotypes in model organisms: Is there a common genetic pathway? *Trends in Genetics, 19,* 588–593.

Wilkie, A. O., Tang, Z., Elanko, N., Walsh, S., Twigg, S. R., et al. (2000). Functional haploinsufficiency of the human homeobox gene MSX2 causes defects in skull ossification. *Nature Genetics, 24*(4), 387–390.

Winter, R., & Baraitser, M. (1996). *London dysmorphology database (1) [Compact Disc].* London: Oxford Medical Databases.

Wyszynski, D. F., Zeiger, J., Tilli, M. T., Bailey-Wilson, J. E., & Beaty, T. H. (1998). Survey of genetic counselors and clinical geneticists regarding recurrence risks for families with nonsyndromic cleft lip with or without cleft palate. *American Journal of Medical Genetics, 79*(3), 184–190.

Problems Associated with Clefts and Craniofacial Anomalies

CHAPTER

5

FEEDING PROBLEMS OF INFANTS WITH CLEFTS OR CRANIOFACIAL ANOMALIES

CLAIRE K. MILLER, PH.D.

ANN W. KUMMER, PH.D.

CHAPTER OUTLINE

INTRODUCTION

Feeding is the one the most immediate challenges parents face following the birth of a baby born with a cleft palate. In fact, parents report that obtaining appropriate instructions about effective feeding methods is a high priority during the first few weeks (Bessell et al., 2011; Chuacharoen, Ritthagol, Hunsrisakhun, & Nilmanat, 2009; Young, O'Riordan, Goldstein, & Robin, 2001). Fortunately, most feeding problems due to a cleft can be easily resolved using certain feeding adaptations and other therapeutic interventions.

An open palate can affect an infant's ability to feed in many ways. First, it can have a profound effect on the oral-motor mechanics and the ability to generate the necessary negative intraoral pressure for effective sucking. In addition, the open palate may cause difficulty with coordination of sucking, swallowing, and respiration during feeding. Inadequate airway protection during swallowing has significant implications in regard to respiratory health (Arvedson & Brodsky, 2002; Boesch et al., 2006). Finally, parental frustration due to difficulty in feeding their child can have a negative effect on the parent–infant bonding process (Johansson & Ringsberg, 2004).

Generally, the more extensive the cleft of the palate is, the greater the chance will be for significant feeding problems and poor oral intake. Because the volume of intake must be sufficient for adequate weight gain before the surgical repair of lip or palatal clefts, early identification and treatment of feeding problems must be made so that the infant can receive adequate nutrition for growth.

This chapter focuses upon the disruptions in the normal feeding process that occur secondary to clefts and other craniofacial anomalies. Assessment of feeding difficulties and the options for individualizing feeding modifications are discussed.

INFANT FEEDING AND EARLY DEVELOPMENT

The primary purpose of feeding is to satisfy the infant's hunger and provide adequate nourishment for normal growth and development. However, the process of feeding is also important for the infant's neuromotor development and sense of well-being (Miller, 2009).

The act of feeding serves to provide the infant with both oral-sensory and oral-motor stimulation. The nipple's tactile input to the mouth initiates the sucking reflex in neurologically intact infants. This sensory input represents the first step in initiation of the suck–swallow–breathe synchrony that is central to the infant feeding process.

Of course feeding is accomplished exclusively by sucking in early infancy. However, the active use of the lower jaw, cheeks, lips, and tongue during sucking provides a basis for the development of more mature feeding skills later on (Morris & Klein, 1987). These oral movements also help to develop skills for speech production.

In addition to nutrition and stimulation, the reflexive activity of both nutritive and nonnutritive sucking facilitates state regulation and helps the infant to maintain homeostasis. The infant quickly learns to use sucking for calming and self-regulation.

Finally, the activity of feeding serves as a very important part of the bonding process between the caregiver and infant. The caregiver spends time holding and cuddling the infant during the feeding process, and learns to identify the infant's cues. In addition, there is mutual eye contact and vocalizations between the caregiver and infant. The behaviors of both the caregiver and infant during feeding have been shown to contribute significantly to the overall success of the feeding and even the bonding process (Meyer et al., 1994).

In summary, the infant's early experiences with feeding form the foundation for important developmental functions. Because a cleft has the potential to interrupt the normal feeding process, this can have significant implications not only for nutrition but also for other functions that are important to the infant's development.

ANATOMY AND PHYSIOLOGY RELEVANT TO INFANT FEEDING

The oral, pharyngeal, and laryngeal anatomy of an infant is very different from that of an adult (Figure 5–1). There are differences not only in the size of the structures but also in their relative positions in the vocal tract. There are also significant differences in feeding physiology in that an infant's mode of feeding is through sucking and is dependent on an efficient suck–swallow–breathe synchrony.

Anatomy Relevant to Infant Feeding

The oral cavity of a newborn infant is small, and the tongue is relatively large (although only half the size of the adult tongue). As such, the tongue completely fills the oral cavity. The infant's *buccal pads* (encapsulated fat masses inside the cheek) are also relatively large and stabilize the lateral walls of the oral cavity. Because the infant has not yet developed teeth, the effective vertical dimension of the oral cavity is reduced in size, causing the tongue to rest in a more anterior position than is typically seen in the adult. The tongue tip protrudes past the alveolar ridge and maintains contact

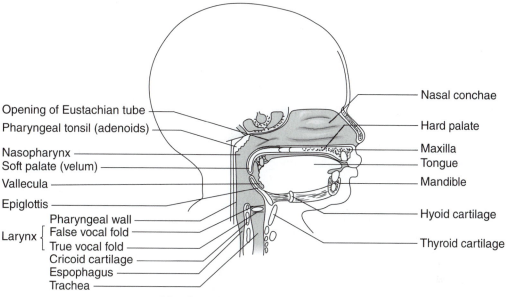

Opening of Eustachian tube

Pharyngeal tonsil (adenoids)

Nasopharynx

Soft palate (velum)

Vallecula

Epiglottis

Pharyngeal wall

Larynx {

False vocal fold

True vocal fold

Cricoid cartilage

Espophagus

Trachea

Nasal conchae

Hard palate

Maxilla

Tongue

Mandible

Hyoid cartilage

Thyroid cartilage

Mouth and pharynx of an newborn

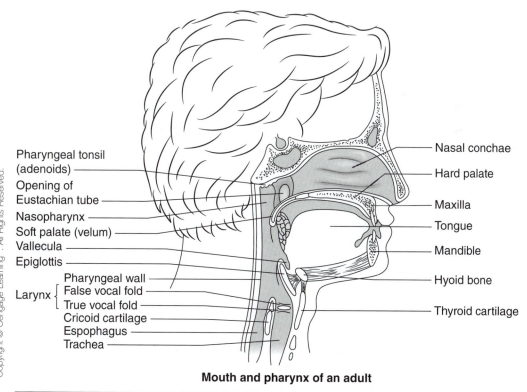

Pharyngeal tonsil (adenoids)

Opening of Eustachian tube

Nasopharynx

Soft palate (velum)

Vallecula

Epiglottis

Pharyngeal wall

Larynx {

False vocal fold

True vocal fold

Cricoid cartilage

Espophagus

Trachea

Nasal conchae

Hard palate

Maxilla

Tongue

Mandible

Hyoid bone

Thyroid cartilage

Mouth and pharynx of an adult

FIGURE 5–1 Anatomy of the head and neck as it relates to feeding in an infant as compared with an adult.

with the lower lip. The temporomandibular joint does not allow much movement of jaw because of undeveloped connective tissue, causing the mouth opening to be smaller in the infant than in the adult. All of these oral characteristics facilitate early *suckling*, characterized by extension–retraction movements of the tongue, as well as the development of more mature up–down tongue movements that are characteristic of true sucking (Arvedson & Brodsky, 2002; Miller, 2009; Morris & Klein, 1987; Wolf & Glass, 1992).

The pharynx of the newborn is short so that the tongue base, soft palate, and pharyngeal walls are all in close approximation. The inferior border of the velum rests just in front of the epiglottis, and the velum has a large area of contact with the tongue.

The size of the infant's larynx is one-third the size of an adult's larynx. It is high in the hypopharynx, residing adjacent to cervical vertebrae C-l through C-3. For comparison, the larynx of an adult is located at the C-6 to C-7 vertebral level. The high position of the infant larynx causes the epiglottis to pass superiorly to the free margin of the soft palate and project into the nasopharynx. The epiglottis is tubular, proportionally narrow, and more vertical in the infant as compared with the adult (Myer, Cotton, & Shott, 1995). The pharyngeal anatomy is well suited for the suck–swallow–breathe synchrony.

Physiology Relevant to Infant Feeding

The infant's feeding process is dependent on smooth synchronization of sucking, swallowing, and breathing. Sucking and swallowing occur in phases generally described as the oral, pharyngeal, and esophageal stages of swallowing.

Oral Phase

The oral phase of swallowing in infants is composed of rhythmic sucking, during which the oral structures work together to stabilize the nipple, create pressure gradients for fluid flow, and control the bolus before swallowing initiation. The presence of the rooting reflex aids in the search for the nipple and the subsequent lip seal around the nipple. The sucking reflex is initiated as the tongue elevates to squeeze the nipple against the alveolar ridge and hard palate. The compression of the nipple against this bony surface creates positive pressure within the nipple and causes the release of a small amount of fluid. The infant then initiates sucking, which requires a rhythmic forward–backward motion of the tongue. The tongue is cupped around the nipple, and a depression in the center of the tongue forms a groove. As the tongue moves backward during sucking, the infant's jaw drops, thus enlarging the space in the oral cavity. This action generates negative pressure, resulting in suction and expression of fluid from the nipple into the infant's oral cavity. Therefore, both nipple compression and the generation of negative pressure are essential for normal infant sucking (Figure 5–2).

Pharyngeal Phase

The pharyngeal phase of swallowing is initiated once the fluid bolus is channeled by the tongue into the pharynx. When the liquid reaches the posterior oral cavity, the tongue base, velum, and posterior pharyngeal wall all work together to provide the driving force for bolus transfer through the pharynx. The velum elevates (partly due to the backward movement of the tongue), and the velopharyngeal valve closes to completely separate the nasal cavity from the oral cavity. As the posterior aspect of the tongue moves downward and the sealed oral cavity is enlarged, negative pressure and suction are

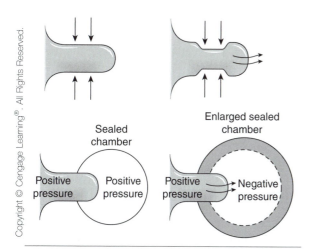

FIGURE 5–2 Comparison of positive pressure (compression) and negative pressure (suction) components during sucking.

created, propelling the fluid bolus to the pharynx. The bolus diverts around the epiglottis as the pharynx fills and contracts sequentially for swallowing (Newman, Cleveland, Blickman, Hillman, & Jaramillo, 1991). During swallowing, the larynx is closed by adduction of the true and false vocal folds, the forward and medial movement of the arytenoids, and the subsequent retroversion of the epiglottis (Ardran & Kemp, 1956; Koenig, Davies, & Thach, 1990; Mathew, 1991).

Throughout the sucking action, the infant continues to maintain nasal breathing. To facilitate this, the epiglottis is positioned around the back of the velum, which keeps the pharynx open and allows the nasal cavity to be in direct contact with the glottis for a continuous patent airway. However, at the time of swallow initiation, respiration ceases.

Esophageal Phase

The bolus moves through the pharynx and into the esophagus, where the esophageal phase of swallowing is initiated. The upper part of the esophagus, commonly referred to as the *upper*

esophageal sphincter (UES), is normally closed but stretches open as the bolus travels through the hypopharynx and into the esophagus. The *lower esophageal sphincter* (LES) relaxes to allow the bolus to enter the stomach. After each swallow occurs, the velum drops down to the base of the tongue and in front of the epiglottis, the tongue returns to an anterior position, sucking and breathing resume, and both the upper and lower esophageal sphincters maintain a closed position.

Synchrony of Sucking, Swallowing, and Respiration

Because the pharynx serves as a conduit for food as well as respiratory air, precise coordination of sucking, swallowing and breathing is crucial to prevent *aspiration* (entry of material into the airway) (Figure 5–3). The suck–swallow–breathe ratio during feeding is generally considered to be 1:1:1 or 2:1:1. Some variations to this pattern occur, particularly

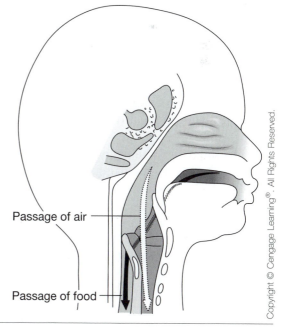

Passage of air

Passage of food

FIGURE 5–3 The pharynx as a conduit of food and air.

during the initial 2 to 3 minutes of feeding when the sucking rate is often higher (Bu'Lock, Woolridge, & Baum, 1990; Mathew, 1991; Wolf & Glass, 1992). Although additional respiratory effort is necessary to support the work of feeding, the intact infant is able to tolerate the decreased ventilation during feeding. This may not be the case in infants presenting with borderline respiratory reserve (Glass & Wolf, 1999; Mathew, 1988b; Mathew, Clark, Pronske, Luna-Solarzano, & Peterson, 1985).

Changes with Growth and Maturation

The size and anatomic relationships of the oral, pharyngeal, and laryngeal structures change significantly during the first 2 to 3 years of life (Figure 5–1). As a result, the process of feeding and swallowing changes as the infant grows and matures.

The oral cavity becomes larger, with concurrent mandibular growth and dental eruption. The tongue begins to descend and move back into the mouth, with the tip becoming positioned under the alveolar ridge. This increased oral space facilitates the development of more refined oral-motor skills for cup drinking, chewing, and speech production.

At the same time, the pharynx elongates and the larynx begins its gradual descent from C-3 to C-6, which is complete by age 3 (Sasaki, Levine, Laitman, Phil, & Crelin, 1977). Neuromuscular maturation, in addition to increased cartilage and connective tissue, results in increased mobility of the hyoid and larynx to elevate and provide sphincteric closure during swallowing. This allows maintenance of airway protection that was previously facilitated by the proximity of structures (Bosma, 1985; Bosma & Donner, 1980).

FEEDING PROBLEMS CAUSED BY CLEFTS AND OTHER CRANIOFACIAL ANOMALIES

The feeding problems of infants who have a cleft depend on the type of cleft (lip or palate) and the severity of the cleft (unilateral or bilateral; incomplete or complete).

Cleft Lip and Alveolus Only

Infants with a cleft of the primary palate (lip and alveolus) only usually do not have significant problems with feeding, especially if the cleft is unilateral. They may have initial problems in achieving an adequate lip seal on the nipple in order to generate effective negative pressure for sucking. With breastfeeding, however, the breast tends to conform to and fill in the cleft area. When bottle feeding, the use of a soft, wide-based nipple, as depicted in Figure 5–4, will close the area of the cleft and allow suction generation. The mother can also assist with lip closure by gently holding the upper lip together while the baby sucks. Infants with cleft lip and alveolus may

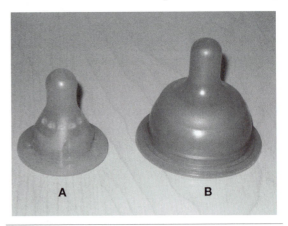

FIGURE 5–4 Basic categories of nipples. (A) Round cross-section. (B) Broad, flat cross-section.

Courtesy Claire K. Miller, Ph.D./Cincinnati Children's Hospital Medical Center & University of Cincinnati College of Medicine

also have initial difficulty in latching on to the nipple. However, once the nipple is placed intraorally, the infant's tongue and jaw movements are usually sufficient to produce compression of the nipple against the intact part of the alveolus and palate for effective sucking.

Cleft Palate Only

Infants with a small cleft of the velum only are often able to feed without special modifications. In fact, in some cases, the infant is able to occlude the cleft with the back of the tongue during part of the sucking movement, so that negative pressure can be obtained (Glass & Wolf, 1999).

Infants with a cleft that extends through the velum and hard palate have much more difficulty feeding for several reasons. The cleft palate results in an open cavity with oral and nasal coupling. Therefore, the infant is unable to generate negative pressure for suction. Infants with a complete cleft of the soft and hard palate are usually not able to breastfeed due to the fact that they will simply be unable to create negative pressure for suction. The use of a supplemental nursing system, such as the Medela Supplemental Nursing System™, may be of some benefit in supporting breastfeeding; however, the infant's growth and hydration status should be closely monitored. Supplemental or exclusive transition to bottle feeding is highly likely.

Depending on the extent of the cleft, the infant may also be unable to find a hard palatal surface for compression of the nipple. If placement cannot be achieved against an area of hard palate, the nipple will be pushed into the area of the cleft.

The open palate often results in *nasal regurgitation*, which is reflux of fluids into the nasopharyngeal and nasal cavities. This can cause discomfort and disorganization with breathing and feeding. In addition, the open cleft allows air to continue to flow in through the nose and then the mouth during feeding. This can result in an excessive intake of air and may cause the infant to become bloated or have episodes of frequent spitting up.

The difficulty with oral feeding can cause excessive expenditure of energy, and thus calories, during feeding. In addition, nasal regurgitation must be subtracted from total intake of formula. Therefore, weight gain and adequate nutrition during the early months of infancy is a primary concern for infants with cleft palate (Glass & Wolf, 1999; Jones, 1988; Redford-Badwal, Mabry, & Frassinelli, 2003). A full-term newborn infant generally needs 2 to 3 ounces of breast milk or formula per pound of body weight per day in order to gain weight appropriately (Butte, 2005; The Cleft Palate Foundation, 1998). Therefore, an infant who weighs 10 pounds requires between 20 and 30 ounces per day—a significant amount for an infant having feeding difficulty. As the infant gains weight, his or her daily intake should increase accordingly.

A final concern is for the parents. Most intact infants can complete a feeding within 20 to 30 minutes. The infant with a cleft palate usually takes much longer to feed. The lengthy feeding times due to the feeding difficulty can be very stressful for both the infant and caretaker, thus affecting the normally pleasurable bonding experience (Carlisle, 1998).

Fortunately, there are several effective methods for bottle-feeding an infant with cleft palate, using special bottles and nipples. These feeding devices allow the feeder to assist with the delivery of formula or breast milk. The use of assisted feeding techniques has been shown to be effective in mitigating the above problems for infants with clefts, although continued outcomes research is needed (Bessell et al., 2011; Shaw, Bannister, & Roberts, 1999).

Cleft Lip and Palate

The infant presenting with a cleft of the lip and palate generally has significant difficulty with all aspects of feeding because of the inability to achieve an anterior seal with the lips, inability to compress the nipple due to the open palate, and failure to generate negative pressure suction (Masarei, Sell, Habel, et al., 2007). Significant nasopharyngeal reflux of liquid secondary to the open nasopharynx is also present. Breastfeeding is usually not possible in this group of infants. As with infants with cleft palate only, the use of assisted feeding techniques is usually necessary for successful feeding.

After the Cleft Lip and Palate Repair

Postoperative feeding recommendations following cleft lip and palate repair vary among centers and remain a controversial topic (Katzel, Basile, Koltz, Marcus, & Firotto, 2009; Skinner, Arvedson, Jones, Spinner, & Rockwood, 1997). Immediate unrestricted feeding is allowed by some groups, whereas others recommend a restricted approach to facilitate good healing. For example, some centers discourage sucking following cleft lip and palate repair, and recommend the use of a cup or a spoon instead. Other centers may recommend supplemental tube feeding for a period of 7–10 days. In contrast, for a number of years some centers have implemented immediate, unrestricted feeding after the cleft repair without problems.

Other Craniofacial Anomalies

In addition to cleft lip and palate, there are other anomalies of the oral cavity, pharynx, or larynx that can cause or contribute to a feeding or swallowing problem. These anomalies include *micrognathia* (small mandible) and *macroglossia* (large tongue), which can interfere with the oral-motor mechanics of feeding and swallowing. Pharyngeal *stenosis* (narrowing) and vascular anomalies can cause compression in the esophagus or airway. A laryngeal cleft or tracheoesophageal fistula can result in aspiration during feeding secondary to communication between the esophagus and trachea. Cortical or cranial nerve involvement, resulting in hypotonia, hypertonia, or generalized oral-motor dysfunction, may affect the neuromuscular coordination required for sucking and swallowing. Finally, conditions that can cause airway compromise, such as *glossoptosis* (posterior displacement of the tongue in the pharynx), midface retrusion, congenital heart or lung disease, or *choanal atresia* (congenital closure of the opening to the pharynx from the back of the nose) can interfere with the suck–swallow–breathe sequence. Many of these anomalies are seen in craniofacial syndromes or conditions.

One such condition is Pierre Robin sequence, which includes micrognathia, glossoptosis, and cleft palate. Pierre Robin sequence can be isolated or can be part of certain syndromes, including Treacher Collins syndrome, Stickler's syndrome, and velocardiofacial syndrome. The characteristic micrognathia and retracted tongue position of Pierre Robin sequence can affect the infant's ability to compress the nipple adequately against the alveolar ridge to express breast milk or formula. In addition, the overall coordination of the suck–swallow–breathe triad may be disrupted (Lehman, Fishman, & Neiman, 1995; Miller, 2009; Shprintzen, 1992; van den Elzen et al., 2001). Glossoptosis, which is typical with Pierre Robin sequence, can cause chronic airway obstruction. This exacerbates the respiratory effort of feeding and can disrupt the sequential chain of suck–swallow–breathe sequences (Miller & Willging, 2007; Nassar, Marques, Trindade, & Bettiol, 2006; Shprintzen & Singer, 1992). Therefore, a patent airway must be confirmed before attempts at oral feeding (Bath & Buil, 1997). Some patients may require placement of a nasopharyngeal (NP) airway, although oral feedings can be done with the NP tube in place (Wagener, Rayatt, Tatman, Gornall, & Slator, 2002). Finally, if the infant has the typical U-shaped cleft palate, problems with generation of negative pressure also contribute to feeding difficulty.

Despite the problems, feeding modifications can be made to help the infant with Pierre Robin sequence feed successfully (Nassar et al., 2006; Kochel et al., 2011). If medical clearance is given for oral feedings, prone (on the tummy) or side-lying (on the side) positioning may help to position the tongue anteriorly and facilitate tongue movements during feeding (Arvedson & Brodsky, 2002; Glass & Wolf, 1999). However, if the infant has a cleft palate, prone positioning is generally not helpful, as the infant is not able to move the milk to the back of the mouth for swallowing. A standard, semi-reclined feeding position helps to minimize gravitational pull on the tongue. Side-lying positioning may be an option with use of a modified bottle. Despite these modifications, supplemental feedings are often necessary (Glass & Wolf, 1999).

Micrognathia and upper airway obstruction are treated in a variety of ways, including positioning, tracheotomy, tongue–lip adhesion, and mandibular distraction (Al-Samkari, Kane, Molter, & Vachharajani, 2010; Chigurupati & Myall, 2005; Izadi et al., 2003; Kochel et al., 2011; Mandell, Yellon, Bradley, Izadi & Gordon, 2004; Schaefer, Stadier, & Gosain, 2004; Tibesar, Price, & Moore, 2006; Zim, 2007).

Infants who undergo mandibular distraction to improve posterior airway space are unable to orally feed during the distraction procedure, as their jaws are immobilized and they are unable to suck. During that time, they are usually fed through a nasogastric (NG) tube. However, once the distraction procedure is completed, oral feeding can be resumed as before.

Moebius syndrome is another condition that affects infant feeding. Moebius syndrome is a genetic disorder that involves absence or underdevelopment of the abducent nerve (VI) and the facial nerve (VII). Affected individuals have weakness or lack of movement in the lips, which limits the infant's ability to achieve and maintain an adequate seal on the nipple. In addition, there may be a chronic open-mouth posture with limited range of movement in the jaw and tongue. A high palatal vault may cause difficulty in establishing an adequate tongue–palate seal. All of these conditions can have a profound effect on the oral-motor mechanics necessary for efficient sucking (Arvedson & Brodsky, 2002; Broussard & Borazjani, 2008). Excessive drooling and anterior loss of formula also commonly occur. Modified presentation of fluid is necessary for infants with Moebius syndrome due to the significantly restricted range of movement in the jaw, lips, and tongue. The use of feeder-assisted squeezing or presentation by a specialized feeding nipple or bottle is likely necessary.

Hemifacial microsomia results in various degrees of mandibular hypoplasia and facial weakness and is usually unilateral but actually can be bilateral (Stromland et al., 2007). This generally results in limitations to the range of motion in the jaw, lips, and tongue on one side. Utilization of the stronger side of the mouth during feeding while stabilizing the weaker side can reduce the feeding problems (Arvedson & Brodsky, 2002).

FEEDING METHODS, MODIFICATIONS, AND FACILITATION TECHNIQUES

With simple modifications, most infants with a cleft are able to feed with relative ease and obtain an adequate amount of nutrition in a reasonable amount of time. There is no single feeding method that will be successful for infants with different types of clefts or craniofacial abnormalities. Instead, the infant's performance during the initial feedings determines which feeding method and technique is most appropriate for that child (Miller, 2009; Miller, 2011; Wolf & Glass, 1992).

General feeding tips are summarized in Appendix 5–1. Also, the American Cleft Palate–Craniofacial Association (ACPA) has a video and online resources for parents and caregivers on how to feed a baby with a cleft (ACPA, 2012).

Breastfeeding

Most pediatricians and health care providers agree that breast milk is best for the newborn infant for several reasons. It contains the mother's antibodies against illnesses and therefore can provide the infant with some immunity. In addition, early food allergies can be avoided through the use of breast milk. It also has been suggested that feeding with breast milk offers some protection from otitis media (Aniansson, Svensson, Becker, & Ingvarsson, 2002; Paradise, Eister, & Tan, 1994). However, opinions regarding the feasibility of breastfeeding a child with a cleft vary across centers (Alexander-Doelle, 1997; Biancuzzo, 1998; Crossman, 1998; Darzi, Chowdri, & Blat, 1996; Kogo et al., 1997; Mei, Morgan, & Reilly, 2009; Reilly, Reid, & Skeat, 2007). As with other feeding methods, the success of breastfeeding depends on the location and severity of the cleft. If the mother wishes to breastfeed her infant with a cleft, consultation with a certified lactation consultant is advisable.

In general, breastfeeding is usually not a problem for the infant who has only a cleft lip because the infant should still be able to achieve adequate suction. Even with a cleft in the lip and alveolus, the breast tends to fill the opening by molding to the shape of the oral cavity. Upright positioning while attempting breastfeeding is generally recommended. Supplemental bottle-feeding or a complete switch to the bottle may be necessary if difficulties with breastfeeding are immediately apparent.

As noted previously, breastfeeding an infant with a cleft palate is very challenging because the infant is unable to generate negative pressure for suction. This can be a particular disappointment for new mothers. If the mother of a child with cleft palate wishes to try breastfeeding, she should confer with a feeding specialist or lactation consultant who has experience feeding infants with cleft palate. Monitoring weight gain closely during a trial period of breastfeeding will provide both objective evidence regarding its feasibility and definitive information as to whether a supplementary feeding method is needed. Future research investigations that monitor the success of breastfeeding, document the efficacy of management strategies, and follow overall infant feeding outcomes are needed to establish generalized clinical protocols (Reilly, Reid, & Skeat, 2007).

If a trial of breastfeeding proves unsuccessful and the mother still wishes to continue breastfeeding, a supplemental nursing system may be an option (Wolf & Glass, 1992). The supplemental nursing system utilizes a reservoir that is filled with formula or milk that the mother has expressed. A thin tube, connected to the reservoir, is taped above the mother's breast and nipple. As the infant latches onto the breast for feeding, the mother supplements the breast milk with milk that is squeezed manually from the reservoir through the tube. The flow of milk needs to be simultaneous with the baby's efforts at sucking. With this method, the baby is supplemented at the breast while maintaining the important physical contact for the infant and mother. In addition, this method stimulates the breast to continue to produce and maintain the milk supply. Drawbacks to the use of supplemental nursing systems include the potential for difficulty in maintaining the proper flow rate, though adjustable flow rate systems are available on some supplemental nursing systems. There is also the possibility that the baby will reject intraoral placement of the tube during breastfeeding.

After attempting breastfeeding with modifications, some mothers may find that using a modified bottle and/or a modified nipple is easier and more efficient. These mothers can still use breast milk, but in this case, the breast milk is given via the modified bottle or nipple.

Breast milk can be expressed through the use of a breast pump, which can be purchased or rented through a local home health supplier. In some cases, breast pumps are covered by insurance, but this usually requires a prescription in the baby's name and a letter from the physician describing the special circumstances that make this equipment necessary.

There are several kinds of breast pumps, including manual pumps, battery-operated pumps, and electric pumps. The electric pumps tend to be more efficient and faster than the manual pumps. As such, they allow both breasts to be pumped at the same time, thus reducing the amount of time required to express the milk.

Modified Nipples

If problems with feeding are immediately apparent, a variety of specialized nipples are available, as described in Table 5–1. Instructions for feeding using adapted nipples are described in Appendix 5–2. When choosing a nipple for enhancement of sucking, there are five basic characteristics to consider with the nipple: pliability shape, size, hole type, and hole size (Mathew, 1988a; Miller, 2011).

Pliability

The nipple must be pliable enough to release breast milk or formula, with limited compression and suction. At the same time, the nipple has to be firm enough to provide an appropriate degree of proprioceptive input to stimulate sucking. A soft nipple tends to have a higher flow rate than a firmer nipple and thus requires less compression effort and suction. The degree of pliability must match the infant's strength of sucking and provide an appropriate flow rate to allow the baby to coordinate the suck–swallow–breathe sequence. For example, nipples designed for premature infants ("preemie" nipples) or the specialized Pigeon nipple® (Figure 5–5) may be used for infants with cleft palate because they are very soft and pliable. A standard nipple can also be softened through boiling.

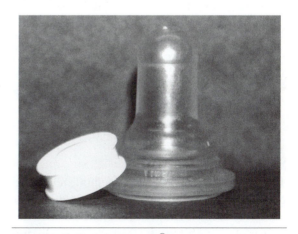

FIGURE 5–5 Pigeon nipple®.
Courtesy Claire K. Miller, Ph.D./Cincinnati Children's Hospital Medical Center & University of Cincinnati College of Medicine

---

TABLE 5–1 Commercially Available Nipples and Bottles

Nipples

- **Orthodontic Nipple:** This style nipple is wide based and has a fast flow rate. It can be used with a squeeze bottle for infants who show good ability to rapidly coordinate the suck–swallow–breath sequence.

- **Pigeon Nipple® (Pigeon Corporation, Chuo-ku, Tokyo, Japan):** The pigeon nipple® has a thick side that is placed against the roof of the mouth and a thin side that enables the infant to express milk through a suckling motion. Due to its thin wall, it does not vent rapidly and therefore has a tendency to collapse. The pigeon nipple® can be used with any type of bottle, including bottles designed to prevent excessive air intake, such as the Playtex Ventair® or Dr. Brown® bottle. The feeder can squeeze the bottle to assist with fluid flow.

- **Ross® Premature Nipple:** This nipple is smaller, thinner, and softer than a standard nipple, making suction easier. This is a fast-flow nipple that should be used only by those infants who have demonstrated tolerance for the increased respiratory effort associated with fast fluid flow.

- **Standard Traditional Nipple:** This nipple (widely available) has a narrow base and has been shown to be effective when used in conjunction with a squeeze bottle while feeding infants who have demonstrated the ability to develop some suction independently. A slight enlargement of the nipple hole may be necessary.

Specialized Nipple and Bottle Systems

- **Mead Johnson Cleft Lip/Palate Nurser (Mead Johnson Nutrition, Glenview, Illinois):** This is a soft bottle that is easily squeezed and also has a long, soft, crosscut nipple. A standard nipple will also fit onto the Mead Johnson bottle. The caregiver can help to regulate the liquid through assistive squeezing. The use of either the crosscut nipple or a standard nipple with a modified hole depends on the oral-motor skills of the infant.

- **Ross Cleft Palate Nurser:** This bottle has a long, thin nipple that requires assistive squeezing to deliver milk to the posterior part of the oral cavity. The long length may cause gagging in some infants. In addition, the small diameter of this nipple does not facilitate tongue movements for sucking. Fluid flow is steady and rapid, but this can be difficult for infants who cannot tolerate a rapid flow rate. In fact, the rapid rate could result in disorganization of airway protection and possible aspiration.

- **SpecialNeeds® Feeder (formerly the Haberman and Mini-Haberman Feeder™):** This specialized nipple and bottle system is designed to allow the release of milk through the infant's compressions alone, without the need for suction. There is a soft nipple that is filled with breast milk or formula. The nipple has a one-way valve that limits the intake of air. It also prevents rapid fluid flow because it only opens when the infant sucks. In addition, the nipple has raised markings that indicate the position of the slit valve in the infant's mouth; the longer the raised mark, the greater the flow. To adjust the rate of flow, the feeder is turned so that the required line (minimum, medium, or maximum) points toward the baby's nose. Light finger pressure can be applied on the nipple to assist with fluid flow as needed. The Mini SpecialNeeds® Feeder is a smaller version of the feeder that is designed for smaller or premature babies with cleft palate or other special feeding problems.

- **Medela SoftCup® Feeder and Bottle:** The SoftCup Feeder is designed to be used with the Medela 80 ml polypropylene bottle. Other bottles can be used, but some leakage may occur in the collar area. The SoftCup Feeder does not require the infant to actively suck because fluid is delivered via a small flexible cup-like reservoir. The feeder controls the flow rate.

© Cengage Learning 2014

Shape

The shape of the nipple has to facilitate adequate contact between the nipple and the tongue for compression. The shape also should enhance the oral-motor patterns desired during sucking (Wolf & Glass, 1992). Nipple shapes basically fall into two categories: traditional nipples and orthodontic nipples (Figure 5–4). The traditional nipple has a straight configuration, which gradually tapers to a flared base. The orthodontic nipple has a broad, flat bulb-type end that flares to a large, wide base. This style is perhaps best known as the NUK® nipple; however, many manufacturers, including Gerber and Playtex, now make nipples shaped similarly to the original NUK style. These nipples are generally advantageous for infants with cleft lip and alveolus as they may conform to the cleft and reduce air leakage while sucking.

Length

The length of the nipple should be based on what is needed to provide adequate contact between the nipple and tongue. Nipple length can vary substantially with regard to the type of base and the distance from the tip to the base, especially for those nipples that have tapered bases. The strength of the infant's suck, the degree of lip closure around the nipple, and the control the feeder provides to maintain the nipple position are other factors that should be considered.

Hole Type

Both the type and the size of the nipple hole determine flow rate (Mathew, 1990). Nipples include either a standard round hole or a crosscut hole, which is basically an "X" configuration. A standard nipple hole can be modified to a crosscut with a single-edged sterile razor blade. The crosscut configuration allows the milk to flow only when the infant compresses the nipple, which makes the crosscut open. This allows the infant to control the milk flow with the normal rhythm of sucking and swallowing and prevents the infant from getting too much liquid, which can cause problems with coordinating sucking, swallowing, and airway protection during feeding.

Hole Size

The size of the nipple hole can vary widely across different styles of nipples. A nipple with a traditional hole should have an opening that is large enough so that when the bottle is held upside down, the liquid drips out but does not run out rapidly. A standard nipple can be enlarged or slit to increase the fluid flow rate; however, the increased flow may cause the infant to have difficulty with coordination of swallowing and breathing.

Table 5–2 compares the characteristics of the commonly used nipples. The type of nipple chosen should be based on the type of cleft and the baby's oral-motor/feeding skills as determined by the initial feeding evaluation.

TABLE 5–2 Characteristics of Commonly Used Nipples

Nipple Type	Pliability	Flow Rate	Shape	Hole Type
SpecialNeeds® Feeder	Soft	Feeder regulated	Slit	
Mead Johnson	Soft	Feeder regulated	Crosscut	
Orthodontic	Soft	Fast	Broad, flat	Hole on top surface of tip
Premature	Soft	Medium, Fast	Traditional	Hole and crosscut
Ross Cleft	Soft	Fast	Long, thin	Large hole
Traditional	Medium	Low	Traditional	Hole and crosscut, several holes

Flexible Bottles and Assisted Fluid Delivery

Specialized bottle and nipple systems are commercially available for infants with cleft palate. Instructions for feeding using specialized bottle systems are described in Appendix 5–2.

The Mead Johnson™ Cleft Palate Nurser (Figure 5–6) is a flexible bottle that allows the feeder to express the milk as needed by squeezing the bottle. This helps the infant to conserve energy and reduce calorie expenditure during feeding. This nurser comes with a specialized nipple, but other nipples can be used with this flexible bottle. Even use of a simple plastic bottle liner in conjunction with a variety of nipples can be effective for providing assistance with breast milk or formula flow. The feeder can apply intermittent pressure to the liner to push fluid out as the infant compresses the nipple (Barone & Tallman, 1998). Pushing the air out of the liner before the feeding reduces excess intake of air. Similarly, the SpecialNeeds® Feeder allows feeder-assisted delivery of the milk. In this case, the longer nipple allows the feeder to compress it to express the milk as needed (Figure 5–7).

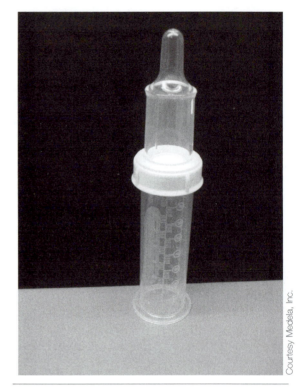

FIGURE 5–7 SpecialNeeds® Feeder by Medela.

Regardless of the device used, the pressure applied to a squeeze bottle, plastic liner, or nipple reservoir must be in rhythm with the infant's suck and swallow efforts to ensure that the infant does not become discoordinated with the suck–swallow–breathe synchrony. An inappropriately rapid rate or continuous squeezing will result in an increased rate of swallowing, which will decrease available breathing time. This may cause the infant to have problems maintaining an appropriate respiratory rate and could cause aspiration into the airway.

Positioning the Infant

Placing the infant in a horizontal position during feeding is a common mistake. This position increases the potential for nasal regurgitation, coughing, and sneezing. In addition, there may be

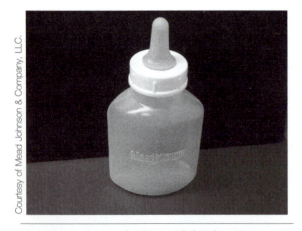

FIGURE 5–6 Mead Johnson Cleft Palate Nurser.

flooding of the Eustachian tube and reflux into the middle ear, causing middle ear effusion. A semi-upright position (of at least 60 degrees) is best for feeding because it facilitates control of jaw, cheek, lip, and tongue movements for sucking and swallowing coordination (Morris & Klein, 1987). This position also allows gravity to assist with swallowing, and it helps to prevent nasal regurgitation (Wolf & Glass, 1992). The baby's head should be supported in a neutral anterior–posterior alignment with the shoulders symmetric and forward, trunk in midline, and the hips flexed. The use of a bottle with an angled neck provides a downward flow of milk and simplifies feeding the infant in upright positioning.

Positioning the Nipple

Finding the optimal intraoral position for the nipple is critical for feeding success. The difference in nipple placement of only a few millimeters can affect feeding success (Clarren, Anderson, & Wolf, 1987). It is important to position the nipple under the bone of the palate to provide a base for nipple compression. Using the right nipple size and shape, based on the patient's cleft, facilitates proper intraoral positioning.

Pacing Intake

The feeder should carefully pace the flow rate during feeding by providing fluid in rhythm with the infant's sucking compressions (Law-Morstatt, Judd, Snyder, Baier, & Dhanireddy, 2003). Flow can be regulated by tilting the nipple slightly upward or partially removing the nipple from the oral cavity. The feeder should modify the pace when there are signs of stress, including eye widening, changes in facial expression, a decrease in alertness, or subtle avoidance of feeding. If the infant begins feeding rapidly and then shows signs of swallowing disorganization, such as coughing

or choking, the feeder should slow the pace of fluid presentation. If the infant begins to slow down or stop sucking during the feeding, this suggests that the infant has tired and needs a pause before continuing feeding. The infant may show signs of excessive air intake and need a pause in feeding to allow burping. Although the feeder must be able to deliver enough nutrition before the infant becomes tired, allowing enough time to facilitate safe feeding is vital to feeding success. Consulting a dietitian about the use of a higher calorie formula preparation with a lower volume intake requirement will allow the infant to spend less time feeding and to use a slower pace of intake while still ingesting an adequate amount of calories for growth (Butte, 2005; Kovar, 1997).

Oral Facilitation Strategies

As a result of an oral-motor/feeding assessment, oral facilitation techniques, such as jaw and cheek support, may be recommended to increase the infant's oral control during feeding (Hwang, Lin, Coster, Bigsby, & Vergara, 2010). The type of bottle used can support the use of certain strategies to increase oral control. For example, the use of a small diameter bottle, such as the infant Volu-Feed Disposable™ Nurser (60 ml capacity), allows the feeder to use hand and finger positioning to facilitate support to the jaw and cheeks during feeding (Miller, 2011; Morris & Klein, 1987).

Preventing Excessive Air Intake

Because the infant with a cleft palate takes in an increased amount of air during feeding, the feeder may need to increase the frequency of burping. As a general rule of thumb, the infant should be burped after every ounce to prevent the discomfort associated with the intake of air that inevitably occurs with each feeding.

Case Report

Appropriate Positioning and Placement

Lydia was born with Pierre Robin sequence with the characteristic micrognathia, glossoptosis, and wide, bell-shaped cleft palate. The potential for upper airway obstruction secondary to the posterior placement of the tongue was analyzed by continuous oxygen saturation monitoring and a formal sleep study. The results of the sleep study were within normal limits, and oxygen saturation levels were maintained except during the mother's initial attempts at oral feedings. Lydia was described as being a poor feeder with little sucking, frequent gasping, and oxygen desaturations. Despite the mother's best efforts, Lydia's intake was minimal (5–10 ml) before she would completely "shut down" and fall asleep, usually 10 minutes into the feeding.

A speech pathology oral-motor/feeding consultation was requested. The results of the evaluation indicated normal oral reflexes with appropriate rooting, as well as the ability to initiate and sustain a rhythmical nonnutritive sucking pattern. The mother explained that she had tried numerous nipples and bottles without success, including two types of cleft palate nipple and bottle systems.

Observation was then made of the mother as she demonstrated the methods she had been using to feed her baby. She positioned Lydia in a semi-reclined, cradled position as she offered her a standard nipple, which had been slit to assist with a faster milk delivery. Upon presentation of the nipple, Lydia made a few tentative sucking attempts as the milk rapidly flowed from the nipple. She coughed, sputtered, and pulled away from the nipple. An oxygen desaturation event was documented. The mother attempted to place the nipple intraorally again and had difficulty placing the nipple onto the tongue body. She continued with these attempts, but the baby continued with the same pattern of resistance and intermittent oxygen desaturations. Lydia then fell asleep after struggling to achieve intake of only 10 ml. The remainder of the feeding was then presented via oral gavage.

During the next feeding time, the speech-language pathologist implemented several interventional techniques. First, Lydia was placed in a more upright position as opposed to the semi-reclined cradle position. This helped Lydia avoid further posterior displacement of her tongue during her efforts at feeding and reduced nasal regurgitation into the nasal cavity. Nonnutritive oral stimulation was provided with Lydia in the upright position to help increase her alertness and to stimulate nonnutritive oral movements. The SpecialNeeds® Feeder was then presented intraorally, with positioning of the nipple slit valve to minimum flow. The longer size of this nipple made placement onto the tongue easier. In addition, the lack of liquid flow from the nipple before active sucking allowed Lydia to become accustomed to the presence of the nipple without being flooded by formula. Once Lydia began sucking, a gentle assistive squeeze was given to deliver a small amount of formula in synchrony with her sucking attempts. Lydia was able to successfully transfer this small amount of formula without any clinical signs of swallowing dysfunction. A cycle of approximately eight assistive squeezes was completed before Lydia showed some disorganization by again pulling away from the nipple. After a brief pause, additional feeding trials revealed that Lydia could handle approximately five sequences of assistive squeezes for completion of suck–swallow before requiring a pause for breathing. Repetition of the cycles with pause intervals was done for approximately 20 minutes, resulting in an intake of approximately 30 ml. Over a 3-week time period, the volume of her oral intake gradually increased with the use of intermittent assistive squeezing and pause intervals during feedings. Eventually the transition to complete oral feedings was accomplished with maintenance of appropriate oxygen saturation levels.

Managing Nasal Regurgitation

Infants with a cleft palate often experience nasal regurgitation. When this occurs, the feeder should stop and allow the infant time to cough or sneeze to clear the nasal passage. If nasal regurgitation occurs frequently during feeding, the caregiver should ensure that the infant is in an upright position that allows gravity to assist with downward flow of liquid. If coughing occurs frequently in conjunction with the nasal regurgitation, the feeder should consider using a slower flow nipple. Also, slowing the presentation of fluid helps to reduce the nasal regurgitation.

Consistency of Method

Consistency in how the baby is fed contributes to overall feeding success. The baby should be fed in the same position, with the same nipple and bottle and with the same technique during each feeding. The feeder must learn how to easily position the baby, how much of an assistive squeeze is required, how long to keep feeding, how often to burp the baby, and how to read the baby's cues related to feeding. If several different nipples and bottles are intermittently tried, and varying positions and different rates of assistive squeezing by a range of feeders are used, it is almost certain that feeding confusion and a poor feeding outcome will result. Fortunately, normal maturation and increased feeding experience of the infant and caregiver helps to gradually improve the feeding process in spite of variations in method which may occur.

Use of Feeding Obturators

A *feeding obturator* a prosthetic appliance that can be used in the first few months of life to assist the infant with cleft palate in feeding (refer to Figures 5–8A and 5–8B). It is retained in the crevices of the cleft and provides a partial seal between the mouth and the nasal cavity. The obturator keeps the tongue from resting inside the cleft, and it provides a solid

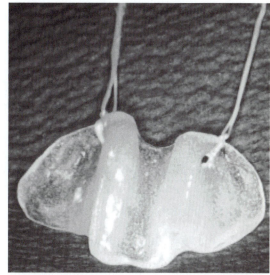

Courtesy Claire K. Miller, Ph.D./Cincinnati Children's Hospital Medical Center & University of Cincinnati College of Medicine

A

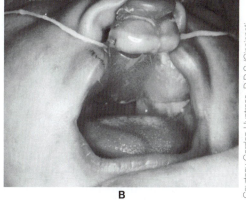

Courtesy Gordon Huntress, D.D.S./Cincinnati Children's Hospital Medical Center & University of Cincinnati College of Medicine

B

FIGURE 5–8 (A and B) (A) An infant-feeding obturator. (B) An infant-feeding obturator in place. This type of obturator provides a separation of the nasal cavity from the oral cavity, which helps to eliminate the regurgitation of liquids into the nose. The feeding appliance also keeps the tongue from resting inside the cleft, and it provides a solid surface so that the tongue can achieve compression of the nipple in order to express the milk.

surface so that the tongue can achieve compression of the nipple against the plate. A pediatric dentist or prosthodontist is the professional who can construct the feeding appliance and check it frequently so that it can be modified periodically as the child grows.

There are differing views regarding the use of feeding obturators for infants with cleft palate (Choi, Kleinheinz, Joos, & Komposch, 1991; Crossman, 1998; Delgado, Schaaf, & Emrich, 1992; Kogo et al., 1997; Kochel et al., 2011; Masarei, Wade, Mars, Sommerlad, & Sell, 2007; Osuji, 1995; Savion & Huband, 2005; Sultana, Rahman, Nessa, & Alam, 2011). Some craniofacial centers use feeding obturators routinely, believing that the appliance improves the ability of the infant to compress the nipple (Crossman, 1998), which can lead to better weight gain (Balluff & Udin, 1986). Obturators do not improve the generation of negative pressure, however (Choi et al., 1991).

Most craniofacial centers do not routinely use these appliances because they feel that with modifications of the nipple or bottle, correct positioning, and appropriate feeding techniques, the obturator simply is not necessary. In fact, research has shown on significant difference in feeding abilities for infants fitted with a maxillary plate compared to those without a plate (Glenny et al., 2004). In addition, there are certain disadvantages to using an obturator, including the expense and need for periodic replacement to accommodate growth. Retention of the obturator can be challenging because the infant has no teeth to stabilize it. Finally, there can be irritation of the oral tissues, and the obturator can cause hygiene concerns.

Oral Hygiene

With all infants, it is important to maintain good oral hygiene. Although the mouths of infants tend to be self-cleaning, it is particularly important to attend to oral hygiene if the infant has a cleft. This is because the open cleft allows fluid to enter the cleft area and nose, even with an upright feeding position. The fluid can mix with mucous secretions from the mouth and nose and form a hard crust, which can become infected, causing irritation and soreness.

For good oral hygiene, the caregiver should cleanse the cleft and surrounding areas following feedings. This can be done by gently wiping the mucous membrane in the oral cavity using a washcloth, a small piece of gauze, or a toothette®, which is soft and spongy. These can be moistened with plain water or water with hydrogen peroxide. Although the caregiver should be careful not to cause discomfort or injury during the cleansing process, it should be remembered that the cleft is not a wound, and therefore it will not be sore to touch during gentle cleansing.

Transitioning to a Cup

Most infants are ready to transition to the cup by 8 or 9 months of age, although some show readiness as early as 6 to 8 months of age (Lang, Lawrence, & Orme, 1994). The initial response to the cup is generally sucking, with tongue protrusion and loss of liquid from the mouth. The infant's oral skills for cup drinking gradually increase so that she is able to take one or two sip-swallows as the caregiver holds the cup. It is often beneficial initially to use a slightly thickened liquid to slow the liquid flow during early cup training.

There are many cup options for weaning the infant from a bottle to a cup. Selecting a cup that does not promote continued sucking is important. A small open cup without a spout, straw, or valve is generally the best option for transitioning away from sucking and toward

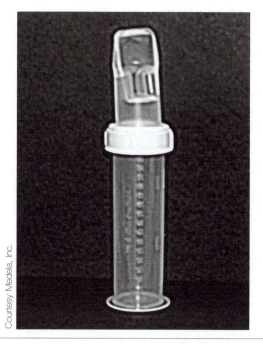

Courtesy Medela, Inc.

FIGURE 5–9   The Medela SoftCup® feeder. This can be used as an alternative during the transitional period between a bottle and cup.

true cup-drinking skills. Using the Medela SoftCup® Feeder is an alternative during the transitional period (Figure 5–9). Milk or breast milk is delivered through a narrow, flexible cup reservoir, facilitating development of oral skills for handling small amounts of liquid from a cup.

Most surgeons recommend weaning the infant from the bottle before palate repair because sucking may cause a breakdown of the repair. Therefore, weaning an infant with cleft palate from bottle to cup drinking should be done sometime before 9 or 10 months of age, which is the typical time for the palate repair.

Introduction of Solid Foods

Solid foods can be introduced to the baby with an unrepaired cleft palate at the same time as with any infant. The timing of solid food introduction is usually dependent on the preferences of the pediatrician and parent. Usually, rice cereals and strained foods are presented around 6 months of age. The baby will respond to the spoon-feedings at first by suckling. This may result in food being pushed into the nasal cavity. As the baby becomes more skilled in eating and begins to use more mature tongue patterns, this occurs less often. Mixing the pureed fruit with the cereal provides a degree of thickness that can reduce the tendency for nasal reflux. The feeder can assist the transition to solids by using appropriate positioning, small boluses, and a slow pace, and by alternating food with liquid to assist with clearance. The slow rate of presentation is particularly important because it allows the baby to gradually learn how to direct the food around the area of the cleft. The feeder should watch the baby for cues to know when to present the next bite. The baby's cues include leaning forward or opening the mouth in anticipation of the spoon. Placing the spoon onto the baby's tongue encourages the baby to close his or her lips on the spoon and stimulate active tongue movements to transfer the food for swallowing. This is especially important following the surgery for cleft lip repair. Rapid spoon-feeding or presentation of large spoonfuls can cause more frequent nasal regurgitation as well as disorganized swallowing.

The transition to more textured foods, including easily dissolvable and later bite-sized, easy-to-manage table foods, also can be introduced in the same sequence as for other children. Foods should initially be offered, with assistance of the feeder, with the baby seated in an upright position to reduce nasal regurgitation. When developmentally appropriate, the baby should be provided with guided opportunities to practice finger feeding with small pieces of crunchy but very easily dissolvable solid foods such as toddler crackers and cookies, as well as soft, easy-to-manage food items such as bite-sized pieces of soft fruits, shredded cheese, or pasta pieces. This helps to develop independence with self-feeding, gives the baby practice with the tongue movements around the cleft, and increases the efficiency of skills needed for mastication. If food is observed passing from the nose or becomes lodged in the area of the cleft, it should be removed gently with either a finger or a swab. Foods that are acidic or spicy should be avoided because the lining of the nose is particularly sensitive to this kind of food. As the baby's oral-motor skills become more proficient, the baby will learn to efficiently manage transfer of solids for swallowing.

ASSESSMENT AND MANAGEMENT OF COMPLEX FEEDING PROBLEMS

Weight gain of infants with demonstrated feeding problems should be monitored closely by the pediatrician. If there is any evidence of inadequate weight gain, the pediatrician may consider the need for further assessment of feeding. In addition, some infants present with complex feeding problems that are not easily resolved with simple modifications. Signs of significant feeding dysfunction or airway protection problems include the inability to establish and maintain a coordinated suck–swallow–breathe sequence, coughing or choking, color change during or after feeding, increased respiratory rate, and oxygen desaturations during feedings. The infant with significant feeding problems may respond to feeding attempts by arching or refusing to accept the nipple. If the infant has these clinical signs or takes 45 minutes or longer to feed, with clearly increased effort and relatively little intake, then a clinical oral-motor/feeding evaluation and/or instrumental swallowing examination is indicated.

Clinical Assessment

A clinical assessment of feeding should be performed by a feeding specialist (i.e., a qualified speech-language pathologist or occupational therapist). In addition, imaging studies of swallowing should be considered to assess the infant's ability to safely feed and to determine the effect of compensatory strategies on the infant's feeding performance. By assessing the infant's structures, specific oral-motor strengths and weaknesses, and responsiveness to compensatory strategies, the clinician may be able to determine an effective way to maximize the child's ability to feed orally. The ultimate goal is to find and implement a feeding method for the infant that results in adequate nutrition and weight gain, while facilitating the suck–swallow–breathe synchrony for safe and efficient feeding.

Videofluoroscopic Swallowing Study (VFSS)

A *videofluoroscopic swallowing study*, also referred to as a *modified barium swallow*, is generally performed by a radiologist and a speech-language pathologist. The videofluoroscopic study allows an overall view of the oral, pharyngeal, and esophageal phases of swallowing as well as the interactions between the phases. Swallowing function, as well as the infant's ability to maintain airway protection during swallowing, is carefully assessed. The degree of nasopharyngeal reflux and the occurrence of penetration or aspiration during swallowing can be documented. The infant's protective reaction to aspirated material can also be assessed. Compensatory strategies, such as positional adaptations, different nipples, and pacing of presentations, can be tested to determine their effect on improving the feeding process (Arvedson & Brodsky, 2002; Kramer, 1985; Newman et al., 1991). Disadvantages of the videofluoroscopic study include radiation to the infant as well as the feeder during the study, the necessity of adding barium contrast to the formula (which increases the viscosity and results in an unfamiliar taste), and the fact that the swallows viewed represent a relatively small sample of feeding overall.

Fiberoptic Endoscopic Evaluation of Swallowing (FEES)

Pediatric *fiberoptic endoscopic evaluation of swallowing* (FEES) involves the transnasal passage of an endoscope for viewing of the pharyngeal and laryngeal structures (Willging, 1995). The focus of this study is on assessing the integrity of airway protection during swallowing. FEES also provides information regarding sensory threshold in the pharynx and larynx (Willging & Thompson, 2005; Aviv et al., 1998). Advantages of the FEES procedure include the ability to clearly visualize pharyngeal and laryngeal structures as well as the spontaneous swallowing of secretions. Feeding can be assessed using the infant's customary bottle and nipple and the usual formula. Small amounts (< 1 ml) of green food coloring or liquid AquADEKs™ (multivitamin and mineral supplement) are added to enhance visualization of the bolus during the study. Compensatory swallowing strategies can be tried during the FEES study without the time limitations of fluoroscopy. Disadvantages include the

temporary loss of view that occurs as the velopharyngeal valve closes around the scope during the swallow. This is generally not a problem with single swallows as the structures quickly return to their resting position, thus restoring the view. This is a disadvantage when viewing rapid chain swallowing sequences, which are characteristic of early infancy, because the view is obscured with more frequency.

Interdisciplinary Feeding Team Evaluation

In severe cases, an evaluation by a team of feeding specialists is indicated. Typically, an interdisciplinary feeding team consists of a core group of medical professionals that may include a gastroenterologist, nutritionist, nurse, speech-language pathologist, occupational therapist, behavioral psychologist, otolaryngologist, pulmonologist, and consulting radiologist. The composition of interdisciplinary feeding teams varies among centers (Lefton-Greif & Arvedson, 1997; Miller et al., 2001; Rudolph, 1994). With the coordinated assessment of these specialists, management and long-term planning for treatment of complicated feeding problems can be accomplished.

Alternative Feeding Methods for Severe Cases

When the feeding problem is not easily resolved with modifications of the nipple or bottle, supplemental feeding through an *orogastric* or *nasogastric (NG) tube* may be required for a period of time. During this time period, treatment strategies for improving oral-motor function for feeding are provided, as appropriate. If the feeding problems persist for a period of time and cannot be adequately resolved with other measures, *gastrostomy (G) tube* feeding may be considered. This is particularly indicated if the infant presents with abnormal oral reflexes or shows poor ability to coordinate airway protection with swallowing during a videofluoroscopic or endoscopic swallowing study. A gastrostomy tube is inserted in the stomach through a surgical procedure and may remain in place for an extended period of time. The tube is removed if and when the infant shows signs of considerable progress with oral feeding skill development and oral intake volume (Rudolph, 1994).

SUMMARY

Whatever feeding method is chosen, it is important that the feeding process be relatively easy and efficient. Overall, the feeding method should allow the infant to receive an adequate amount of intake for nutrition and weight gain. It should be easy enough so that the infant can conserve energy and efficient enough so that it does not cause lengthy feeding times and eventual frustration for the caregiver. Consistency of nipple and bottle use is as important as the consistency of the feeder's method. The feeding system should allow the infant to experience some sucking to support and encourage normal oral-motor skill development. The option chosen should be relatively inexpensive and readily available.

Finally, it is important that the feeding process is made to be a pleasurable experience for both the infant and the caregiver. It should not be forgotten that the time spent in feeding serves as an important part of the bonding process as well as the foundation for early sensorimotor and developmental experiences.

FOR REVIEW AND DISCUSSION

1. Describe the normal swallowing process and how it changes with growth.

2. What are the reasons that cleft palate causes feeding difficulty? Why is there less of a problem with cleft lip?

3. What are some reasons that breastfeeding is particularly difficult for a baby with cleft palate? How would you counsel the mother about alternative feeding methods?

4. What modifications can be made to a nipple in order to assist the baby with a cleft palate in feeding?

5. Describe different types of bottles that are commercially available for infants with cleft palate.

6. Discuss some feeding facilitation techniques that may be helpful for a child with feeding difficulties.

7. What are the reasons that an upright feeding position is preferable to a supine position?

8. How would you counsel the caregiver to deal with oral hygiene for the infant with a cleft?

REFERENCES

Alexander-Doelle, A. (1997). Breastfeeding and cleft palates. *AWHONN Lifelines, 1*(4), 27.

Al-Samkari, H. T., Kane, A. A., Molter, D. W., & Vachharajani, A. (2010). Neonatal outcomes of Pierre Robin Sequence: An institutional experience. *Clinical Pediatrics, 49*(12), 1117–1122.

American Cleft Palate–Craniofacial Association (ACPA). (2012). Feeding your baby. Accessed May 28, 2012, from http://www.cleftline.org/parents-individuals/feeding-your-baby/.

Aniansson, G., Svensson, H., Becker, M., & Ingvarsson, L. (2002). Otitis media and feeding with breast milk of children with cleft palate. *Scandinavian Journal of Plastic and Reconstructive Surgery, 36,* 9–15.

Ardran, G. M., & Kemp, F. H. (1956). Closure and opening of the larynx during swallowing. *British Journal of Radiology, 29,* 205–208.

Arvedson, J., & Brodsky, L. (Eds.). (2002). *Pediatric swallowing and feeding: Assessment and management* (2nd ed.). San Diego, CA: Singular Publishing Group.

Aviv, J. E., Kim, T., Thomson, J. E., Sunshine, S., Kaplan, S., & Close, L. G. (1998). Fiberoptic endoscopic evaluation of swallowing with sensory testing (FEESST) in healthy controls. *Dysphagia, 13*(2), 87–92.

Balluff, M. A., & Udin, R. D. (1986). Using a feeding appliance to aid the infant with a cleft palate. *Ear, Nose, and Throat Journal, 65*(7), 316–320.

Barone, C. M., & Tallman, L. L. (1998). Modification of Playtex nurser for cleft palate patients. *Journal of Craniofacial Surgery, 9*(3), 271–274.

Bath, A. P., & Buil, P. D. (1997). Management of upper airway obstruction in Pierre Robin sequence. *Journal of Laryngology and Otology, 111*(12), 1155–1157.

Bessell, A., Hooper, L., Shaw, W. C., Reilly, S., Reid, J., & Glenny, A. M. (2011) Feeding interventions for growth and development in infants with cleft lip, cleft palate, or cleft lip and palate (Review). *The Cochrane Database of Systematic Reviews,* 2011, Issue 2. Art. No.: CD003315.

Biancuzzo, M. (1998). Clinical focus on clefts. Yes! Infants with clefts can breastfeed. *AWHONN Lifelines, 2*(4), 45–49.

Boesch, R. P., Daines, C., Willging, J. P., Kaul, A., Cohen, A. P., Wood, R. E., & Amin, R. S. (2006). Advances in the diagnosis and management of chronic pulmonary aspiration in children. *European Respiratory Journal, 24*(4), 847–861.

Bosma, J. D. (1985). Postnatal ontogeny of performances of the pharynx, larynx, and mouth. *American Review of Respiratory Disorders, 131,* S10–S15.

Bosma, J. D., & Donner, M. W. (1980). *Physiology of the pharynx.* Philadelphia: W. B. Saunders.

Broussard, A. B., & Borazjani, J. G. (2008). The faces of Moebius Syndrome: Recognition and anticipatory guidance. *The American Journal of Maternal-Child Nursing, 33*(5), 272–278.

Bu'Lock, F., Woolridge, M. W., & Baum, J. D. (1990). Development of coordination of sucking, swallowing and breathing: Ultrasound study of term and preterm infants. *Developmental Medical Child Neurology, 32*(8), 669–678.

Butte, N. F. (2005). Energy requirements of infants. *Public Health Nutrition, 8*(7a), 953–967.

Carlisle, D. (1998). Feeding babies with cleft lip and palate. *Nursing Times, 94*(4), 59–60.

Chigurupati, R., & Myall, R. (2005). Airway management in babies with micrognathia: The case against early distraction. *Journal of Oral Maxillofacial Surgery, 63,* 1209–1215.

Choi, B. H., Kleinheinz, J., Joos, U., & Komposch, G. (1991). Sucking efficiency of early orthopaedic plate and teats in infants with cleft lip and palate. *International Journal of Oral Maxillofacial Surgery, 20*(3), 167–169.

Chuacharoen, R., Ritthagol, W., Hunsrisakhun, J., & Nilmanat, K. (2009). Felt needs of parents who have a 0–3-month-old child with a cleft lip and palate. *Cleft Palate–Craniofacial Journal, 46*(3), 252–257.

Clarren, S. K., Anderson, B., & Wolf, L. S. (1987). Feeding infants with cleft lip, cleft palate, or cleft lip and palate. *Cleft Palate Journal, 24*(3), 244–249.

The Cleft Palate Foundation. (1998). *Feeding an infant with a cleft.* Chapel Hill, NC: Author.

Crossman, K. (1998). Breastfeeding a baby with a cleft palate: A case report. *Journal of Human Lactation, 14*(1), 47–50.

Darzi, M. A., Chowdri, N. A., & Bhat, A. N. (1996). Breast feeding or spoon feeding after cleft lip repair: A prospective, randomised study. *British Journal of Plastic Surgery, 49*(1), 24–26.

Delgado, A. A., Schaaf, N. G., & Emrich, L. (1992). Trends in prosthodontic treatment of cleft palate patients at one institution: A twenty-one year review. *Cleft Palate–Craniofacial Journal, 29*(5), 425–428.

Glass, R. P., & Wolf, L. S. (1999). Feeding management of infants with cleft lip and palate and micrognathia. *Infants and Young Children, 12*(1), 70–81.

Glenny, A. M., Hooper, L., Shaw, W. C., Reilly, S., Kasem, S., & Reid, J. (2004). Feeding interventions for growth and development in infants with cleft lip, cleft palate or cleft lip and palate. *The Cochrane Database of Systematic Reviews* (3), CD003315

Hwang, Y., Lin, C. Coster, W., Bigsby, R., & Vergara, E. (2010). Effectiveness of cheek and jaw support to improve feeding performance of preterm infants. *The American Journal of Occupational Therapy, 66*(6), 886–894.

Izadi, K., Yellon, R., Mandell, D., Smith, M., Song, S., Bidic, S., & Bradley, J. (2003). Correction of upper airway obstruction in the newborn with internal mandibular distraction osteogenesis. *Journal of Craniofacial Surgery, 14*(4), 493–499.

Johansson, B., & Ringsberg, K. C. (2004). Parents' experiences of having a child with cleft lip and palate. *Journal of Advanced Nursing, 47*(2), 165–173.

Jones, W. B. (1988). Weight gain and feeding in the neonate with cleft: A three-center study. *Cleft Palate Journal, 25*(4), 379–384.

Katzel, E., Basile, P., Koltz, P., Marcus, J., & Firotto, J. (2009). Current surgical practices in cleft care: cleft palate repair techniques and postoperative care. *Plastic & Reconstructive Surgery, 124*(3), 899–906.

Kochel, J., Meyer-Marcotty, P., Wirbelauer, J., Böohm, H., Kochel, M., Thomas, W., Hebestreit, H., et al. (2011). Treatment modalities of infants with upper airway obstruction-review of the literature and presentation of novel orthopedic appliances. *Cleft Palate–Craniofacial Journal, 48* (1), 44–55.

Koenig, J. S., Davies, A. M., & Thach, B. T. (1990). Coordination of breathing, sucking, and swallowing during bottle feedings in human infants. *Journal of Applied Physiology, 69,* 1623–1629.

Kogo, M., Okada, G., Ishii, S., Shikata, M., Iida, S., & Matsuya, T. (1997). Breast feeding for cleft lip and palate patients, using the Hotz-type plate. *Cleft Palate–Craniofacial Journal, 34*(4), 351–353.

Kovar, A. J. (1997). Nutrition assessment and management in pediatric dysphagia. *Seminars in Speech and Language, 18*(1), 39–49.

Kramer, S. S. (1985). Special swallowing problems in children. *Gastrointestinal Radiology, 10*, 241–250.

Lang, S., Lawrence, C. J., & Orme, R. L. (1994). Cup feeding: An alternative method of infant feeding. *Archives of Diseases in Childhood, 71*(4), 365–369.

Law-Morsatt, L., Judd, D. M., Snyder, P., Baier, R. J., & Dhanireddy, R. (2003). Pacing as a treatment strategy for transitional sucking patterns. *Journal of Perinatology, 23*, 483–488.

Lefton-Greif, M. A., & Arvedson, J. C. (1997). Pediatric feeding/swallowing teams. *Seminars in Speech and Language, 18*(1), 5–11; Quiz 12.

Lehman, J. A., Fishman, J. R., & Neiman, G. S. (1995). Treatment of cleft palate associated with Robin sequence: Appraisal of risk factors. *Cleft Palate–Craniofacial Journal, 32*(1), 25–29.

Mandell, D., Yellon, R., Bradley, J., Izadi, K., & Gordon, C. (2004). Mandibular distraction for micrognathia and severe upper airway obstruction. *Archives of Otolaryngology-Head & Neck Surgery, 130*(3), 344–348.

Masarei, A. G., Sell, D., Habel, A., Mars, M., Sommerlad, B. C., & Wade, A. (2007). The nature of feeding infants with unrepaired cleft lip and/or palate compared with healthy noncleft infants. *Cleft Palate–Craniofacial Journal, 44*(3), 321–328.

Mathew, O. P. (1988a). Nipple units for newborn infants: A functional comparison. *Pediatrics, 81*(5), 688–691.

Mathew, O. P. (1988b). Respiratory control during nipple feeding in preterm infants. *Pediatric Pulmonology, 5*(4), 220–224.

Mathew, O. P. (1990). Determinants of milk flow through nipple units: Role of hole size and nipple thickness. *American Journal of Diseases of Children, 144*(2), 222–224.

Mathew, O. P. (1991). Science of bottle feeding. *Journal of Pediatrics, 119*(4), 511–519.

Mathew, O. P., Clark, M. L., Pronske, M. L., Luna-Solarzano, H. G., & Peterson, M. D. (1985). Breathing pattern and ventilation during oral feeding in term newborn infants. *Journal of Pediatrics, 106*(5), 810–813.

Mei, C., Morgan, A., & Reilly, S. (2009). Benchmarking clinical practice against best evidence: An example from breastfeeding infants with cleft lip and/or palate. *Evidence-based Communication Assessment and Intervention, 3*(1), 48–66.

Meyer, E. C., Coll, C. T., Lester, B. M., Boukydis, C. F., McDonough, S. M., & Oh, W. (1994). Family-based intervention improves maternal psychological well-being and feeding interaction of preterm infants. *Pediatrics, 93*(2), 241–246.

Miller, C., Burklow, K., Santoro, K., Kirby, E., Mason, D., & Rudolph, C. (2001). An interdisciplinary team approach to the management of pediatric feeding and swallowing disorders. *Children's Health Care, 30*(3), 201–218.

Miller, C. K. (2009). Updates on pediatric feeding and swallowing problems. *Current Opinion in Otolaryngology & Head & Neck Surgery, 17*(3), 194–199.

Miller, C. K. (2011). Feeding issues and interventions in infants and children with clefts and craniofacial syndromes. *Seminars in Speech and Language, 32*(2), 115–126.

Miller, C. K., & Willging, J. P. (2007). The implications of upper-airway obstruction on successful infant feeding. *Seminars in Speech and Language, 28*(3), 190–203.

Morris, S. E., & Klein, M. D. (1987). *Prefeeding skills: A comprehensive resource for feeding development.* Tucson, AZ: Therapy Skill Builders.

Myer, C. M., Cotton, R. T., & Shott, S. R. (1995). *The pediatric airway: An interdisciplinary approach.* Philadelphia: J. B. Lippincott.

Nassar, E., Marques, I. L., Trindade, A. S., & Bettiol, H. (2006). Feeding-facilitating techniques for the nursing infant with Robin sequence. *Cleft Palate–Craniofacial Journal, 43*(1), 55–60.

Newman, L. A., Cleveland, R. H., Blickman, J. G., Hillman, R. E., & Jaramillo, D. (1991). Videofluoroscopic analysis of the infant swallow. *Investigative Radiology, 26*(10), 870–873.

Osuji, O. O. (1995). Preparation of feeding obturators for infants with cleft lip and palate. *Journal of Clinical Pediatric Dentistry, 19*(3), 211–214.

Paradise, J., Eister, B., & Tan, L. (1994). Evidence in infants with cleft palate that breast milk protects against otitis media. *Pediatrics, 94*(6), 853–860.

Redford-Badwal, D. A., Mabry, K., & Frassinelli, J. D. (2003). Impact of cleft lip and/or palate on nutritional health and oral-motor development. *Dental Clinics of North America, 47*(2), 305–317.

Reilly, S., Reid, J., & Skeat, J. (2007). ABM Clinical protocol #17: Guidelines for breastfeeding infants with cleft lip, cleft palate, or cleft lip and palate. *Breastfeeding Medicine, 2*(4), 243–250.

Rudolph, C. D. (1994). Feeding disorders in infants and children. *Journal of Pediatrics, 125*(6, Pt. 2), S116–S124.

Sasaki, C. T., Levine, P. A., Laitman, J. T., Phil, M., & Crelin, E. S. (1977). Postnatal descent of the epiglottis in man. *Archives of Otolaryngology, 103*, 169–171.

Savion, L., & Huband, M. (2005). A feeding obturator for a preterm baby with Pierre Robin sequence. *Journal of Prosthetic Dentistry, 93*(2), 197–200.

Schaefer, R., Stadier, J., & Gosain, A. (2004). To distract or not distract: An algorithm for airway management in isolated Pierre Robin sequence. *Plastic and Reconstructive Surgery, 113*(4), 1113–1125.

Shaw, W., Bannister, R., & Roberts, C. (1999). Assisted feeding is more reliable for infants with clefts: A randomized trial. *Cleft Palate–Craniofacial Journal, 36*(3), 262–268.

Shprintzen, R. J. (1992). The implications of the diagnosis of Robin sequence. *Cleft Palate–Craniofacial Journal, 29*(3), 205–209.

Shprintzen, R. J., & Singer, L. (1992). Upper airway obstruction and the Robin sequence. *International Anesthesiology Clinics of North America, 30*(4), 109–114.

Skinner, J., Arvedson, J. C., Jones, G., Spinner, C., & Rockwood, C. (1997). Post-operative feeding strategies for infants with cleft lip. *International Journal of Pediatric Otorhinolaryngology, 42*, 169–178.

Stromland, K., Miller, M., Sjögreen, L. Johansson, M., Joelsson, B., Billstedt, E., Gillberg, C. et al. (2007). Oculo-auriculovertebral spectrum: associated anomalies, functional deficits, and possible developmental risk factors. *American Journal of Medical Genetics Part A, 143A*, 1317–1325.

Sultana, A., Rahman, M. M., Nessa, J., & Alam, M. S. (2011). A feeding aid prosthesis for a preterm baby with cleft lip and palate. *Mymensingh Medical Journal, 20*(1), 22–27.

Tibesar, R. J., Price, D. L., & Moore, E. J. (2006). Mandibular distraction osteogenesis to relieve Pierre Robin upper airway obstruction. *American Journal of Otolaryngology—Head and Neck Surgery, 27*, 436–439.

van den Elzen, A., Semmekrot, B., Bongers, E., Huygen, P., & Marres, H. (2001). Diagnosis and treatment of Pierre Robin sequence: Results of a retrospective clinical study and review of literature. *European Journal of Pediatrics, 160*, 47–53.

Wagener, S., Rayatt, S. S., Tatman, A. J., Gornall, P., & Slator, R. (2003). Management of infants with Pierre Robin sequence. *Cleft Palate–Craniofacial Journal, 40*(2), 180–185.

Willging, J. P. (1995). Endoscopic evaluation of swallowing in children. *International Journal of Pediatric Otorhinolaryngology, 32* (Suppl.), S107–S108.

Willging, J. P., & Thompson, D. M. (2005). Pediatric FEESST: Fiberoptic Endoscopic Evaluation of Swallowing with Sensory Testing. *Current Gastroenterology Reports, 7*(3), 240–243.

Wolf, L. S., & Glass, R. P. (1992). Feeding and swallowing disorders in infancy: Assessment and management. Tucson, KL: Therapy Skill Builders.

Young, J., O'Riordan, M., Goldstein, J., & Robin, N. (2001). What information do parents of newborns with cleft lip, palate, or both want to know? *Cleft Palate–Craniofacial Journal, 38*(1), 55–58.

Zim, S. (2007). Treatment of upper airway obstruction in infants with micrognathia using mandibular distraction osteogenesis. *Facial Plastic Surgery, 23*(2), 107–112.

General Feeding Tips for Parents

By Claire K. Miller, Ph.D

Relax

Most parents report feeling anxious about learning how to feed their baby with a cleft but find the problems to be fewer than expected and easy to overcome when using the right type of nipple, bottle, and technique.

Feeding Equipment and Methods

A particular method of feeding is usually recommended shortly after birth by a nurse, speech-language pathologist, or occupational therapist. Try to use the adapted nipples, bottles, and feeding methods that are recommended, and be sure not to hesitate to call the nurse or speech-language pathologist if any questions arise about how to use the equipment.

Using Appropriate Positioning

Feeding a baby with cleft palate in an upright position as opposed to the traditional cradle or reclined position reduces the amount of liquid that can escape up into the nose during feeding. Try using a pillow or small foam wedge to support the baby against you in an upright position.

Dealing with Nasal Regurgitation

If milk does have a tendency to come from the baby's nose even while using an upright position, the flow of the liquid may be too fast. Try using a nipple with a slower flow rate, such as one with a smaller crosscut or slit.

Feeding Refusal

- The baby may seem to be refusing to breast- or bottle-feed. Try to problem-solve what might be happening by considering the length of time between feedings. If the feedings are too close together, the baby may not be hungry enough to be motivated to feed.

- Consider the size of the nipple hole and whether the baby is working too hard to extract the fluid. This is a common problem. Explore using a nipple that either has a faster flow rate or that is flexible enough to allow assistive squeezing if necessary.

- If breastfeeding, the baby may be overwhelmed with the initial milk letdown during feeding and demonstrate avoidance. Experiment with hand-expressing some milk before beginning to breastfeed.

- Experiment with the temperature of the formula if bottle-feeding. Although not proven by research, many infants seem to prefer warm formula as opposed to room temperature.

- Try to be consistent with the method being used for feeding. Train others who may be feeding the baby to use the same positioning, the same feeding equipment, and the same type of strategies you use when feeding your baby. For example, demonstrate how to use assistive squeezing or how often you give the baby breaks for resting or burping during a feeding.

Managing Air Intake during Feeding

Babies with clefts will tend to swallow some extra air while feeding. After intake of every ounce (or so), giving the baby a pause from feeding and chance to burp may help to alleviate discomfort associated with excessive air intake.

Persistent Oral Feeding Problems

Most feeding problems can be easily resolved. If your baby continues to have trouble feeding and you are concerned, consult your pediatrician for a referral to a speech-language pathologist or occupational therapist experienced with the special feeding issues associated with cleft lip/palate or other craniofacial anomalies.

Feeding Infants with Clefts Using Adapted Nipples and Bottles

By Claire K. Miller, Ph.D.

Bottle Feeding Using the Mead Johnson™ Cleft Palate Nurser

- Position baby in a semi-upright position in your lap. Hold the Mead Johnson bottle in your right hand, using your left arm/hand to support the baby's head and shoulders.

- The Mead Johnson nipple or nipple of choice (pigeon nipple®, standard nipple, orthodontic nipple, etc.) can be used with the Mead Johnson flexible bottle.

- Use the nipple to touch the corner of the baby's lip to help stimulate mouth opening. When the baby's mouth opens, take care to place the nipple onto the body of the tongue, not in the space in front of the tongue.

- If the baby has a cleft lip and palate, allow the baby to try sucking the nipple first before beginning to provide a gentle assistive squeeze of the bottle.

- Begin with one gentle squeeze of the bottle, watching the baby's reaction.

- Try to squeeze in a rhythmic manner in time to the baby's sucking.

- Avoid using a continuous squeezing motion, as this will overwhelm the baby.

- Use regular squeezing at the beginning of the feeding when the baby is eating vigorously; slow the rate toward the middle and end of the feeding when the baby's sucking rate slows down.

Bottle Feeding Using the SpecialNeeds® Feeder

- The SpecialNeeds® Feeder has several parts: bottle, nipple, disc, collar, and valve membrane.

- Begin assembling the feeder by pressing the valve membrane onto the upper side of the disc (the stud should go through the center hole).

- Fill the bottle compartment with breast milk or formula. Put the valve membrane into the nipple, and then use the collar to put all the parts together onto the bottle. Squeeze the nipple compartment while the feeder is upright. Then turn the feeder upside down, releasing the nipple compartment. This allows the formula to enter the nipple reservoir.

- Position the baby in a semi-upright position on your lap, holding the bottle in one hand and supporting the baby with your other arm/hand.

- Begin by lining up the shortest line (minimum flow) on the nipple reservoir with the baby's nose.

- Touch the nipple to the corner of the baby's mouth, and when the mouth opens, gently advance the nipple onto the baby's tongue.

- Try to position the nipple under any intact part of the palate.

- Allow the baby some time to begin sucking.

- The nipple will release fluid as the baby compresses it with sucking.

- Based on the baby's sucking efforts, rotate the nipple until the medium line (medium flow) or longest line (maximum flow) is under the baby's nose—determine flow rate based upon baby's response.

- If needed, you may compress the reservoir to give extra assistance with fluid expression every second or third suck.

Bottle Feeding Using the Pigeon Nipple®

- The pigeon nipple® has a Y-shaped opening. Rub a soft clean cloth over the opening to loosen it before using.

- Use the nipple with a flexible bottle such as the Mead Johnson.

- Find the "V" in the base of the nipple. This is the air vent that should be placed on the top of the nipple, under the infant's nose while feeding.

- Position the nipple on the infant's tongue. The infant's sucking motion will activate the flow.

Feeding with the Medela SoftCup® Feeder

- The SoftCup Feeder has a silicone reservoir, one disc, one valve membrane, and a collar.

- The valve should be pressed onto the upper side of the disc so that the stud goes completely through the center hole.

- Slip the reservoir into the collar.

- Put the assembled valve into the reservoir, making sure that the valve and the high rim of the disc are facing the inside of the reservoir.

- Place the reservoir over the bottle, and tighten the collar to make a good seal.

- Hold the feeder upright and squeeze below the pads of the reservoir.

- Keep squeezing and tip the feeder upside down.

- Release the pads and some fluid will flow into the reservoir; repeat until almost filled.

- Position the baby and present the soft cup to the lips; the baby's mouth will slightly open.

- Present small amounts of the fluid, allowing time for the baby to transfer and swallow each small amount given.

C H A P T E R

6

DEVELOPMENTAL ASPECTS: SPEECH, LANGUAGE, AND COGNITION

CHAPTER OUTLINE

INTRODUCTION

Children with a history of cleft palate are at risk for delays in the acquisition of speech skills and may be at risk for delays in early language development. It is obvious that children with a cleft palate will be behind their unaffected peers in the acquisition of early developmental phonemes because of the open palate. This delay persists until the palate is repaired and often for some time postoperatively.

The articulation problems secondary to velopharyngeal insufficiency/incompetence (VPI) have been well documented in the literature. There is a good understanding of how the abnormal structure and function of the velopharyngeal valve can affect speech, frequently causing obligatory and compensatory errors (Kummer, 2011; Trost-Cardamone, 1997). How the presence of orofacial anomalies can affect language and cognitive development is less clear. Of course, significant difficulties with speech production may cause expressive language skills to appear delayed due to the difficulty with production. However, there are many more subtle factors that may affect development in this population.

Children with craniofacial syndromes are at greatest risk for speech and language disorders. This is due not only to the orofacial anomalies but also to neurological disorders and resulting cognitive problems that commonly occur with craniofacial syndromes.

This chapter outlines what is known about the development of children with clefts and craniofacial conditions, particularly in the area of language. It is hoped that the reader will learn to be attentive to all aspects of development, including language and learning, when evaluating a child from one of these populations. Developmental delays are particularly important to recognize and remediate during the critical period of brain development in order for the child to reach his or her full potential.

FACTORS IMPORTANT FOR NORMAL SPEECH, LANGUAGE, AND COGNITIVE DEVELOPMENT

Unlike other primates, humans have the innate ability to learn to communicate through spoken or verbal language. The ability to learn is the key factor and is dependent on the individual's *cognition*. (Cognition is the ability to engage in conscious intellectual activities that are important for learning.) Although cognition is important for language learning, the development of language further enhances the development of cognitive skills (Dowling, 2004). In fact, language is a tool for thought and problem solving.

Speech, language, and cognitive development are dependent on some basic prerequisites, including brain structure and function, environmental stimulation, hearing, motivation, and attending skills. Normal anatomy and physiology of the speech mechanism are also important for expressive language and speech development. When one considers the basic prerequisites for normal speech and language learning, it is easy to understand why some children with orofacial anomalies are at risk for delayed development.

This section describes these basic prerequisites for language learning and how these prerequisites may be affected by the occurrence of a cleft or craniofacial condition.

Brain Structure and Function

The brain determines an individual's intelligence, which includes the ability to perceive, comprehend, assimilate, analyze, categorize, imitate, and learn. When intelligence is significantly below normal, there are usually generalized delays that affect function in all aspects of development, including cognition, language, and speech. Intelligence and cognitive function are totally dependent on the structure of the brain and the function of the central nervous system. Therefore, normal brain structure and function are necessary requirements for the development of both speech and language.

Relatively recent research suggests that individuals with clefts may also have structural differences in the brain and are at risk for brain abnormalities. Using magnetic resonance imaging (MRI) technology, Nopoulos and colleagues (Nopoulos et al., 2001; Nopoulos et al., 2005; Nopoulos, Berg, Canady, et al., 2002; Nopoulos, Berg, Van Demark, et al., 2002; Richman & Nopoulos, 2009) have found, structural abnormalities in the brain morphology of men with a history of nonsyndromic clefts of the lip and/or palate. These authors reported finding midline anomalies, enlarged regions of the cerebrum, decreased volumes of the posterior cerebrum and cerebellum, and abnormalities in the frontal lobe. More recently, Rosen and colleagues (Rosen et al., 2011) reported finding brain abnormalities in 6.3% of fetuses with cleft lip and/or palate, through prenatal MRI imaging. These findings suggest that there may be a relationship between facial development and brain development.

Neurologic dysfunction is a particular risk for children with a history of cleft palate only (CPO), especially those who have other congenital anomalies (Broder, Richman, & Matheson, 1998; Goodstein, 1961; Richman, 1980; Richman, Eliason, & Lindgren, 1988; Strauss & Broder, 1993). This is due to the fact that isolated cleft palate often occurs as part of a syndrome that may include neurologic dysfunction and low intelligence as phenotypic features. In fact, there are many craniofacial syndromes, some that include clefts and some that do not, that include a form of neurological dysfunction as a phenotypic feature. Shprintzen (1998) listed the following craniofacial conditions that can include cognitive dysfunction: Apert syndrome, BBB (Opitz) syndrome, Beckwith-Wiedemann syndrome, Carpenter syndrome, CHARGE association, Down syndrome, Cornelia de Lange syndrome, fetal alcohol syndrome, fetal hydantoin, holoprosencephaly sequence, Noonan syndrome, otopalatodigital syndrome, Rubinstein-Taybi syndrome, Shprintzen-Goldberg I syndrome, Shprintzen-Goldberg II syndrome (Shprintzen et al., 1978), velocardiofacial syndrome, Weaver syndrome, and Williams syndrome.

Intellectual impairment is one of the most commonly expressed phenotypic features of velocardiofacial syndrome (VCFS) (also known as 22qll.2 deletion syndrome or DiGeorge syndrome) (D'Antonio, Scherer, Miller, Kalbfleisch, & Bartley, 2001; Persson et al., 2006; Scherer, D'Antonio, & Kalbfleisch, 1999;

Scherer, D'Antonio, & Rodgers, 2001). In addition, several authors have shown that patients with VCFS demonstrate significant brain abnormalities, including reduced brain volume of both white and grey matter (Eliez, Antonarakis, Morris, Dahoun, & Reiss, 2001; Eliez, Schmitt, White, & Reiss, 2000; Eliez, Blasey, et al., 2001; Kates et al., 2001, 2004; van Amelsvoort et al., 2004), cerebellar hypoplasia (Devriendt, Van Thienen, Swillen, & Fryns, 1996; Lynch et al., 1995; van Amelsvoort et al., 2004; Yamagishi, 2002), larger corpus callosum area (Antshel, Conchelos, Lanzetta, Fremont, & Kates, 2005), and Chiari malformation (Hultman et al., 2000). These findings certainly have implications for cognitive, social, and language development in the VCFS population.

Some syndromes and conditions do not have cognitive or neurological dysfunction as typical phenotypic features, but have the potential for causing impairment in intellectual or neurological function. For example, in craniofrontonasal dysplasia, intellect is generally normal unless there are also midline defects of the brain. In Crouzon syndrome, cognition is also typically within normal limits. However, hydrocephalus with increased intracranial pressure may occur due to the craniosynostosis. If left untreated, this can have a permanent effect on intelligence and cognitive function.

Environmental Stimulation

Environmental stimulation and environmental experience are important factors in language development. Just as is the case with adults learning a foreign language, children learning their first language need to be constantly exposed to language for efficient learning to take place. In addition, they must have experiences with the environment before words about the environment are meaningful to them. Therefore, children who live in a language-rich environment are likely to develop language skills faster and have a more extensive vocabulary than children with little language stimulation. Language learning is easier under the age of 5 during the period of critical brain development (Dowling, 2004). Therefore, stimulation during this period of time is particularly important.

Children with a history of cleft or craniofacial condition are usually not different from other children in the amount of stimulation that they receive from their environment. In one study, the language input of mothers of children with clefts was found to be similar to the input of mothers of noncleft children (Chapman & Hardin, 1991). In some cases, children with a cleft or craniofacial condition may actually have an advantage over their unaffected peers. This is because most of these children are followed by a cleft palate or craniofacial anomaly team, and the speech-language pathologist on the team usually counsels the parents on methods of language stimulation in the home. (See Handout Section for a sample home program for parents to use in stimulating language.) In addition, some parents are so concerned about the potential effect of the anomalies on their child's development that they become particularly diligent in providing speech and language stimulation. Affected children may have another advantage in that they often qualify for enrollment in an early intervention program, most of which are geared toward the development of cognitive and language skills.

Although some affected children may have some advantages in early stimulation, others are not as fortunate. Children with significant anomalies and serious medical conditions may undergo many surgical procedures and frequent hospitalizations in the early years. Unfortunately, a hospital room is usually not a language-rich environment. Additionally, the severely affected child may not have as many opportunities to interact with others as his or her unaffected or less affected peers because of the compromised medical condition and possibly also the child's appearance. Social isolation can certainly have a negative effect on the process of language learning.

Hearing and Vision

It is through sensory perception that we learn about the world around us and develop a method for communicating with each other. Both speech and language learning is done through the use of audition and vision.

Children with a history of cleft palate are at high risk for chronic middle ear effusion and conductive hearing loss due to Eustachian tube malfunction. In addition, many craniofacial syndromes include conductive or sensorineural hearing loss as a phenotypic feature. For example, a primary phenotypic feature of Waardenburg syndrome is congenital sensorineural hearing loss that is usually severe and bilateral. Sensorineural hearing loss can also be found in hemifacial microsomia (also known as Goldenhar syndrome, facioauriculovertebral malformation sequence, and oculoauriculovertebral dysplasia), CHARGE association, Stickler syndrome, Treacher Collins syndrome, Turner syndrome, and others.

Even a mild, fluctuating conductive hearing loss can temporarily affect the acquisition of oral language skills. Speech development can be affected by the inability to adequately perceive high-frequency, low-intensity sounds. Language development can be affected by the strain required for hearing. Making that constant effort to hear is exhausting, so the child may respond by not listening. Consequently, less language is heard, perceived, analyzed, and learned.

A severe hearing loss or deafness affects the child's ability to perceive and thus imitate speech sounds. A child with a severe hearing impairment has difficulty learning all aspects of language. Even resonance is affected by the inability to monitor and therefore modulate velopharyngeal function. Overall, verbal communication is extremely difficult, if not impossible, to acquire without adequate hearing.

Hearing loss is suspected to be a primary reason that children with history of cleft often score lower on verbal performance measures than their noncleft peers in the early years (Broen, Devers, Doyle, Prouty, & Moller, 1998; Jocelyn, Penko, & Rode, 1996; Kritzinger, Louw, & Hugo, 1996; Lamb et al., 1973). Additional support for hearing loss as a factor in early measures of intelligence comes from the studies that show that these differences in intelligence disappear with age or with the insertion of pressure-equalizing (PE) tubes (Musgrave, McWilliams, & Mathews, 1975; Paradise, 1998).

The need for adequate auditory skills for normal speech and language development is fairly obvious. However, vision is also important. We learn speech by watching faces. We learn meaning by watching expressions and body gestures. In addition, we use language to "code" our world through the association of auditory words with the visual perception of words that represent nouns, verbs, adjectives, and so on. Some craniofacial syndromes affect the eyes and thus vision. This can therefore cause a delay in language development.

Motivation

The next prerequisite for language development is motivation. Although many new skills can be learned passively, a skill will be acquired much more rapidly if there is a need and desire to learn the skill. This general principle certainly holds true for language learning (Syal, 2011).

In most cases, young children are motivated to talk because this is the best way to communicate. However, if a caregiver or an older sibling anticipates the child's needs and wants, there is little reason to learn to talk, particularly under the age of 2, when gestures are effective for what the child needs to communicate. It is only when the child wants to communicate something more than the "here and now" that this gestural system is no longer effective. With an increase in the need to communicate, there is a corresponding increase in the motivation to communicate and the development of verbal language.

For the most part, children with a history of cleft are no different from their unaffected peers in communicating their needs through gestures during the first year (Long & Dalston, 1982a). During the second year, the child begins to use verbal language and discontinues the use of gestures because verbal language is usually a more effective form of communication.

One problem is that some parents of children with clefts tend to overprotect their child, especially during times of surgery or medical appointments. In doing so, they may provide for the child's needs without requiring verbal communication from the child. Although this is understandable at times, persistent overprotection reduces the child's need to communicate verbally, and this can have a detrimental effect on the child's expressive language development.

Another issue with motivation occurs if the child has difficulty with speech sound production. When speech intelligibility is poor, verbal language may be an ineffective means of communication (Grunwell & Russell, 1988). Therefore, the child may revert back to using gestures, at least to augment speech. In addition, the child may compensate by keeping utterance length short. On the surface, this may appear to be an expressive language disorder due to the telegraphic nature of the speech. Instead, it is a compensatory strategy because shorter utterances are easier to produce clearly and easier for the listeners to understand. If intelligibility continues to be poor as the child gets older, this can cause the child to be less assertive when engaging in conversational skills as compared with others (Chapman, Graham, Gooch, & Visconti, 1998; Frederickson, Chapman, & Hardin-Jones, 2006). As an adult, the individual may continue to use shorter utterances to improve intelligibility (Pannbacker, 1975).

Attention

Another prerequisite for language learning is the ability to attend to the environment and particularly to the verbal communication of others. *Attention deficit-hyperactivity disorder* (ADHD) refers to a cluster of behavioral characteristics that involve impaired attention, impulsivity, distractibility, and hyperactivity (American Psychiatric Association [APA], 2004). It has been estimated that 3% to 5% of elementary school-aged children have this disorder, making it the most prevalent psychiatric disorder of childhood (APA, 2004). ADHD is five to nine times more prevalent in boys than in girls (Lecendreuz, Konofal, & Faraone, 2010).

When a child has a significant attention deficit, distractibility, and a high activity level, the stimulation from the environment may not be adequately perceived or processed, and language learning is affected as a result. In addition, the child with ADHD is less likely to participate in language-enriching activities, such as reading, listening to a story, or playing a game. Children with ADHD are often diagnosed with learning disabilities (Cantwell & Baker, 1991; Cherkes-Julkowski, 1998; Sidoti, Marsh, Marty-Grames, & Noetzel, 1996; Tirosh, Berger, Cohn-Ophir, Davidovitch, & Cohen, 1998) and language disorders (Cantwell & Baker, 1991; Cherkes-Julkowski, 1998; Damico, Damico, & Armstrong, 1999; Fergusson & Horwood, 1992; Love & Thompson, 1988; Purvis & Tannock, 1997; Tirosh et al., 1998; Tirosh & Cohen, 1998; Wright, 1982). One study found that 30% of children with speech and language impairments also had ADHD (Beitchman, Hood, Rochon, & Peterson, 1989).

Although ADHD is usually diagnosed in children with no identified neurological lesion, the same characteristics are commonly seen in individuals with documented brain damage or neurological deficits (Max et al., 1998; Niemann, Ruff, & Kramer, 1996). Children with craniofacial syndromes that include neurological dysfunction are at significant risk for difficulties with attention and concentration. As an example, attention deficits and difficulty with concentration are typical problems with velocardiofacial syndrome (Heineman-de Boer, Van Haelst, Cordia-de Haan, & Beemer, 1999; Swillen et al., 1997, 1999).

Vocal Tract Anatomy and Physiology

There are many physical prerequisites that are important for speech production. There must be structural integrity of the entire vocal tract. In addition, the physiology must be normal for respiration, phonation, velopharyngeal function, articulation, and neurological function. Clefts and craniofacial conditions may include a variety of structural abnormalities, including dental malocclusion and velopharyngeal dysfunction. The effects of these abnormalities on speech are covered in the next three chapters.

DEVELOPMENT OF CHILDREN WITH CLEFTS AND CRANIOFACIAL SYNDROMES

The literature on the developmental status of children with clefts and craniofacial anomalies is often contradictory and difficult to interpret. This is partly because these are very heterogeneous populations. They can differ not only in the type and severity of the cleft or craniofacial condition but also with respect to other medical conditions such as chronic middle ear effusion and hearing loss; the number of hospitalizations; the type and effectiveness of the surgical repairs; parental attitudes and involvement; and even environmental factors. Children with clefts and craniofacial anomalies may show deficits when compared to a peer group but still score well within the normal range (Hardin-Jones, 2011). Finally, deficits that are noted early in development may no longer be noted in later years. Therefore, it is very difficult to determine the characteristics of "typical" development for children affected by clefts.

Language and Cognitive Development

Several authors have reported that children with nonsyndromic clefts show some early deficits in prelanguage skills during the first 3 years of life (Fox, Lynch, & Brookshire, 1978; Hentges et al., 2011; Kapp-Simon & Krueckeberg, 2000; Neiman & Savage, 1997; (Scherer, Williams, & Proctor-Williams, 2008; Snyder & Scherer, 2004; Speltz et al., 2000; Starr, Chinski, Canter, & Meier, 1977). In addition, some studies have found that children with clefts have lower scores in verbal performance than nonverbal performance on standardized tests (Broen et al., 1998; Estes & Morris, 1970;

Lamb, Wilson, & Leeper, 1973; Ruess, 1965; Wirls, 1971). In contrast, other studies have found no verbal–nonverbal differences in the cleft population (Leeper, Pannbacker, & Roginski, 1980; McWilliams & Matthews, 1979). One study showed no differences in comprehension as compared to unaffected peers (Long & Dalston, 1983). Some studies have reported that children with clefts have immature syntactic development, short utterance length, and overall delays in expressive language as compared with their unaffected peers (Hom, 1972; Morris, 1962; Smith & McWilliams, 1968; Spriestersbach, Darley, & Morris, 1958; Whitcomb, Ochsner, & Wayte, 1976). Others have found the linguistic abilities of children with repaired clefts to be within the normal range. One study found that children with clefts who demonstrate compensatory articulation productions had a higher frequency of language delays than those without compensatory productions (Pamplona, Ysunza, Gonzalez, Ramirez, & Patino, 2000).

Considering the cognitive development of children with nonsyndromic clefts, there is not yet a great deal of research in this area. However, there are a few studies that show that children with clefts are at risk for minor delays in cognitive development when compared to their unaffected peers, particularly in the early years (Hardin-Jones & Chapman, 2011; Kapp-Simon & Krueckeberg, 2000; Neiman & Savage, 1997; Snyder & Scherer, 2004; Speltz et al., 2000). This is consistent with the studies on language development. There is also some research to show that children with clefts have a higher rate of reading disability than their peers (Broder et al., 1998; Richman et al., 1988).

Although children with nonsyndromic clefts may be at risk for early delays in both language and cognitive development, these delays seem to disappear with time (Broen et al., 1998; Collett, 2010; Jocelyn, 1996; Musgrave et al., 1975; Neiman & Savage, 1997; Richman, 2009; Shames & Rubin, 1979; Zimmerman & Canfield, 1968). This may be due to the cleft palate repair, the resolution of middle ear disease that can cause fluctuant hearing loss, and/or the correction of velopharyngeal insufficiency that can impact expressive language development.

The prognosis for language and cognition is not as good for children with isolated cleft palate or syndromic clefts. McWilliams and Matthews (1979) found that in a population of 108 children with isolated cleft palate and other anomalies, 51% had a full-scale IQ of 89 or below, and 37% had IQs of 69 or below. Language and learning disabilities, which can further affect language, are commonly found in individuals with craniofacial syndromes (Broder et al., 1998; Richman et al., 1988; Strauss & Broder, 1993). An example of this is velocardiofacial syndrome (VCFS) (Glaser et al., 2002; Kok & Solman, 1995; Motzkin, Marion, Goldberg, Shprintzen, & Saenger, 1993; Scherer, D'Antonio, & Kalbfleisch, 1999; Shprintzen, 1998; Shprintzen et al., 1978; Swillen et al., 1999; Vantrappen et al., 1999). Children with a craniofacial syndrome are also more likely to exhibit other characteristics that can affect language and cognitive development, including sensorineural hearing loss, velopharyngeal dysfunction, malocclusion, attention deficits, frequent hospitalizations, and even social isolation (Elfenbein, Waziri, & Morris, 1981; Mossey, Little, Munger, Dixon, & Shaw, 2009; Peterson, 1973).

Speech Sound Development

Early sound production in the form of cooing and babbling is an important part of normal speech development. By associating the physical movement of sound production with the auditory results through a tactile-kinesthetic-auditory feedback loop, infants are able to learn to produce sounds volitionally. Infants with cleft palate, however, have an inadequate sound production mechanism, and they frequently have an impaired auditory system due to hearing loss. With these factors alone, they are at risk for delays in speech sound development, even after the palate is repaired (Jones et al., 2003; O'Gara & Logemann, 1988).

Certainly, infants with unrepaired clefts have less variety in speech sound production than their unaffected peers, and they may even vocalize less, at least until the palate is repaired (Long & Dalston, 1982b). Infants with an unrepaired cleft palate demonstrate an alteration in the manner of production with a predominant use of nasal phonemes (/m/, /n/) for most oral sounds. The use of nasal phonemes for oral sounds are *obligatory distortions* (caused by abnormal structure only) due to oral-nasal cavity coupling. Additionally, *compensatory errors* (errors in production in response to abnormal structure) can occur due to structural constraints that restrict phonemic development (Harding & Grunwell, 1996; Kummer, 2011; O'Gara & Logemann, 1988). As a result, infants with an open cleft may begin to use glottal stops rather than the oral plosives (/p/, /b/, /t/, /d/, /k/, /g/) that are typical of a normal babbling pattern (Chapman, 1991; Smith & Kuehn, 2007).

The open palate can also affect the infant's place of articulation. Unaffected infants use anterior sounds in prespeech productions (Roug, Landberg, & Lundberg, 1989; Smith & Oller, 1981; Stoel-Gammon, 1985). In contrast, infants with clefts, regardless of type, babble with a predominant use of posterior consonants, particularly glottal stops and velars (Hardin-Jones, Chapman, & Schulte, 2003; Lohmander-Agerskov, Soderpalm, Friede, Persson, & Lilja, 1994; Russell, 1991; Willadsen & Albrechtsen, 2006). One study showed better speech sound development in children treated with infant orthopedics during the first year than in those who were not (Konst, Rietveld, Peters, & Kuijpers-Jagtman, 2003).

The infant's abnormal speech sound development as a result of the open palate can persist into early speech (Estrem & Broen, 1989; Hardin, 1991; O'Gara, Logemann, & Rademaker, 1994). In addition, if the palate is unrepaired when the child begins to use single words, then he or she will be able to say *mama*, but *dada* will be replaced with *nana* (Lynch, Fox, & Brookshire, 1983).

Although early articulatory patterns persist for some time after palate repair, several investigators have found that within the first few years, glottal productions gradually decrease and oral productions increase. As a result, the speech of those with a successful palate repair may gradually become similar to noncleft peers by the age of 4 or 5 (Chapman, 1993; Chapman & Hardin, 1992; O'Gara & Logemann, 1988; O'Gara, Logemann, & Rademaker, 1994).

How quickly children with repaired clefts are able to acquire oral sounds and "catch up" with their unaffected peers after the palate repair has been a subject of several investigations. One factor that may affect the acquisition of articulation skills is the age of palate repair. Many authors have suggested that children who undergo early palate repair demonstrate better overall speech than those with a later repair (Dorf & Curtin, 1990; Grobbelaar, Hudson, Fernandes, & Lentin, 1995; McWilliams, Morris, & Shelton, 1990; O'Gara & Logemann, 1988; Peterson-Falzone, 1996). Considering the critical period for brain development for speech sound production (Dowling, 2004), it makes sense that the longer the palate remains unrepaired, the harder it is to correct the child's speech. Another factor is regular otologic care, which can prevent hearing loss and help mitigate the risk for delayed speech development. A final factor is the effect of early intervention. Through early intervention, speech-language pathologists can do a great deal to lessen the effects of the cleft on developing communication skills. In particular, working on the production of oral sounds and oral airflow can be helpful. Speech (and language) stimulation at this age is often best done by training the parents to work with the child frequently during each day between speech therapy sessions.

Once the palate is repaired, most children have adequate structure for speech sound production. However, even if the palate is repaired by 9–10 months, the child will have missed the developmental stage where plosives are usually produced and practiced through normal babbling, usually around 6 months. As a result, some of these infants continue to show deficits in the production of certain early developmental sounds for some time after the palate is repaired (Jones, Chapman, & Hardin-Jones, 2003).

If the child has significant velopharyngeal insufficiency (short velum or velar defect) following palate repair, this limits the oral consonants that can be produced. As the child's expressive language increases, a wider range of consonants is needed for intelligibility. In this situation, many children with VPI either decrease their language output by shortening utterance length or increase their consonant repertoire by developing compensatory articulation productions, where articulation is primarily produced in the pharynx or larynx. Harding and Grunwell (1996) reported that around 30 months of age, the nasal fricative (a compensatory production) became prevalent in the speech of their patients with a repaired cleft. This may be because at this point in speech sound development, there is a need for a fricative-plosive contrast, and a normal fricative may be difficult to produce when

there is VPI and a lack of intraoral air pressure as a result. Once acquired and habituated, compensatory productions usually persist, even after the VPI is corrected.

Although compensatory productions can usually be corrected with speech therapy, delays in correcting the structure can have a serious impact on the time it takes to correct the errors, and long delays can even affect the ultimate prognosis. Just as the ability to learn a new language after the age of 6 years is decreased—and after puberty is almost impossible without retaining an accent—the ability to correct faulty speech patterns is also reduced as the child passes the critical period for brain development and speech/language learning (Dowling, 2004).

Another factor that may affect the speech development of children with craniofacial syndromes is oral-motor dysfunction, particularly in the form of apraxia. Children with velocardiofacial syndrome often demonstrate mild to severe apraxia in addition to obligatory and compensatory productions due to VPI (Kummer, Lee, Stutz, Maroney, & Brandt, 2007).

SUMMARY

Based on the existing research, it appears that children with nonsyndromic clefts are at risk for mild delays in development during the first 3 years of life. These delays may be secondary to factors such as fluctuating conductive hearing loss or VPI (McWilliams et al., 1990; Mossey, Little, Munger, Dixon, & Shaw, 2009). These delays, when they occur, are usually mild and tend to improve with early intervention and time. Ultimately, the child usually catches up with his or her noncleft peers.

The risk for developmental delay is greatest for children with a known craniofacial syndrome or those with history of cleft palate only (which is often indicative of a syndrome). The language deficits found in many craniofacial syndromes have more complex etiologies than those found in the cleft population. Therefore, these children should be carefully evaluated at an early age so that intervention can be initiated as soon as possible if needed.

In considering speech sound development, children with an unrepaired cleft palate necessarily acquire speech sounds differently than their unaffected peers. Once the palate is repaired, the rate of this development varies and is affected by the child's age at the time of the repair. Even though the prognosis for normal speech development is fairly good once the palate is repaired, the child remains at risk for persistent articulation errors, compensatory productions, and abnormal resonance due to malocclusion and VPI. Therefore, speech and resonance, in addition to language, should be carefully monitored throughout preschool and early school years.

FOR REVIEW AND DISCUSSION

1. What populations of children with clefts are at particular risk for developmental delays? Why is this?

2. In what cases could there be a concern about brain structure when there is a cleft lip and/or palate?

3. What recent evidence could explain the language disorders and neurological dysfunction in children with velocardiofacial syndrome?

4. Why do you think some children with craniofacial conditions actually receive more language stimulation than unaffected children? Why do some affected children receive less language stimulation than the norm?

5. Why do you think that children with a history of cleft palate may seem delayed in development in the early years but seem to catch up by the time they are in school? What do you think could be done to mitigate these initial delays?

6. What is the effect of an open palate on speech sound acquisition? Why do children still demonstrate abnormal speech after the palate is repaired?

7. How would you explain to a physician that early palate repair is better for speech development and ultimate speech outcome than later palate repair?

8. Describe how you would counsel the parent of an infant about speech and language stimulation. In addition to regular stimulation techniques, what additional instructions would you give to the parent of a child with a cleft? What should be done differently after the palate repair?

REFERENCES

American Psychiatric Association. (2004). *Diagnostic and statistical manual of mental disorders* (4th ed.). Washington, DC: Author.

Antshel, K., Conchelos, J., Lanzetta, G., Fremont, W., & Kates, W. R. (2005). Behavioral and corpus callosum morphology relationships in velocardiofacial syndrome

(22qll.2 deletion syndrome). *Psychiatry Research*, *138*, 235–245.

Beitchman, J. H., Hood, J., Rochon, J., & Peterson, M. (1989). Empirical classification of speech/language impairments in children: II. Behavioral characteristics. *Journal of the American Academy of Child and Adolescent Psychiatry*, *28*, 118–123.

Broder, H. L., Richman, L. C., & Matheson, P. B. (1998). Learning disability, school achievement, and grade retention among children with cleft: A two-center study. *Cleft Palate-Craniofacial Journal*, *35*(2), 127–131.

Broen, P. A., Devers, M. C., Doyle, S. S., Prouty, J. M., & Moller, K. T. (1998). Acquisition of linguistic and cognitive skills by children with cleft palate. *Journal of Speech, Language, and Hearing Research*, *41*(3), 676–687.

Cantwell, D. P., & Baker, L. (1991). Association between attention deficit-hyperactivity disorder and learning disorders. *Journal of Learning Disabilities*, *24*(2), 88–95.

Chapman, K. L. (1991). Vocalizations of toddlers with cleft lip and palate. *Cleft Palate-Craniofacial Journal*, *28*(2), 172–178.

Chapman, K. L. (1993). Phonologic processes in children with cleft palate. *Cleft Palate-Craniofacial Journal*, *30*(1), 64–72.

Chapman, K. L., Graham, K. T., Gooch, J., & Visconti, C. (1998). Conversational skills of preschool and school-age children with cleft lip and palate. *Cleft Palate-Craniofacial Journal*, *35*(6), 503–516.

Chapman, K. L., & Hardin, M. A. (1991). Language input of mothers interacting with their young children with cleft lip and palate. *Cleft Palate-Craniofacial Journal*, *28*(1), 78–85; Discussion 85–86.

Chapman, K. L., & Hardin, M. A. (1992). Phonetic and phonological skills of two-year-olds with cleft palate. *Cleft Palate-Craniofacial Journal*, *29*(5), 435–443.

Cherkes-Julkowski, M. (1998). Learning disability, attention-deficit disorder, and language impairment as outcomes of prematurity: A longitudinal descriptive study. *Journal of Learning Disabilities*, *31*(3), 294–306.

Damico, J. S., Damico, S. K., & Armstrong, M. B. (1999). Attention-deficit hyperactivity disorder and communication disorders: Issues and clinical practices. *Child and Adolescent Psychiatric Clinics of North America*, *8*(1), 37–60.

D'Antonio, L. L., Scherer, N. J., Miller, L. L., Kalbfleisch, J. H., & Bartley, J. A. (2001). Analysis of speech characteristics in children with velocardiofacial syndrome (VCFS) and children with phenotypic overlap without VCFS. *Cleft Palate-Craniofacial Journal*, *38*(5), 455–467.

Devriendt, K., Van Thienen, M., Swillen, A., & Fryns, J. (1996). Cerebellar hypoplasia in a patient with velocardiofacial syndrome. *Developmental Medicine and Neurology*, *38*, 945–949.

Dorf, D. S., & Curtin, J. W. (1990). Early cleft repair and speech outcome: A ten-year experience. In J. Bardach & H. L. Morris (Eds.), *Multidisciplinary management of cleft lip and palate* (pp. 341–348). Philadelphia: W. B. Saunders.

Dowling, J. E. (2004). *The great brain debate: Nature or nurture?* Washington, DC: Joseph Henry Press.

Elfenbein, J. L., Waziri, M., & Morris, H. L. (1981). Verbal communication skills of six children with craniofacial anomalies. *Cleft Palate Journal*, *18*(1), 59–64.

Eliez, S., Antonarakis, S. E., Morris, M. A., Dahoun, S. P., & Reiss, A. L. (2001). Parental origin of the deletion 22qll.2 and brain development in velocardiofacial syndrome: A preliminary study. *Archives of General Psychiatry, 58,* 64–68.

Eliez, S., Blasey, C. M., Schmitt, E. J., White, C. D., Hu, D., & Reiss, A. L. (2001). Velocardiofacial syndrome: Are structural changes in the temporal and mesial temporal regions related to schizophrenia? *American Journal of Psychiatry, 158,* 447–453.

Eliez, S., Schmitt, J. E., White, C. D., & Reiss, A. L. (2000). Children and adolescents with velocardiofacial syndrome. *American Journal of Psychiatry, 157,* 409–415.

Estes, R. E., & Morris, H. L. (1970). Relationships among intelligence, speech proficiency, and hearing sensitivity in children with cleft palates. *Cleft Palate Journal, 7,* 763–773.

Estrem, T., & Broen, P. A. (1989). Early speech production of children with cleft palate. *Journal of Speech and Hearing Research, 32*(1), 12–23.

Fergusson, D. M., & Horwood, L. J. (1992). Attention deficit and reading achievement. *Journal of Child Psychology and Psychiatry and Allied Disciplines, 33*(2), 375–385.

Frederickson, M. S., Chapman, K. L., & Hardin-Jones, M. (2006). Conversational skills of children with cleft lip and palate: A replication and extension. *The Cleft Palate–Craniofacial Journal, 43*(2), 179–188.

Glaser, B., Mumme, D. L., Blasey, C., Morris, M. A., Dahoun, S. P., et al. (2002). Language skills in children with velocardiofacial syndrome (deletion 22qll.2). *Journal of Pediatrics, 140*(6), 753–758.

Goodstein, L. D. (1961). Intellectual impairment in children with cleft palates. *Journal of Speech and Hearing Research, 4,* 287–294.

Grobbelaar, A. O., Hudson, D. A., Fernandes, D. B., & Lentin, R. (1995). Speech results after repair of the cleft soft palate. *Plastic and Reconstructive Surgery, 95*(7), 1150–1154.

Grunwell, P., & Russell, V. J. (1988). Phonological development in children with cleft palate. *Clinical Linguistics and Phonetics, 2,* 75–95.

Hardin, M. A. (1991). Cleft palate: Intervention. *Clinics in Communication Disorders, 1*(3), 12–18.

Harding, A., & Grunwell, P. (1996). Characteristics of cleft palate speech. *European Journal of Disorders of Communication, 31,* 331–357.

Hardin-Jones, M., & Chapman, K. L. (2011). Cognitive and language issues associated with cleft lip and palate. *Seminars in Speech and Language, 32*(2), 127–140.

Hardin-Jones, M., Chapman, K., & Scherer, N. J. (2006, June 13). Early intervention in children with cleft palate. *The ASHA Leader, 11*(8), 8–9, 32.

Hardin-Jones, M., Chapman, K. L., & Schulte, J. (2003). The impact of cleft type on early vocal development in babies with cleft palate. *Cleft Palate-Craniofacial Journal, 40*(5), 453–459.

Heineman-de Boer, J. A., Van Haelst, M. J., Cordia-de Haan, M., & Beemer, F. A. (1999). Behavior problems and personality aspects of 40 children with velocardiofacial syndrome. *Genetic Counseling, 10*(1), 89–93.

Hentges, F., Hill, J., Bishop, D. V., Goodacre, T., Moss, T., & Murray, L. (2011). The effect of cleft lip on cognitive development in school-aged children: A paradigm for examining sensitive period effects. *Journal of Child Psychology and Psychiatry, 52*(6), 704–712.

Hom, L. (1972). Language development of the cleft palate child. *Journal of South African Speech and Hearing Association, 19*(1), 17–29.

Hultman, C. S., Riski, J. E., Cohen, S. R., Burstein, F. D., Boydston, W. R., Hudgins, R. J., Grattin-Smith, D., et al. (2000). Chiari malformation, cervical spine anomalies, and neurologic deficits in velocardiofacial syndrome. *Plastic and Reconstructive Surgery, 106*(1), 16–24.

Jocelyn, L. J., Penko, M. A., & Rode, H. L. (1996). Cognition, communication, and hearing in young children with cleft lip and palate and in control children: A longitudinal study. *Pediatrics, 97*(4), 529–534.

Jones, C. E., Chapman, K. L., & Hardin-Jones, M. A. (2003). Speech development of children with cleft palate before and after palatal surgery. *Cleft Palate-Craniofacial Journal, 40*(1), 19–31.

Kapp-Simon, K. A., & Krueckeberg, S. (2000). Mental development in infants with cleft lip and/or palate. *Cleft Palate-Craniofacial Journal, 37*(1), 65–70.

Kates, W. R., Burnette, C. P., Bessette, B. A., Folley, B. S., Strunge, L., et al. (2004). Frontal and caudate alterations in velocardiofacial syndrome (deletion at chromosome 22qll.2). *Journal of Child Neurology, 19*(5), 337–342.

Kates, W. R., Burnette, C. P., Jabs, E. W., Rutberg, J., Murphy, A. M., Grados, M., et al. (2001). Regional cortical white matter reductions in velocardiofacial syndrome: A volumetric MRI analysis. *Biological Psychiatry, 49*(8), 677–684.

Kok, L. L., & Solman, R. T. (1995). Velocardiofacial syndrome: Learning difficulties and intervention. *Journal of Medical Genetics, 32*(8), 612–618.

Konst, E. M., Rietveld, T., Peters, H. F., & Kuijpers-Jagtman, A. M. (2003). Language skills of young children with unilateral cleft lip and palate following infant orthopedics: A randomized clinical trial. *Cleft Palate-Craniofacial Journal, 40*(4), 356–362.

Kritzinger, A., Louw, B., & Hugo, R. (1996). Early communication functioning of infants with cleft lip and palate. *South African Journal of Communication Disorders-die Suid-Afrikaanse Tydskrif vir Kommunikasieafwykings, 43*, 77–84.

Kummer, A. W. (2011). Disorders of resonance and airflow secondary to cleft palate and/or velopharyngeal dysfunction. *Seminars in Speech and Language, 32*(2), 141–149.

Kummer, A. W., Lee, L., Stutz, L., Maroney, A., & Brandt, J. W. (2007). The prevalence of apraxic characteristics in patients with velocardiofacial syndrome as compared to other populations. *Cleft Palate-Craniofacial Journal, 44*(2), 175–181.

Lamb, M., Wilson, F., & Leeper, H. (1973). The intellectual function of cleft palate children compared on the basis of cleft type and sex. *Cleft Palate Journal, 10*, 367–377.

Lecendreux, M., Konofal, E., & Faraone, S. V. (2010). Prevalence of attention deficit hyperactivity disorder and associated features among children in France. *Journal of Attention Disorders, 15*(6), 516–524.

Leeper, H. A., Jr., Pannbacker, M., & Roginski, J. (1980). Oral language characteristics of adult cleft-palate speakers compared on the basis of cleft type and sex. *Journal of Communication Disorders, 13*(2), 133–146.

Lohmander-Agerskov, A., Soderpalm, E., Friede, H., Persson, E. C., & Lilja, J. (1994). Pre-speech in children with cleft lip and palate or cleft palate only: Phonetic analysis related to morphologic and functional factors. *Cleft Palate-Craniofacial Journal, 31*(4), 271–279.

Long, N. V., & Dalston, R. M. (1982a). Gestural communication in twelve-month-old cleft lip and palate children. *Cleft Palate Journal, 19*(1), 57–61.

Long, N. V., & Dalston, R. M. (1982b). Paired gestural and vocal behavior in one-year-old cleft lip and palate children. *Journal of Speech and Hearing Disorders, 47*(4), 403–406.

Long, N. V., & Dalston, R. M. (1983). Comprehension abilities of one-year-old infants with cleft lip and palate. *Cleft Palate Journal, 20*(4), 303–306.

Love, A. J., & Thompson, M. G. (1988). Language disorders and attention deficit disorders in young children referred for psychiatric services: Analysis of prevalence and a conceptual synthesis. *American Journal of Orthopsychiatry, 58*(1), 52–64.

Lynch, D. R., McDonald-McGinn, D. M., Zackai, E. H., Emanuel, B. S., Driscoll, D. A., Whitaker, L. A., & Fischbeck, K. H. (1995). Cerebellar atrophy in a patient with velocardiofacial syndrome. *Journal of Medical Genetics, 32*(7), 561–563.

Lynch, J. L., Fox, D. R., & Brookshire, B. L. (1983). Phonological proficiency of two cleft palate toddlers with school-age follow-up. *Journal of Speech & Hearing Disorders, 48*(3), 274–285.

Max, J. E., Arndt, S., Castillo, C. S., Bokura, H., Robin, D. A., Lundgren, S. D., Smith, W. L., et al. (1998). Attention-deficit hyperactivity symptomatology after traumatic brain injury: A prospective study. *Journal of the American Academy of Child Adolescent Psychiatry, 37*(8), 841–847.

McWilliams, B. J., & Matthews, H. P. (1979). A comparison of intelligence and social maturity in children with unilateral complete clefts and those with isolated cleft palates. *Cleft Palate Journal, 16*, 363–372.

McWilliams, B. J., Morris, H. L., & Shelton, R. L. (1990). Language disorders. In B. J. McWilliams, H. L. Morris, & R. L. Shelton (Eds.), *Cleft palate speech* (vol. 2, pp. 236–246). Philadelphia: B. C. Decker.

Morris, H. L. (1962). Communication skills of children with cleft lip and palate. *Journal of Speech and Hearing Research, 5*, 79–90.

Mossey, P. A., Little, J., Munger, R. G., Dixon, M. J., & Shaw, W. C., (2009). Cleft lip and palate. *Lancet, 374*(9703), 1773–1785.

Motzkin, B., Marion, R., Goldberg, R., Shprintzen, R., & Saenger, P. (1993). Variable phenotypes in velocardiofacial syndrome with chromosomal deletion. *Journal of Pediatrics, 123*(3), 406–410.

Musgrave, R. H., McWilliams, B. J., & Matthews, H. P. (1975). A review of the results of two different surgical procedures for the repair of clefts of the soft palate only. *Cleft Palate Journal, 12*, 281–290.

Neiman, G. S., & Savage, H. E. (1997). Development of infants and toddlers with clefts from birth to three years of age. *Cleft Palate-Craniofacial Journal, 34*(3), 218–225.

Niemann, H., Ruff, R. M., & Kramer, J. H. (1996). An attempt towards differentiating attentional deficits in traumatic brain injury. *Neuropsychological Review, 6*(1), 11–46.

Nopoulos, P., Berg, S., Canady, J., Richman, L., Van Demark, D., & Andreasen, N. C. (2002). Structural brain abnormalities in adult males with clefts of the lip and/or palate. *Genetics in Medicine, 4*(1), 1–9.

Nopoulos, P., Berg, S., Van Demark, D., Richman, L., Canady, J., & Andreasen, N. C. (2001). Increased incidence of a midline brain anomaly in patients with nonsyndromic clefts of the lip and/or palate. *Journal of Neuroimaging, 11*(4), 418–424.

Nopoulos, P., Berg, S., Van Demark, D., Richman, L., Canady, J., & Andreasen, N. C. (2002). Cognitive dysfunction in adult males with nonsyndromic clefts of the lip and/or palate. *Neuropsychologia, 40*(12), 2178–2184.

Nopoulos, P., Choe, L., Berg, S., Van Demark, D., Canady, J., & Richman, L. (2005). Ventral frontal cortex morphology in adult males with isolated orofacial clefts: Relationship to abnormalities in social function. *Cleft Palate-Craniofacial Journal, 42*(2), 138–144.

O'Gara, M. M., & Logemann, J. A. (1988). Phonetic analyses of the speech development of babies with cleft palate. *Cleft Palate Journal, 25*(2), 122–134.

O'Gara, M. M., Logemann, J. A., & Rademaker, A. W. (1994). Phonetic features by babies with unilateral cleft lip and palate. *Cleft Palate-Craniofacial Journal, 31*(6), 446–451.

Pamplona, M. C., Ysunza, A., Gonzalez, M., Ramirez, E., & Patino, C. (2000). Linguistic development in cleft palate patients with and without compensatory articulation disorder. *International Journal of Pediatric Otorhinolaryngology, 54*(2–3), 81–89.

Pannbacker, M. (1975). Oral language skills of adult cleft palate speakers. *Cleft Palate Journal, 12*(1), 95–106.

Paradise, J. L. (1998). Otitis media and child development: Should we worry? *Pediatric Infectious Disease Journal, 17*(11), 1076–1083; Discussion 1099–1100.

Persson, C., Niklasson, L., Oskarsdottir, S., Johansson, S., Jonsson, R., & Soderpalm, E. (2006). Language skills in 5–8-year-old children with 22q11 deletion syndrome. *International Journal of Language and Communication Disorders, 41*(3), 313–333.

Peterson, S. J. (1973). Speech pathology in craniofacial malformations other than cleft lip and palate. *ASHA Reports, 8,* 11–131.

Peterson-Falzone, S. J. (1996). The relationship between timing of cleft palate surgery and speech outcome: What have we learned, and where do we stand in the 1990s? *Seminars in Orthodontics, 2*(3), 185–191.

Purvis, K. L., & Tannock, R. (1997). Language abilities in children with attention deficit hyperactivity disorder, reading disabilities, and normal controls. *Journal of Abnormal Child Psychology, 25*(2), 133–144.

Richman, L. C. (1980). Cognitive patterns and learning disabilities of cleft palate children with verbal deficits. *Journal of Speech and Hearing Research, 23*(2), 447–456.

Richman, L. C., Eliason, M. J., & Lindgren, S. D. (1988). Reading disability in children with clefts. *Cleft Palate Journal, 25*(1), 21–25.

Richman, L. C., & Nopoulos, P. (2009). Neuropsychological and neuroimaging aspects of cleft lip and palate. In J. E. Losee & R. E. Kirschner (Eds.), *Comprehensive cleft care* (pp. 991–1000). New York: McGraw-Hill.

Rosen, H., Chiou, G. J., Stoler, J. M., Mulliken, J. B., Tarui, T., Meara, J. G., & Estroff, J. A. (2011). Magnetic resonance imaging for detection of brain abnormalities in fetuses with cleft lip and/or cleft palate. *Cleft Palate-Craniofacial Journal, 48*(5), 619–622.

Roug, L., Landberg, L., & Lundberg, L. J. (1989). Phonetic development in early infancy: A study of four Swedish children during the first eighteen months of life. *Journal of Child Language, 16*(1), 19–40.

Ruess, A. L. (1965). A comparative study of cleft palate children and their siblings. *Journal of Clinical Psychology, 21,* 354–360.

Russell, V. J. (1991). *Speech development in children with cleft lip and palate.* Unpublished doctoral dissertation, Leicester Polytechnic, Leicester, UK.

Scherer, N. J., Williams, A. L., & Proctor-Williams, K. (2008). Early and later vocalization skills in children with and without cleft palate. *International Journal of Pediatric Otorhinolaryngology*, 72(6), 827–840.

Scherer, N. J., D'Antonio, L. L., & Kalbfleisch, J. H. (1999). Early speech and language development in children with velocardiofacial syndrome. *American Journal of Medical Genetics*, 88(6), 714–723.

Scherer, N. J., D'Antonio, L. L., & Rodgers, J. R. (2001). Profiles of communication disorder in children with velocardiofacial syndrome: Comparison to children with Down syndrome. *Genetics in Medicine*, 3(1), 72–78.

Shames, C., & Rubin, H. (1979). Psycholinguistic measures of language and speech. In K. R. Bzoch (Ed.), *Communicative disorders related to cleft lip and palate* (pp. 202–223). Boston: Little, Brown.

Shprintzen, R. J. (1998). Complex craniofacial disorders. In S. E. Gerber (Ed.), *Etiology and prevention of communicative disorders* (*vol. 2*, pp. 147–199). San Diego, CA: Singular Publishing Group.

Shprintzen, R. J., Goldberg, R. B., Lewin, M. L., Sidoti, E. J., Berkman, M. D., Argamaso, R. V., & Young, D. (1978). A new syndrome involving cleft palate, cardiac anomalies, typical facies, and learning disabilities: Velocardiofacial syndrome. *Cleft Palate Journal*, 15(1), 56–62.

Sidoti, E. J., Jr., Marsh, J. L., Marty-Grames, L., & Noetzel, M. J. (1996). Long-term studies of metopic synostosis: Frequency of cognitive impairment and behavioral disturbances. *Plastic and Reconstructive Surgery*, 97(2), 276–281.

Smith, B. E., & Kuehn, D. P. (2007). Speech evaluation of velopharyngeal dysfunction. *The Journal of Craniofacial Surgery*, 18(2), 251–261.

Smith, B. L., & Oller, D. K. (1981). A comparative study of premeaningful vocalizations produced by normally developing and Down's syndrome infants. *Journal of Speech and Hearing Disorders*, 46(1), 46–51.

Smith, R. M., & McWilliams, B. J. (1968). Psycholinguistic abilities of children with clefts. *Cleft Palate Journal*, 5, 238–249.

Snyder, L. E., & Scherer, N. (2004). The development of symbolic play and language in toddlers with cleft palate. *American Journal of Speech-Language Pathology*, 13(1), 66–80.

Speltz, M. L., Endriga, M. C., Hill, S., Maris, C. L., Jones, K., & Omnell, M. L. (2000). Cognitive and psychomotor development of infants with orofacial clefts. *Journal of Pediatric Psychology*, 25(3), 185–190.

Spriestersbach, D. C., Darley, F., & Morris, H. L. (1958). Language skills in children with cleft palate. *Journal of Speech and Hearing Research*, 1, 279–285.

Stoel-Gammon, C. (1985). Phonetic inventories, 15–24 months: A longitudinal study. *Journal of Speech & Hearing Research*, 28(4), 505–512.

Strauss, R. P., & Broder, H. (1993). Children with cleft lip/palate and mental retardation: A subpopulation of cleft-craniofacial team patients. *Cleft Palate-Craniofacial Journal*, 30(6), 548–556.

Swillen, A., Devriendt, K., Legius, E., Eyskens, B., Dumoulin, M., Gewillig, M., & Fryns, J. P. (1997). Intelligence and psychosocial adjustment in velocardiofacial syndrome: A study of 37 children and adolescents with VCFS. *Journal of Medical Genetics*, 34(6), 453–458.

Swillen, A., Devriendt, K., Legius, E., Prinzie, P., Vogels, A., Ghesquiere, P., & Fryns, J. P. (1999). The behavioural phenotype in velo-cardio-facial syndrome (VCFS): From infancy to adolescence. *Genetic Counseling*, 10(1), 79–88.

Tirosh, E., Berger, J., Cohen-Ophir, M., Davidovitch, M., & Cohen, A. (1998). Learning disabilities with and without attention-deficit hyperactivity disorder: Parents' and teachers' perspectives. *Journal of Child Neurology, 13*(6), 270–276.

Tirosh, E., & Cohen, A. (1998). Language deficit with attention-deficit disorder: A prevalent comorbidity. *Journal of Child Neurology, 13*(10), 493–497.

Trost-Cardamone, J. E. (1997). Diagnosis of specific cleft palate speech error patterns for planning therapy of physical management needs. In K. R. Bzoch (Ed.), *Communicative disorders related to cleft lip and palate* (*vol. 4*, pp. 313–330). Austin, TX: Pro-Ed.

van Amelsvoort, T., Daly, E., Henry, J., Robertson, D., Ng, V., Owen, M., Murphy, K. C., et al. (2004). Brain anatomy in adults with velocardiofacial syndrome with and without schizophrenia: Preliminary results of a structural magnetic resonance imaging study. *Archives of Genera! Psychiatry, 61*, 1085–1096.

Vantrappen, G., Devriendt, K., Swillen, A., Rommel, N., Vogels, A., Eyskens, B., Gewillig, M., et al. (1999). Presenting symptoms and clinical features in 130 patients with the velocardiofacial syndrome. The Leuven experience. *Genetic Counseling, 10*(1), 3–9.

Whitcomb, L., Ochsner, G., & Wayte, R. (1976). A comparison of expressive language skills of cleft-palate and non-cleft-palate children: A preliminary investigation. *Journal of the Oklahoma Speech and Hearing Association, 3*, 25–28.

Willadsen, E., & Albrechtsen, H. (2006). Phonetic description of babbling in Danish toddlers born with and without unilateral cleft lip and palate. *Cleft Palate-Craniofacial Journal, 43*(2), 189–200.

Wirls, C. J. (1971). Psychosocial aspects of cleft lip and palate. In W. C. Grabb, S. W. Rosenstein, & K. Bzoch (Eds.), *Cleft lip and palate* (pp. 119–129). Boston: Little, Brown.

Wright, G. F. (1982). Attention deficit disorder. *Journal of School Health, 52*(2), 119–120.

Yamagishi, H. (2002). The 22q11.2 deletion syndrome. *The Keio Journal of Medicine, 52*(2), 77–88.

Zimmerman, J., & Canfield, W. (1968). Language and speech development. In R. Stark (Ed.), *Cleft palate: A multidiscipline approach* (pp. 220–242). New York: Harper and Row.

CHAPTER

7

RESONANCE DISORDERS AND VELOPHARYNGEAL DYSFUNCTION (VPD)

CHAPTER OUTLINE

INTRODUCTION

During normal speech production, sound is generated by the vocal folds. The sound then changes as it travels through the cavities of the vocal tract. Both the laryngeal sound and the resonance of the vocal tract provide the quality and uniqueness of each individual's voice.

It is important that both the sound energy and the airflow within the vocal tract are directed through the pharynx without obstruction. Once through the pharynx, the velopharyngeal valve plays a key role in directing the sound and airflow into the appropriate cavity for each speech sound.

Resonance disorders are common in individuals with a history of cleft lip and palate or other craniofacial anomalies. Resonance disorders can be due to a form of velopharyngeal dysfunction, or they can be due to obstruction in one or more cavities of the vocal tract. Velopharyngeal dysfunction can not only cause a resonance disorder (hypernasality), but it can also cause nasal emission of the air stream. When there is significant nasal emission due to a large velopharyngeal opening, several other speech characteristics can occur as a result of inadequate oral airflow and air pressure for consonants.

The purpose of this chapter is to acquaint the reader with different types of resonance disorders and the speech characteristics of velopharyngeal dysfunction. The various types and causes of velopharyngeal dysfunction are also described.

NORMAL VOICE AND RESONANCE

Speech production requires both airflow and sound. Airflow from the lungs is converted into air pressure by the articulators. Air pressure is particularly important for *pressure-sensitive phonemes*, which include plosives, fricatives, and affricates. On the other hand, sound is needed for voiced consonants and all vowels. The sound that originates from vocal fold vibration is modified as it travels through the vocal tract by the natural resonances of the cavities. See Figure 7–3 for a schema of speech production using both airflow and sound.

In physics, *resonance* is described as the tendency of a system to vibrate (oscillate) with a larger amplitude at some frequencies than at others. Resonance, as it relates to speech, is the modification of phonated sound through selective enhancement of certain formant frequencies as opposed to others. This modification is determined by the size and shape of the cavities of the vocal tract (Kummer, 2011a).

To further describe resonance, it makes sense to begin with phonation. To initiate *phonation* (voicing), the vocal folds close through muscular forces. Positive air pressure from the lungs builds, forcing the vocal folds to open. The high velocity air produces a lowered pressure within the *glottis* (space between the vocal folds), which then brings the lower edges of the vocal folds back together (called the *Bernoulli effect*). The elasticity of the tissue then brings the upper edge of the vocal folds together. This completes one vibratory cycle of the vocal folds (Titze, 1980,

2000). The vibration of the vocal folds (due to rapid cycles of opening and closing) causes oscillation of the air stream, thus producing the sound of voicing.

The intensity (loudness) of the voice can be increased by increasing both the airflow from the lungs and the resistance of the vocal folds. With increased airflow, the vocal fold edges have greater lateral displacement. With increased resistance, they recoil with greater force. These factors increase the amplitude of the sound pressure wave, which is perceived as increased volume.

The frequency (pitch) of the voice is a function of the length, thickness, and elasticity of the vocal folds. All objects have a frequency or set of frequencies with which they naturally vibrate when set in motion. The vocal folds are no exception. They naturally vibrate in response to the driving force of subglottic air pressure. The most commonly occurring frequency at which they vibrate is known as the *fundamental frequency*, which is the lowest frequency of a periodic waveform. In addition, the tissue that is considered the cover of each vocal fold is disturbed in three dimensions by airflow. These disturbances create additional frequencies called harmonics. The *harmonics* are component frequencies of the signal that are whole number multiples of the fundamental frequency.

As the sound from the vocal folds travels through the cavities of the vocal tract, the various frequencies that make up this complex sound are selectively enhanced as a function of the shape and size of the cavities. As a rule of thumb (and of physics), when a complex sound passes through a short or small cavity, the higher frequencies in that sound will be enhanced. If that same complex sound passes through a longer or larger cavity, the lower frequencies in that sound will be enhanced.

The effect of cavity size on resonance can be illustrated several ways. For example, if you blow across a bottle that is half full, you will hear a certain pitch. If you pour out some of the liquid and blow again, the pitch will be perceived as lower, despite the same sound source. This is because as the bottle is emptied, the resonating cavity becomes bigger, thus enhancing more of the lower formant frequencies. The same principle applies to wind instruments. A longer chamber results in perception of a lower sound than a shorter chamber. Therefore, resonance for speech is directly related to the size and shape of the resonating cavities of the vocal tract (pharyngeal cavity, oral cavity, and nasal cavity). Smaller cavities of the vocal tract enhance higher frequencies, whereas larger cavities enhance lower frequencies and result in a richer sound.

When considering the effects of vocal fold vibration and vocal cavity size on pitch and resonance, it is easy to understand why the voice of a child is perceived as higher than the voice of an adult. In comparison, a child has a smaller larynx than an adult, and thus a faster vocal fold vibration rate plus higher harmonics. In addition, the pharynx is shorter and the oral cavity is smaller. Therefore, more of the higher harmonics are enhanced during speech as compared to an adult with a larger pharyngeal and oral cavity. In addition, it has been shown that adult males and females differ not only in the length and thickness of the vocal folds but also with respect to oral and pharyngeal cavity sizes. These differences affect the resonant frequencies that influence the overall perception of voice quality and pitch (Ikeda, Matsuzaki, & Aomatsu, 2001). Overall, both phonation and resonance combine to provide the unique qualities of each individual's voice.

During connected speech, normal speakers use *prosody*, which is a combination of changes in frequency, intensity, rate, and stress. The variation of pitch is used for emphasis, to express emotions, to ask a question, to differentiate meaning, and for many other functions. These pitch changes occur as a result of changes in vocal fold length and mass, and alterations in pharyngeal cavity size. For example, for higher pitches, the vocal folds are lengthened and tensed, with decreased mass. In addition, the larynx raises, which shortens the pharynx, and the lateral pharyngeal walls contract, which narrows the pharynx (Ikeda et al., 2001). The decrease in the size of the pharynx further enhances the higher frequencies produced by the vocal folds.

Although there is sound energy in the oral cavity for all oral sounds, there are subtle differences in resonance between various voiced phonemes. Because the larynx, pharynx, mandible, tongue, and velum are all interconnected by the hyoid muscle group, the height of the velum and the configuration of the pharynx are affected by tongue position during the production of different speech phonemes (Tom, Titze, Hoffman, & Story, 2001). As a result, movement of the tongue or velum can alter the size and shape of the pharynx and/or oral cavity (Hiiemae & Palmer, 2003).

Resonance is a component of all voiced phonemes, but it is particularly important for vowels. In fact, it can be said that vowels are "resonance sounds," because they are produced by manipulating the resonance in the oral cavity. The acoustic properties of each distinct vowel are determined by the position of the tongue, mandible, and lips, which affects the size and shape of the oral cavity. Altering the position of one of these structures changes the selective enhancement of the formant frequencies and thus changes the vowel.

Despite the fact that vowels are generally considered oral sounds, normal speech is characterized by a slight degree of nasal resonance on each vowel. This can be shown through nasometry (see Chapter 14). A high vowel, such as /i/, consistently has more nasal

resonance than a low vowel, such as /ɑ/. A working theory is that the velum is like a heavy curtain. As such, some sound is transmitted through the velum during vowel production. There may be more nasal resonance on high vowels as compared to low vowels because with a high tongue position there is more oral impedance and more oral pressure (Jones, 2005). Both of these factors can result in more transpalatal transmission of the sound (Gildersleeve-Neumann & Dalston, 2001).

RESONANCE DISORDERS

A *resonance* disorder is characterized by abnormal transmission of sound energy through the oral, nasal, and/or pharyngeal cavities of the vocal tract during speech production (Kummer, 2011a). This causes the perception of what some people generally call "nasality." Resonance disorders include hypernasality (too much sound energy in the nasal cavity), hyponasality (too little sound in the nasal cavity), cul-de-sac resonance (blocked sound in one of the cavities), or a mixture of these types. Causes of resonance disorders include dysfunction of the velopharyngeal valve, an opening or fistula in the palate, obstruction in one or more of the vocal cavities, and even misarticulation (Smith & Kuehn, 2007). Anything that disrupts the transmission of sound in the cavities of the vocal tract will cause abnormal resonance.

Resonance disorders, particularly hypernasality, are often labeled as "voice disorders." This is an inappropriate categorization because resonance disorders are not laryngeal in origin. Therefore, most specialists consider resonance disorders to be distinct from voice disorders (Riski & Verdolini, 1999).

The following sections describe the types and causes of resonance disorders in more detail.

Hypernasality

Hypernasality is a resonance disorder that occurs when there is abnormal nasal resonance during the production of oral sounds. This is due to abnormal *coupling* (sharing of acoustic energy) of the oral and nasal cavities during speech. Hypernasality is often described as just "nasal," muffled, or characterized by mumbling. This is due to the *damping* (sound absorption) effect as the sound goes through the pharyngeal cavity and turbinates of the nasal cavity (Buder, 2005). In addition to the video samples with this text, there are audio samples of various degrees of hypernasality in children, men, and women on the website of the American Cleft Palate–Craniofacial Association (2006).

Because hypernasality is due to abnormal resonance of sound (as opposed to air), it is always associated with voiced, rather than voiceless, speech sounds (Cassassolles et al., 1995). Hypernasality is particularly perceptible on vowels, because they are voiced, relatively long in duration, and are typically not substituted with a different placement. Hypernasality is more noted on high vowels than low vowels (Andrews & Rutherford, 1972; Lee, Wang, & Fu, 2009). This is due to the high tongue position, which reduces oral resonance space and causes partial impedance of sound coming through the oral cavity. The relatively narrow space as a result of the high tongue position also causes an increase in sound pressure, which can result in increased transmission of sound through the velum (Awan, Omlor, & Watts, 2011; Gildersleeve-Neumann & Dalston, 2001). If the velum is thin, due to a submucous cleft, for example, this can significantly add to the perception of hypernasality, even in the absence of velopharyngeal dysfunction.

When there is moderate to severe hypernasality, *nasalization of oral phonemes* is common. For example, it makes sense that when the velopharyngeal valve remains at least partially open during the attempted production of a voiced plosive, the acoustic product will be closer to the nasal cognate of that oral sound (e.g., m/b, n/d, and ŋ/g). Nasalization can occur on any voiced oral sound. In addition, nasal sounds may even be substituted for voiceless sounds (e.g., n/s) as a compensatory strategy. Therefore, with moderate to severe hypernasality, the speech may consist primarily of nasal sounds (/m/, /n/, and /ŋ/). Hypernasality on vowels and nasalization of consonants often increase with utterance length, speed, or phonemic complexity due to the additional demands on the velopharyngeal mechanism.

Hypernasality is usually caused by a fairly large velopharyngeal opening (Kummer, Briggs, & Lee, 2003; Kummer, Curtis, Wiggs, Lee, & Strife, 1992). However, it can also occur in patients with normal velopharyngeal function, but a thin velum due to a submucous cleft. Hypernasality can be due to a large oronasal fistula in patients with a history of cleft palate repair (Figure 7–1). Finally, hypernasality can even be phoneme specific due to

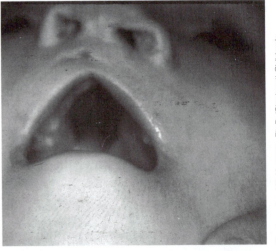

Courtesy Ann W. Kummer, Ph.D./Cincinnati Children's Craniofacial Team

FIGURE 7–1 A very large palatal fistula that would cause significant hypernasality.

nasal articulation on certain oral sounds (e.g., ŋ/l, ŋ/r). This type of hypernasality is considered phoneme specific and is due to mislearning. (Causes of velopharyngeal dysfunction are further discussed in a section below.)

Hypernasality should not be confused with a nasal twang, which has been described as a characteristic of certain dialects. This quality has been found to occur with pharyngeal area narrowing and vocal tract shortening (Story, Titze, & Hoffman, 2001; Titze, Bergan, Hunter, & Story, 2003; Yanagisawa, Estill, Mambrino, & Talkin, 1991; Yanagisawa, Kmucha, & Estill, 1990). It may also be related to the high posterior tongue position on certain vowels, as is common with a southern dialect.

Hyponasality and Denasality

Hyponasality occurs when there is a reduction in normal nasal resonance during speech caused by obstruction in the nasopharynx or nasal cavity. The overall perceptual feature is that the individual sounds "stuffed up." The term *denasality* typically refers to abnormal resonance due to total upper airway obstruction. Because it is impossible to know whether there is total blockage of the nasal cavity through a perceptual assessment alone, the term hyponasality is more commonly used.

Hyponasality particularly affects the production of the nasal consonants (/m/, /n/, /ŋ/). When nasal resonance is reduced, nasal consonants sound similar to their oral phoneme cognates (b/m, d/n, g/ŋ). Hyponasality can also affect the quality of vowels if it is severe. This is due to the fact that all vowels, particularly high vowels, have some nasal resonance caused by transmission of sound through the velum.

The cause of hyponasality is almost always obstruction somewhere in the nasopharynx or nasal cavity. Upper airway obstruction can cause symptoms other than hyponasality,

including a chronic open mouth posture, mouth breathing, loud snoring, and even sleep apnea. It has even been shown that nasal obstruction can reduce lip closing force (Sabashi et al., 2011).

Common causes of upper airway obstruction in a general population include swelling of the nasal passages secondary to allergic rhinitis or the common cold, adenoid hypertrophy, or even hypertrophic tonsils that intrude into the pharynx (Scott, Moldan, Tibesar, Lander, & Sidman, 2011). Upper airway obstruction causing hyponasality may also be due to congenital structural abnormalities (Adil, Huntley, Choudhary, & Carr, 2011). In fact, hyponasality and even obstructive sleep apnea are very common in individuals with a history of cleft palate or craniofacial conditions (Maclean, Waters, Fitzsimons, Hayward, & Fitzgerald, 2009; Muntz, Wilson, Park, Smith, & Grimmer, 2008; Robison & Otteson, 2011a). Common causes in the cleft population include a deviated septum (particularly with unilateral clefts), choanal stenosis or atresia, a stenotic naris, or maxillary retrusion that restricts the pharyngeal and nasal cavity space. Maxillary retrusion with midface deficiency is common in individuals with clefts and is also a phenotypic feature of several craniofacial syndromes, such as Crouzon syndrome, Apert syndrome, and Pfeiffer syndrome. Maxillary advancement can often decrease hyponasality and improve characteristics of airway obstruction (Demetriades, Chang, Laskarides, & Papageorge, 2010; Jakobsone, Stenvik, & Espeland, 2011; Pourdanesh, Sharifi, Mohebbi, & Jamilian, 2012; Schendel, Powell, & Jacobson, 2011).

Hyponasality may actually be more common than hypernasality in adolescents and adults with clefts. One reason for this is that velopharyngeal insufficiency (VPI) is usually corrected in the preschool or early school years so that hypernasality is no longer present as the individual gets older. However, because the surgical procedures that are designed to correct VPI narrow or reduce the size of the nasopharyngeal space, hyponasality is a common complication of the surgery (de Serres et al., 1999; Hall, Golding-Kushner, Argamaso, & Strauch, 1991; Witt, 2009).

Because the cause of hyponasality is almost always obstruction somewhere in the nasal cavity or pharynx, treatment involves either medical or surgical intervention. The only exception is when characteristics of hyponasality occur inconsistently due to apraxia of speech.

Cul-de-Sac Resonance

Cul-de-sac resonance occurs when the acoustic energy enters a cavity of the vocal tract but is blocked from exiting at the cavity's normal outlet. The sound is therefore trapped in this blind pouch, and some of the sound is absorbed by the soft tissues. As a result, the speech is perceived as muffled and low in volume. Like hyponasality, *cul-de-sac resonance* is due to obstruction, but in this case the place of obstruction is at the cavity's exit point rather than at the entrance or within the nasal cavity.

There are three types of cul-de-sac resonance, depending on the location of the blockage (Kummer, 2011a). All are defined by blockage at the cavity's exit point.

Oral cul-de-sac resonance is noted if the sound is partially blocked from exiting the oral cavity during speech. This can occur due to *microstomia* (a small mouth opening). It is also what is heard with mumbling or speaking without opening the mouth normally.

Nasal cul-de-sac resonance is noted if the sound is partially blocked from exiting the nasal cavity during speech. This is most noticeable when there is a combination of VPI (which would otherwise cause hypernasality), but also a blockage in the anterior part of the nose. Nasal cul-de-sac resonance is commonly found in individuals with a history of cleft palate with VPI, and also a stenotic naris or a deviated septum. Nasal cul-de-sac resonance can be simulated by either imitating hypernasality or producing a series of nasal phonemes (e.g., ma, ma, ma, ma, ma) while pinching the nose closed.

Pharyngeal cul-de-sac resonance occurs when most of the sound remains in the oropharynx during speech. This is typically caused by large tonsils that block the exit of the oropharynx and thus the entrance to the oral cavity (Kummer, Billmire, & Myer, 1993; Shprintzen et al., 1987). As with other types of cul-de-sac resonance, this blockage causes speech to be low in volume and muffled in quality. Pharyngeal cul-de-sac resonance has been described in the literature as "potato-in-the-mouth" speech (Finkelstein, Bar-Ziv, Nachmani, Berger, & Ophir, 1993). This is actually a great description because a speaker with a potato in the mouth is likely to have these same speech characteristics! Although enlarged tonsils are the most common cause of pharyngeal cul-de-sac resonance, it can also occur due to scar tissue or other forms of obstruction on the pharyngeal wall of the hypopharynx or oropharynx (Figure 7–2).

Cul-de-sac resonance is always due to a structural abnormality causing a blockage of one of the resonating cavities. Therefore, this type of resonance disorder cannot be corrected with speech therapy. Instead, correction requires medical or surgical intervention. However, the speech-language pathologist (SLP) is often the person to identify the cause of the abnormal resonance and therefore refer for appropriate intervention.

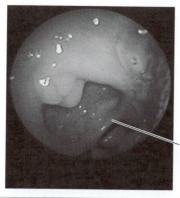

Scar tissue in
the hypopharynx

FIGURE 7–2 Scar band on the posterior pharyngeal wall. This can impede the transmission of sound energy through the pharynx, thus causing cul-de-sac resonance.

Courtesy Ann W. Kummer, Ph.D./Cincinnati Children's Hospital Medical Center & University of Cincinnati College of Medicine

Mixed Resonance

Mixed resonance is any combination of hypernasality (with or without nasal emission), hyponasality, and cul-de-sac resonance. Although hypernasality and hyponasality cannot occur simultaneously, they can occur at different times in the connected speech of the same speaker. For example, there can be hypernasality on oral sounds and hyponasality on nasal sounds.

Mixed resonance is common in individuals with apraxia. If the individual has difficulty coordinating anterior articulation with velopharyngeal articulation, there may be inappropriate upward movement of the velum on nasal sounds and downward movement of the velum on oral sounds (Ogar et al., 2006). In connected speech, there is usually more hypernasality than hyponasality, because moving the velum up for closure is harder than keeping it in the rest position.

Mixed resonance can also be caused by a combination of VPI and blockage in the pharynx. For example, there can be a short velum causing inadequate velopharyngeal closure on oral sounds, but also enlarged adenoids that block the sound from entering the nasal cavity on nasal sounds.

In addition to mixed resonance, some individuals demonstrate hyponasality and nasal emission, which has the same cause as hypernasality. Again, this does not occur simultaneously, but on different speech sounds. A common cause for this combination is enlarged, yet irregular, adenoid tissue. During the production of oral sounds, the velum closes against the adenoid pad, but a tight velopharyngeal seal cannot be obtained due to the irregular tissue. As a result, there is nasal emission. On the other hand, when the velum goes down for the production of nasal sounds, the adenoid pad is large enough that it obstructs the transmission of sound into the nasal cavity, thus causing hyponasality.

Effect of Surgery on Resonance

A discussion of resonance would not be complete without a mention of how resonance can change as a result of surgical alteration of the structures. In some cases, adenoidectomy can improve hyponasality if there was obstruction. In other cases, it can make speech worse by causing velopharyngeal insufficiency with hypernasality (and nasal emission). Tonsillectomy can eliminate cul-de-sac resonance by removing the blockage at the entrance of the oral cavity (see Chapter 8). Surgery to correct hypernasality (e.g., pharyngeal flap or sphincter pharyngoplasty) can be unsuccessful, resulting in residual hypernasality, or it can cause hyponasality due to over-correction (see Chapter 18). In addition, if the pharyngeal flap or sphincter (surgery for hypernasality) is placed too low in the pharynx, this can effectively shorten the resonating tube, causing an unwanted change in resonance (Smith, & Kuehn, 2007). Basically, anything that changes the length or shape of the resonating cavities can affect the quality of the voice.

Treatment of Resonance Disorders

It is important to emphasize again that resonance disorders are *almost always* caused by structural anomalies, and therefore resonance disorders *almost always* require medical or surgical intervention. Hypernasality is usually due to a structural or neurophysiological disorder that interferes with the function of the velopharyngeal valve. This can only be corrected or improved with surgery or a prosthetic device (if surgery is not an option). Hyponasality and cul-de-sac resonance are usually due to a blockage in one or more of the cavities of the vocal tract. Again, this is treated with medical or surgical intervention.

The *only* time that speech therapy is indicated for a resonance disorder is when the abnormal resonance is phoneme-specific due to faulty articulation placement. This may include the use of a nasal sound consistently for an oral sound, or an abnormally high tongue position during production of vowels. This can even be noted after surgical intervention due to the preoperative development of compensatory productions. Correction of the structure should be done first, and then speech therapy can be effective in correction of abnormal function that developed as a compensatory strategy.

NASAL EMISSION AND EFFECTS ON SPEECH

Speech production begins with the lungs. It is the air from the lungs that provides the initiating force for phonation (see Figure 7–3). Once

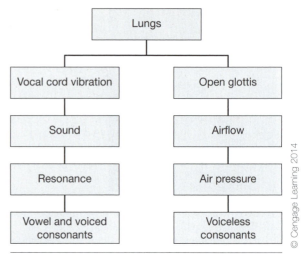

FIGURE 7–3 Schema of Speech Production

© Cengage Learning 2014

released from the glottis, the airflow courses superiorly through the pharynx. For nasal sounds, the airflow continues its upward movement to be released through the nasal cavity along with the nasal sound. For oral sounds however, the velopharyngeal valve closes to redirect the airflow (along with the sound) into the oral cavity. Intraoral airflow is converted into air pressure when the flow is blocked or restricted by the articulators (tongue, teeth, and lips) (Kummer, 2011a).

Velopharyngeal dysfunction (and an oronasal fistula) can cause a leak of the airflow into nasal cavity during speech. This leak can cause audible nasal emission and can affect several other aspects of speech, which are described next.

Types of Nasal Emission

Nasal emission occurs when there is an attempt to build up intraoral air pressure for the production of consonants while there is a leak in the system (velopharyngeal valve or oronasal fistula). As a result, some of the airflow is released through the nose, causing a disruption in the aerodynamic process of speech. Nasal emission occurs on *pressure-sensitive phonemes* (plosives, fricatives, and affricates). It is most noticed on voiceless phonemes because they are associated with more air pressure than their voiced counterparts, where the adduction of the vocal folds attenuates the air pressure somewhat. Nasal emission often occurs with hypernasality, but can also occur with normal resonance.

There are four basic types of nasal emission: inaudible nasal emission, audible nasal emission, nasal rustle (often called nasal turbulence), and finally, phoneme-specific nasal emission (PSNE). The type of nasal emission has to do with the relative size of the opening (which affects the acoustic properties of both nasal airflow and resonance) and its cause (i.e., abnormal structure or abnormal function).

Inaudible nasal emission occurs with a relatively large opening. Although there is a significant loss of airflow through the opening, this type of nasal emission is inaudible because there is very little impedance (and thus friction) to the flow. In addition, a large opening also causes hypernasality, which would mask the sound of nasal emission. Although the nasal emission is not audible, there is evidence that it is there because it causes secondary characteristics, including weak or omitted consonants, short utterance length, a nasal grimace, and even compensatory articulation productions. (See following for more information.)

Audible nasal emission occurs when there is a medium-sized velopharyngeal opening. In this cause, there is greater resistance to the flow, making the nasal emission more audible. In addition, there is less pronounced hypernasality. There still may be some of the other secondary characteristics due to a leak of airflow.

Nasal rustle (also called *nasal turbulence*) is due to a small velopharyngeal opening. Despite its size, a small opening can actually cause more speech distortion than an opening that is a little larger. This is because as the air goes through a small opening, the pressure of the airflow increases. As this pressurized air is released on the nasal side of the opening, it causes very audible bubbling of the nasal secretions (Kummer et al., 2003; Kummer et al., 1992; Mason & Grandstaff, 1971). The bubbling of a nasal rustle can be seen easily through *nasopharyngoscopy* (a nasal endoscopic procedure), and can even be seen through videofluoroscopy when there is a good coating of barium. Because the nasal rustle is due to bubbling of secretions, nasal congestion can make this distortion even more noticeable. When it occurs, a nasal rustle can be very loud. As such, it can mask the sound of the consonants, thus affecting not only the quality of speech but also the intelligibility.

Because it is due to a small velopharyngeal opening, a nasal rustle tends to be somewhat inconsistent, and in some speech conditions (e.g., single words and short sentences) it may not be heard at all. This is because with short utterances or with effort, the individual may be able to achieve velopharyngeal closure. However, with an increase in utterance length, speed, phonemic complexity, or even fatigue, the nasal emission often becomes more consistent. This is why nasal rustle cannot be corrected with speech therapy. The gains that are made in the therapy room are usually not maintained outside of therapy.

Phoneme-specific nasal emission (PSNE) is when the nasal emission occurs only on certain pressure-sensitive sounds and is due to faulty articulation of these phonemes in the pharynx. PSNE most commonly occurs on the /s/ and /z/ phonemes but can occur on all sibilant sounds (/s/, /z/, /ʃ/, /ʒ/, /ʧ/, /ʤ/). PSNE is due to mislearning (abnormal function rather than abnormal structure) and is further discussed later in this chapter.

Obligatory Distortions and Compensatory Errors

Whenever there are structural anomalies within the vocal tract (e.g., dental or occlusal anomalies, an oronasal fistula, or velopharyngeal insufficiency), the individual's speech may be characterized by obligatory distortions and/or compensatory errors (Trost-Cardamone, 1990). *Obligatory distortions*, sometimes called *passive speech characteristics* (Harding & Grunwell, 1996, 1998), occur when the articulation placement is normal, but an abnormality of the structure or physiology causes distortion of speech. In contrast, *compensatory errors*, sometimes called *active speech characteristics* (Harding & Grunwell, 1996, 1998), are misarticulations that occur in response to abnormal structure (or abnormal speech physiology).

A distinction between obligatory distortions and compensatory errors is important to make because the compensatory characteristics are under the patient's control and can therefore be corrected with speech therapy once the structure is corrected. Obligatory distortions are purely the result of abnormal structure (or physiology) and require surgical or prosthetic intervention for correction.

Obligatory distortions secondary to significant VPI or a large oronasal fistula include hypernasality and nasal emission. Additional obligatory distortions due to a fairly large opening include the following:

- *Weak or omitted consonants*: When air is leaked through the velopharyngeal valve, it reduces the amount of airflow that is available in the oral cavity for the production of consonants. This causes the consonants to be weak in intensity and pressure or to be omitted completely. There is a direct inverse relationship between nasal emission and oral airflow. Therefore, the greater the nasal emission, the weaker the consonants tend to be.

- *Short utterance length*: A leak of airflow through the nose reduces the oral airflow available for connected speech. Therefore, more frequent breaths are required during speech for replacement of the airflow. This causes utterance length to be shortened and connected speech to be choppy. It has been shown that individuals with a large velopharyngeal opening attempt to raise intraoral pressure by increasing airflow rate during consonant production. As a result, they may produce respiratory volumes that are twice that of normal speakers (Huber & Stathopoulos, 2003). This increased effort makes speech physically difficult and can cause the individual to become fatigued during speech.

- *Nasalization of oral consonants:* When voiced plosives are produced in the presence of significant VPI or a large oronasal fistula, these oral phonemes sound more like their nasal cognates (e.g., m/b, n/d, and ŋ).

- *Nasal grimace*: A nasal grimace can be seen as muscle contractions just above the nasal bridge and/or at the side of the nares (Figure 7–4). Just as muscle contractions can be noted in the face when a person is trying to lift something heavy, the nasal grimace seems to be an overflow muscle reaction that occurs with extreme effort to achieve velopharyngeal closure. Once velopharyngeal function is corrected, these facial contractions during speech usually disappear spontaneously.

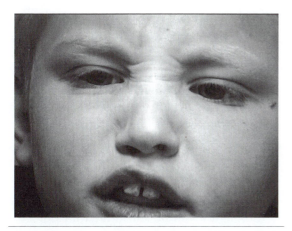

FIGURE 7–4 Nasal grimace during speech. Note the contraction above the nose and at the side of the nose. This is due to the extra effort of trying to achieve velopharyngeal closure.

Courtesy Ann W. Kummer, Ph.D./Cincinnati Children's Hospital Medical Center & University of Cincinnati College of Medicine

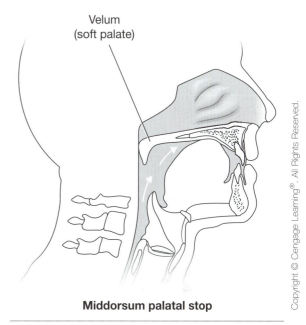

Velum
(soft palate)

Middorsum palatal stop

FIGURE 7–5 Diagram of the tongue position for a palatal-dorsal production (middorsum palatal stop).

There are a few compensatory articulation productions that individuals may use when there is a large symptomatic oronasal fistula. The productions are developed to close either the fistula with the tongue or the valve behind the fistula before the airflow is lost. These compensatory productions include the following:

- *Palatal-dorsal production* (aka *middorsum palatal stop*): This stop-plosive is produced with the dorsum of the tongue against the middle of the hard palate (Trost, 1981) (Figure 7–5). It is often substituted for the lingual-alveolar sounds (/t/, /d/, /n/, /l/) if the fistula is in the area of the alveolus. It may also be used to occlude a fistula in the palate during speech. Because the place of production is between that for lingual-alveolars and velars, the boundaries for distinguishing the two placements are lost, and the acoustic product sounds like a cross between the two placements. (A palatal-dorsal placement is also seen as a compensatory production for anterior oral cavity crowding that occurs due to dental malocclusion. This is discussed in Chapter 9.)

- *Velar plosive:* When there is a large oronasal fistula in the hard palate, the substitution of velar sounds (/k/ and /g/) for anterior oral sounds allows the individual to impound the airflow behind the fistula, before the airflow is lost through it (Ainoda, Yamashita, & Tsukada, 1985; Powers, 1962; Trost-Cardamone, 1997). The airflow is then released and flows horizontal to the fistula, thus reducing the amount of nasal emission. In some cases, velars sounds are actually *co-articulated* (produced at the same time) with the intended anterior sounds (lingual-alveolars and bilabials) (Gibbon, Ellis, & Crampin, 2004). Backing of phonemes can sometimes occur as a compensation for VPI, because the back of the tongue can help to push the velum upward to assist with velopharyngeal closure as a compensatory strategy (Brooks, Shelton, & Youngstrom, 1965).

- *Velar fricative/affricate:* A velar fricative is produced with the back of the tongue slightly elevated so that it is in the same position as a /j/ (as in "yellow") sound (Figure 7–6). It is produced by forcing air through the narrow passage that is created between the tongue and the velum. A velar affricate is produced with a combination of a velar plosive and a velar fricative. Both of these sounds can be voiced or voiceless. They are typically substituted for sibilants. In most cases, they are used to compensate for a large oronasal fistula because they are produced behind the area where the fistula is usually located.

When the compensatory productions are used in response to VPI, the manner of production is usually maintained, but the place of production is moved posteriorly to the pharynx. This allows the individual to take advantage of the airflow that is available in the pharynx before it is reduced because of the velopharyngeal opening. The following are compensatory articulation productions that are sometimes used when there is a VPI:

- *Pharyngeal plosive:* The pharyngeal plosive can be voiced or voiceless and is produced with the back of the tongue articulating against the pharyngeal wall (Figure 7–7). Although it can be substituted for other consonants, a pharyngeal plosive is typically substituted for velar plosives (/k/, /g/). During production of this sound, the entire tongue moves posteriorly in order to articulate against the posterior pharyngeal wall, thus taking advantage of the airflow in the pharynx. The airflow is then released through the velopharyngeal valve. An increase in pharyngeal activity can often be

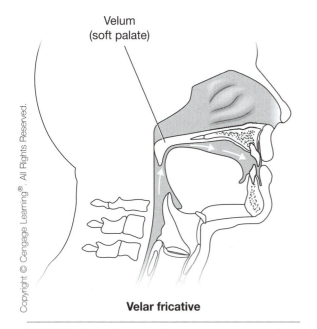

Velar fricative

FIGURE 7–6 Diagram of the tongue position for a velar fricative.

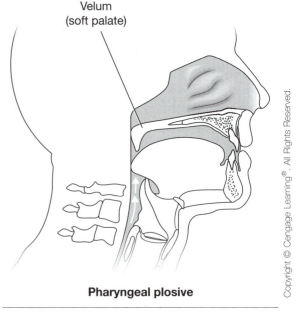

Pharyngeal plosive

FIGURE 7–7 Diagram of the tongue position for a pharyngeal plosive.

noted by observing the throat area. Due to the difficulty of producing this phoneme, there is often a longer duration between the consonant and the following vowel than is typically noted with other consonant placements.

- *Pharyngeal fricative/affricate:* A pharyngeal fricative can be voiced or voiceless and is produced by retracting the base of the tongue so that it approximates, but does not touch, the pharyngeal wall (Figure 7–8). As the airflow is forced through the narrow opening that is created between the base of the tongue and pharyngeal wall, the fricative (friction) sound occurs. A pharyngeal affricate can also be voiced or unvoiced and is produced by a combination of a pharyngeal plosive and pharyngeal fricative. Because these sounds are produced in the pharynx, the airflow is released through the velopharyngeal valve

as nasal emission. Pharyngeal fricatives and affricates are usually substituted for sibilant sounds. As with the other pharyngeal compensatory productions, an increase in pharyngeal activity can be noted in the throat area during speech.

- *Posterior nasal fricative:* A posterior nasal fricative is usually voiceless and is produced by elevating the back of the tongue so that it articulates against the velum, just like an /ŋ/ placement. As the air flows upward through the pharynx, the back of the tongue blocks the entrance into the oral cavity. Therefore, the air is forced through the closed velopharyngeal valve, causing a small opening (Figure 7–9). This production results in very audible nasal emission (Trost, 1981) called a nasal rustle (turbulence). The posterior nasal fricative may be used as a substitution for any of the pressure-sensitive phonemes, but it is typically used for sibilants.

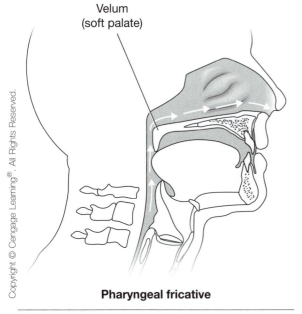

Pharyngeal fricative

FIGURE 7–8 Diagram of the tongue position for a pharyngeal fricative.

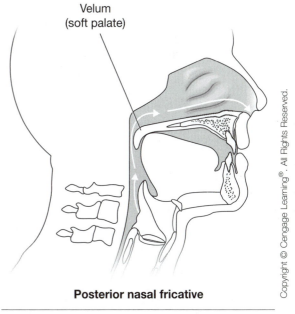

Posterior nasal fricative

FIGURE 7–9 Diagram of the tongue position for a posterior nasal fricative.

- *Nasal snort:* The nasal snort is produced by a forcible emission of air through the nose that results in a noisy, sneeze-like sound. The nasal snort is typically associated with the production of /s/ blends. It often occurs concurrently with a nasal grimace.

- *Nasal sniff:* The nasal sniff is not a common compensatory articulation production, but it does occur in some cases. It is produced by a forcible inspiration through the nose, and therefore it is the opposite of nasal emission. The nasal sniff is usually substituted for sibilant sounds, particularly the /s/. Due to the difficulty in coordinating the inspiration of the nasal sniff and expiration for other sounds, the nasal sniff typically occurs only in the final word position, rather than in all word positions.

- *Glottal stop:* A glottal stop is a voiced plosive that is produced by adduction of the vocal folds, a buildup of subglottic air pressure, and then sudden separation of the vocal folds to release the airflow (Figure 7–10). This results in a grunt-type sound. A glottal stop is often produced in normal speech for a /t/ sound when followed by an /n/ sound (e.g., "mitten," "button," "Clinton," etc.). When there is significant VPI, glottal stops are often substituted for plosive sounds, but they may also be substituted for fricatives and affricates, especially if the child has not yet developed the fricative manner in his or her phonemic repertoire. Glottal stops can be co-articulated with other phonemes. This co-articulation is characterized by one manner of production with simultaneous valving at two places of production (Bispo et al., 2011; Trost-Cardamone, 1997). For example, the child can co-articulate a /b/ sound with a glottal stop. Visually, it appears as if the individual is producing

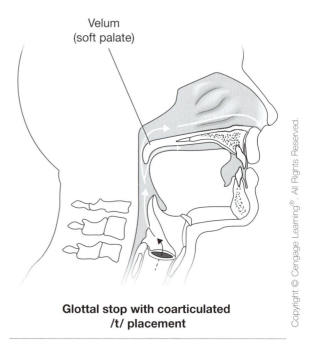

Velum (soft palate)

Glottal stop with coarticulated /t/ placement

FIGURE 7–10 Diagram of the tongue position for a glottal stop with a co–articulated /t/.

the sound correctly with appropriate oral placement, even though the plosive production is actually produced at the level of the glottis. Glottal stops can be seen as increased laryngeal activity in the throat area. Because air pressure is released at the glottis, there is no need for velopharyngeal closure, so glottal stops often appear to be associated with a significant velopharyngeal opening (Henningsson & Isberg, 1986).

- *Glottal fricative (/h/):* The /h/ sound is actually a glottal fricative. As such, it can be substituted for oral fricatives when there is VPI, because it is produced below the level of the velopharyngeal leak (Harding & Grunwell, 1998; Proctor, Shadle, & Iskarous, 2010).

- *Breathiness:* Breathiness is a vocal quality where the vocal cords are held further apart than normal so that a larger volume of air escapes between them. A breathy vocal quality can be used as a compensatory strategy for VPI because a breathy voice can mask the perception of hypernasality (which depends on voicing) because there is less sound in the nasal cavity. In addition, with an open glottis there is less air pressure and therefore less audible nasal emission through the velopharyngeal valve.

DYSPHONIA

Dysphonia is characterized by breathiness, hoarseness, low intensity, and/or glottal fry during phonation. Children with a history of craniofacial anomalies or VPI may have an increased risk for dysphonia for several reasons, although further research is needed (D'Antonio, Muntz, Province, & Marsh, 1988; McWilliams, Lavorato, & Bluestone, 1973; Robison & Otteson, 2011b).

One common finding is a hyperfunctional voice disorder in individuals with mildly impaired velopharyngeal valving. This is because when there is increased respiratory and muscular effort to close the velopharyngeal port, it can also result in hyperadduction of the vocal folds. Chronic hyperadduction can cause thickening and edema of the vocal folds, which ultimately leads to the formation of vocal nodules (Figure 7–11). *Vocal nodules* are small callus-like masses that typically occur symmetrically on both vocal folds and are due to chronic abuse, misuse, or overuse of the folds. Speech therapy to increase oral airflow when there is VPI is not only ineffective, but it can also cause or exacerbate vocal fold pathology.

Other causes of dysphonia in these populations include congenital laryngeal anomalies, which are more common in individuals with congenital craniofacial syndromes. Dysphonia can even be secondary to complications from

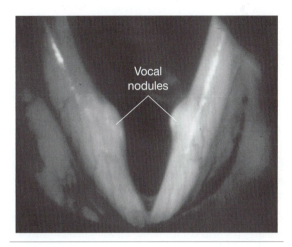

FIGURE 7–11 Bilateral vocal nodules as seen through endoscopy.

Courtesy Ann W. Kummer, Ph.D./Cincinnati Children's Hospital Medical Center & University of Cincinnati College of Medicine

long-term tracheostomy (e.g., tracheal stenosis). As previously noted, low intensity and breathiness may occur as a compensatory strategy to mask the hypernasality and nasal emission. Finally, when there is VPI, the lack of adequate oral acoustic energy in combination with the absorption of sound energy by the pharyngeal tissues results in a damping effect, causing the voice to be low in intensity (Bernthal & Beukelman, 1977).

VELOPHARYNGEAL DYSFUNCTION

The function of the velopharyngeal valve is thoroughly described in Chapter 1. As noted previously, the velopharyngeal valve must close completely for the production of oral sounds and open completely for the production of nasal sounds. To do this effectively, there must be normal velopharyngeal structure (anatomy), and normal velopharyngeal function (neurophysiology). In addition, the speaker must open or close the velopharyngeal valve as appropriate for each speech sound, which requires learning. Velopharyngeal function can be defective due to a problem in any one of these three areas.

Velopharyngeal dysfunction (VPD) refers to a condition where the velopharyngeal valve does not close consistently and completely during the production of oral sounds (D'Antonio et al., 1988; Folkins, 1988; Jones, 1991; Loney & Bloem, 1987; Marsh, 1991; Morris, 1992; Netsell, 1988; Penfold, 1997; Witt et al., 1997). This term is also used when the velopharyngeal valve does not open consistently and completely during the production of nasal sounds due to apraxia. Velopharyngeal dysfunction is used as a broad term that encompasses all disorders that affect the velopharyngeal valve (Witt, 2009).

Unfortunately, the literature is full of inconsistencies in the use of terminology for disorders of the velopharyngeal valve. Some authors and clinicians use the common terms *velopharyngeal inadequacy, velopharyngeal impairment, velopharyngeal insufficiency, velopharyngeal incompetence,* and *velopharyngeal dysfunction* interchangeably; whereas others use these terms in a specific way to suggest etiology (Kummer, 2011b; Loney & Bloem, 1987; Trost, 1981; Trost-Cardamone, 1981, 1989). Specificity in terminology is felt to be important by this author because each of these categories of velopharyngeal dysfunction has a different underlying cause that has an impact on appropriate treatment. Therefore, the terminology proposed by Trost-Cardamone is used in this text as follows:

The term *velopharyngeal insufficiency (VPI)* is used to describe an anatomical or structural defect that prevents adequate velopharyngeal closure. Velopharyngeal insufficiency is the most common type of VPD because it includes a short or defective velum, which is common in children with a history of cleft palate (Figure 7–12). *Velopharyngeal incompetence (VPI)* is used to refer to a neurophysiological

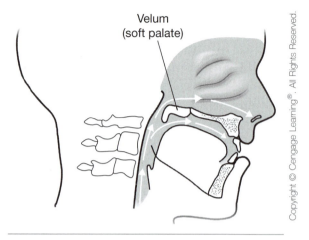

FIGURE 7–12 Velopharyngeal insufficiency. In this case, the velum is too short to achieve velopharyngeal closure during speech.

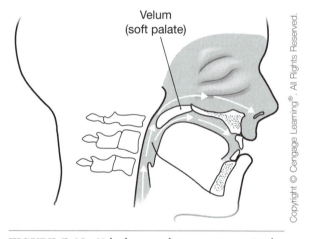

FIGURE 7–13 Velopharyngeal incompetence. In this case, the velum doesn't move well enough to achieve velopharyngeal closure during speech.

disorder that results in poor movement of the velopharyngeal structures (Figure 7–13). VPI (for velopharyngeal insufficiency or incompetence) is used for disorders that are medically based and therefore require physical management. Hence, VPI is not a condition that can be corrected with speech therapy.

In contrast to VPI, *velopharyngeal mislearning* is an articulation disorder that includes the substitution of certain nasal or pharyngeal sounds for oral sounds. This results in an open velopharyngeal valve during the production of those particular speech sounds. For example, if the child substitutes a pharyngeal fricative for an /s/ sound, the velopharyngeal valve will necessarily be open during the production of this pharyngeal sound. Velopharyngeal mislearning may be secondary to VPI or may occur with no history of VPI. It is corrected with speech therapy.

Causes of Velopharyngeal Dysfunction

Normal velopharyngeal closure for speech requires normal structure, normal physiology, and normal (learned) function. There are many types and causes of abnormal structure, abnormal physiology, and abnormal function that can affect the velopharyngeal valve, resulting in velopharyngeal dysfunction. Some of these are described here.

Velopharyngeal Insufficiency (VPI)

As noted above, velopharyngeal insufficiency (VPI) refers to a structural defect that causes the velum to be too short or too irregular to obtain a tight closure against the posterior pharyngeal wall during speech. There are many causes of discrepancies between the length of the velum and the needed length for firm velopharyngeal contact. The following is a list of some of these causes.

History of Cleft Palate

Velopharyngeal insufficiency occurs most commonly in individuals with a history of cleft palate. Although surgeons attempt to achieve as much velar length during the cleft palate repair as possible, 20% to 30 % of patients with a history of cleft palate demonstrate velopharyngeal insufficiency following the cleft repair.

Velopharyngeal insufficiency following cleft palate repair is often because the velum is too short (Figure 7–12). In some cases, an irregularity at the posterior border of the velar eminence, usually in midline, can cause a velopharyngeal gap. In addition, there may be an abnormality of the levator sling. Although the surgeon may attempt to repair the orientation and connection of the levator veli palatini muscles, it does not guarantee that these paired muscles will function normally for speech. Even scar tissue in a repaired cleft palate may affect movement.

Submucous Cleft Palate

The characteristics of a submucous cleft are described in Chapter 2. Although the vast majority of individuals with submucous cleft have normal speech, some have characteristics of velopharyngeal insufficiency (Gosain & Hettinger, 2009; McWilliams, 1991). Velopharyngeal insufficiency can occur with a submucous cleft due to a small notch in the posterior border of the velum, hypoplasticity of musculus uvulae muscles, or anterior orientation of the levator veli palatini muscles. Because a submucous cleft is a malformation, the velopharyngeal gap will most likely be in the midline. If the submucous cleft extends through the velum and hard palate, the levator veli palatini muscle inserts into the hard palate, as if there had been an overt cleft palate (refer to Figure 2–14 in Chapter 2). This renders these muscles useless in elevating the velum for speech.

One characteristic of a submucous cleft is a zona pellucida, which is an area of thin mucosa and little, if any, underlying muscle. Because the velum is thin, there is more transpalatal transmission of sound energy through it to the nasal cavity. Therefore, even if the velopharyngeal valve is functioning normally, there may be hypernasality due to this defect.

Deep Pharynx

The velum may be normal in morphology, but it may be unable to reach the posterior pharyngeal wall due to an abnormally deep pharynx. Linear growth of the cranial base, rather than flexion, can elongate the pharynx, and abnormal curvature of the cervical spine can also increase the anterior–posterior dimensions of the pharynx (Haapanen, Heliovaara, & Ranta, 1991; Leveau-Geffroy, Perrin, Khonsari, & Mercier, 2011). This can be seen in some craniosynostosis syndromes. As will be noted in Chapter 12, the relative length of the velum and depth of the pharynx cannot be determined by an intraoral examination because velopharyngeal contact occurs above the level of an oral view.

Adenoid Atrophy

In the early years, most children actually have veloadenoidal closure because the adenoids are in the place of normal velar contact. Adenoid tissue is most prominent in very young children but begins to slowly atrophy around the age of 6. With the onset of puberty, there can be significant, and sometimes sudden, atrophy of the adenoid tissue, causing an increase in the distance between the velum and posterior pharyngeal wall. If the velum is normal, it stretches to accommodate the difference in the depth of the pharynx; thus, normal velopharyngeal closure is maintained.

Children with a repaired cleft palate or with a submucous cleft may demonstrate normal resonance and velopharyngeal function during the preschool and early school years. However, they may experience gradual deterioration in velopharyngeal closure as they reach adolescence. This is because the velum may not be capable of stretching sufficiently to accommodate the difference in pharyngeal depth because of the involution of the adenoid tissue (Handelman & Osborne, 1976; Mason & Warren, 1980; Morris, Wroblewski, Brown, & Van Demark, 1990; Shapiro, 1980; Siegel-Sadewitz & Shprintzen, 1986). When this occurs, parents often report that their child has begun to mumble, doesn't speak loud enough, or has become "lazy" with speech.

Irregular Adenoids

As noted in Chapter 1, children usually have veloadenoidal closure. Therefore, it is important for the velum to close firmly against the adenoid pad during speech. Although it is not commonly recognized, irregular adenoids can cause velopharyngeal insufficiency in some cases (Ren, Isberg, & Henningsson, 1995). If the adenoid pad has indentations in the surface, this can make it impossible for the velum to close tightly against it (Figure 7–14A and 7–14B), which results in a small velopharyngeal (actually veloadenoidal) opening (Figure 7–14B). Even adenoidal protrusions can affect closure by causing a lateral gap on either side (Figure 7–14C). Because the opening is usually small, it rarely causes hypernasality. In fact, there may be hyponasality if the adenoid tissue is large. However, this opening causes nasal emission. Ironically, irregularity of the adenoid pad commonly occurs after an adenoidectomy. This is because with adenoidectomy the capsule deep to the adenoid pad is left in place, as it protects the underlying bone of the skull base. Therefore, some regrowth of the adenoid can occur over time.

Hypertrophic Tonsils

The (faucial) tonsils are located in the oral cavity between the anterior and posterior faucial pillars (see Chapter 1 and Chapter 8). As such, they usually do not have any effect on

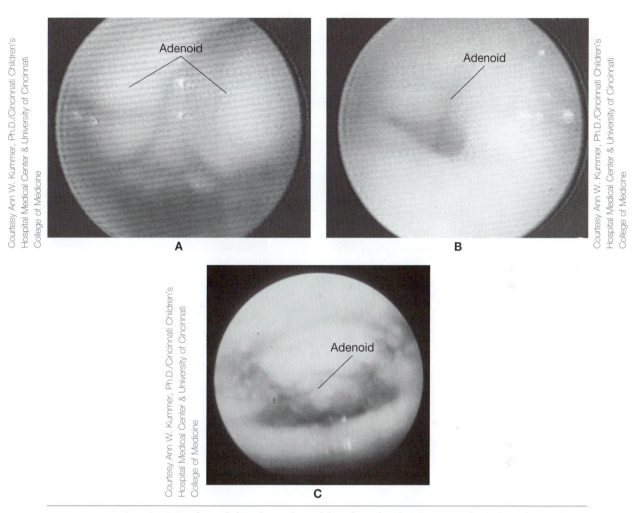

FIGURE 7–14 (A–C) (A) A deep cleft in the surface of the adenoid pad. (B) As a result of adenoid irregularity, the velum is unable to achieve a tight seal against the adenoid, resulting in nasal air emission. (C) A protrusive adenoid pad, which causes a leak on each side during velar closure.

velopharyngeal function because they are well below and anterior to the velopharyngeal valve. On rare occasions, however, hypertrophic tonsils can cause mechanical interference with the function of the velopharyngeal valve and also affect resonance.

As tonsils become hypertrophic, they can expand anteriorly, medially, or posteriorly. If they expand posteriorly, they can often be seen

through nasopharyngoscopy in the oropharynx and even in the nasopharynx. Tonsils that are in the pharynx can affect the medial movement of the lateral pharyngeal walls during speech by pushing against the posterior faucial pillars. When a tonsil is so large that its upper pole projects into the pharynx, it can also become positioned between the velum and posterior pharyngeal wall, thus preventing the velum

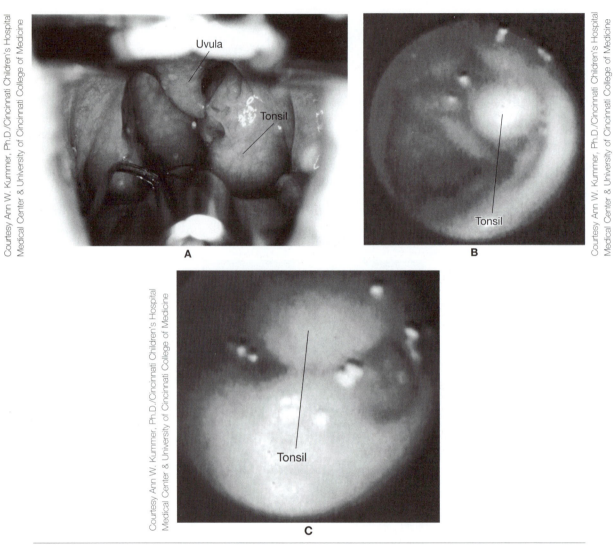

FIGURE 7–15 (A–C) (A) Large tonsil on the right (patient's left). The uvula can be seen to deviate toward the large tonsil, which indicates that it is pushing on the posterior faucial pillar and is intruding into the pharynx. (B) The same tonsil in the pharynx, as seen through nasopharyngoscopy. (C) The tonsil can be seen between the velum and posterior pharyngeal wall during velopharyngeal closure. Because there is not a tight seal, a small opening can be seen just to the left of the tonsil. There is a bubble in this area due to nasal air emission.

from achieving an adequate velopharyngeal seal during speech (Abdel-Aziz, 2012; Finkel-stein, Nachmani, & Ophir, 1994; Henningsson & Isberg, 1988; Kummer, Billmire, et al., 1993; MacKenzie-Stepner, Witzel, Stringer, & Laskin, 1987; Maryn, Van Lierde, De Bodt, & Van Cauwenberge, 2004; Shprintzen, Sher, & Croft, 1987) (Figure 7–15, A–C). This can result in a small velopharyngeal gap, causing nasal emission. In addition, the tonsil in the pharynx can also obstruct sound transmission into both the oral and nasal cavities, causing a mixture of hyponasality and cul-de-sac resonance. If one tonsil is much larger than the other, it will often push the velum upward on that side. Because of the pulling and stretching of the velum on that side, the uvula will deviate and appear to point toward the large tonsil.

If the tonsils expand medially, they will not affect velopharyngeal function. However, as noted previously, they can cause a pharyngeal cul-de-sac resonance by blocking the sound from entering the oral cavity. Tonsils that expand anteriorly may affect oral resonance and can also cause difficulty with articulation of posterior sounds, particularly velars (k, g) (Henningsson & Isberg, 1988).

Otolaryngologists commonly perform tonsillectomies for chronic tonsillitis and/or airway obstruction. If there are speech and resonance issues secondary to hypertrophic tonsils, the primary care physician and otolaryngologist should be made aware of this. A recommendation for tonsillectomy to correct these issues would be appropriate.

Adenoidectomy

A well-known and well-documented risk of an adenoidectomy is postoperative velopharyngeal insufficiency (Andreassen, Leeper, & MacRae, 1991; Croft, Shprintzen, & Ruben, 1981; Donnelly, 1994; Fernandes, Grobbelaar, Hudson, & Lentin, 1996; Kummer, Myer, Smith, & Shott, 1993; Parton & Jones, 1998; Ren, Isberg, & Henningsson, 1995; Robinson, 1992; Seid, 1990; Witzel, Rich, Margar-Bacal, & Cox, 1986; Maryn et al., 2004; Saunders,

---

CASE REPORT

Hypertrophic Tonsils

Ellen was a 9-year-old child with a history of normal speech and language development. She had never had speech therapy. However, her speech had gradually become nasal and hard to understand over about a 2-year period. The parents reported that Ellen had also begun to snore loudly at night.

Upon examination, Ellen was noted to have an open mouth posture with an anterior tongue position at rest. An evaluation of speech revealed normal articulation, but nasal emission during the production of pressure-sensitive phonemes. Resonance was characterized by hyponasality and a cul-de-sac quality.

An intraoral examination revealed a hypertrophic tonsil on the right side. It extended medially beyond the point of the midline of the oropharynx. The left tonsil was of normal size. A nasopharyngoscopy assessment showed the tonsil to be in the nasopharynx and between the velum and posterior pharyngeal wall during velopharyngeal closure. Because of the interference of the tonsil, there was a small velopharyngeal opening on either side of the tonsil during velopharyngeal closure, resulting in nasal emission. The large tonsil in the pharynx interfered with the transmission of sound energy into the nasal cavity, thus causing hyponasality on nasal sounds. The size of the tonsil also blocked the sound energy from entering the oral cavity, thus causing cul-de-sac resonance on oral sounds.

Given these findings, the obvious treatment was a tonsillectomy. Once this was done, resonance returned to normal, and nasal emission was no longer noted. Ellen was able to maintain a closed mouth posture, and snoring was no longer noted at night.

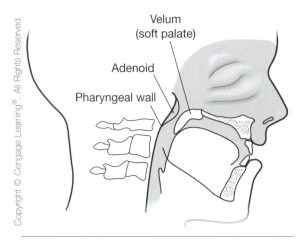

Velum
(soft palate)

Adenoid

Pharyngeal wall

FIGURE 7–16   Position of the adenoid in the pharynx. The adenoid pad can help with closure in many cases. In many young children, there is veloadenoidal closure rather than velopharyngeal closure.

Hartley, Sell, & Sommerlad, 2004; Stewart, Ahmad, Razzell, & Watson, 2002). This is because young children with a prominent adenoid pad usually achieve veloadenoidal closure rather than velopharyngeal closure (Figure 7–16). Removal of the adenoids results in a deeper nasopharynx and a greater distance for the velum to stretch in order to achieve closure. (For more information regarding adenoids, see Chapter 8.)

Hypernasality or nasal emission following adenoidectomy can occur in individuals with no velar defect. However, this is typically short-lived, lasting from a few hours to as long as 6 to 8 weeks. Certain compensations occur in the velopharyngeal mechanism to adapt to the changes in the pharyngeal dimension. These compensations include an increase in velar mobility, an increase in velar height during closure, an increase in velar stretch, and increased movement of the pharyngeal walls (Neiman & Simpson, 1975). Therefore, in most cases, the speech returns to normal once these adaptations are made.

The risk for permanent velopharyngeal insufficiency following adenoidectomy has been estimated to be between 1:1500 and 1:3000 (Donnelly, 1994; Stewart, Ahmed, Razzell, & Watson, 2002). The biggest risk factor is a history of cleft palate. Patients with a repaired cleft palate may have tenuous velopharyngeal closure preoperatively, scarring of the velum, and the lack of muscle reserve to stretch postoperatively (Parton & Jones, 1998). Presence of a submucous cleft palate is also a major risk factor for similar reasons. In fact, many patients with velopharyngeal insufficiency following adenoidectomy are found through nasopharyngoscopy to have an occult submucous cleft after the fact (Parton & Jones, 1998; Saunders, Hartley, Sell, & Sommerlad, 2004; Schmaman, Jordaan, & Jammine, 1998). Other risk factors include a family history of cleft palate or hypernasality, sucking difficulties as an infant, and oral-motor dysfunction or other neuromuscular problems.

Adenoidectomy is usually contraindicated for patients with a history of cleft palate, submucous cleft, or other risk factors. However, if the patient has upper airway obstruction due to the adenoid pad or the adenoid tissue blocking the opening to the Eustachian tube, a conservative superior half-adenoidectomy can be performed (Finkelstein, Wexler, Nachmani, & Ophir, 2002). With this procedure, the airway obstruction is relieved while maintaining enough tissue inferiorly for the velum to continue to close against the adenoid pad for speech. (It should be noted that VPI post-adenoidectomy cannot be corrected with speech therapy because it is caused by a structural defect.)

Tonsillectomy

As noted previously, the tonsils reside in the oral cavity (not in the nasopharynx, where the adenoids are located). Therefore, unlike adenoidectomy, tonsillectomy is highly unlikely to cause problems with speech. There are possible exceptions, however. First, significant scarring of the posterior faucial pillar postoperatively could potentially affect lateral pharyngeal wall movement. There may be a particular concern for individuals who are prone to forming *keloids*, which is excessive scar tissue formed during healing. In addition, lesions of branches of the vagus and glossopharyngeal nerves can affect velopharyngeal function (Haapanen, Ignatius, Rihkanen, & Ertama, 1994).

Finally, although it is rare, velopharyngeal incompetence can be a learned protection response after the surgery. Tonsillectomy can result in significant pain for a week or 10 days after the procedure. Opening and closing the velopharyngeal valve for swallowing and speech can exacerbate the pain.

Postoperative avoidance of velopharyngeal closure can become habituated in some patients, resulting in severe velopharyngeal dysfunction following the surgery (Gibb & Stewart, 1975). This is treated as a learned compensatory strategy.

Maxillary Advancement

Class III malocclusion with midface retrusion is particularly common in patients with a history of cleft lip and palate, but it can also occur in individuals without a history of cleft. These patients can benefit from maxillary advancement, which is done through either *orthognathic surgery* (surgery that involves the bones of the maxilla and mandible) or *distraction osteogenesis* (a method of gradually lengthening a bone) (see Chapter 19). The purpose of maxillary advancement is to correct

CASE REPORT

Velopharyngeal Dysfunction following Tonsillectomy

Ashley was a 12-year-old who was referred for evaluation of severe hypernasality after a tonsillectomy. The tonsillectomy had been done 1 month previously for upper airway obstruction. Ashley had had an adenoidectomy at the age of 5, with no effect on speech.

The tonsillectomy was done with no complications. However, Ashley refused to swallow for several days postoperatively. As a result, she was kept in the hospital for 3 days on IV fluids. She rarely spoke for 9–10 days after the surgery, complaining that it hurt too much to talk. Once she began to talk, her speech was severely hypernasal. In addition, she experienced significant nasal regurgitation of fluids if her head was turned down even slightly.

Nasopharyngoscopy showed very little velopharyngeal movement during speech or with swallowing. In addition, the tongue base was held in an anterior position during both speech and swallowing. It was hypothesized that this occurred initially to avoid pain during velopharyngeal movement and then became habituated after the pain resolved.

Ashley was seen for six sessions of speech therapy over a 4-week period of time. As a result of the therapy, speech and swallowing returned to normal.

A lesson to be learned from this case is that even when severe velopharyngeal incompetence is noted perceptually and through nasopharyngoscopy, it reflects only what the individual is currently doing with the velopharyngeal mechanism. It does not reflect what the individual is capable of doing.

midface deficiency in order to normalize the occlusion and the facial profile.

Maxillary advancement can result in many positive changes for the patient. There is typically a dramatic improvement in facial profile and overall aesthetics as a result of this surgery. In addition, the normalization of occlusion often results in elimination of speech distortion, particularly on sibilant sounds, without intervening speech therapy (Guyette, Polley, Figueroa, & Smith, 2001; Kummer et al., 1989; Lee, Whitehill, Ciocca, & Samman, 2002; Maegawa, Sells, & David, 1998; Mason, Turvey, & Warren, 1980; McCarthy, Coccaro, & Schwartz, 1979; Trindade, Yamashita, Sugui-moto, Mazzottini, & Trindade, 2003; Vallino, 1990; Ward, McAuliffe, Holmes, Lynham, & Monsour, 2002). (It should be noted that this improvement only occurs with *obligatory distortions*, where tongue position during articulation was normal before the surgery, but the structure was abnormal, causing speech sound distortion.) Finally, maxillary advancement can reduce or eliminate nasal obstruction or hyponasality, which is common in these patients, by increasing the nasal cavity space.

Although maxillary advancement results in many benefits for the patient, it can have a negative effect on velopharyngeal function (Haapanen, Kalland, Heliovaara, Hukki, & Ranta, 1997; Heliovaara, Hukki, Ranta, & Haapanen, 2004; Heliovaara, Ranta, Hukki, & Haapanen, 2002; Janulewicz et al., 2004; Kummer, Strife, Grau, Creaghead, & Lee, 1989; Maegawa et al., 1998; Mason et al., 1980; Niemeyer, Gomes Ade, Fukushiro, & Genaro, 2005; Okazaki et al., 1993; Satoh et al., 2004). With this procedure, the anterior movement of the maxilla also causes anterior movement of the posterior border of the hard palate, with its soft palate attachments. This results in an increase in the pharyngeal depth. If there is only tenuous velopharyngeal closure preoper-

atively or if the velum is scarred due to a previous velar repair, it may not be able to stretch adequately following the surgery to span the entire pharyngeal depth. It would seem that the gradual nature of maxillary advancement through distraction might allow for the velopharyngeal mechanism to adapt to its new situation and minimize post-advancement hypernasality. Studies have shown, however, that even with distraction patients with borderline velopharyngeal closure can develop velopharyngeal insufficiency (Chanchareon-sook, Whitehill, & Samman, 2007; Guyette, Polley, Figueroa, & Smith, 2001; Ko, Figueroa, Guyette, Polley, & Law, 1999; Nohara, Tachimura, & Wada, 2006; Satoh et al., 2004; Trindade et al., 2003).

The exact risk of velopharyngeal insufficiency following maxillary advancement is not known, but it is not a common occurrence in individuals who have no history of cleft palate or velar abnormality. In fact, the velopharyngeal mechanism normally makes the same types of adaptations following maxillary advancement as it does following normal adenoid atrophy or adenoidectomy (Kummer et al., 1989). Therefore, most individuals do not experience a long-term problem with velopharyngeal function postoperatively. Those at greatest risk for hypernasality following maxillary advancement are the individuals who often can benefit the most from the procedure, particularly patients with a history of cleft palate (Janulewicz et al., 2004; Haapanen, Kalland, Heliovaara, Hukki, & Ranta, 1997; Kummer et al., 1989; Maegawa et al., 1998; Mason et al., 1980; McCarthy et al., 1979; Okazaki et al., 1993). The risk appears to be somewhat related to the amount of advancement, so those with the greatest maxillary movement are at greatest risk for velopharyngeal dysfunction postoperatively (Maegawa et al., 1998; Phillips, Klaiman, Delorey, & MacDonald, 2005). If speech and velopharyngeal function deteriorate after maxillary advancement, secondary surgery for speech is usually done (see Chapter 18).

Treatment of Oral, Nasal, and Pharyngeal Cavity Tumors

Oral, nasal, and pharyngeal cavity tumors occur in both children and in adults. In children, the most common tumor is a *hemangioma*, which is a congenital anomaly in which a proliferation of blood vessels results in a large mass. In adults, malignant tumors of the oral cavity are more commonly seen.

When a tumor or growth interferes with function or becomes life threatening, it is usually treated by *resection* (surgical removal). Resections of areas of the oral cavity can affect the integrity of the separation of the nasal and oral cavities and the function of the velopharyngeal valve (Bodin, Lind, & Arnander, 1994; Brown, Zuydam, Jones, Rogers, & Vaughan, 1997; Myers & Aramany, 1977; Yoshida, Michi, Yamashita, & Ohno, 1993). This is particularly a concern if tissue is taken from the hard palate, velum, or pharyngeal walls.

The use of radiation for oral or pharyngeal tumors can also affect the function of the velopharyngeal valve. Radiation can cause shrinkage of not just the tumor but also of the adjacent structures, including the velum and pharyngeal walls. When this occurs, surgical correction is often not possible due to the tissue damage. Therefore, prosthetic intervention is often used (see Chapter 20).

Velopharyngeal Incompetence (VPI)

Velopharyngeal incompetence refers to a neurophysiological disorder that results in poor movement of the velopharyngeal structures. Velopharyngeal incompetence is characterized by poor elevation and inadequate "knee action" of the velum during speech (Figure 7–13). On lateral videofluoroscopy, the velum often appears to be below the level of the hard palate during speech, and the *velar eminence* (high point of the velum as it bends) is not significant. Lateral pharyngeal wall motion may also be very poor so that there is minimal medial movement to assist with closure.

Velopharyngeal incompetence can be due to neurological injury (e.g., traumatic brain injury, cerebral palsy, stroke), neuromuscular diseases (e.g., muscular dystrophy, myasthenia gravis, etc.), or cranial nerve damage. Velopharyngeal incompetence is often associated with hypotonia, dysarthria, and apraxia of speech. The causes and associations of velopharyngeal incompetence are further discussed as follows.

Hypotonia

Hypotonia is a state of low muscle tonicity and sometimes reduced muscle strength. It is caused by different diseases and disorders of the brain that affect the motor nerve control or muscle strength. Generalized hypotonia can affect the strength and consistency of movement of the entire velopharyngeal valve, including the pharyngeal walls. Hypotonia affecting velopharyngeal function is a common characteristic of velocardiofacial syndrome.

It should be noted, however, that extensive lateral wall motion is normally noted only in the sagittal pattern of closure, which is the least common pattern found in both normal and abnormal speakers (Witzel & Posnick, 1989). Therefore, when lateral wall motion is limited, it may not be the result of a physiological defect (Finkelstein, Talmi, Nachmani, Hauben, & Zohar, 1992; Shprintzen, Rakof, Skolnick, & Lavorato, 1977; Siegel-Sadewitz & Shprintzen, 1982; Skolnick, Shprintzen, McCall, & Rakoff, 1975; Witzel & Posnick,

1989). In addition, posterior pharyngeal wall motion is limited, even in normal speakers. Therefore, the observation of a lack of lateral or posterior pharyngeal wall motion in an abnormal speaker is not particularly significant.

Dysarthria

Dysarthria is an oral-motor disorder that affects all the subsystems of speech, including respiration, phonation, resonance, and articulation. It is characterized by abnormalities of strength, range of motion, speed, accuracy, and tonicity of the speech muscles due to central and/or peripheral nervous system impairment. Velopharyngeal incompetence causes many of the speech characteristics that are typical of dysarthria, including hypernasality, weak or omitted consonants, short utterance length, and decreased volume (Netsell, 1969; Vijayalakshmi & Reddy, 2006; Yorkston, Beukelman, & Traynor, 1988).

Dysarthria with hypernasality can be secondary to either upper or lower motor neuron lesions and has been associated with a variety of neurological conditions. Some of these conditions include cerebral palsy, multiple schlerosis, myasthenia gravis, myotonic dystrophy, neurofibromatosis, Parkinson's disease, and cerebral or brainstem tumors. Dysarthria with hypernasality has been associated with mental retardation or developmental delay (Heller, Gens, Moe, & Lewin, 1974; Kline & Hutchinson, 1980). It can also be secondary to acquired neurological damage due to traumatic brain injury (TBI) or cerebral vascular accident (CVA). Any disorder that causes cerebral, cerebellar, or brainstem damage can cause dysarthria with hypernasality.

Apraxia of Speech

Apraxia of speech is a motor speech disorder that causes difficulty combining and sequencing oral-motor movements. When it occurs in children and affects speech development, it is also called *childhood apraxia of speech (CAS)* or *developmental apraxia.* In children, the exact cause is usually not known. When it occurs in adults or after speech has been developed, it is usually due to a neurological injury and may be called *verbal apraxia, dyspraxia,* or just *apraxia.*

Apraxia of speech is characterized by difficulty executing volitional oral movements and sequencing oral movements for connected speech. Although we typically think of apraxia as affecting the anterior articulators (lips, tongue, and jaws), it can also affect the posterior articulators (velopharyngeal valve) and other subsystems of speech (respiration and phonation) (Bradley, 1997; Sealey & Giddens, 2010; Trost-Cardamone, 1989).

Apraxia causes inconsistent velopharyngeal incompetence due to the difficulty in coordinating anterior articulation with velopharyngeal movement for connected speech. Due to the problem with coordination, the velum may stay down inappropriately for oral sounds (causing hypernasality) and go up inappropriately for nasal sounds (causing hyponasality). The speaker may produce both correct and incorrect productions of each phoneme, even within a single utterance. The timing of closure may also be affected so that closure does not occur until after the initiation of phonation, when it is too late (Warren, Dalston, & Mayo, 1993; Warren, Dalston, Trier, & Holder, 1985).

All errors, including those of resonance, tend to increase in severity with an increase in utterance length and phonemic complexity. With longer utterances, the velum may appear to pulse up and down erratically. It may even stay down in a resting position because of difficulty coordinating velopharyngeal closure with anterior articulation of oral sounds. Therefore, although there will be mixed resonance with apraxia, the predominant feature, particularly in longer utterances, is hypernasality.

CASE REPORT

Hypernasality Secondary to Dysarthria

Brandon was a 20-year-old college student when he had a cerebral hemorrhage secondary to an arterial venous (AV) malformation. This affected his speech, swallowing, the movement of the right side of his body, his walking, and vision. Fortunately, there was no cognitive loss. Brandon had received speech therapy for characteristics of dysarthria.

Brandon was referred to our VPI clinic because one of his primary concerns was hypernasality, low volume, poor breath support, and increased effort to talk. He had already tried a palatal lift, which was helpful, but he was interested in a more permanent solution.

At the time of the evaluation, Brandon was found to have normal articulatory placement, but characteristics of dysarthria including slow rate, imprecise movements, difficulty with initiation of movements for sound production, and labored movement. Articulation was affected by weak consonants due to significant nasal emission. In addition, there was poor breath support, short utterance length, glottal fry, aphonia at the ends of utterances, and severe hypernasality.

Nasopharyngoscopy showed inconsistent velar elevation, with occasional touch closure of the velum against the posterior pharyngeal wall at midline. The velum was noted to tire easily, however, and drop down inappropriately. There was also poor lateral pharyngeal wall motion.

Because Brandon no longer wanted to use a palatal lift, surgical intervention (specifically a pharyngeal flap) was offered as an option. Brandon was told that the goals of the surgery would be to improve the quality and clarity of speech while decreasing the effort to produce speech. Brandon was counseled that although improvement could be expected, this would not result in normal speech. He was also informed of the potential risks of the surgery, including the possibility of airway obstruction and even sleep apnea. After weighing the potential risks and benefits, Brandon and his family decide to pursue the surgery.

Brandon was seen for a reassessment 6 weeks after placement of the pharyngeal flap. At that time, he demonstrated significantly improved speech. The hypernasality was reduced to a mild degree, and the nasal air emission was only slight. Of most significance was the increase in oral pressure and thus speech sound clarity and intensity. Because Brandon no longer needed to take frequent breaths to replenish lost airflow due to nasal emission, his utterance length was much longer. In fact, he was able to count to 23 on one breath rather than to 4 as he had preoperatively.

Although the pharyngeal flap did not result in a total correction of speech, it did result in significant improvement in the quality and clarity of speech. It also made speech less effortful. Brandon and his family were very pleased with the result.

Of note, Brandon was seen again about 10 years later with a complaint about chronic aspiration with swallowing. In the interim, he had completed both his bachelor's and master's degrees. His speech remained clear and very acceptable, although mild dysarthria was still noted.

Velar Paralysis or Paresis

Individuals with either congenital or acquired lower motor neuron damage may demonstrate specific velopharyngeal paralysis or *paresis* (partial loss of movement or weakness) of the velum or pharyngeal musculature (Rousseaux,

Lesoin, & Quint, 1987). This can occur with involvement of the glossopharyngeal nerve (CN IX), the vagus nerve (CN X), or the hypoglossal nerve (CN XII). The paralysis or paresis is usually unilateral and can occur in the absence of other oral-motor deficits. When the vagus nerve (CN X) is involved, there may also be unilateral involvement of the larynx and vocal fold on the same side.

A unilateral velar paralysis or paresis typically causes a unilateral velopharyngeal opening on that side. When this is observed from an intraoral perspective, the velum can be seen to droop on the affected side during phonation. On the other hand, the uvula will be noted to deviate to the side with better movement. Unilateral paralysis or paresis of the velum is commonly observed in individuals with hemifacial microsomia (Tan & Chen, 2009).

Stress Incompetence and Velar Fatigue

Playing a wind instrument requires more intraoral air pressure and more velopharyngeal strength and stamina than speech. Because of this, velopharyngeal incompetence secondary to stress on the velopharyngeal valve sometimes occurs in musicians when playing wind instruments, even though they have no characteristics of velopharyngeal incompetence in speech (Bennett & Hoit, 2012; Conley, Beecher, & Marks, 1995; Evans, Driscoll, & Ackermann, 2011; Gordon, Astrachan, & Yanagisawa, 1994; Malick, Moon, & Canady, 2007; Shanks, 1990). For professional musicians or students who wish to become professionals, this is more than a minor inconvenience. Stress VPI has also been noted with singers, particularly those with less experience. The opening that often occurs with stress incompetence can be small. How-

ever, this results in a loud nasal rustle, which is certainly unwanted when playing music.

Stress incompetence is evaluated through nasopharyngoscopy to determine the location of the opening and possible cause. (The location of the opening cannot be clearly seen through videofluoroscopy.) Depending on the size, location, and cause of the opening, a prosthetic device (particularly a palatal lift) can be used. For a more permanent correction, surgical correction can be considered. Usually, only a minor procedure is needed, such as a collagen injection. In more severe cases, a unilateral or bilateral sphincter pharyngoplasty or even pharyngeal flap could be considered.

If velar fatigue begins to occur during speech or if there is a gradual onset of hypernasality, the person should be monitored over a period of time because these symptoms may indicate the onset of a progressive neurological disorder.

Velopharyngeal Mislearning

As noted previously, velopharyngeal mislearning is an articulation disorder that includes the substitution of certain nasal or pharyngeal sounds for oral sounds. This placement results in an open velopharyngeal valve, causing nasal emission or hypernasality during the production of those particular speech sounds. Although the speech characteristics may sound just like those of individuals with velopharyngeal insufficiency or incompetence, individuals with velopharyngeal mislearning are not candidates for surgical or prosthetic intervention. Instead, speech therapy is successful in correcting these functional speech characteristics (Kummer, 2011b). It is critically important to make a differential diagnosis between misarticulations caused by mislearning alone versus those caused by VPI so that the patient receives the appropriate treatment.

Compensatory Productions

Compensatory productions due to VPI are also learned misarticulations. These compensatory productions continue after surgical correction of the VPI because the individual's articulation pattern has usually become habituated by the time this surgery is done. In addition, hypernasality and nasal emission may continue to persist until the patient learns to actually use the new structures. Because changing structure does not change function, speech therapy is usually required to change those abnormal speech patterns once the structural defects have been corrected.

Other Learned Misarticulations

Although learned misarticulations occur as compensatory errors due to VPI or other structural anomalies, they can also occur as misarticulations in children with normal structures. If the misarticulations are produced in the pharynx or nasal cavity rather than the oral cavity, there will be phoneme-specific nasal emission or phoneme-specific hypernasality on these selected consonants (Kummer, 2011b).

Phoneme-specific nasal emission (*PSNE*) occurs when the individual uses a pharyngeal fricative or posterior nasal fricative as a substitution for oral fricatives (and sometimes affricates). As a result of the pharyngeal placement, nasal emission occurs on these misarticulated phonemes. These misarticulations resulting in PSNE usually occur on sibilant sounds, particularly /s/ and /z/.

Phoneme-specific hypernasality occurs when the individual consistently substitutes a nasal sound for an oral sound (e.g., ŋ/l or ŋ/r). Phoneme-specific hypernasality can also occur on vowels, particularly high vowels, if the back

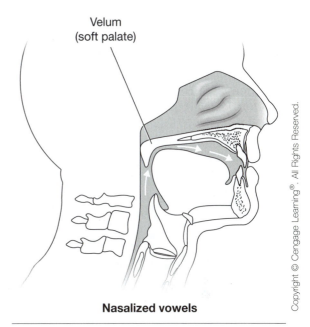

Velum
(soft palate)

Nasalized vowels

FIGURE 7–17 Diagram of the tongue position for nasalized vowels.

of the tongue is too high during production (Falk & Kopp, 1968; Gibbon, Smeaton-Ewins, & Crampin, 2005) (Figure 7–17). Although velopharyngeal closure is normal, the resonance is perceived as hypernasal because of the increase in oral impedance (Karnell, Schultz, & Canady, 2001) and the increase in transpalatal transmission of the sound (Gildersleeve-Neumann & Dalston, 2001).

Abnormal Resonance due to Hearing Loss or Deafness

Velopharyngeal function is learned through imitation and auditory feedback. For individuals with severe hearing impairment or deafness, the lack of hearing and auditory feedback affects the ability to learn to use the velopharyngeal valve for speech. Although affected individuals can learn to produce consonant sounds, there is no visual or tactile-kinesthetic feedback for resonance or velopharyngeal movements. Therefore, individuals with severe hearing impairment or deafness typically demonstrate abnormal resonance that can be a mixture of hypernasality, hyponasality, and cul-de-sac resonance (Abdullah, 1988; Fletcher & Daly, 1976; Subtelny, Whitehead, & Samar, 1992; Ysunza & Vazquez, 1993). Cochlear implants hold promise for not only increasing understanding of speech but also improving the resonance of oral speakers in the future (Hassan et al., 2011).

FACTORS THAT IMPACT SPEECH CHARACTERISTICS AND SEVERITY

The severity of VPI can vary from a very small pinhole-sized opening to a very large opening that includes the entire velopharyngeal port. However, the size of the velopharyngeal opening does not correlate well with the severity of the speech disorder and the effect on intelligibility (Jones, 2005). The lack of a one-to-one correlation is due to several factors, including the separate effects of gap size on acoustics versus aerodynamics, the consistency of closure, and the confounding effects of altered articulation and phonation.

Size of the Velopharyngeal Opening

If the effects of articulation and phonation are factored out or if both are normal, there still would be a poor correlation between the size of the velopharyngeal opening and the severity of the speech distortion. However, specific speech characteristics can be predictors of the approximate size of the opening (Table 7–1). This has to do with basic principles of physics and the acoustic effects of forcing air and sound through various sized openings.

One basic law of physics is that any type of flow (water, air, or sound) will continue in the same direction unless it is blocked by another force. In normal speech, airflow and sound energy move in a superior direction from the glottis through the pharynx. With closure of the velopharyngeal valve, the flow is redirected anteriorly into the oral cavity. When there is a velopharyngeal opening during speech, the flow is only partially redirected anteriorly. Because the airflow is perpendicular to the opening, even a very small opening results in some form of nasal escape (Kummer et al., 2003; Kummer et al., 1992).

If the velopharyngeal opening is large, air and sound will go through the opening without much resistance. The movement of air is unobstructed, turbulence is low, and nasal emission is not very audible. Instead, hypernasality is most noticeable. Oral sounds may be "nasalized" in that they will sound similar to nasal phonemes at the same placement (e.g., /m/ for bilabials, /n/ for lingual-alveolars, and /ŋ/ for velars). Oral sounds may also be substituted by compensatory productions (pharyngeal phonemes or glottal stops) due to the lack of sufficient intraoral air pressure. Because there is a significant amount of nasal emission (although not very audible), any attempted oral consonants will be very weak in intensity and pressure. In addition, utterance length is short due to the need to take more frequent breaths to compensate for the loss of air pressure.

If the velopharyngeal opening is moderate in size, there are similar characteristics as for a large opening. However, hypernasality is less severe and nasal emission is more audible. This is because with a smaller opening, there is more resistance to the flow of air as it comes through the valve, causing a turbulence sound. Also, there is more intraoral air pressure, so consonants are stronger and utterance length is less affected than with a larger opening.

TABLE 7–1 Perceptual Characteristics of Speech as a Prediction of Velopharyngeal Gap Size

Perceptual Characteristics	Predict	Relative Gap Size
Severe hypernasality Inaudible nasal emission Weak consonants Short utterance length Compensatory productions	⟹	⬭ (large)
Moderate hypernasality Audible nasal emission Slightly weak consonants May be compensatory productions	⟹	⬭ (medium)
Mild hypernasality Audible nasal emission	⟹	⬭ (small)
Nasal rustle (turbulence)	⟹	⬭ (smallest)

© Cengage Learning 2014

Small openings are typically characterized by normal speech and resonance. However, as noted before, a small opening usually causes a very loud and distracting nasal rustle (nasal turbulence) (Kummer et al., 2003; Kummer et al., 1992). The nasal rustle can be loud enough to mask the oral sound that is being articulated, which also affects the intelligibility of speech. Therefore, the speech quality from a small opening may be judged to be more severely affected than the speech quality from a larger opening.

Individuals who demonstrate a small, yet consistent velopharyngeal gap have been termed the *almost-but-not-quite* (ABNQ) group by Morris (1984). These individuals are generally not stimulable for improvement through auditory discrimination training or articulation therapy. This is because an underlying structural or physiological disorder precludes complete velopharyngeal closure. Therefore, surgical or prosthetic management is more appropriate. Correction is indicated, even though the opening is small, because this size of opening often results in more severely affected speech than a larger opening.

Inconsistency of Velopharyngeal Closure

If velopharyngeal closure is inconsistent, the quality of speech may also be variable.

Inconsistent velopharyngeal closure is most common in individuals who have a small velopharyngeal opening. Morris (1984) termed this subgroup of individuals the *sometimes-but-not-always* (SBNA) group. Individuals in this group may be able to achieve total closure with effort. However, just as it is difficult to carry a 50-pound weight for long, it is difficult for these individuals to continue to exert enough effort to maintain closure for a prolonged period of time. Closure may be complete for single words or short utterances but may break down with the motoric demands of connected speech. Speech may be best at the beginning of the day but become noticeably worse as the day goes on and the individual becomes fatigued. Inconsistencies in velopharyngeal closure can result in significant variations in the quality of speech and perception of resonance.

Abnormal Articulation and Phonation

Another factor that affects the intelligibility of speech and judgments of severity is the status of articulation. If the individual has developed good articulation skills and has preserved the appropriate place of articulation, the overall intelligibility of speech will be better than that of a person with the same size of opening who has poor articulation skills. If the individual uses compensatory articulation productions for either VPI or malocclusion, these errors will affect the overall intelligibility of speech and the judgment of severity.

The quality of phonation is a final factor that affects judgments of severity. The use of a breathy voice may reduce the perception of nasal emission and hypernasality. In addition, increased vocal effort may temporarily increase velopharyngeal function and decrease gap size for improved resonance (McHenry, 1997). On the other hand, low volume and other dysphonic characteristics, such as hoarseness and glottal fry, can have a negative effect on the overall intelligibility of the speech.

SUMMARY

Resonance depends on the size and shape of the cavities of the vocal tract and the function of the velopharyngeal valve. Resonance disorders can be caused by velopharyngeal dysfunction or by blockage in the vocal tract. Velopharyngeal dysfunction can cause not only hypernasality but also nasal emission, which affects several aspects of speech production.

Although resonance disorders and VPI (velopharyngeal insufficiency and incompetence) are not directly treated by the speech-language pathologist, it is this professional's responsibility to make a differential diagnosis based on the speech characteristics and to determine the probable cause. It is critical to determine whether the cause is abnormal structure versus abnormal function. This information is used to ensure that the individual receives appropriate treatment.

Speech therapy is never appropriate for hypernasality or nasal emission caused by VPI. Instead, surgery or prosthetic management is indicated. However, speech therapy is appropriate for correction of compensatory errors secondary to VPI after the physical correction. Therapy is also appropriate for correction of placement errors that cause nasal emission or hypernasality that is phoneme specific.

FOR REVIEW AND DISCUSSION

1. What is resonance as it relates to speech? Discuss factors relating to the vocal tract that can alter resonance. Why is resonance primarily associated with vowels rather than consonants?

2. How is a resonance disorder similar to a voice disorder? How is it different?

3. How are velopharyngeal insufficiency, velopharyngeal incompetence, and velopharyngeal mislearning similar? How are they different? Why do you think making a distinction between these types of velopharyngeal dysfunctions is an important part of an evaluation of abnormal resonance?

4. Describe the basic characteristics of hyponasality, hypernasality, cul-de-sac resonance, and mixed resonance. What are the possible causes of each? Try to imitate each type of abnormal resonance.

5. Describe the difference between hypernasality and nasal emission with speech. What other speech characteristics can occur with significant nasal emission, and why? Try to imitate these characteristics.

6. What is the difference between an obligatory articulation error and a compensatory articulation error? Give examples of each. Why do you think it is important to make a distinction between the two types of errors?

7. What are some of the causes of dysphonia in children with either a history of cleft palate or another craniofacial condition?

8. How does the size of the velopharyngeal gap affect speech characteristics? Why do you think it is important to understand this relationship? Why do you think the relationship between the size of the gap and the speech characteristics is not always the same when comparing different individuals?

9. List some of the causes of velopharyngeal insufficiency, velopharyngeal incompetence, and velopharyngeal mislearning. How do you think some of these causes could be treated?

REFERENCES

Abdel-Aziz, M. (2012). Hypertrophied tonsils impair velopharyngeal function after palatoplasty. *The Laryngoscope, 122*(3), 528–532.

Abdullah, S. (1988). A study of the results of speech language and hearing assessment of three groups of repaired cleft palate children and adults. *Annals of the Academy of Medicine of Singapore, 17*(3), 388–391.

Adil, E., Huntley, C., Choudhary, A., & Carr, M. (2011). Congenital nasal obstruction: Clinical and radiologic review. *European Journal of Pediatrics, 171*(4), 641–650.

Ainoda, N., Yamashita, K., & Tsukada, S. (1985). Articulation at age 4 in children with early repair of cleft palate. *Annals of Plastic Surgery, 15*(5), 415–422.

American Cleft Palate–Craniofacial Association (ACPA) (2006). Accessed January 8, 2013, from http://www.acpa-cpf.org/education/educational_resources/speech_samples/.

Andreassen, M. L., Leeper, H. A., & MacRae, D. L. (1991). Changes in vocal resonance and nasalization following adenoidectomy in normal children: Preliminary findings. *Journal of Otolaryngology, 20*(4), 237–242.

Andrews, J. R., & Rutherford, D. (1972). Contribution of nasally emitted sound to the perception of hypernasality of vowels. *Cleft Palate Journal, 9*, 147–156.

Awan, S. N., Omlor, K., & Watts, C. R. (2011). Effects of computer system and vowel loading on measures of nasalance. *Journal of Speech Language Hearing Research, 54*(5), 1284–1294.

Bennett, K., & Hoit, J. D. (2012). Stress Velopharyngeal Incompetence (SVPI) in Collegiate Trombone Players. [In press.] *Cleft Palate-Craniofacial Journal.* doi: 10.1597/11-181.

Bernthal, J. E., & Beukelman, D. R. (1977). The effect of changes in velopharyngeal orifice area on vowel intensity. *Cleft Palate Journal, 14*(1), 63–77.

Bispo, N. H., Whitaker, M. E., Aferri, H. C., Neves, J. D., Dutka Jde, C., & Pegoraro-Krook, M. I. (2011). Speech therapy for compensatory articulations and velopharyngeal function: A case report. *Journal of Applied Oral Science, 19*(6), 679–684.

Bodin, I. K., Lind, M. G., & Arnander, C. (1994). Free radial forearm flap reconstruction in surgery of the oral cavity and pharynx: Surgical complications, impairment of speech and swallowing. *Clinics in Otolaryngology, 19*(1), 28–34.

Bradley, D. P. (1997). Congenital and acquired velopharyngeal inadequacy. In K. R. Bzoch (Ed.), *Communicative disorders related to cleft lip and palate* (vol. 4, pp. 223–243). Austin, TX: Pro-Ed.

Brooks, A. R., Shelton, R. L., & Youngstrom, K. A. (1965). Compensatory tongue-palate-posterior pharyngeal wall relationships in cleft palate. *Journal of Speech and Hearing Disorders, 30,* 166.

Brown, J. S., Zuydam, A. C., Jones, D. C., Rogers, S. N., & Vaughan, E. D. (1997). Functional outcome in soft palate reconstruction using a radial forearm free flap in conjunction with a superiorly based pharyngeal flap. *Head & Neck, 19*(6), 524–534.

Buder, E. H. (2005). The acoustics of nasality: Steps towards a bridge to source literature. *Perspectives on Speech Science and Orofacial Disorders, 15*(1), 9–14.

Cassassolles, S., Paulus, C., Ajacques, J. C., Berger-Vachon, C., Laurent, M., & Perrin, E. (1995). Acoustic characterization of velar insufficiency in young children. *Revue de Stomatologie et de Chirurgie Maxillofaciale, 96*(1), 13–20.

Chanchareonsook, N., Whitehill, T. L., & Samman, N. (2007). Speech outcome and velopharyngeal function in cleft palate: Comparison of Le Fort I maxillary osteotomy and distraction osteogenesis–early results. *Cleft Palate–Craniofacial Journal, 44*(1), 23–32.

Conley, S. F., Beecher, R. B., & Marks, S. (1995). Stress velopharyngeal incompetence in an adolescent trumpet player. *Annals of Otology, Rhinology and Laryngology, 104*(9 Pt. 1), 715–717.

Croft, C. B., Shprintzen, R. J., & Ruben, R. J. (1981). Hypernasal speech following adenotonsillectomy. *Otolaryngology—Head & Neck Surgery, 89*(2), 179–188.

D'Antonio, L. L., Muntz, H. R., Province, M. A., & Marsh, J. L. (1988). Laryngeal/voice findings in patients with velopharyngeal dysfunction. *Laryngoscope, 98*(4), 432–438.

de Serres, L. M., Deleyiannis, F. W., Eblen, L. E., Gruss, J. S., Richardson, M. A., & Sie, K. C. (1999). Results with sphincter pharyngoplasty and pharyngeal flap. *International Journal of Pediatric Otorhinolaryngology, 48*(1), 17–25.

Demetriades, N., Chang, D. J., Laskarides, C., & Papageorge, M. (2010). Effects of mandibular retropositioning, with or without maxillary advancement, on the oro-naso-pharyngeal airway and development of sleep-related breathing disorders. *Journal of Oral and Maxillofacial Surgery, 68*(10), 2431–2436.

Donnelly, M. J. (1994). Hypernasality following adenoid removal. *Irish Journal of Medical Science, 163*(5), 225–227.

Evans, A., Driscoll, T., & Ackermann, B. (2011). Prevalence of velopharyngeal insufficiency in woodwind and brass students. *Occupational Medicine Journal (London), 61*(7), 480–482.

Falk, M. L., & Kopp, G. A. (1968). Tongue position and hypernasality in cleft palate speech. *Cleft Palate Journal, 5*(3), 228–237.

Fernandes, D. B., Grobbelaar, A. O., Hudson, D. A., & Lentin, R. (1996). Velopharyngeal incompetence after adenotonsillectomy in noncleft patients. *British Journal of Oral and Maxillofacial Surgery, 34*(5), 364–367.

Finkelstein, Y., Bar-Ziv, J., Nachmani, A., Berger, G., & Ophir, D. (1993). Peritonsillar abscess as a cause of transient velopharyngeal insufficiency. *Cleft Palate–Craniofacial Journal, 30*(4), 421–428.

Finkelstein, Y., Nachmani, A., & Ophir, D. (1994). The functional role of the tonsils in speech. *Archives of Otolaryngology—Head & Neck Surgery, 120*(8), 846–851.

Finkelstein, Y., Talmi, Y. P., Nachmani, A., Hauben, D. J., & Zohar, Y. (1992). On the variability of velopharyngeal valve anatomy and function: A combined peroral and nasendoscopic study. *Plastic and Reconstructive Surgery, 89*(4), 631–639.

Finkelstein, Y., Wexler, D. B., Nachmani, A., & Ophir, D. (2002). Endoscopic partial adenoidectomy for children with submucous cleft palate. *Cleft Palate–Craniofacial Journal, 39*(5), 479–486.

Fletcher, S. G., & Daly, D. A. (1976). Nasalance in utterances of hearing-impaired speakers. *Journal of Communication Disorders, 9*(1), 63–73.

Folkins, J. W. (1988). Velopharyngeal nomenclature: Incompetence, inadequacy, insufficiency, and dysfunction. *Cleft Palate Journal, 25*(4), 413–416.

Gibb, A. G., & Stewart, I. A. (1975). Hypernasality following tonsil dissection—Hysterical aetiology. *Journal of Laryngology and Otology, 89*(7), 779–781.

Gibbon, F., Smeaton-Ewins, P., & Crampin, L. (2005). Tongue-palate contact during selected vowels in children with cleft palate. *Folia Phoniatrica Logopaedica, 57*(4), 181–192.

Gibbon, F. E., Ellis, L., & Crampin, L. (2004). Articulatory placement for /t/, /d/, /k/ and /g/ targets in school age children with speech disorders associated with cleft palate. *Clinical Linguistic and Phonetics, 18*(6–8), 391–404.

Gildersleeve-Neumann, C. E., & Dalston, R. M. (2001). Nasalance scores in noncleft individuals: Why not zero? *Cleft Palate–Craniofacial Journal, 38*(2), 106–111.

Gordon, N. A., Astrachan, D., & Yanagisawa, E. (1994). Videoendoscopic diagnosis and correction of velopharyngeal stress incompetence in a bassoonist. *Annals of Otology, Rhinology and Laryngology, 103*(8 Pt. 1), 595–600.

Gosain, A. K., & Hettinger, P. C. (2009). Submucous cleft Palate. In J. E. Lossee & R. E. Kirschner (Eds.), *Comprehensive Cleft Care* (pp. 361–369). New York: McGraw-Hill.

Guyette, T. W., Polley, J. W., Figueroa, A., & Smith, B. E. (2001). Changes in speech following maxillary distraction osteogenesis. *Cleft Palate–Craniofacial Journal, 38*(3), 199–205.

Haapanen, M. L., Heliovaara, A., & Ranta, R. (1991). Hypernasality and the nasopharyngeal space. A cephalometric study. *Journal of Craniomaxillofacial Surgery*, 19(2), 77–80.

Haapanen, M. L., Ignatius, J., Rihkanen, H., & Ertama, L. (1994). Velopharyngeal insufficiency following palatine tonsillectomy. *European Archives of Oto-Rhino-Laryngology*, 251(3), 186–189.

Haapanen, M. L., Kalland, M., Heliovaara, A., Hukki, J., & Ranta, R. (1997). Velopharyngeal function in cleft patients undergoing maxillary advancement. *Folia Phoniatrica et Logopedica*, 49(1), 42–47.

Hall, C. D., Golding-Kushner, K. J., Argamaso, R. V., & Strauch, B. (1991). Pharyngeal flap surgery in adults. *Cleft Palate–Craniofacial Journal*, 28(2), 179–182; Discussion 182–183.

Handelman, C. S., & Osborne, G. (1976). Growth of the nasopharynx and adenoid development from one to eighteen years. *Angle Orthodontist*, 46(3), 243–259.

Harding, A., & Grunwell, P. (1996). Characteristics of cleft palate speech. *European Journal of Disorders of Communication*, 31(4), 331–357.

Harding, A., & Grunwell, P. (1998). Active versus passive cleft-type speech characteristics. *International Journal of Language and Communication Disorders*, 33(3), 329–352.

Hassan, S. M., Malki, K. H., Mesallam, T. A., Farahat, M., Bukhari, M., & Murry, T. (2012). The Effect of Cochlear Implantation on Nasalance of Speech in Postlingually Hearing-Impaired Adults. *Journal of Voice*, 26(5), 669 e17–22.

Heliovaara, A., Hukki, J., Ranta, R., & Haapanen, M. L. (2004). Cephalometric pharyngeal changes after Le Fort I osteotomy in different types of clefts. *Scandinavian Journal of Plastic and Reconstructive Surgery and Hand Surgery*, 38(1), 5–10.

Heliovaara, A., Ranta, R., Hukki, J., & Haapanen, M. L. (2002). Cephalometric pharyngeal changes after Le Fort I osteotomy in patients with unilateral cleft lip and palate. *Acta Odontologica Scandinavica*, 60(3), 141–145.

Heller, J. C., Gens, G. W., Moe, D. G., & Lewin, M. L. (1974). Velopharyngeal insufficiency in patients with neurologic, emotional, and mental disorders. *Journal of Speech and Hearing Disorders*, 39(3), 350–359.

Henningsson, G. E., & Isberg, A. M. (1986). Velopharyngeal movement patterns in patients alternating between oral and glottal articulation: A clinical and cineradiographical study. *Cleft Palate Journal*, 23(1), 1–9.

Henningsson, G., & Isberg, A. (1988). Influence of tonsils on velopharyngeal movements in children with craniofacial anomalies and hypernasality. *American Journal of Orthodontics and Dentofacial Orthopedics*, 94(3), 253–261.

Hiiemae, K. M., & Palmer, J. B. (2003). Tongue movements in feeding and speech. *Critical Reviews in Oral Biology & Medicine*, 14(6), 413–429.

Huber, J. E., & Stathopoulos, E. T. (2003). Respiratory and laryngeal responses to an oral air pressure bleed during speech. *Journal of Speech Language Hearing Research*, 46(5), 1207–1220.

Ikeda, T., Matsuzaki, Y., & Aomatsu, T. (2001). A numerical analysis of phonation using a two-dimensional flexible channel model of the vocal folds. *Journal of Biomechanical Engineering*, 123(6), 571–579.

Jakobsone, G., Stenvik, A., & Espeland, L. (2011). The effect of maxillary advancement and impaction on the upper airway after bimaxillary surgery to correct Class

III malocclusion. *American Journal of Orthodontics and Dentofacial Orthopedics, 139*(4 Suppl.), e369–376.

Janulewicz, J., Costello, B. J., Buckley, M. J., Ford, M. D., Close, R., & Gassner, R. (2004). The effects of Le Fort I osteotomies on velopharyngeal and speech functions in cleft palate patients. *Journal of Oral and Maxillofacial Surgery, 62*(3), 308–314.

Jones, D. L. (1991). Velopharyngeal function and dysfunction. *Clinics in Communication Disorders, 1*(3), 19–25.

Jones, D. L. (2005). Perceptual aspects of nasality. *Perspectives on Speech Science and Orofacial Disorders, 15*(1), 9–14.

Karnell, M. P., Schultz, K., & Canady, J. (2001). Investigations of a pressure-sensitive theory of marginal velopharyngeal inadequacy. *Cleft Palate–Craniofacial Journal, 38*(4), 346–357.

Kline, L. S., & Hutchinson, J. M. (1980). Acoustic and perceptual evaluation of hypernasality of mentally retarded persons. *American Journal of Mental Deficiency, 85*(2), 153–160.

Ko, E. W., Figueroa, A. A., Guyette, T. W., Polley, J. W., & Law, W. R. (1999). Velopharyngeal changes after maxillary advancement in cleft patients with distraction osteogenesis using a rigid external distraction device: A 1-year cephalometric follow-up. *Journal of Craniofacial Surgery, 10*(4), 312–320; Discussion 321–322.

Kummer, A. W. (2011a). Disorders of resonance and airflow secondary to cleft palate and/or velopharyngeal dysfunction. *Seminars in Speech and Language, 32*(2), 141–149.

Kummer, A. W. (2011b). Types and causes of velopharyngeal dysfunction. *Seminars in Speech and Language, 32*(2), 150–158.

Kummer, A. W., Billmire, D. A., & Myer, C. M., III. (1993). Hypertrophic tonsils: The effect on resonance and velopharyngeal closure. *Plastic and Reconstructive Surgery, 91*(4), 608–611.

Kummer, A. W., Briggs, M., & Lee, L. (2003). The relationship between the characteristics of speech and velopharyngeal gap size. *Cleft Palate–Craniofacial Journal, 40*(6), 590–596.

Kummer, A. W., Curtis, C., Wiggs, M., Lee, L., & Strife, J. L. (1992). Comparison of velopharyngeal gap size in patients with hypernasality, hypernasality and nasal emission, or nasal turbulence (rustle) as the primary speech characteristic. *Cleft Palate–Craniofacial Journal, 29*(2), 152–156.

Kummer, A. W., Myer, C. M. L., Smith, M. E., & Shott, S. R. (1993). Changes in nasal resonance secondary to adenotonsillectomy. *American Journal of Otolaryngology, 14*(4), 285–290.

Kummer, A. W., Strife, J. L., Grau, W. H., Creaghead, N. A., & Lee, L. (1989). The effects of Le Fort I osteotomy with maxillary movement on articulation, resonance, and velopharyngeal function. *Cleft Palate Journal, 26*(3), 193–199.

Lee, G. S., Wang, C. P., & Fu, S. (2009). Evaluation of hypernasality in vowels using voice low tone to high tone ratio. *Cleft Palate–Craniofacial Journal, 46*(1), 47–52.

Leveau-Geffroy, S., Perrin, J. P., Khonsari, R. H., & Mercier, J. (2011). [Cephalometric study of the velocardiofacial syndrome: Impact of dysmorphosis on phonation]. *Revue de Stomatologie et de Chirurgie Maxillofaciale, 112*(1), 11–15.

Loney, R. W., & Bloem, T. J. (1987). Velopharyngeal dysfunction: Recommendations for use of nomenclature. *Cleft Palate Journal,* *24*(4), 334–335.

MacKenzie-Stepner, K., Witzel, M. A., Stringer, D. A., & Laskin, R. (1987). Velopharyngeal insufficiency due to hypertrophic tonsils. A report of two cases. *International Journal of Pediatric Otorhinolaryngology, 14*(1), 57–63.

Maclean, J. E., Waters, K., Fitzsimons, D., Hayward, P., & Fitzgerald, D. A. (2009). Screening for obstructive sleep apnea in preschool children with cleft palate. *Cleft Palate–Craniofacial Journal, 46*(2), 117–123.

Maegawa, J., Sells, R. K., & David, D. J. (1998). Speech changes after maxillary advancement in 40 cleft lip and palate patients. *Journal of Craniofacial Surgery, 9*(2), 177–182; Discussion 183–184.

Malick, D., Moon, J., & Canady, J. (2007). Stress velopharyngeal incompetence: Prevalence, treatment, and management practices. *Cleft Palate–Craniofacial Journal, 44*(4), 424–433.

Marsh, J. L. (1991). Cleft palate and velopharyngeal dysfunction. *Clinics in Communication Disorders, 1*(3), 29–34.

Maryn, Y., Van Lierde, K., De Bodt, M., & Van Cauwenberge, P. (2004). The effects of adenoidectomy and tonsillectomy on speech and nasal resonance. *Folia Phoniatrica Logopaedica, 56*(3), 182–191.

Mason, R. M., & Grandstaff, H. L. (1971). Evaluating the velopharyngeal mechanism in hypernasal speakers. *Language, Speech, and Hearing Services in the Schools, 2*(4), 53–61.

Mason, R., Turvey, T. A., & Warren, D. W. (1980). Speech considerations with maxillary advancement procedures. *Journal of Oral Surgery, 38*(10), 752–758.

Mason, R. M., & Warren, D. W. (1980). Adenoid involution and developing hyper-

nasality in cleft palate. *Journal of Speech and Hearing Disorders, 45*(4), 469–480.

McCarthy, J. G., Coccaro, P. J., & Schwartz, M. D. (1979). Velopharyngeal function following maxillary advancement. *Plastic and Reconstructive Surgery, 64*(2), 180–189.

McHenry, M. A. (1997). The effect of increased vocal effort on estimated velopharyngeal orifice area. *American Journal of Speech-Language Pathology, 6*(4), 55–61.

McWilliams, B. J. (1991). Submucous clefts of the palate: How likely are they to be symptomatic? *Cleft Palate–Craniofacial Journal, 28*(3), 247–249; Discussion 250–251.

McWilliams, B. J., Lavorato, A. S., & Bluestone, C. D. (1973). Vocal cord abnormalities in children with velopharyngeal valving problems. *Laryngoscope, 83*, 1745.

Morris, H. L. (1984). Types of velopharyngeal incompetence. In H. Winitz (Ed.), *Treating articulation disorders: For clinicians by clinicians* (p. 211). Baltimore: University Park Press.

Morris, H. L. (1992). Some questions and answers about velopharyngeal dysfunction during speech. *American Journal of Speech-Language Pathology, 1*(3), 26–28.

Morris, H. L., Wroblewski, S. K., Brown, C. K., & Van Demark, D. R. (1990). Velarpharyngeal status in cleft palate patients with expected adenoidal involution. *Annals of Otology, Rhinology, and Laryngology, 99*(6, Pt. 1), 432–437.

Muntz, H., Wilson, M., Park, A., Smith, M., & Grimmer, J. F. (2008). Sleep disordered breathing and obstructive sleep apnea in the cleft population. *The Laryngoscope, 118*(2), 348–353.

Myers, E. N., & Aramany, M. A. (1977). Rehabilitation of the oral cavity following resection of the hard and soft palate.

Transactions of the American Academy of Ophthalmology and Otolaryngology, 84(5), 941–951.

Neiman, G. S., & Simpson, R. K. (1975). A roentgencephalometric investigation of the effect of adenoid removal upon selected measures of velopharyngeal function. *Cleft Palate Journal, 12,* 377–389.

Niemeyer, T. C., Gomes Ade, O., Fukushiro, A. P., & Genaro, K. F. (2005). Speech resonance in orthognathic surgery in subjects with cleft lip and palate. *Journal of Applied Oral Science, 13*(3), 232–236.

Netsell, R. (1969). Evaluation of velopharyngeal function in dysarthria. *Journal of Speech and Hearing Disorders, 34*(2), 113–122.

Netsell, R. (1988). Velopharyngeal dysfunction. In D. Yoder & R. Kent (Eds.), *Decision-making in speech-language pathology* (pp. 150–151). Toronto: B. C. Decker.

Nohara, K., Tachimura, T., & Wada, T. (2006). Prediction of deterioration of velopharyngeal function associated with maxillary advancement using electromyography of levator veli palatini muscle. *Cleft Palate–Craniofacial Journal, 43*(2), 174–178.

Ogar, J., Willock, S., Baldo, J., Wilkins, D., Ludy, C., & Dronkers, N. (2006). Clinical and anatomical correlates of apraxia of speech. *Brain and Language; 97*(3), 343–350.

Okazaki, K., Satoh, K., Kato, M., Iwanami, M., Ohokubo, F., & Kobayashi, K. (1993). Speech and velopharyngeal function following maxillary advancement in patients with cleft lip and palate. *Annals of Plastic Surgery, 30*(4), 304–311.

Parton, M. J., & Jones, A. S. (1998). Hypernasality following adenoidectomy: A significant and avoidable complication. *Clinical Otolaryngology, 23*(1), 18–19.

Penfold, C. N. (1997). Management of velopharyngeal dysfunction. *British Journal of Oral and Maxillofacial Surgery, 35*(6), 454.

Phillips, J. H., Klaiman, P., Delorey, R., & MacDonald, D. B. (2005). Predictors of velopharyngeal insufficiency in cleft palate orthognathic surgery. *Plastic Reconstructive Surgery, 115*(3), 681–686.

Pourdanesh, F., Sharifi, R., Mohebbi, A., & Jamilian, A. (2012). Effects of maxillary advancement and impact on nasal airway function. *International Journal of Oral and Maxillofacial Surgery, 41*(11), 1350–1352.

Powers, G. R. (1962). Cinefluorographic investigation of articulatory movements of selected individuals with cleft palates. *Journal of Speech and Hearing Research, 5,* 59.

Proctor, M. I., Shadle, C. H., & Iskarous, K. (2010). Pharyngeal articulation in the production of voiced and voiceless fricatives. *Journal of the Acoustical Society of America, 127*(3), 1507–1518.

Ren, Y. F., Isberg, A., & Henningsson, G. (1995). Velopharyngeal incompetence and persistent hypernasality after adenoidectomy in children without palatal defect. *Cleft Palate–Craniofacial Journal, 32*(6), 476–482.

Riski, J. E., & Verdolini, K. (1999). Is hypernasality a voice disorder? *ASHA, 41*(1), 10–11.

Robinson, J. H. (1992). Association between adenoidectomy, velopharyngeal incompetence, and submucous cleft. *Cleft Palate–Craniofacial Journal, 29*(4), 385.

Robison, J. G., & Otteson, T. D. (2011a). Increased prevalence of obstructive sleep apnea in patients with cleft palate. *Archives of Otolaryngology—Head & Neck Surgery, 137*(3), 269–274.

Robison, J. G., & Otteson, T. D. (2011b). Prevalence of hoarseness in the cleft palate population. *Archives of Otolaryngology—Head & Neck Surgery, 137*(1), 74–77.

Rousseaux, M., Lesoin, F., & Quint, S. (1987). Unilateral pseudobulbar syndrome with limited capsulothalamic infarction. *European Neurology, 27*(4), 227–230.

Sabashi, K., Washino, K., Saitoh, I., Yamasaki, Y., Kawabata, A., Mukai, Y., & Kitai, N. (2011). Nasal obstruction causes a decrease in lip-closing force. *Angle Orthodontist, 81*(5), 750–753.

Satoh, K., Nagata, J., Shomura, K., Wada, T., Tachimura, T., Fukuda, J., & Shiba, R. (2004). Morphological evaluation of changes in velopharyngeal function following maxillary distraction in patients with repaired cleft palate during mixed dentition. *Cleft Palate–Craniofacial Journal, 41*(4), 355–363.

Saunders, N. C., Hartley, B. E., Sell, D., & Sommerlad, B. (2004). Velopharyngeal insufficiency following adenoidectomy. *Clinical Otolaryngology & Allied Sciences, 29*(6), 686–688.

Schendel, S., Powell, N., & Jacobson, R. (2011). Maxillary, mandibular, and chin advancement: Treatment planning based on airway anatomy in obstructive sleep apnea. *Journal of Oral and Maxillofacial Surgery, 69*(3), 663–676.

Schmaman, L., Jordaan, H., & Jammine, G. H. (1998). Risk factors for permanent hypernasality after adenoidectomy. *South African Medical Journal, 88*(3), 266–269.

Scott, A. R., Moldan, M. M., Tibesar, R. J., Lander, T. A., & Sidman, J. D. (2011). A theoretical cause of nasal obstruction in patients with repaired cleft palate. *American Journal of Rhinology and Allergy, 25*(1), 58–60.

Sealey, L. R., & Giddens, C. L. (2010). Aerodynamic indices of velopharyngeal function in childhood apraxia of speech. *Clinical Linguistics & Phonetics, 24*(6), 417–430.

Seid, A. B. (1990). Velopharyngeal insufficiency versus adenoidectomy for obstructive apnea: A quandary. *Cleft Palate Journal, 27*(2), 200–202.

Shanks, J. C. (1990). Velopharyngeal incompetence manifested initially in playing a musical instrument. *Journal of Voice, 4*(2), 169–171.

Shapiro, R. S. (1980). Velopharyngeal insufficiency starting at puberty without adenoidectomy. *International Journal of Pediatric Otorhinolaryngology, 2*(3), 255–260.

Shprintzen, R. J., Rakof, S. J., Skolnick, M. L., & Lavorato, A. S. (1977). Incongruous movements of the velum and lateral pharyngeal walk *Cleft Palate Journal, 14*(2), 148–157.

Shprintzen, R. J., Sher, A. E., & Croft, C. B. (1987). Hypernasal speech caused by tonsillar hypertrophy. *International Journal of Pediatric Otorhinolaryngology, 14*(1), 45–56.

Siegel-Sadewitz, V. L., & Shprintzen, R. J. (1982). Nasopharyngoscopy of the normal velopharyngeal sphincter: An experiment of biofeedback. *Cleft Palate Journal, 19*(3), 194–200.

Siegel-Sadewitz, V. L., & Shprintzen, R. J. (1986). Changes in velopharyngeal valving with age. *International Journal of Pediatric Otorhinolaryngology, 11*(2), 171–182.

Skolnick, M. L., Shprintzen, R. J., McCall, G. N., & Rakoff, S. (1975). Patterns of velopharyngeal closure in subjects with repaired cleft palate and normal speech: A multi-view videofluoroscopic analysis. *Cleft Palate Journal, 12*, 369–376.

Smith, B. E, & Kuehn, D. P. (2007). Speech evaluation of velopharyngeal dysfunction. *The Journal of Craniofacial Surgery, 18*(2), 251–261.

Stewart, K. J., Ahmed, R. E., Razzell, R. E., & Watson, A. C. H. (2002). Altered speech following adenoidectomy: A 20-year experience. *British Journal of Plastic Surgery, 55,* 469–473.

Story, B. H., Titze, I. R., & Hoffman, E. A. (2001). The relationship of vocal tract shape to three voice qualities. *Journal of the Acoustical Society of America, 109*(4), 1651–1667.

Subtelny, J. D., Whitehead, R. L., & Samar, V. J. (1992). Spectral study of deviant resonance in the speech of women who are deaf. *Journal of Speech & Hearing Research, 35*(3), 574–579.

Tan, Y. C., & Chen, P. K. (2009). Hemipalatal hypoplasia. *The Journal of Craniofacial Surgery, 20*(4), 1150–1153.

Titze, I. R. (1980). Comments on the myoelastic-aerodynamic theory of phonation. *Journal of Speech and Hearing Research, 23*(3), 495–510.

Titze, I. R. (2000). Principles of Voice Production (2nd ed.). National Center for Voice and Speech, University of Iowa, Iowa City.

Titze, I. R., Bergan, C. C., Hunter, E. J., & Story, B. (2003). Source and filter adjustments affecting the perception of the vocal qualities twang and yawn. *Logopedics, Phoniatrics, Vocology, 28*(4), 147–155.

Tom, K., Titze, I. R., Hoffman, E. A., & Story, B. H. (2001). Three-dimensional vocal tract imaging and formant structure: Varying vocal register, pitch, and loudness. *Journal of the Acoustical Society of America, 109*(2), 742–747.

Trindade, I. E., Yamashita, R. P., Suguimoto, R. M., Mazzottini, R., & Trindade, A. S., Jr. (2003). Effects of orthognathic surgery on speech and breathing of subjects with cleft lip and palate: Acoustic and aerodynamic assessment. *Cleft Palate–Craniofacial Journal, 40*(1), 54–64.

Trost, J. E. (1981). Articulatory additions to the classical description of the speech of persons with cleft palate. *Cleft Palate Journal, 18*(3), 193–203.

Trost-Cardamone, J. E. (1989). Coming to terms with VPI: A response to Loney and Bloem. *Cleft Palate Journal, 26*(1), 68–70.

Trost-Cardamone, J. E. (1990). Speech in the first year of life: A perspective on early acquisition. In D. E. Kernahan & S. W. Rosenstein (Eds.), *Cleft lip and palate: A system of management* (pp. 91–103). Baltimore: Williams & Wilkins.

Trost-Cardamone, J. E. (1997). Diagnosis of specific cleft palate speech error patterns for planning therapy of physical management needs. In K. R. Bzoch (Ed.), *Communicative disorders related to cleft lip and palate* (vol. 4, pp. 313–330). Austin, TX: Pro-Ed.

Vallino, L. D. (1990). Speech, velopharyngeal function, and hearing before and after orthognathic surgery. *Journal of Oral & Maxillofacial Surgery, 48*(12), 1274–1281.

Vijayalakshmi, P., & Reddy, M. R. (2006). Assessment of dysarthric speech and an analysis on velopharyngeal incompetence. Conference Proceedings, *IEEE English Medical and Biological Society, 1,* 3759–3762.

Ward, E. C., McAuliffe, M., Holmes, S. K., Lynham, A., & Monsour, F. (2002). Impact of malocclusion and orthognathic reconstruction surgery on resonance and articulatory function: An examination of variability in five cases. *British Journal of Oral Maxillofacial Surgery, 40*(5), 410–417.

Warren, D. W., Dalston, R. M., & Mayo, R. (1993). Hypernasality in the presence of "adequate" velopharyngeal closure. *Cleft Palate–Craniofacial Journal, 30*(2), 150–154.

Warren, D. W., Dalston, R. M., Trier, W. C, & Holder, M. B. (1985). A pressure-flow technique for quantifying temporal patterns of palatopharyngeal closure. *Cleft Palate Journal, 22*(1), 11–19.

Witt, P. D. (2009). Velopharyngeal dysfunction. In J. E. Lossee & R. E. Kirschner (Eds.), *Comprehensive Cleft Care* (pp. 627–640). New York: McGraw-Hill.

Witt, P. D., O'Daniel, T. G., Marsh, J. L., Grames, L. M., Muntz, H. R., & Pilgram, T. K. (1997). Surgical management of velopharyngeal dysfunction: Outcome analysis of autogenous posterior pharyngeal wall augmentation. *Plastic and Reconstructive Surgery, 99*(5), 1287–1296; Discussion 1297–1300.

Witzel, M. A., & Posnick, J. C. (1989). Patterns and location of velopharyngeal valving problems: Atypical findings on video nasopharyngoscopy. *Cleft Palate Journal, 26*(1), 63–67.

Witzel, M. A., Rich, R. H., Margar-Bacal, F., & Cox, C. (1986). Velopharyngeal insufficiency after adenoidectomy: An 8-year review. *International Journal of Pediatric Otorhinolaryngology, 11*(1), 15–20.

Yanagisawa, E., Estill, J., Mambrino, L., & Talkin, D. (1991). Supraglottic contributions to pitch raising. Videoendoscopic study with spectroanalysis. *Annals of Otolology, Rhinolology, and Laryngology, 100*(1), 19–30.

Yanagisawa, E., Kmucha, S. T., & Estill, J. (1990). Role of the soft palate in laryngeal functions and selected voice qualities. Simultaneous velolaryngeal videoendoscopy. *Annals of Otology, Rhinology, and Laryngology, 99*(1), 18–28. [Published erratum appears in *Annals of Otology, Rhinology, and Laryngology*, 99(6, Pt. 1), 431.]

Yorkston, K. M., Beukelman, D. R., & Traynor, C. D. (1988). Articulatory adequacy in dysarthric speakers: A comparison of judging formats. *Journal of Communication Disorders, 21*(4), 351–361.

Yoshida, H., Michi, K., Yamashita, Y., & Ohno, K. (1993). A comparison of surgical and prosthetic treatment for speech disorders attributable to surgically acquired soft palate defects. *Journal of Oral and Maxillofacial Surgery, 51*(4), 361–365.

Ysunza, A., & Vazquez, M. C. (1993). Velopharyngeal sphincter physiology in deaf individuals. *Cleft Palate–Craniofacial Journal, 30*(2), 141–143.

CHAPTER

8

FACIAL, ORAL, AND PHARYNGEAL ANOMALIES

J. PAUL WILLGING, M.D.

ANN W. KUMMER, PH.D.

CHAPTER OUTLINE

INTRODUCTION

Cleft palate and craniofacial anomalies can have a significant impact on the various functions. In addition, the typical disease processes that exist in the general population are often found with increased prevalence in patients with these anomalies.

The purpose of this chapter is to review the congenital anomalies and acquired disorders of the face, oral cavity, and pharyngeal cavity. Because the ear, nose, and throat are important for speech production, abnormalities of these structures can particularly affect the quality and intelligibility of speech.

THE EAR

Children born with craniofacial anomalies may have associated malformations of the external or middle ear. Abnormalities of the inner ear are less commonly encountered but can occur. Malformations of the ear can affect aesthetics and can cause hearing loss that ultimately affects the ability to communicate.

External Ear

Figure 8–1A shows a normal pinna. Patients with craniofacial anomalies, especially those with syndromes, often have *microtia*, which is a malformation of the pinna (Alasti & Van Camp, 2009; Brent, 1999; Luquetti, Heike, Hing, Cunningham, & Cox, 2011) (Figure 8–1B and C). The more severely malformed the pinna is, the greater the chances are for significant problems within the middle ear or the ossicles (Kountakis, Helidonis, & Jahrsdoerfer, 1995). When there is microtia of the external ear, it is not uncommon to also find *aural atresia* (also called *auditory atresia*), which is a closure or absence of the external auditory canal. This is commonly found in Treacher Collins syndrome, hemifacial microsomia, or Nager syndrome. Aural atresia results in a *conductive hearing loss* because the sound energy cannot travel directly through the external auditory canal to the tympanic membrane and therefore cannot reach the inner ear.

Children with bilateral aural atresia require bone conduction hearing aids. These may be conventional aids that make contact with the skull by means of a headband, or they may be bone-anchored hearing aids that are implanted (*osseointegrated*) into the bone of the skull for a rigid attachment. Bone conduction hearing aids directly vibrate the end organ within the cochlea. Children with unilateral aural atresia generally do not require a hearing aid if their hearing is normal in the unaffected ear. It is of interest that children with aural atresia rarely experience ear infections. The explanation for this is not known.

Reconstruction of the auditory canal (in addition to the middle ear structures of the tympanic membrane and ossicular chain) can be done in the early school years. Patients with bilateral aural atresia benefit from reconstruction, with an improvement in hearing. Patients with unilateral atresia are often reconstructed, but the benefits are less easily quantifiable. The risk of this surgical procedure lies in the potential damage to CN VII (Chang, Lee, Choi, & Song, 2007), which is the facial nerve that controls motion on each side of the face. Damage to the nerve can cause partial or

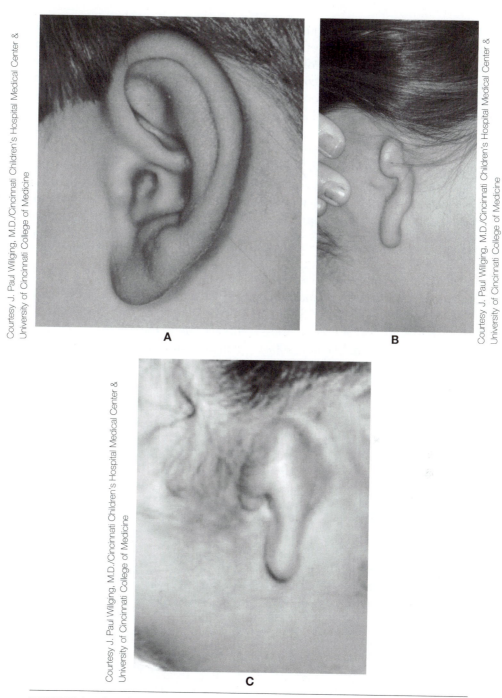

A

B

C

FIGURE 8–1 (A–C) (A) A normal pinna. The pinna is composed of fibroelastic cartilage covered by a thin layer of skin. The delicate folding of the cartilage provides the normal shape of the ear. (B–C) Two patients with microtia. Microtia is the result of abnormal development of the external ear. The more severe the external deformity, the more likely it is that the middle ear cannot be reconstructed, despite the fact that the external ear and middle ear develop from different sites of origin.

complete paralysis that may be temporary or permanent, depending on the degree of injury. Computed tomography (CT) scans of the temporal bone can be used to predict the course of the facial nerve in atretic ears, but these scans are not always of value. A rating scale has been developed to predict the outcome of the surgical correction of the external auditory canal and tympanic membrane, based on the overall development of the middle ear space, the size and position of the ossicles, the presence of the stapes, and the position of the facial nerve.

Middle Ear

When malformations are found in the external ear, there are often malformations or anomalies of the middle ear structures as well (Kosling, Omenzetter, & Bartel-Friedrich, 2009; Shea-han, Miller, Earley, Sheahan, & Blayney, 2004) (Figure 8–2). For example, abnormal formation

of the ossicles, in addition to external ear malformations, is common in Crouzon, Apert, and Goldenhar syndromes. In some cases, there is fusion of the ossicles to the surrounding bone. When the ossicles are abnormally formed or fused, this affects the transmission of sound to the inner ear, causing a conductive hearing loss.

As noted above, surgical correction of abnormalities of the middle ear, including the tympanic membrane and ossicles, can be done in the early school years. In addition, bone conduction hearing aids allow correction of most kinds of conductive hearing loss.

Eustachian Tube

Eustachian tube connects the middle ear with the nasopharynx. This tube is closed at rest and opens when the tensor veli palatini muscle, which is attached directly to the cartilage of the Eustachian tube, contracts in the act of

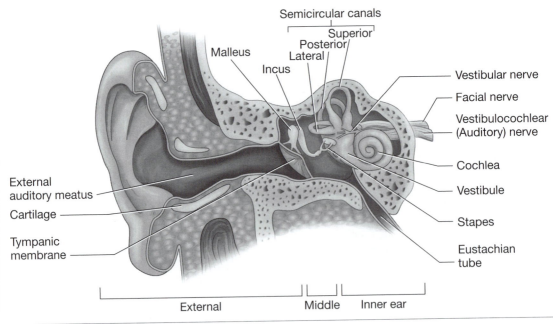

FIGURE 8–2 The external, middle, and inner ear. Note the angulation of the Eustachian tube, as is typical of an adult. The angulation of the Eustachian tube changes with growth and development. In the young child, the Eustachian tube ascends up to the middle ear at a 10-degree angle. In the adult, this angle changes to 45 degrees. The orientation of the musculature around the Eustachian tube also changes over time, improving the ability to ventilate the middle ear with age.

swallowing and yawning. As the Eustachian tube opens, it provides ventilation for the middle ear and mastoid cavities, which is important for normal function. Eustachian tube opening also results in equalization of middle ear pressure with the pressure of the environment. Finally, it allows fluids to drain out of the middle ear space.

When the Eustachian tube fails to function normally, fluids collect within the middle ear space due to the negative pressure, resulting in *middle ear effusion*. If the Eustachian tube begins to function, the fluids will be absorbed by the lymphatics in the middle ear mucosa, and the normal condition will be restored. If the Eustachian tube continues to malfunction, however, the middle ear effusion will persist. Bacteria can ascend the Eustachian tube and grow in this effusion, leading to an ear infection called *acute otitis media* (Figure 8–3).

Acute otitis media is a common disease process in children. In fact, all young children, even those without ear anomalies, are at risk for middle ear disease, and half of children under the age of 3 will have at least one episode of acute otitis media. This is because in children under around the age of 6, the Eustachian tubes lie in a horizontal plane between the nasopharynx and the middle ear. This horizontal plane impairs middle ear drainage and allows for reflux of secretions from the pharynx into the tube. In addition, the Eustachian tubes are oriented in such a way that the tensor veli palatini muscles, which open the tubes, are directed at an unfavorable angle for this function. Both of these anatomic relationships predispose children to a tendency for ear infections. As growth and development occur, the skull base flexes upon itself, moving the origin of the Eustachian tube musculature into a more favorable orientation for the opening of the tube. The palate also drops over time in relation to the ear, resulting in a 45° angulation of the Eustachian tube up to the middle ear. This angulation prevents some of the reflux of nasopharyngeal secretions into the Eustachian tube and thereby minimizes the incidence of infections (Figure 8–2).

In addition to the normal risk for middle ear disease in the early years, children with cleft palate or other craniofacial anomalies are at increased risk for recurrent otitis media or persistent middle ear effusions (Alper et al., 2011; Alper et al., 2012; da Silva, Collares, & da Costa, 2010; Sapci, Mercangoz, Evcimik, Karavus, & Gozke, 2008; Sheahan et al., 2004). A cleft palate or any abnormality that affects the soft palate, and therefore the tensor veli palatini muscle, may have an adverse effect on Eustachian tube function, and thus the middle ear. Patients with a cleft palate also have abnormally shaped Eustachian tube cartilages with abnormal attachment to the tensor veli palatini muscle, thus adding to the risk for chronic middle ear disease (da Silva, Collares, & da Costa, 2010; Durr & Shapiro, 1989; Heller, Gens, Croft, & Moe, 1978; Paradise, 1976; Paradise et al., 1974; Paradise & Bluestone, 1974; Trujillo, 1994).

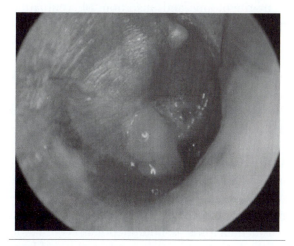

FIGURE 8–3 Acute otitis media treated with a myringotomy. The infected middle ear fluid can be seen exuding from the hole created in the eardrum.

Courtesy J. Paul Willging, M.D./Cincinnati Children's Hospital Medical Center & University of Cincinnati College of Medicine

Acute otitis media usually causes a high fever and severe ear pain. As a result, the affected child is often inconsolable. Occasionally, the tympanic membrane ruptures due to both the increased pressure produced by the inflammatory process in the middle ear and the toxic effect of the bacterial infection.

In addition to causing discomfort and pain, otitis media causes a conductive hearing loss because of the diminished mobility of the tympanic membrane in vibrating against the ossicles in the middle ear. The extent of the conductive hearing loss is variable, ranging from 5 to 55 decibels, according to the physical nature of the effusion.

One serious potential complication of otitis media is *mastoiditis*, which is an infection of the mastoid process of the temporal bone. This infection is essentially a closed-space abscess that can cause erosion of the bone, leading to potentially life-threatening complications. The infection often extends laterally behind the ear, causing the ear to protrude from the side of the head. It can also erode medially, causing meningitis or brain abscess.

Sensorineural hearing loss is another potential serious complication of repeated ear infections. The toxins produced by the bacteria may enter the cochlea through the delicate membranes in the middle ear. With repeated exposure to these toxins, the hair cells of the cochlea may be damaged, leading to a permanent hearing loss.

Acute otitis media is treated with oral antibiotics that sterilize the middle ear effusion and result in rapid resolution of the child's ear symptoms. Antibiotics treat the infection, but do not make the fluid dissipate. The middle ear fluid persists in children after the infection has been resolved for about 1 month in 40% of patients, up to 2 months in 20% of patients, and about 3 months in 5% of patients (Liu, Sun, & Zhao, 2001; Teele, Klein, & Rosner, 1980).

Although the fluid is in the middle ear space, a mild conductive hearing loss is present. Once the Eustachian tube begins to function normally, allowing a return to normal middle ear pressure and normal aeration function, the fluid in the middle ear is absorbed. In the meantime, antibiotics may help prevent additional infections from developing, but have no effect in speeding the resolution of the effusion.

The treatment for recurrent acute otitis media often includes multiple courses of antibiotics. However, the potential for the development of antibiotic-resistant bacteria increases with the number of antibiotics prescribed and the total duration of antibiotic treatment. Chronic antibiotic use in the treatment of *noninfected* middle ear effusion has been one of the major factors in the development of antibiotic-resistant bacteria.

Surgical intervention is recommended if the child has had six or more episodes of otitis or a middle ear effusion that persists for 3 months or longer and is associated with a conductive hearing loss. Recurrent acute otitis media and persistent middle ear effusions are treated with a myringotomy and insertion of ventilation tubes (American Academy of Family Physicians, American Academy of Otolaryngology Head and Neck Surgery, & American Academy of Pediatrics Subcommittee on Otitis Media with Effusion, 2004; Rosenfeld et al., 2004). A *myringotomy* is a small, surgical incision that is made in the tympanic membrane to allow for drainage of middle ear fluid. *Ventilation tubes*, also called *pressure-equalizing (PE) tubes* (Figure 8–4), are surgically inserted in the eardrum to provide an alternate route for air to enter the middle ear when the Eustachian tube is nonfunctional. Ventilation tubes do not correct the underlying problems related to recurrent otitis media. Instead, they bypass the Eustachian tube function until growth and development have progressed to

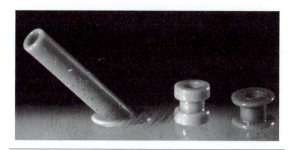

FIGURE 8–4   Examples of types of pressure-equalizing (PE) tubes.

Courtesy J. Paul Willging, M.D./Cincinnati Children's Hospital Medical Center & University of Cincinnati College of Medicine

the point where normal Eustachian tube function can be achieved. If normal pressures can be established in the middle ear, the effusion will resolve and not recur. In addition, the irritative effect of the effusion on the mucosa reverses leading to a normal middle ear system. The conductive hearing loss due to the effusion also disappears returning hearing to normal.

Ventilation tubes typically remain in the eardrum for a length of time determined by their size. The longer the flanges of the tube, the longer their retention will be. The tubes generally extrude within 1 to 2 years. As the tube is expelled, the tympanic membrane heals. Ventilation tubes are generally required only once in the majority (80%) of patients requiring their placement. If recurring ear infections are again encountered after the ventilation tubes have extruded, another set of tubes can be inserted.

An adenoidectomy is often considered in conjunction with the second set of tubes. The Eustachian tubes open on either side of the nasopharynx, with the adenoid lying between these openings. If the adenoid is enlarged, or is frequently infected, mucosal edema or the adenoid tissue itself may obstruct the Eustachian tube openings, contributing to continued middle ear pathology (Nguyen, Manoukian, Yoskovitch, & Al-Sebeih, 2004). Therefore, an adenoidectomy can be beneficial in establishing improved

Eustachian tube function (Gates, Avery, Prihoda, & Cooper, 1987; Grimmer, & Poe, 2005).

A particularly aggressive approach to the management of recurrent ear infections is required for patients with cleft palate and other craniofacial anomalies, given their increased risk. This includes early insertion of ventilation tubes. In fact, those children who have a cleft lip and palate often have ventilation tubes inserted prophylactically at the time of the lip repair. Children with craniofacial anomalies should have their hearing tested by 6 months of age and should have repeat testing performed as necessary. Following palatoplasty, Eustachian tube function usually improves, and the incidence of ear infections decreases. The incidence rates of recurrent otitis media among children with a history of a cleft palate never reach that of a child born with a normal palate, but approach it over time.

Inner Ear

Structural malformations of the inner ear arise from abnormal development of the otic capsule within the temporal bone. Abnormalities of the inner ear are uncommon but may be associated with craniofacial anomalies, especially with certain syndromes (Stickler, Treacher Collins, hemifacial microsomia, etc.). Inner ear abnormalities typically cause a *sensorineural hearing loss*, which is a problem with the creation of nerve impulses within the inner ear or the transmission of the nerve impulse through the brainstem to the auditory cortex. A hearing aid for one or both ears is often effective. Cochlear implants are offered as a means to treat sensorineural hearing loss in patients who derive no benefit from conventional hearing aids (Moores, 2005).

Audiologic Care

Because children born with clefts or other craniofacial anomalies often have congenital abnormalities of the auditory structures, they are at increased risk for ear disease and hearing loss. Hearing loss may occur intermittently or become permanent. It can range from mild to severe. Hearing loss can significantly affect speech and language development, education, social interactions, and even vocational opportunities. Therefore, children with craniofacial anomalies should be followed by an audiologist and otolaryngologist for periodic evaluations and treatment as necessary.

The American Cleft Palate–Craniofacial Association has specific recommendations for audiologic management of children born with a cleft lip/palate or other craniofacial anomalies (ACPA, 2009). They are as follows:

- Each child should have an appropriate assessment of hearing sensitivity for each ear within the first 3 months of age.

- The timing of audiological follow-up examinations should be determined on the basis of the child's history of ear disease or hearing loss. Audiological follow-up examinations should continue through adolescence.

- Acoustic-immittance (tympanometric) measures should be obtained as a part of each audiological evaluation to monitor middle ear status.

- All children undergoing myringotomies and placement of ventilating tubes should be seen pre- and postoperatively for audiologic assessment.

- When a persistent hearing loss is identified, amplification (hearing aids, auditory training systems) should be considered.

- When hearing loss occurs in the presence of microtia or atresia, whether unilateral or bilateral, bone conduction amplification should be considered, depending upon degree of loss; an implantable bone conduction aid may be a treatment option.

- Once amplification has been provided, a regular follow-up schedule is needed to monitor hearing thresholds and the function of the amplification system.

- For any child with a documented hearing loss, referral should be made to the child's school district for appropriate educational services as soon as the hearing loss is identified.

- In the absence of a positive history of otologic disease or hearing loss, audiologic examination or screening should still be carried out at least yearly through the age of 6 years to assure adequate monitoring of hearing.

SPEECH NOTES

It is unlikely that mild hearing loss will cause speech and language difficulties, but it is likely that diminished hearing can aggravate an underlying tendency for the development of articulation errors and can disrupt speech and language acquisition (Baudonck, Van Lierde, Dhooge, & Corthals, 2011; Coez et al., 2010; Ertmer, 2011; Fitzpatrick, Crawford, Ni, & Durieux-Smith, 2011; Moeller, McCleary et al., 2010). Auditory stimulation is particularly important during the first year of life. During this time, the neurons in the auditory brainstem are maturing, and the neural connections are being formed (Sininger, Doyle, & Moore, 1999). If sensory input to the auditory nervous system is interrupted during early development, this can have a detrimental effect on speech and language learning (Rvachew, Slawinski, Williams, & Green, 1999). Hearing must always be evaluated in the presence of speech and language difficulties to ensure normal auditory function before initiation of therapeutic intervention for speech and language disorders.

FACIAL STRUCTURES

Every year, thousands of children are born with cleft lip (and/or cleft palate) or other anomalies of the facial structures. Facial anomalies affect overall aesthetics and can result in a certain amount of stigma for the individual. In addition, many facial anomalies can impair vital functions of daily life (e.g., speech, hearing, vision, feeding, etc.). The following section describes some of the more common facial anomalies and their potential effect on function.

Nose

Anomalies of the nose include severe external deformities (facial clefting), abnormalities of the nasal base (cleft of the primary palate), and internal derangement (deviated nasal septum). Many nasal anomalies can affect breathing and resonance.

A deviated nasal septum may occur as a result of a cleft palate where there is inadequate structural support for the cartilaginous septum to remain in the midline. This is particularly common with unilateral cleft lip and palate. The septum generally deflects into the cleft side of the nose due to a lack of support from the floor of the nose on that side. A deviated septum may also occur as a result of birth trauma, when the nose of the neonate is forced against the pelvis during delivery, causing the septum to slip off the maxillary crest.

Some children experience chronic sinus problems. When this occurs, evaluation of the sinuses is typically done through a computed tomography (CT) scan, as can be seen in Figure 8–5. Unlike acute sinusitis, which may resolve with medication, chronic sinusitis often requires surgery.

There are several anomalies that affect the anterior or posterior openings of the nasal cavity. The anterior opening of the nasal cavity occurs through the paired nares. These openings can be narrowed by overgrowth of the maxilla, an anomaly known as *pyriform aperture stenosis* (Brown, Myer, & Manning, 1989; Visvanathan & Wynne, 2012). There can also be stenosis of one naris or both nares secondary to a cleft lip repair. The nasal cavity opens posteriorly through the choanae, which communicate with the nasopharynx. The choanae may be narrowed in a condition known as *choanal stenosis*, or completely blocked, as in *choanal atresia*. These abnormalities can be either unilateral or bilateral. The choanae can also be blocked by enlarged adenoids.

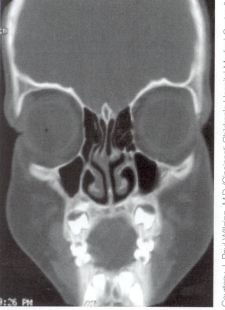

Courtesy J. Paul Willging, M.D./Cincinnati Children's Hospital Medical Center & University of Cincinnati College of Medicine

FIGURE 8–5 Computed tomography scan of the nose and paranasal sinuses. This scan shows the nasal cavities separated by the nasal septum. The turbinates are the small bones arising from the lateral aspect of the nasal cavity. The sinuses are air-filled spaces that are found in the cheeks and between the eyes.

Neonates are obligate nasal breathers. When neonates with bilateral choanal atresia attempt nasal respiration and it is unsuccessful, they become fussy and eventually begin to cry. The infants breathe well while crying, but as they settle down, they again attempt nasal respiration unsuccessfully, only to repeat the process. Without early surgical intervention, this cyclical *cyanosis* (bluish skin color due to a lack of oxygen) can lead to death from exhaustion. Choanal atresia occurs more commonly in females and has an incidence of 1:8000 births (Kubba, Bennett, & Bailey, 2004). It is associated with other congenital abnormalities in 50% of patients.

Maxilla

Maxillary retrusion (also known as *midface deficiency*) is characterized by a small upper jaw (maxilla) relative to the lower jaw (mandible). This is a common anomaly in individuals with repaired cleft lip and palate. It is felt to be due to an inherent deficiency in the maxilla from the cleft and also due to the possible restriction in maxillary growth with the surgical repair (Kawakami, Yagi, & Takada, 2002). With maxillary retrusion, there is usually at least an anterior crossbite and often a *Class III malocclusion*, where the maxilla is retrusive relative to the mandible (see Chapter 9).

Maxillary retrusion can affect the size of the nasal cavity (because the maxilla forms the floor of the nose) and the depth of the pharynx. This can have a negative effect on the pharyngeal and nasal airway.

Facial Nerve

Facial paralysis may occur as a result of an injury (surgical or traumatic), infection (as in *Bell's palsy*), or may be due to congenital abnormalities of the nerve or associated muscles (Chen & Wong, 2005; Peitersen, 1992; Shen, Zhang, Zhao, & Shen, 2009; Terzis & Anesti, 2011; Yetter, Ogren, Moore, & Yonkers, 1990). The paralysis may be partial, as in hemifacial microsomia, or may be complete and bilateral, as in Moebius syndrome. Bilateral facial paralysis may result in a mask-like facies.

THE ORAL CAVITY

The oral cavity extends from the lips anteriorly to the faucial pillars posteriorly. Anomalies of the oral cavity are common and can have a significant effect on speech. Dental anomalies are discussed in Chapter 9 and are therefore not covered in this chapter.

Lips

The lips function in eating, speech, and prevention of *sialorrhea* (drooling). A common problem following a cleft lip repair is a short upper lip. The lip may be deficient in tissue due to the basic dysmorphology from the cleft lip, and it may also be shortened secondary to the contractile effects of the scar from the cleft lip repair. If the premaxilla is protrusive, the relative shortening of the lip is further increased.

SPEECH NOTES

Facial paralysis causes a lack of facial expression and lip movement, which affects feeding and speech (Goldberg, DeLorie, Zuker, & Manktelow, 2003; Meyerson & Foushee, 1978). Facial paralysis also affects the ability to produce bilabial and even labiodental phonemes. Tongue movement is usually unaffected. The individual may learn to compensate by producing bilabial sounds with the tongue tip. Some individuals become very adept at producing the sound in a way that is acoustically similar to the labial sound.

SPEECH NOTES

When the upper lip is short and/or the premaxilla is protrusive, there may be *bilabial incompetence*, which is the inability to close the lips naturally at rest. If lip closure is difficult to accomplish at rest, it makes sense that there will also be difficulties with the production of bilabial sounds (/p/, /b/, /m/) with speech. As a result, the individual may compensate by producing these sounds with labiodental placement. This usually results in little auditory distortion, but can be visually distracting to the listener.

There are several additional anomalies of the upper lip that can occur following a cleft lip repair, including vermilion tissue above the white roll, asymmetry of the lip, and a flattening of Cupid's bow. If the orbicularis oris muscle around the lips is not approximated during the lip repair, the discontinuity of these muscle bundles may be apparent over time. These particular lip anomalies are cosmetic and do not affect speech or function.

Mouth

Congenital abnormalities of the size and shape of the mouth can occur, especially with some syndromes. The suffix *"stomia"* is used for the word "mouth." This is not to be confused with the suffix *"somia"* which refers to body.

Macrostomia refers to an excessively large mouth opening. This is particularly common with hemifacial microsomia, where one corner of the mouth can extend into the cheek, making the mouth opening on that particular side large and distorted in appearance. On the other hand, *microstomia* refers to a small mouth opening. Microstomia more often results from acquired injuries, such as electrical burns sustained after a child chews on an electrical cord. Severe contractures of the mouth are possible secondary to scarring.

Tongue

Lingual (tongue) anomalies are associated with certain syndromes. *Macroglossia* is a condition in which the tongue is abnormally large, and it is one of the main characteristics of Beckwith-Wiedemann syndrome (Figure 8–6). Because the tongue is too large to fit in the oral cavity, it protrudes past the alveolar ridge, causing an open-mouth posture. The chronic open-mouth posture can also contribute to excessive drooling. As the dentition develops, an anterior open bite may occur because the tongue is in the area where the teeth are erupting. The biggest concern, however, at least initially, is the effect that it can have on the airway.

SPEECH NOTES

Macrostomia does not usually cause speech problems. On the other hand, if the microstomia is severe enough to affect mouth opening, it can affect articulation and cause oral cul-de-sac resonance (see Chapter 7 for more information).

SPEECH NOTES

Macroglossia can affect the production of lingual-alveolar phonemes and can cause either a frontal or a lateral distortion of sibilants (Topouzelis, Iliopoulos, & Kolokitha, 2011; Van Borsel, Van Snick, & Leroy, 1999). It can also contribute to the use of palatal-dorsal articulation, especially if the tongue tip rests anterior to the alveolar ridge. Macroglossia also affects resonance. Because the tongue fills most of the oral cavity, there is little space for normal resonance of the sound. This results in an oral cul-de-sac resonance.

In contrast to macroglossia, *microglossia* is a relatively small tongue for the oral cavity space. It usually has no detrimental effect on speech.

A lobulated tongue may or may not affect lingual mobility. However, if mobility is affected, speech will be affected as well.

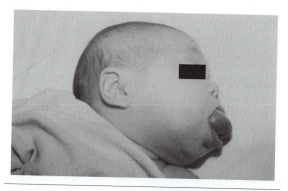

FIGURE 8–6 Macroglossia secondary to Beckwith-Wiedemann syndrome. Beckwith-Wiedemann syndrome is a congenital disorder characterized by macroglossia, omphalocele, hypoglycemia, and abnormalities of the kidneys, pancreas, and adrenal cortex. This photo demonstrates macroglossia with severe discrepancy between the size of the oral cavity and the size of the tongue.

Courtesy J. Paul Willging, M.D./Cincinnati Children's Hospital Medical Center & University of Cincinnati College of Medicine

Other lingual anomalies include a *lobulated tongue*, which is common in orofaciodigital (OFD) syndrome (refer to Figure 13–20 in Chapter 13). The tongue may appear to have multiple lobes, with fissures between each lobe.

Finally, a discussion of lingual anomalies would not be complete without a discussion of ankyloglossia. *Ankyloglossia*, commonly referred to as *"tongue-tie,"* is a congenital condition that causes restriction of tongue tip movement. This can occur because either the lingual frenulum is congenitally short and/or it is attached close to the tip of the tongue rather than a third of the way back, as is normally seen (Figure 8–7). True ankyloglossia is defined as a condition where the frenulum restricts tongue movement to the extent that the person cannot elevate the tongue tip sufficiently to touch the roof of the mouth, with the mouth open, and cannot protrude the tongue tip past the mandibular gingival ridge or incisors. With protrusion, the tongue tip has a midline indentation in the tip, which appears as a heart-shaped notch. *Ankylosis* (immobility due to restriction) of the tongue can also occur after radical oral surgery, causing the same limitations in tongue tip movement.

The lingual frenulum is frequently short in newborns, but it tends to correct itself as the child grows (Garcia Pola, Gonzalez Garcia, Garcia Martin, Gallas, & Seoane Leston,

SPEECH NOTES

Ankyloglossia has less effect on speech than most lay people (and even some professionals) assume. This is because very little tongue tip excursion is needed for normal speech production (Kummer, 2005; Moller, 1994). In English, the farthest that the tongue needs to protrude is against the back of the maxillary incisors for a /θ/ and /ð/ sounds. The most it needs to elevate is to the alveolar ridge (without the mouth widely open) for the /l/ sound. The lingual trill, as in a Spanish /r/, may be affected by ankyloglossia in some cases however. Because ankyloglossia rarely causes problems with speech, frenulectomy is usually not indicated for speech, except perhaps if there is oral-motor dysfunction. However, it may be indicated for the reasons noted above, particularly for feeding problems.

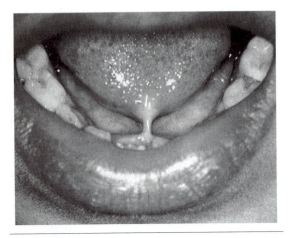

FIGURE 8–7 Ankyloglossia. Ankyloglossia is a condition describing the attachment of the lingual frenulum to the anterior tongue tip. It may impede normal tongue mobility but rarely requires intervention for speech purposes.

Courtesy J. Paul Willging, M.D./Cincinnati Children's Hospital Medical Center & University of Cincinnati College of Medicine

2002). However, it can affect the newborn infant's ability to latch on to the nipple and therefore affect the infant's ability to feed. Later in life, ankyloglossia can affect the person's ability to move a bolus in the mouth, particularly if the bolus is in the *buccal sulcus* (area between the teeth and the cheeks [Kern, 1991]). Infrequently, the short lingual frenulum can pull the gingiva away from bottom teeth between the mandibular incisors. Ankyloglossia can affect aesthetics, making some

affected individuals self-conscious. It can even affect "French kissing."

Palate

Palatal arch anomalies are common, particularly in individuals with a history of cleft palate or other craniofacial syndromes. There may be abnormalities in the height, width, and configuration of the palatal arch. The palatal vault may be low and flat due to collapsed lateral palatal segments, or it may be very high and narrow, causing crowding of the teeth and tongue. A narrow, high-arched palate is often seen in children who have had an endotracheal tube at birth.

A *fistula* (pl. *fistulae* or *fistulas*) is an abnormal opening or passageway between two epithelialized organs that do not normally connect. A palatal fistula (also called an *oronasal fistula*), is an opening that leads from the oral surface of the palate and/or velum to the nasal cavity. Fistulas occur as an unintentional postoperative breakdown of the cleft repair due to inadequate healing. In addition, maxillary advancement, and sometimes growth, can cause a small, asymptomatic fistula to open further and become symptomatic.

Although fistulas can occur anywhere along the palatal suture lines, a common site for a fistula is at the junction of the hard and soft palate. If there was a bilateral complete cleft of the lip and

SPEECH NOTES

Whenever the palatal arch is low, flat, or narrow, it restricts the oral cavity space, which may cause the tongue to protrude. As the tongue protrudes, the tongue tip is in an abnormal position for tongue-tip articulation so that distortion of speech is inevitable. This can cause a fronting of anterior lingual sounds. On the other hand, the individual may try to compensate by retracting the tongue and using a palatal-dorsal placement. This typically results in a lateral distortion of sibilants and even lingual-alveolar phonemes.

SPEECH NOTES

A nasolabial fistula does not affect speech because it is located under the lip and out of the way of the airflow and speech sound articulation.

The effect of an oronasal fistula on speech depends on both its size and its location. A small palatal fistula is usually not symptomatic, because during production of most speech phonemes the course of the airflow is horizontal to the fistula opening. If the fistula is in the area of the incisive foramen, however, nasal emission on lingual-alveolar sounds may be noted because as the tongue tip elevates for the sound production, it may push the airstream into the fistula. A medium-sized fistula can cause consistent nasal air emission on all sounds, particularly anterior sounds. There may also be compensatory productions to either close the fistula with the tongue or produce the sound behind the fistula before the air leak. A very large fistula causes hypernasality, in addition to nasal emission.

Research has shown that an anterior leak of air through an open fistula can affect the function of the velopharyngeal valve as well (Isberg & Henningsson, 1987; Tachimura, Hara, Koh, & Wada, 1997). Therefore, evaluation of velopharyngeal function must be done with this in mind.

If the fistula is causing both nasal emission and hypernasality, it is best to close it as soon as possible for the sake of speech development. However, the surgical results are better if it is closed with the bone graft, which is timed with the eruption of teeth. Therefore, a large symptomatic fistula may be left open for several years. If this is the case, an obturator can be used for speech purposes until the fistula can be surgically repaired.

---

palate, fistulas are also commonly seen at the junction of the premaxilla and lateral segments.

A *nasolabial fistula* is an opening in the alveolus (high in the gum ridge just under the upper lip). It is sometimes called an *intentional fistula*. This is because it is often left deliberately by the surgeon during the initial repair in order to allow for unrestricted maxillary growth for a period of time (Folk, D'Antonio, & Hardesty, 1997). The nasolabial fistula is later closed by an alveolar bone graft when the permanent teeth begin to erupt.

Depending on its location and size, a fistula may be asymptomatic for speech, yet may cause regurgitation of fluids (and sometimes food) into the nasal cavity. In particular, it is common for a nasolabial fistula to cause slight regurgitation of food (particularly chocolate and red sauce) in the corresponding nostril. A large palatal fistula can even cause food to become stuck in the opening and even in the nasal cavity.

TONSILS AND ADENOIDS

The *tonsils* are a collection of lymphoid tissue, known as *Waldeyer's ring*, which surrounds the opening to the oropharynx. The *faucial tonsils* (which are commonly known just as "tonsils") are located on each side of the mouth between the anterior and posterior faucial pillars. The *lingual tonsils* are located at the base of the tongue. The *pharyngeal tonsil*, also known as the *adenoid*, is located in the nasopharynx. Due to its location in the pharynx, the adenoid pad can actually assist with velopharyngeal closure. In fact, young children with a prominent adenoid pad usually have veloadenoidal closure, rather than velopharyngeal closure (Maryn, Van Lierde, De Bodt, & Van Cauwenberge, 2004) (Figure 8–8).

Tonsillar tissue is most important during the child's first 2 years of life. This is because it

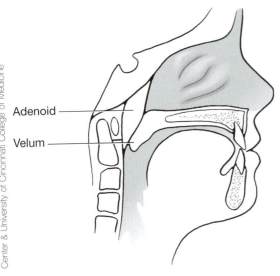

Adenoid

Velum

FIGURE 8–8   The adenoid pad assists in velopharyngeal closure in children. The sudden removal of adenoid tissue during adenoidectomy requires compensation of soft palate motion to maintain proper velopharyngeal closure. If any abnormality exists in the architecture or neurological function of the palate, this compensation may not be successful, which leads to nasal air escape.

serves as part of the body's immune system by developing antibodies against infections (Brodsky, Moore, Stanievich, & Ogra, 1988). As foreign materials enter the body through the nose and mouth, they pass over this specialized tissue. Antigens adhere to the lining of this tissue where this foreign protein is incorporated into the substance of the tonsil to be presented to the mucosal immune system.

Over time, the tonsil and adenoid tissue tends to atrophy, particularly with puberty, so that by around the age of 16 only small remnants of this tissue remain. Fortunately, atrophy (and even surgical removal) of tonsil and/or adenoid tissue has little effect on immunity. This is because there is redundancy in the immune system. In fact, the entire gastrointestinal tract is lined with the same type of tissue as found in the tonsils and adenoid, and as such it serves a similar function.

Tonsil and adenoid tissue is particularly prone to *hypertrophy* (abnormal enlargement of a part of the body caused by enlargement of its constituent cells) in young children. The etiology for the overgrowth of this tissue is unknown but is thought to be secondary to chronic stimulation from infection or allergic sources. Adenoid and/or tonsillar hypertrophy often causes upper airway obstruction and abnormal resonance.

Tonsillar Hypertrophy

Tonsillar hypertrophy (excessive enlargement of the faucial tonsils) is typically graded on a 4-point scale. Tonsils that are 1+ in size are contained within the faucial pillars; tonsils that are 2+ extend minimally beyond the faucial pillars; tonsils that are 3+ obstruct the oropharyngeal inlet to a moderate degree; and finally, tonsils that are 4+ in size touch in the midline (Figure 8–9A). Occasionally, one tonsil will be significantly larger than the other (Figure 8–9B). This abnormal growth pattern can be a cause of concern and should be further investigated.

Tonsils that are excessively large (grade 3+ or larger) may expand anteriorly, medially, or posteriorly. If they expand posteriorly, they may intrude into the oropharynx. In severe cases, they may even expand upward into the nasopharynx, thus interfering with velopharyngeal function.

Adenoid Hypertrophy

Adenoid hypertrophy (excessive enlargement of the adenoid pad) can obstruct the nasopharyngeal airway and can even block the choanal opening to the back of the nasal cavity (Figure 8–10). This can cause upper airway obstruction, characterized by mouth breathing, snoring, and even sleep apnea.

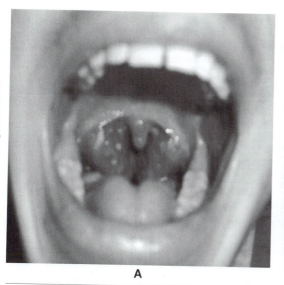

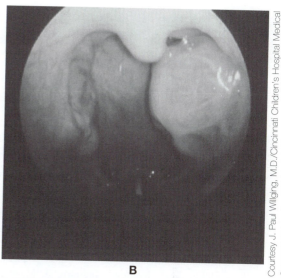

A

B

FIGURE 8–9 (A and B) (A) Large (grade 4+) tonsils bilaterally. (B) A large tonsil on the patient's left side. Asymmetric tonsils are a cause for concern, as a tumor may be causing the abnormal growth pattern. In this example, the left tonsil is a grade 4, whereas the right tonsil is a grade 1.

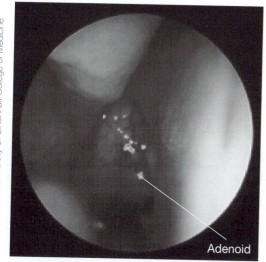

Adenoid

FIGURE 8–10 Adenoid tissue blocking the choana. The adenoid is a collection of lymphoid tissue in the nasopharynx. It has the capacity to enlarge and block nasal respiration. At times, the adenoid tissue can grow into the posterior aspect of the nose, completely blocking the posterior choanae.

Lingual Tonsil Hypertrophy

Lingual tonsil hypertrophy (abnormal enlargement of the lingual tonsil at the base of the tongue) occurs infrequently but can be a particular problem for children with Down syndrome (Al-Shamaa et al., 2003; Donnelly, Shott, LaRose, Chini, & Amin, 2004) (Figure 8–11).

Adenotonsillar hypertrophy is the enlargement of both the tonsil and adenoid tissue. Adenotonsillar hypertrophy may be relative in that it can occur with normal-sized tonsils and adenoid tissue, but with relatively small adjacent structures. For example, patients with midface hypoplasia, as in Crouzon, Apert, and Down syndromes, may have an adenoid pad situated in a relatively small nasopharynx, creating the obstructive symptoms. A similar problem may occur in patients with retrognathia (as is common in Pierre Robin sequence), where normal tonsil and adenoid tissue, combined with a narrow oropharyngeal inlet and glossoptosis, can create upper airway obstruction.

SPEECH NOTES

Enlarged tonsils can affect speech and resonance in several ways.

- If the tonsils expand toward midline resulting in "kissing tonsils," they will block the entrance to the oral cavity, causing pharyngeal cul-de-sac resonance.

- If one tonsil (or both of the tonsils) pushes against the posterior faucial pillar, this can limit the function of the palatopharyngeus muscle and therefore affect lateral pharyngeal wall movement. This typically causes a small velopharyngeal opening so nasal emission is the result.

- If the tonsils expand posteriorly so that they are in the pharynx, this can affect the transmission of sound into the nasal cavity, resulting in hyponasality.

- Occasionally, a tonsil extends into the pharynx and then upward so that it is between the velum and posterior pharyngeal wall during velopharyngeal closure. This usually results in an incomplete velopharyngeal seal with small gaps on either side of the interfering tonsil. As noted previously, a small gap typically causes nasal emission/rustle (see Figure 7-15A and Figure 7-15B in Chapter 7) (Finkelstein, Nachmani, & Ophir, 1994; Kummer, Billmire, & Myer, 1993; MacKenzie-Stepner, Witzel, Stringer, & Laskin, 1987; Shprintzen, Sher, & Croft, 1987).

- If the tonsils expand anteriorly, articulation of posterior sounds (e.g., /k/ and /g/) can be affected. As a result, the individual may compensate by fronting.

- If there is airway obstruction with tonsillar hypertrophy, regardless of the direction of expansion, the tongue is often displaced down and forward in order to open the airway. This can cause fronting of sibilants and even fronting of lingual-alveolar sounds.

Overall, hypertrophic tonsils can cause a mixture of hyponasality, pharyngeal cul-de-sac resonance, nasal emission, and abnormal articulation—sometimes in the same patient (Al-Shamaa, Jefferson, & Ball, 2003; Feilberg, Sorensen, & Eriksen, 1993; Oulis, Vadiakas, Ekonomides, & Dratsa, 1994; Singh, Gathwala, Pathania, Singh, & Yadav, 1994) (see Chapter 7 for more information). In addition, they can cause difficulty with swallowing due to the blockage at the back of the oral cavity. The treatment for these speech, resonance, and swallowing characteristic is tonsillectomy.

SPEECH NOTES

Enlarged adenoids can also affect speech in several ways.

- Adenoid hypertrophy can interfere with sound transmission into the nasal cavity during speech, causing hyponasality.

- If the adenoid pad is irregular in configuration, this can affect the firmness of the veloadenoidal seal during speech. This typically causes nasal emission or rustle (see Chapter 7 for more information).

- Large adenoids can obstruct the opening to the Eustachian tube, thus disrupting middle ear function and potentially causing conductive hearing loss.

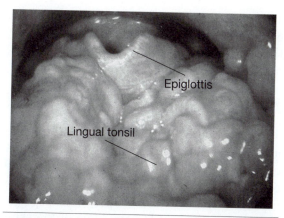

FIGURE 8–11 Lingual tonsils. Lingual tonsils are located in the base of the tongue. They can enlarge to the point that the airway is partially obstructed, leading to breathing difficulties. The larynx cannot be seen in this photograph due to the enlargement of the lingual tonsils. The valleculla is completely filled with lingual tonsil tissue.

Courtesy J. Paul Willging, M.D./Cincinnati Children's Hospital Medical Center & University of Cincinnati College of Medicine

UPPER AIRWAY OBSTRUCTION: EFFECTS AND TREATMENT

As noted above, upper airway obstruction in children is commonly caused by tonsillar and/or adenoid hypertrophy. Evidence of airway obstruction is often visible on the child's face. The typical *adenoid* facies (which can be seen with tonsillar hypertrophy as well) is charac-terized by an open-mouth posture, anterior tongue position, the forward and downward position of the mandible, facial elongation, *suborbital coloring* ("black eyes"), puffy eyes, and the appearance of pinched nostrils. Symptoms of airway obstruction due to ade-noid and/or tonsillar hypertrophy may also include *stertorous* (a heavy snoring sound) breathing, chronic mouth breathing, loud snoring, and even obstructive sleep apnea.

Obstructive sleep apnea (OSA) is a disorder that is characterized by long pauses in breath-ing during sleep due to upper airway obstruc-tion. An obstructive sleep apnea event is a period when the person is exerting muscular forces to inspire but is unsuccessful in moving air into the lungs due to a blockage in the upper airway. The obstructed airway is further compromised during deep sleep by general-ized hypotonia that causes collapse of the hypopharyngeal structures. In a supine posi-tion, the tongue base retrodisplaces, causing further compromise of the airway. Common characteristics of sleep apnea include rest-lessness during sleep and constant tossing and turning to find a position where breathing requires less effort. When observed in chil-dren, this is significant and requires attention. *Polysomnography* (an overnight sleep study) is used to diagnosis sleep disturbances in order to determine appropriate treatment.

SPEECH NOTES

The lingual tonsils are rarely large enough to require removal. However, when lingual hypertrophy occurs, it can affect both resonance and the upper airway.

- The lingual tonsil may block the sound energy from entering the oral cavity, causing a pharyngeal cul-de-sac resonance.

- If the airway is affected, the tongue may be forced into an anterior position, causing fronting of anterior consonants during speech.

The diagnosis of obstructive sleep apnea is a confirmation that the individual's sleep is inadequate, causing the person to be tired during the day. This can impair concentration, memory, and daily function at school (or work). It can also cause hyperactivity and learning problems in children. Sleep apnea contributes to a long-term risk for weight issues, cardiovascular disease, heart attack, stroke, hypertension, and depression. Because of the short-term and long-term effects that sleep apnea can have on learning, the quality of life, and on long-term health, it should be considered in all children with craniofacial anomalies, and actively treated whenever it is diagnosed (Carter & Watenpaugh, 2008; Jayaraman, Sharafkhaneh, Hirshkowitz, & Sharafkhaneh, 2008).

Tonsillectomy

Tonsillectomy is indicated for hypertrophic tonsils that are causing upper airway obstruction or affecting speech and resonance. Tonsillectomy is also indicated for recurrent tonsillitis or peritonsillar abscess. Because the tonsils reside in the oral cavity, they do not contribute to velopharyngeal function. Therefore, tonsillectomy is *not* contraindicated for patients with cleft palate, submucous cleft, or velopharyngeal insufficiency (D'Antonio, Snyder, & Samadani,

1996; Paulson, Macarthur, Beaulieu, Brockman, & Milczuk, 2012). When a tonsillectomy is done, the tonsils are removed in their entirety, including the capsule deep under the tonsil.

Adenoidectomy

The indications for adenoidectomy include airway obstruction, hyponasality, and in some cases intractable middle ear effusion (Darrow & Siemens, 2002). With adenoidectomy, the capsule deep to the adenoid pad is left in place, as it protects the underlying bone of the skull base. Because the capsule is left in place, some regrowth of the adenoid can occur over time. Adenoid regrowth often results in a very irregular surface (Figure 8–11).

Tracheostomy

A *tracheostomy* is a surgical procedure that is done to relieve conditions that cause life-threatening airway obstruction. The tracheostomy procedure is done by making a vertical incision in the midline of the neck overlying the trachea. The trachea is then incised vertically, usually through the third and fourth rings, creating an opening in the anterior wall of the trachea. A tracheostomy tube is then inserted into the tracheal opening, and the

SPEECH NOTES

Despite the change in the oral anatomy with a tonsillectomy, this results in either no effect on speech or a positive effect. The positive effect may be the elimination of cul-de-sac resonance by removing the blockage at the entrance to the oral cavity. Despite this, hypernasality has been reported following tonsillectomy in a few rare cases (Gibb & Stewart, 1975; Haapanen, Ignatius, Rihkanen, & Ertama, 1994; Mora et al., 2009; Subramaniam & Kumar, 2009). This can be due to either an abnormal scarring of the faucial pillars, which can restrict lateral or pharyngeal wall movement or a postoperative "protection response" secondary to the pain of the procedure. With this protection response, the patient avoids velopharyngeal movement for both swallowing and speech, and this avoidance can remain as a habit long after the pain is gone. Fortunately, this is easy to correct with only a few speech therapy sessions.

SPEECH NOTES

The irregular surface that occurs with adenoid regrowth after adenoidectomy can affect the firmness of the veloadenoidal seal during speech. This usually causes a small velopharyngeal opening and thus nasal emission. This small velopharyngeal opening may disappear with time as the adenoid pad begins to normally atrophy before puberty. In some cases, however, another partial adenoidectomy to smooth the surface may be considered.

Velopharyngeal insufficiency following adenoidectomy is a risk, although the risk is minimal for most children (Donnelly, 1994; Fernandes, Grobbelaar, Hudson, & Lentin, 1996; Parton & Jones, 1998; Pulkkinen, Ranta, Heliovaara, & Haapanen, 2002; Ren, Isberg, & Henningsson, 1995; Saunders, Hartley, Sell, & Sommerlad, 2004; Witzel, Rich, Margar-Bacal & Cox, 1986). The risk has been estimated to be between 1:1500 and 1:3000 (Stewart, Ahmed, Razzell, & Watson, 2002).

Temporary velopharyngeal insufficiency during the first few weeks following adenoidectomy is very common. With removal of the adenoid pad, the soft palate must extend farther posteriorly, or the lateral walls must extend farther medially, to achieve closure. Most patients are able to accomplish this adjustment in velopharyngeal function within a few days or weeks. If the hypernasality or nasal emission persists beyond 6 to 8 weeks, it is unlikely to resolve spontaneously. Therefore, surgical repair is required to correct the velopharyngeal insufficiency. It should be noted that speech therapy will not correct hypernasality or nasal emission following adenoidectomy because the cause is abnormal structure and not abnormal function.

There are several risk factors for velopharyngeal insufficiency following adenoidectomy. The biggest risk factor is a history of repaired cleft palate or a submucous cleft. In fact, patients who have hypernasality after adenoidectomy are frequently found to have an occult submucous cleft on further inspection (Parton & Jones, 1998; Saunders et al., 2004; Schmaman, Jordaan, & Jammine, 1998). Other risk factors include a family history of cleft palate or hypernasality, sucking difficulties as an infant, and oral-motor dysfunction or other neuromuscular problems. If the patient has upper airway obstruction due to enlarged adenoids, yet has one or more of these risk factors, a conservative superior half adenoidectomy can be performed (Finkelstein, Wexler, Nachmani, & Ophir, 2002). With this procedure, the airway obstruction is relieved while maintaining adequate tissue inferiorly for the velum to close against the pad for speech.

edges of the opening are sutured to the skin in the neck. The *stoma* is the tracheal opening through which the patient can breathe.

Tracheostomy is often indicated for certain congenital anomalies, such as subglottic stenosis, tracheal stenosis, or laryngeal web. Infants born with Pierre Robin sequence are often candidates for tracheostomy due to the airway problems that occur as a result of the small mandible (micrognathia) and glossoptosis (Figure 8–12). Tracheostomy is also indicated for patients who cannot adequately raise secretions

from their airway and therefore need frequent suctioning. This includes patients who are unconscious and those who are unable to cough due to paralysis or significant chest pain.

Uvulopalatopharyngoplasty (UPPP)

In the pediatric population, upper airway obstruction is primarily caused by adenotonsillar hypertrophy and therefore treated by *adenotonsillectomy* (removal of adenoids and

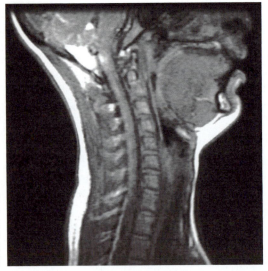

Courtesy J. Paul Wilging, M.D./Cincinnati Children's Hospital Medical Center & University of Cincinnati College of Medicine

FIGURE 8–12 Glossoptosis. The tongue base is too far back in the pharynx, causing significant airway obstruction.

tonsils). In teenagers and adults, however, the tonsils and adenoids are very small and therefore are not likely to cause obstruction. Obstructive sleep apnea in older patients is often secondary to redundant mucosa of the soft palate and posterior pharyngeal wall, causing the oropharyngeal inlet to be small. In these cases, the treatment of the obstruction is a surgical procedure called *uvulopalatopharyngoplasty* (UPPP) (Aneeza et al., 2011; Blythe, Henrich, & Pillsbury, 1995; Croft & Golding-Wood, 1990; Han, Xu, Hu, & Zhang, 2012; Kavey, Whyte, Blitzer, & Gidro-Frank, 1990; Yanagisawa & Weaver, 1997).

As part of the UPPP, the remaining tonsil tissue is removed, and the anterior and posterior tonsillar pillars are sewn together to open the oropharyngeal inlet. The free margin of the soft palate is resected along with the uvula, and the raw edges of the soft palate are sewn together, shortening the soft palate. Although snoring is usually markedly improved as a result of this procedure, the overall effect on the sleep apnea is often disappointing.

There are a few other surgical procedures that can be done for obstructive sleep apnea. These include moving the tongue base anteriorly, reducing the size of the tongue base, or bringing the mandible forward along with the tongue.

Continuous Positive Airway Pressure (CPAP)

Frequently, *continuous positive airway pressure (CPAP)* is required for long-term resolution of the obstructive apnea. The CPAP

SPEECH NOTES

If done properly, uvulopalatopharyngoplasty (UPPP) does not have a negative effect on velopharyngeal function and thus on resonance. This is because the velar tissue that is removed is below the area of normal velar contact with the posterior pharyngeal wall. However, if the surgeon is too aggressive and removes too much of the velum under its bend, this can affect the patient's resonance and also cause nasal regurgitation during swallowing (Rihkanen & Soini, 1992; Salas-Provance & Kuehn, 1990; Tewary & Cable, 1993).

CASE REPORT

Upper Airway Obstruction, Hypernasality, and CPAP

Tam was a Vietnamese male born with bilateral complete cleft lip and palate. The cleft lip was closed in Vietnam, but the palate was left unrepaired. When Tam entered the United States at the age of 21, the palate was still open, and he did not speak any English. Soon after arriving in this country, the palate was repaired, and a pharyngeal flap (to correct velopharyngeal insufficiency) was done. Although the prognosis for correcting speech is guarded when the palate is closed that late, Tam exceeded all expectations. He received several months of speech therapy following his surgery, and he quickly developed oral production of speech sounds and also learned English.

Tam was seen for an evaluation in VPI clinic several years later, at the age of 27. At that time, articulation was normal for the production of all speech sounds. Resonance was found to be mildly hypernasal, and there was barely audible nasal air emission during the production of pressure-sensitive phonemes. Overall, Tam was happy with his speech. However, he reported difficulty with nasal breathing and significant snoring at night, which was the primary reason for his return. A sleep study was done, and this confirmed sleep apnea.

A nasopharyngoscopy (endoscopy) assessment showed the cause of these symptoms. Although the pharyngeal flap was an appropriate width and in good position, the lateral ports (for breathing on either side of the flap) were small for normal nasal breathing. During speech, the right port closed completely, but the left port remained partially open. Therefore, it was determined that the narrow ports restricted nasal breathing, particularly during sleep, but the open left port caused the mild hypernasality and nasal emission with speech.

With this combination of symptoms, determining the appropriate treatment is a challenge. If the left port were narrowed further for speech, it would increase the airway problems. On the other hand, opening the ports to improve nasal breathing would increase the hypernasality. After discussing the options with Tam, he decided to forgo further surgical intervention. Instead, he began using CPAP (continuous positive airway pressure) at night, which resulted in significant improvement in his sleep. With this option, the flap could be left intact for speech, yet the airway was forced open at night for sleep.

equipment consists of a face mask and an air pressure generator. The patient wears the mask over the nose during sleep, and a certain level of continuous positive air pressure, usually in the range of 6–20 cm H_2O, is delivered to the pharynx through the nose. This forces the pharyngeal airway open and prevents pharyngeal collapse during respiration. Although CPAP is effective in overcoming the effects of obstructive sleep apnea, long-term nightly use of the machine leads to a high degree of noncompliance over time.

SUMMARY

The oropharyngeal structures are essential organs for verbal communication. Congenital anomalies of these structures can therefore interfere with the development of articulation and language and the production of normal speech and resonance. Speech-language pathologists, whether working directly with craniofacial anomalies or not, need to form a partnership with otolaryngologists to adequately diagnose these disorders and treat them appropriately.

FOR REVIEW AND DISCUSSION

1. Describe the potential malformations of the ears in patients that have craniofacial anomalies.

2. What is the purpose of Eustachian tube function? Describe normal Eustachian tube function, including the action of the muscle. What happens if the Eustachian tube does not function normally?

3. Why are young children more prone to otitis media than adults? Why are children with a history of cleft palate particularly at risk for chronic middle ear effusion and otitis media? What can be done prophylactically for children who are at particular risk?

4. Describe potential malformations of the nose. How could these malformations affect resonance? If there is abnormal resonance, is the individual a candidate for speech therapy? Why or why not?

5. Describe the purpose and location of the tonsils and adenoids.

6. What are the potential effects of tonsillar hypertrophy? What are the potential effects of adenoid hypertrophy?

7. Describe the potential risks and benefits of tonsillectomy. Describe the potential risks and benefits of adenoidectomy.

8. Why is it important to discuss the tonsils and adenoids separately? Why do you think people confuse the risk and benefits of tonsillectomy versus adenoidectomy?

9. What are treatment options for upper airway obstruction? When is tracheotomy appropriate? When is uvulopalatopharyngoplasty (UPPP) appropriate?

REFERENCES

Alasti, F., & Van Camp, G. (2009). Genetics of microtia and associated syndromes. *Journal of Medical Genetics*, *46*(6), 361–369.

Al-Shamaa, M., Jefferson, P., & Ball, D. R. (2003). Lingual tonsil hypertrophy: Airway management. *Anaesthesia*, *58*(11), 1134–1135.

Alper, C. M., Losee, J. E., Mandel, E. M., Seroky, J. T., Swarts, D. J., & Doyle, W. J. (2011). Post-palatoplasty Eustachian tube function in young children with cleft palate. *Cleft Palate–Craniofacial Journal*, *49*(4), 504–507.

Alper, C. M., Losee, J. E., Mandel, E. M., Seroky, J. T., Swarts, J. D., & Doyle, W. J. (2012). Pre- and post-palatoplasty Eustachian tube function in infants with cleft palate. *International Journal of Pediatric Otorhinolaryngology*, *76*(3), 388–391.

American Academy of Family Physicians, American Academy of Otolaryngology Head and Neck Surgery, & American Academy of Pediatrics Subcommittee on Otitis Media with Effusion. (2004). Otitis media with effusion. *Pediatrics*, *113*(5), 1412–1429.

American Cleft Palate–Craniofacial Association. (2009). Parameters for evaluation and treatment of patients with cleft lip/palate or other craniofacial anomalies. American Cleft Palate–Craniofacial Association homepage. Accessed February 18, 2011, from http://www.acpa-cpf.org.

Aneeza, W. H., Marina, M. B., Razif, M. Y., Azimatun, N. A., Asma, A., & Sani, A. (2011). Effects of uvulopalatopharyngoplasty: A seven year review. *Medical Journal of Malaysia, 66*(2), 129–132.

Baudonck, N., Van Lierde, K., Dhooge, I., & Corthals, P. (2011). A comparison of vowel productions in prelingually deaf children using cochlear implants, severe hearing-impaired children using conventional hearing aids and normal-hearing children. *Folia Phoniatrica et Logopaedica, 63*(3), 154–160.

Blythe, W. R., Henrich, D. E., & Pillsbury, H. C. (1995). Outpatient uvuloplasty: An inexpensive, single-staged procedure for the relief of symptomatic snoring. *Otolaryngology—Head and Neck Surgery, 113* (1), 1–4.

Brent, B. (1999). The pediatrician's role in caring for patients with congenital microtia and atresia. *Pediatric Annals, 28*(2), 374–383.

Brodsky, L., Moore, L., Stanievich, J., & Ogra, P. (1988). The immunology of tonsils in children: The effect of bacterial load on the presence of B- and T-cell subsets. *Laryngoscope, 98*(1), 93–98.

Brown, O. E., Myer, C. M., III, & Manning, S. C. (1989). Congenital nasal pyriform aperture stenosis. *Laryngoscope, 99*(1), 86–91.

Carter, R., III, & Watenpaugh, D. E. (2008). Obesity and obstructive sleep apnea: Or is it OSA and obesity? *Pathophysiology, 15* (2), 71–77.

Chang, S. O., Lee, J. H., Choi, B. Y., & Song, J. J. (2007). Long term results of postoperative canal stenosis in congenital aural atresia surgery. *Acta Otolaryngologica* (558), 15–21.

Chen, W. X., & Wong, V. (2005). Prognosis of Bell's palsy in children—Analysis of 29 cases. *Brain and Development, 27*(7), 504–508.

Coez, A., Belin, P., Bizaguet, E., Ferrary, E., Zilbovicius, M., & Samson, Y. (2010). Hearing loss severity: Impaired processing of formant transition duration. *Neuropsychologia, 48*(10), 3057–3061.

Croft, C. B., & Golding-Wood, D. G. (1990). Uses and complications of uvulopalatopharyngoplasty. *Journal of Laryngology and Otology, 104*(11), 871–875.

D'Antonio, L. L., Snyder, L. S., & Samadani, S. (1996). Tonsillectomy in children with or at risk for velopharyngeal insufficiency: Effects on speech. *Otolaryngology—Head and Neck Surgery, 115*(4), 319–323.

da Silva, D. P., Collares, M. V., & da Costa, S. S. (2010). Effects of velopharyngeal dysfunction on middle ear of repaired cleft palate patients. *Cleft Palate–Craniofacial Journal, 47*(3), 225–233.

Darrow, D. H., & Siemens, C. (2002). Indications for tonsillectomy and adenoidectomy. *Laryngoscope, 112*(8, Suppl. 100, Pt. 2), 6–10.

Donnelly, L. F., Shott, S. R., LaRose, C. R., Chini, B. A., & Amin, R. S. (2004). Causes of persistent obstructive sleep apnea despite previous tonsillectomy and adenoidectomy in children with Down syndrome as depicted on static and dynamic cine MRI. *American Journal of Roentgenology, 183*(1), 175–181.

Donnelly, M. J. (1994). Hypernasality following adenoid removal. *Irish Journal of Medical Science, 163*(5), 225–227.

Durr, D. G., & Shapiro, R. S. (1989). Otologic manifestations in congenital velopharyngeal insufficiency. *American Journal of Diseases of Children, 143*(1), 75–77.

Ertmer, D. J. (2011). Assessing speech intelligibility in children with hearing loss:

Toward revitalizing a valuable clinical tool. *Language, Speech, and Hearing Services in Schools, 42*(1), 52–58.

Feilberg, V. L., Sorensen, J. N., & Eriksen, H. O. (1993). Hypertrophic tonsils, upper airway obstruction and cardiac complications. A combined otological, medical and anesthesiological problem. *Ugeskrift for Laeger, 155*(38), 3003–3005.

Fernandes, D. B., Grobbelaar, A. O., Hudson, D. A., & Lentin, R. (1996). Velopharyngeal incompetence after adenotonsillectomy in noncleft patients. *British Journal of Oral and Maxillofacial Surgery, 34*(5), 364–367.

Finkelstein, Y., Nachmani, A., & Ophir, D. (1994). The functional role of the tonsils in speech. *Archives of Otolaryngology–Head & Neck Surgery, 120*(8), 846–851.

Finkelstein, Y., Bar-Ziv, J., Nachmani, A., Berger, G., & Ophir, D. (1993). Peritonsillar abscess as a cause of transient velopharyngeal insufficiency. *Cleft Palate–Craniofacial Journal, 30*(4), 421–428.

Finkelstein, Y., Wexler, D. B., Nachmani, A., & Ophir, D. (2002). Endoscopic partial adenoidectomy for children with submucous cleft palate. *Cleft Palate–Craniofacial Journal, 39*(5), 479–486.

Fitzpatrick, E. M., Crawford, L., Ni, A., & Durieux-Smith, A. (2011). A descriptive analysis of language and speech skills in 4- to 5-yr-old children with hearing loss. *Ear and Hearing, 32*(5), 605–616.

Folk, S. N., D'Antonio, L. L., & Hardesty, R. A. (1997). Secondary cleft deformities. *Clinics in Plastic Surgery, 24*(3), 599–611.

Garcia Pola, M. J., Gonzalez Garcia, M., Garcia Martin, J. M., Gallas, M., & Seoane Leston, J. (2002). A study of pathology associated with short lingual frenum. *Journal of Dentistry for Children, 69*(1), 59–62.

Gates, G., Avery, C., Prihoda, T., & Cooper, J. J. (1987, December 3). Effectiveness of adenoidectomy and tympanostomy tubes in the treatment of chronic otitis media with effusion. *New England Journal of Medicine, 317*, 1444–1451.

Gibb, A. G., & Stewart, I. A. (1975). Hypernasality following tonsil dissection—Hysterical aetiology. *Journal of Laryngology and Otology, 89*(7), 779–781.

Goldberg, C., DeLorie, R., Zuker, R. M., & Manktelow, R. T. (2003). The effects of gracilis muscle transplantation on speech in children with Moebius syndrome. *Journal of Craniofacial Surgery, 14*(5), 687–690.

Grimmer, J. F., & Poe, D. S. (2005). Update on Eustachian tube dysfunction and the patulous Eustachian tube. *Current Opinion in Otolaryngology & Head and Neck Surgery, 13*(5), 277–282.

Haapanen, M. L., Ignatius, J., Rihkanen, H., & Ertama, L. (1994). Velopharyngeal insufficiency following palatine tonsillectomy. *European Archives of Oto-Rhino-Laryngology, 251*(3), 186–189.

Han, D., Xu, W., Hu, R., & Zhang, L. (2012). Voice function following Han's uvulopalatopharyngoplasty. *Journal of Laryngology and Otology, 126*(1), 47–51.

Heller, J. C., Gens, G. W., Croft, C. B., & Moe, D. G. (1978). Conductive hearing loss in patients with velopharyngeal insufficiency. *Cleft Palate Journal, 15*(3), 246–253.

Isberg, A., & Henningsson, G. (1987). Influence of palatal fistulas on velopharyngeal movements: A cineradiographic study. *Plastic and Reconstructive Surgery, 79*(4), 525–530.

Jayaraman, G., Sharafkhaneh, H., Hirshkowitz, M., & Sharafkhaneh, A. (2008). Pharmacotherapy of obstructive sleep apnea.

Therapeutic Advances in Respiratory Disease, 2(6), 375–386. doi: 10.1177/1753465808098225.

Kavey, N. B., Whyte, J., Blitzer, A., & Gidro-Frank, S. (1990). Postsurgical evaluation of uvulopalatopharyngoplasty: Two case reports. *Sleep, 13*(1), 79–84.

Kawakami, M., Yagi, T., & Takada, K. (2002). Maxillary expansion and protraction in correction of midface retrusion in a complete unilateral cleft lip and palate patient. *Angle Orthodontics, 72*(4), 355–361.

Kern, I. (1991, July 1). Tongue tie. *Medical Journal of Australia, 155*, 33–34.

Kosling, S., Omenzetter, M., & Bartel-Friedrich, S. (2009). Congenital malformations of the external and middle ear. *European Journal of Radiology, 69*(2), 269–279.

Kountakis, S., Helidonis, E., & Jahrsdoerfer, R. (1995). Microtia grade as an indicator of middle ear development in aural atresia. *Archives of Otolaryngology—Head & Neck Surgery, 121*(8), 885–886.

Kubba, H., Bennett, A., & Bailey, C. M. (2004). An update on choanal atresia surgery at Great Ormond Street Hospital for Children: Preliminary results with Mitomycin C and the KTP laser. *International Journal of Pediatric Otorhinolaryngology, 68*(7), 939–945.

Kummer, A. W. (2005, December 27). To clip or not to clip? That's the question. *The ASHA Leader, 10*(17), 6–7, 30.

Kummer, A. W., Billmire, D. A., & Myer, C. M. D. (1993). Hypertrophic tonsils: The effect on resonance and velopharyngeal closure. *Plastic and Reconstructive Surgery, 91*(4), 608–611.

Liu, L., Sun, Y., & Zhao, W. (2001). The effects of otitis media with effusion and hearing loss on the speech outcome after cleft palate surgery. *Zhonghua Kou Qiang Yi Xue Za Zhi, 36*(6), 424–426.

Luquetti, D. V., Heike, C. L., Hing, A. V., Cunningham, M. L., & Cox, T. C. (2011). Microtia: Epidemiology and genetics. *American Journal of Medical Genetics Part A*. doi: 10.1002/ajmg.a.34352.

MacKenzie-Stepner, K., Witzel, M. A., Stringer, D. A., & Laskin, R. (1987). Velopharyngeal insufficiency due to hypertrophic tonsils. A report of two cases. *International Journal of Pediatric Otorhinolaryngology, 14*(1), 57–63.

Maryn, Y., Van Lierde, K., De Bodt, M., & Van Cauwenberge, P. (2004). The effects of adenoidectomy and tonsillectomy on speech and nasal resonance. *Folia Phoniatrica et Logopedica, 56*(3), 182–191.

Meyerson, M. D., & Foushee, D. R. (1978). Speech, language and hearing in Moebius syndrome: A study of 22 patients. *Developmental Medicine & Child Neurology, 20*(3), 357–365.

Moller, K. T. (1994). Dental-occlusal and other oral conditions and speech. In J. E. Bernthal & N. W. Bankson (Eds.), *Child phonology: Characteristics, assessment, and intervention with special populations* (pp. 3–28). New York: Thieme Medical Publishers.

Moores, D. F. (2005). Cochlear implants: An update. *American Annals of the Deaf, 150*(4), 327–328.

Mora, R., Jankowska, B., Mora, F., Crippa, B., Dellepiane, M., & Salami, A. (2009). Effects of tonsillectomy on speech and voice. *Journal of Voice, 23*(5), 614–618.

Nguyen, L. H., Manoukian, J. J., Yoskovitch, A., & Al-Sebeih, K. H. (2004). Adenoidectomy: Selection criteria for surgical cases of otitis media. *Laryngoscope, 114*(5), 863–866.

Oulis, C. J., Vadiakas, G. P., Ekonomides, J., & Dratsa, J. (1994). The effect of hypertrophic adenoids and tonsils on the development of posterior crossbite and oral habits. *Journal of Clinical Pediatric Dentistry, 18*(3), 197–201.

Paradise, J. L. (1976). Management of middle ear effusions in infants with cleft palate. *Annals of Otology, Rhinology, and Laryngology, 85*(2, Suppl. 25, Pt. 2), 285–288.

Paradise, J. L., Alberti, P. W., Bluestone, C. D., Cheek, D. B., Lis, E. F., & Stool, S. E. (1974). Pediatric and otologic aspects of clinical research in cleft palate. *Clinics in Pediatrics (Philadelphia), 13*(7), 587–593.

Paradise, J. L., & Bluestone, C. D. (1974). Early treatment of the universal otitis media of infants with cleft palate. *Pediatrics, 53*(1), 48–54.

Parton, M. J., & Jones, A. S. (1998). Hypernasality following adenoidectomy: A significant and avoidable complication. *Clinics in Otolaryngology, 23*(1), 18–19.

Paulson, L. M., Macarthur, C. J., Beaulieu, K. B., Brockman, J. H., & Milczuk, H. A. (2012). Speech outcomes after tonsillectomy in patients with known velopharyngeal insufficiency. *International Journal of Otolaryngol*, 2012. doi: 10.1155/2012/912767.

Peitersen, E. (1992). Natural history of Bell's palsy. *Acta Oto-Laryngologica, 492* (Suppl.), 122–124.

Pulkkinen, J., Ranta, R., Heliovaara, A., & Haapanen, M. L. (2002). Craniofacial characteristics and velopharyngeal function in cleft lip/palate children with and without adenoidectomy. *European Archives of Oto-Rhino-Laryngology, 259* (2), 100–104.

Ren, Y. F., Isberg, A., & Henningsson, G. (1995). Velopharyngeal incompetence and persistent hypernasality after adenoidectomy in children without palatal defect. *Cleft Palate–Craniofacial Journal, 32*(6), 476–482.

Rihkanen, H., & Soini, I. (1992). Changes in voice characteristics after uvulopalatopharyngoplasty. *European Archives of Otorhinolaryngology, 249*(6), 322–324.

Rosenfeld, R. M., Culpepper, L., Doyle, K. J., Grundfast, K. M., Hoberman, A., Kenna, M. A., Lieberthal, A. S., et al. (2004). Clinical practice guideline: Otitis media with effusion. *Otolaryngology—Head & Neck Surgery, 130*(5, Suppl.), 95–118.

Rvachew, S., Slawinski, E., Williams, M., & Green, C. (1999). The impact of early onset otitis media on babbling and early language development. *Journal of the Acoustical Society of America, 105*(1), 467–475.

Salas-Provance, M. B., & Kuehn, D. P. (1990). Speech status following uvulopalatopharyngoplasty. *Chest, 97*(1), 111–117.

Sapci, T., Mercangoz, E., Evcimik, M. F., Karavus, A., & Gozke, E. (2008). The evaluation of the tensor veli palatini muscle function with electromyography in chronic middle ear diseases. *European Archives of Oto-Rhino-Laryngology, 265* (3), 271–278.

Saunders, N. C., Hartley, B. E., Sell, D., & Sommerlad, B. (2004). Velopharyngeal insufficiency following adenoidectomy. *Clinical Otolaryngology & Allied Sciences, 29*(6), 686–688.

Schmaman, L., Jordaan, H., & Jammine, G. H. (1998). Risk factors for permanent hypernasality after adenoidectomy. *South African Medical Journal, 88*(3), 266–269.

Sheahan, P., Miller, L., Earley, M. J., Sheahan, J. N., & Blayney, A. W. (2004). Middle ear disease in children with congenital velopharyngeal insufficiency. *Cleft Palate—Craniofacial Journal, 41*(4), 364–367.

Shen, Z., Zhang, Y., Zhao, K., & Shen, Y. (2009). Peripheral facial paralysis in temporal bone trauma and cholesteatoma otitis media. *Lin Chung Er Bi Yan Hou Tou Jing Wai Ke Za Zhi, 23*(1), 21–23.

Shprintzen, R. J., Sher, A. E., & Croft, C. B. (1987). Hypernasal speech caused by tonsillar hypertrophy. *International Journal of Pediatric Otorhinolaryngology, 14* (1), 45–56.

Singh, I., Gathwala, G., Pathania, R., Singh, J., & Yadav, S. P. (1994). Hypertrophic tonsils causing articulation defect. *Indian Journal of Pediatrics, 61*(1), 106–107.

Sininger, Y., Doyle, K., & Moore, J. (1999). The case for early identification of hearing loss in children: Auditory system development, experimental auditory deprivation, and development of speech perception and hearing. *Pediatric Clinics of North America, 46*(2), 1–14.

Stewart, K. J., Ahmed, R. E., Razzell, R. E., & Watson, A. C. H. (2002). Altered speech following adenoidectomy: A 20 year experience. *British Journal of Plastic Surgery, 55,* 469–473.

Subramaniam, V., & Kumar, P. (2009). Impact of tonsillectomy with or without adenoidectomy on the acoustic parameters of the voice: A comparative study. *Archives of Otolaryngology–Head & Neck Surgery, 135*(10), 966–969.

Tachimura, T., Hara, H., Koh, H., & Wada, T. (1997). Effect of temporary closure of oronasal fistulae on levator veli palatini muscle activity. *Cleft Palate–Craniofacial Journal, 34*(6), 505–511.

Teele, D., Klein, J., & Rosner, B. (1980). Epidemiology of otitis media in children. *Annals of Otology, Rhinology, and Laryngology, 89*(3, Suppl.), 5–6.

Terzis, J. K., & Anesti, K. (2011). Experience with developmental facial paralysis: Part I. Diagnosis and associated stigmata. *Plastic and Reconstructive Surgery, 128*(5), 488e–497e.

Tewary, A. K., & Cable, H. R. (1993). Speech changes following uvulopalatopharyngoplasty. *Clinical Otolaryngology and Allied Sciences, 18*(5), 390–391.

Topouzelis, N., Iliopoulos, C., & Kolokitha, O. E. (2011). Macroglossia. *International Dental Journal, 61*(2), 63–69.

Trujillo, L. (1994). Prevention of conductive hearing loss in cleft palate patients. *Folia Phoniatrica et Logopedica, 46*(3), 123–126.

Van Borsel, J., Van Snick, K., & Leroy, J. (1999). Macroglossia and speech in Beckwith-Wiedemann syndrome: A sample survey study. *International Journal of Language & Communication Disorders, 34*(2), 209–221.

Visvanathan, V., & Wynne, D. M. (2012). Congenital nasal pyriform aperture stenosis: A report of 10 cases and literature review. *International Journal of Pediatric Otorhinolaryngolohy, 76*(1), 28–30.

Witzel, M. A., Rich, R. H., Margar-Bacal, F., & Cox, C. (1986). Velopharyngeal insufficiency after adenoidectomy: An 8-year review. *International Journal of Pediatric Otorhinolaryngology, 11*(1), 15–20.

Yanagisawa, E., & Weaver, E. M. (1997). An unusual appearance of velopharyngeal closure in a post-uvulopalatopharyngoplasty patient. *Ear Nose and Throat Journal, 76* (1), 14–15.

Yetter, M. F., Ogren, F. P., Moore, G. F., & Yonkers, A. J. (1990). Bell's palsy: A facial nerve paralysis diagnosis of exclusion. *Nebraska Medical Journal, 75*(5), 109–116.

CHAPTER

9

DENTAL ANOMALIES

RICHARD CAMPBELL, D.M.D., M.S.

MURRAY DOCK, D.D.S., M.S.D.

CHAPTER OUTLINE

INTRODUCTION

Children with a history of cleft of the lip and alveolus, or with other craniofacial anomalies, commonly have anomalies of the teeth and jaws (Akcam, Evirgen, Uslu, & Toygar Memikoğlu, 2010; Aljamal, Hazza'a, & Rawashdeh, 2010; Tannure et al., 2012). Their dental problems can include any combination of missing or extra teeth; crowded, impacted, or rotated teeth; or dental crossbite. Jaw problems may range from simple to complex and may include any combination of upper or lower jaw deficiency; upper or lower jaw excess; deep overbite; anterior or posterior openbite; and anterior or posterior crossbite. Both dental and occlusal anomalies have the potential to cause obligatory speech distortion or result in the use of compensatory articulation productions.

Dental management of these patients requires coordination among several dental specialists, including pediatric dentists, orthodontists, oral maxillofacial surgeons, and prosthodontists (Kirschner & LaRossa, 2000; Kuijpers-Jagtman, Borstlap-Engels, Spauwen, & Borstlap, 2000; Mouradian, Omnell, & Williams, 1999; Strong, 2002; Turvey, Vig, & Fonseca, 1996; Vasan, 1999; Wangsrimongkol & Jansawang, 2010). Together, they monitor and treat problems of the developing dentition, occlusion, and facial growth of the patient with cleft lip and/or palate (Strauss, 1998, 1999).

Oral rehabilitation of abnormal structures can be a prolonged process, and throughout it all the speech-language pathologist must correct the functional modifications in speech that occur along the way. Close cooperation between the dental specialists and the speech-language pathologist leads to a more holistic management of speech defects secondary to the dental abnormalities.

A brief review of the dentition and its effect on speech production follows. Oral anatomy was covered in Chapter 1 and is not repeated in this chapter.

NORMAL DENTITION/ OCCLUSION

The dentition has two arches of teeth, the upper (or maxillary) arch and the lower (or mandibular) arch. Each arch consists of a right and left half; thus the teeth are paired with one of each type on either side (Figure 9–1).

In a child's life, there are two sets of teeth. The first set consists of the 20 primary or *deciduous teeth*, 10 in each arch (Figure 9–2). Deciduous teeth are shed and replaced by 32 permanent teeth (16 in each arch).

In the deciduous dentition, there are 10 upper and 10 lower teeth, for a total of 20. In one arch, starting from the midline and moving *distally* (moving away from the center or point of origin), the pairs are central incisors, lateral incisors, canines (cuspids), primary first molars, and primary second molars (Figure 9–2). The central and lateral incisors are in the premaxilla bone. The lateral incisor and canine are situated on either side of the incisive suture, where the premaxilla normally fuses with the lateral segments of the maxilla. Because this is the usual area of clefting, these teeth may be malformed, missing, or duplicated.

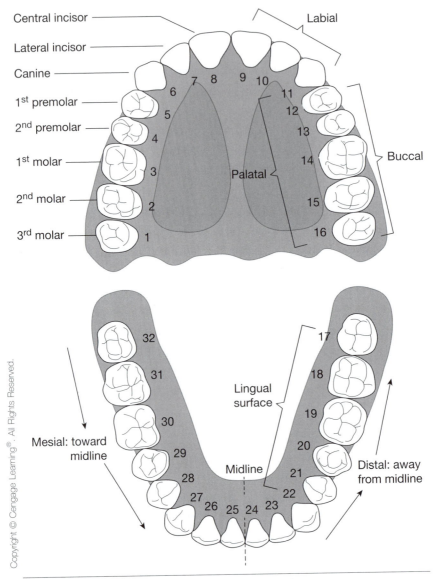

FIGURE 9–1 Occlusal view of all 32 permanent teeth.

In the permanent dentition, there are 16 upper and 16 lower teeth, for a total of 32 (Figure 9–1). In one arch, starting from the midline and proceeding distally, the pairs are central incisors, lateral incisors, canines (cuspids), first premolars (first bicuspids), second premolars (second bicuspids), first molars (6-year molars), second molars (12-year molars), and lastly, third molars (wisdom teeth). In addition to these anatomical names,

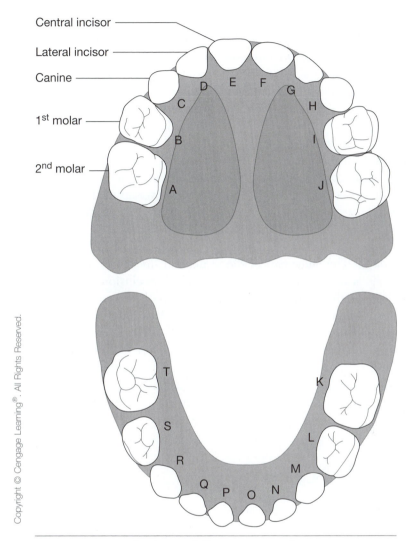

Central incisor

Lateral incisor

Canine

1st molar

2nd molar

FIGURE 9–2 Occlusal view of all 20 primary teeth.

the primary teeth are often lettered A through T, and the permanent teeth are numbered 1 through 32. The term *succedaneous teeth* is sometimes used to describe the 20 permanent teeth that replace the original deciduous teeth.

The incisor teeth are somewhat shovel shaped, and their biting surfaces are thin, knifelike edges. The remaining teeth have rounded points for chewing. The points on the teeth are known as *cusps*. Canines have one point or cusp. Premolars (bicuspids) typically have two cusps, although they may sometimes have three. Cusps are arranged in rows, one to the outside (buccal or labial) and one to the inside (palatal or lingual). Upper molars have four cusps—two buccal and two palatal (or lingual). Lower molars have four or five cusps—two or three buccal and two lingual. This buccal cusp to lingual cusp arrangement creates a valley between the cusps, called the *central fossa*. Variations in the shapes of teeth and the number of cusps do occur but are usually of only academic interest to the clinician.

Many terms are used to describe the position of the teeth in the arch (see Figure 9–1). The dental *midline* is at the apex of the dental arch, where the left and right halves join. The direction toward the midline is *mesial*. The direction away from the midline is *distal*. The outer part of the arch that touches the lip is *labial*. The part of the arch that is posterior to the canine teeth is frequently referred to as *buccal*, for the buccinator muscle that moves the cheeks. The inner part of the upper and lower arch that is in contact with the tongue is referred to as *lingual*. Many clinicians refer to the inner part of the upper arch as *palatal*, because of its proximity to the

surface of the hard palate. *Overjet* is the horizontal (or anterior–posterior) relationship between the incisors. It refers to how far the upper incisor teeth are ahead of the lower incisors. Overjet is typically measured in millimeters from the labial surface of the lower incisor to the labial surface of the upper incisor, with the teeth in occlusion. A normal amount of overjet is about 2 mm, with upper incisors and lower incisors in light contact. *Overbite* refers to the vertical overlap of the upper and lower incisors. Normal overbite is approximately 2 mm, or about 25% of the distance of the lower incisors.

Dental occlusion refers to the bite, or the manner in which the teeth fit together. In normal occlusion, the upper arch partially overlaps the lower arch so that the cusps of one arch fit into the fossae of the opposing arch (Figure 9–3). Normal relationship of the upper to the lower teeth is called a Class I occlusion, as will be further explained here. Normal occlusion is important for aesthetics, biting and chewing, and speech.

SPEECH NOTES

With normal dental occlusion, the maxillary incisors overlap the mandibular teeth. The tongue rests in the mandible. The tongue tip is behind the incisors and just under the alveolar ridge. As a result of this occlusion, the tongue tip is in appropriate placement to be able to move up and down for lingual-alveolar articulation, without interference from the teeth. In addition, the upper and lower lips are approximated, making bilabial and labiodental sounds easy to produce.

Most people believe that the teeth are necessary for normal speech. Actually, this isn't true. Although the teeth are closed for production of *sibilant sounds* (/s/, /z/, /ʃ/, /ʒ/, /ʧ/, /ʤ/), closing the teeth is done to elevate the mandible, which positions the tongue tip just under the alveolar ridge. The fricative sound is not produced between the teeth but is created by the airstream between the tongue tip and the alveolar ridge. Teeth are not even necessary for labiodental sounds (/f/, /v/) because these sounds can be produced with the bottom lip against the top gum ridge. Because teeth are not necessary for normal speech, even edentulous people are usually able to articulate clearly. In addition, when there is premature loss of the deciduous teeth due to decay, this does not tend to affect speech unless there is also maxillary crowding (Gable, Kummer, Lee, Creaghead, & Moore, 1995).

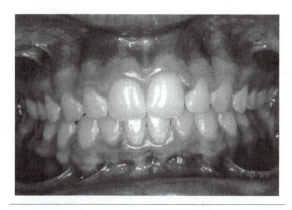

FIGURE 9–3 Normal dental occlusion with the normal overlap of the upper teeth over the lower teeth.

Courtesy Richard Campbell, D.M.D., M.S. & Murray Dock, D.D.S., M.S.D./ Cincinnati Children's Hospital Medical Center & University of Cincinnati College of Medicine

DENTAL ANOMALIES

Abnormal Incisor Relationships

A certain amount of overjet and overbite is normal, as noted above. The *overjet* is abnor-mal when the horizontal (or anterior–posterior) relationship between the incisors exceeds 2 mm when the upper and lower incisors are in light contact (Figure 9–4A and B). *Underjet*, or *anterior crossbite*, refers to a reversal of the normal upper to lower incisor relationships so that the upper incisors are inside (or lingual to) the lower incisors (Figure 9–5). Like overjet, underjet is measured in millimeters. An *overbite* is when there is too much overlap of the upper incisors over the lower incisors. The overbite is considered abnormal when the percentage of coverage of the upper incisors over the lower incisors exceeds 2 mm, or about 25% of the distance of the lower incisors (Figure 9–6). Greater amounts of overbite are associated with a deep overbite, or *deepbite*. If the upper teeth completely overlap the lower or if the lower incisors are in contact with the palate, this would be called a 100% overbite. *Underbite* (deep bite) refers to a vertical overlap of the lower incisors over the upper incisors.

SPEECH NOTES

Although teeth are not necessary for normal speech, they may cause speech problems by interfering with bilabial or lingual sound production (Shprintzen, Siegel-Sadewitz, Amato, & Goldberg, 1985). Many speech sounds can be affected because most consonants are produced in the front of the oral cavity, near the anterior dental arch, the lips, or tongue (Shprintzen et al., 1985). Dental abnormalities most commonly affect the following groups of phonemes: sibilant phonemes (/s/, /z/, /ʃ/, /ʒ/, /tʃ/, /dʒ/), lingual-alveolar phonemes (/t/, /d/, /n/, /l/), bilabial phonemes (/p/, /b/, /m/), and labiodental phonemes (/f/, /v/).

Abnormalities of the dentition or occlusion may affect speech by causing obligatory distortions and/or compensatory errors (Trost-Cardamone, 1997). An *obligatory distortion* occurs when articulation placement is normal, but the structural abnormalities (in this case, the teeth) interfere with the airstream or sound. This results in speech distortion. A *compensatory error* occurs when articulation is altered in order to compensate for structural abnormalities. This results in a substitution error. It's interesting that there does not appear to be a direct relationship between the severity of the malocclusion and the severity of the misarticulations or distortions. Instead, an individual's ability to adapt to structural abnormalities plays a significant role in the amount of speech distortion (Johnson & Sandy, 1999).

SPEECH NOTES

Severe overjet of incisors may affect bilabial competence at rest and alter the production of bilabial sounds during speech. Individuals may attempt to compensate by using a labiodental placement for bilabial sounds.

Underjet, causing an anterior crossbite, can cause the maxillary teeth to interfere with tongue tip placement for sibilants. This may result in an obligatory lateral distortion. If the speaker compensates by opening the teeth, this usually results in a frontal distortion.

Both an overbite and underbite can shorten the vertical dimension of the oral cavity during occlusion, thus affecting production of sibilant sounds. The individual can compensate by opening the teeth slightly to increase the vertical dimension. This usually results in no distortion because sibilant sounds are produced by the tongue tip rather than the teeth.

A diastema is merely a cosmetic concern and has no effect on speech.

A *diastema* is a space or opening between the teeth. It usually refers to a space between the maxillary central incisors (Figure 9–7).

Rotated, Supernumerary, or Ectopic Teeth

Rotated teeth are common in individuals who have had a cleft of the primary palate (see Figure 9–8). Central incisors and lateral incisors, if present, are most often affected and are usually rotated toward the cleft. The incisors may also be fused at the roots.

When there has been a cleft in the alveolar ridge, *supernumerary teeth* (extra teeth) (Figure 9–9A) or *ectopic teeth* (normal teeth that erupt in abnormal positions) (Figure 9–9B) may be displaced palatally or labially, usually in the line of the cleft. These often remain unerupted, although they occasionally erupt partially or even

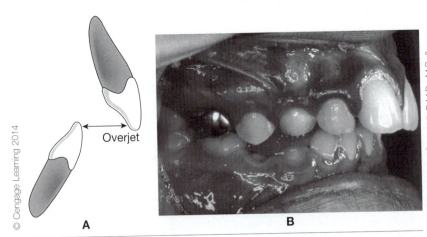

© Cengage Learning 2014

Overjet

A   B

Courtesy Richard Campbell, D.M.D., M.S. & Murray Dock, D.D.S., M.S.D./Cincinnati Children's Hospital Medical Center & University of Cincinnati College of Medicine

FIGURE 9–4 (A and B)   Overjet. (A) Overjet is the horizontal overlap of the incisors. (B) Abnormal overjet from incisor protrusion can be seen in this example.

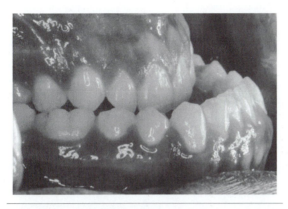

FIGURE 9–5 Underjet. Underjet is when the upper incisors are lingual to the lower incisors, as seen in this case of severe underjet.

Courtesy Richard Campbell, D.M.D., M.S. & Murray Dock, D.D.S., M.S.D./ Cincinnati Children's Hospital Medical Center & University of Cincinnati College of Medicine

completely. If erupted, supernumerary or ectopic teeth may be displaced palatally or labially.

Missing Teeth

Congenitally missing teeth are a frequent finding in patients with cleft of the primary palate (Figure 9–10A–C) (Camporesi et al., 2010). Missing permanent teeth can be replaced with an implant and crown (Figure 9–10D). Even children with a history of submucous cleft have an increased frequency of missing teeth or other dental abnormalities (Heliovaara, Ranta, & Rautio, 2004). The lateral incisor and/or canine (of the maxillary arch) are missing most frequently because these are the teeth border

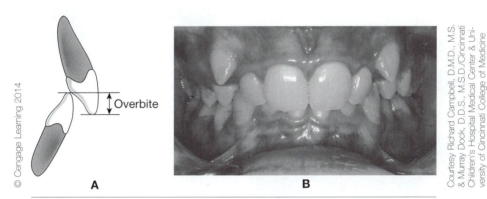

© Cengage Learning 2014

A

Overbite

B

Courtesy Richard Campbell, D.M.D., M.S. & Murray Dock, D.D.S., M.S.D./Cincinnati Children's Hospital Medical Center & University of Cincinnati College of Medicine

FIGURE 9–6 (A and B) Overbite. (A) An overbite is measured as the vertical overlap of the incisors from the incisal edges and is often expressed as a percentage of overbite. (B) In this instance the upper incisors almost completely overlap the lower incisors, making it a deepbite.

SPEECH NOTES

Rotated, supernumerary, or ectopic teeth may interfere with tongue tip movement during speech. Despite normal placement of the tongue tip, the teeth can divert the airstream laterally, causing an obligatory lateral distortion on sibilants, and even lingual-alveolar phonemes. If the individual pulls the tongue back to compensate, this causes the dorsum of the tongue to touch the palate. This placement also diverts the airstream laterally, resulting in a lateral distortion.

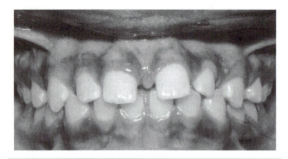

FIGURE 9–7 Diastema. A diastema is a space or opening between any of the teeth. Clinicians commonly use the term "disastema" to indicate the space between the maxillary central incisors, as seen in this case.

Courtesy Richard Campbell, D.M.D., M.S. & Murray Dock, D.D.S., M.S.D./ Cincinnati Children's Hospital Medical Center & University of Cincinnati College of Medicine

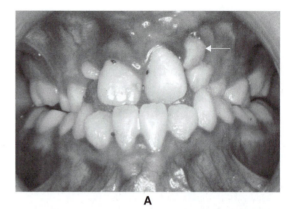

A

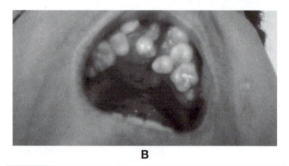

B

FIGURE 9–9 (A and B) Supernumerary and ectopic teeth. (A) An extra tooth may occur in the line of the cleft, as in this case of a supernumerary primary incisor, distal and superior to the patient's maxillary left central incisor (arrow). (B) Multiple ectopic teeth in the area of lingual movement for speech.

Courtesy Richard Campbell, D.M.D., M.S. & Murray Dock, D.D.S., M.S.D./ Cincinnati Children's Hospital Medical Center & University of Cincinnati College of Medicine

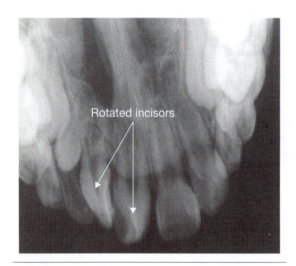

FIGURE 9–8 Rotated teeth in the cleft site. An occlusal X-ray demonstrates that teeth in the line of the cleft are frequently malpositioned or rotated about the long axis of the roots. In this view, the maxillary right central and lateral incisors (arrows) are rotated approximately 90 degrees each so that the lingual surfaces of their crowns are facing each other. By comparison, the maxillary left central and lateral incisors are nearly normal, with almost no rotation (the right side of this view). Note that there is also a supernumerary tooth distal to the rotated incisors.

Courtesy Richard Campbell, D.M.D., M.S. & Murray Dock, D.D.S., M.S.D./ Cincinnati Children's Hospital Medical Center & University of Cincinnati College of Medicine

the incisive suture lines and therefore are in the line of the cleft. Even when present, teeth in the area of the cleft may be smaller than normal, misshapen, or malformed.

Open Bite

Open bite occurs when one or more maxillary teeth fail to occlude with the opposing mandibular teeth (Figure 9–11A–E). Open bites primarily affect the anterior dentition (anterior open bite) and less commonly the posterior dentition (lateral open bite). Causes of open

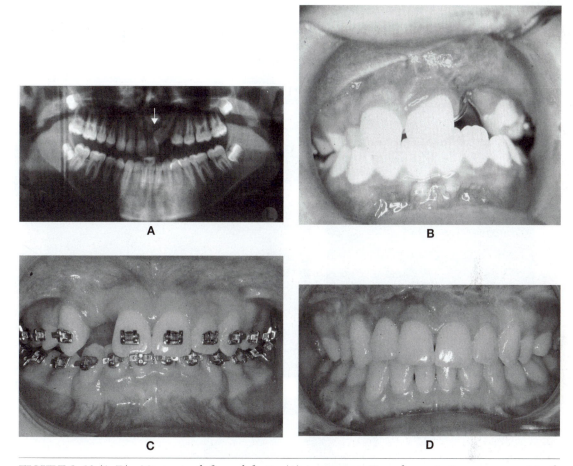

FIGURE 9–10 (A–D)   Missing teeth from cleft site. (A) A panoramic X-ray demonstrating a permanent tooth missing from the cleft site. The upper left lateral incisor (tooth #10) is frequently missing, as it is in this case (see the arrow), and the upper left canine has moved into its place. (B) The lateral incisor and canine are both missing. (C) The lateral incisor is missing. (D) The missing lateral incisor in C is replaced with an implant and crown.

Courtesy Richard Campbell, D.M.D., M.S. & Murray Dock, D.D.S., M.S.D./Cincinnati Children's Hospital Medical Center & University of Cincinnati College of Medicine

bite include missing teeth or poor occlusion due to digit or pacifier sucking habits or skeletal discrepancies. Open bites are sealed by the tongue on swallowing, which is often confused as tongue thrust (Proffit & Fields, 2000).

Crossbite

Crossbite is a common dental abnormality in children with a history of cleft lip and palate.

In crossbite, the normal overlap of the upper teeth to the lower teeth is reversed so that the upper teeth are inside the lower teeth. A crossbite may involve only one upper and one lower tooth, called a *single-tooth crossbite* (Figure 9–12). Multiple-tooth crossbites are described by their position in the dental arch as either anterior or posterior.

An *anterior crossbite*, characterized by the maxillary incisors positioned inside the mandibular incisors, is commonly seen in patients

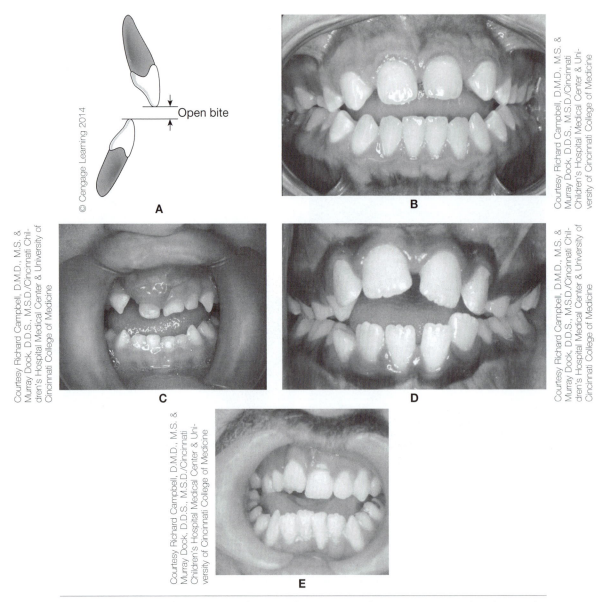

© Cengage Learning 2014

Open bite

A

Courtesy Richard Campbell, D.M.D., M.S. & Murray Dock, D.D.S., M.S.D./Cincinnati Children's Hospital Medical Center & University of Cincinnati College of Medicine

B

Courtesy Richard Campbell, D.M.D., M.S. & Murray Dock, D.D.S., M.S.D./Cincinnati Children's Hospital Medical Center & University of Cincinnati College of Medicine

C

Courtesy Richard Campbell, D.M.D., M.S. & Murray Dock, D.D.S., M.S.D./Cincinnati Children's Hospital Medical Center & University of Cincinnati College of Medicine

D

Courtesy Richard Campbell, D.M.D., M.S. & Murray Dock, D.D.S., M.S.D./Cincinnati Children's Hospital Medical Center & University of Cincinnati College of Medicine

E

Courtesy Richard Campbell, D.M.D., M.S. & Murray Dock, D.D.S., M.S.D./Cincinnati Children's Hospital Medical Center & University of Cincinnati College of Medicine

FIGURE 9–11 (A–E)   Anterior open bite. (A) The anterior teeth are not in contact. (B–E) Examples of an anterior open bite. Open bite is often attributed to tongue thrust, but little evidence exists to support that assumption. Open bite is difficult to treat, often involving orthognathic surgery in conjunction with orthodontics.

with dental or skeletal Class III malocclusion. An anterior crossbite may involve any or all of the anterior teeth, including the central incisors, lateral incisors, or canines (Figure 9–13).

A *lateral (posterior) crossbite* involves any combination of teeth distal (posterior) to the canines and usually occurs because the maxilla is too narrow. Posterior crossbites can be unilateral

SPEECH NOTES

The effect on speech of missing teeth or an open bite depends on the size of the oral cavity. If oral cavity size is normal, there may be no effect on speech because normal speech does not require teeth (Moller, 1994). If the palatal arch is low, flat, or narrow, or if there is maxillary retrusion or macroglossia, this will likely cause oral cavity crowding during occlusion. Oral cavity crowding inhibits tongue movement for the production of sibilant phonemes. To compensate, the individual will either open the dental arch, or the tongue will seek an opening in the dental arch where there are missing teeth.

If there is an anterior opening (due to missing maxillary incisors or an open bite), the tongue may protrude through it, causing fronting of sibilants and even lingual-alveolar sounds. On the other hand, if there is a lateral opening (due to missing teeth in the line of the cleft), the tongue tip may deviate to that opening, redirecting the air stream to the opposite side. This results in a lateral distortion.

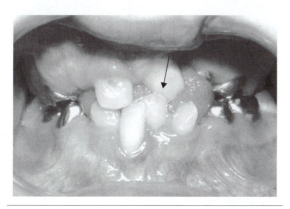

FIGURE 9–12 Single-tooth crossbite. A crossbite involving only one tooth may be referred to as a single-tooth crossbite. Often a maxillary central or lateral incisor is involved, as in this case of the upper left central incisor being displaced lingually to the lower left central incisor (see the arrow).
Courtesy Richard Campbell, D.M.D., M.S. & Murray Dock, D.D.S., M.S.D./ Cincinnati Children's Hospital Medical Center & University of Cincinnati College of Medicine

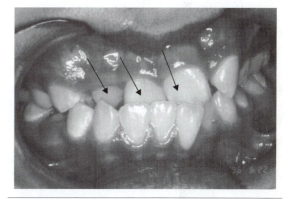

FIGURE 9–13 Anterior crossbite. When most of the incisors are involved in crossbite, an anterior crossbite is said to have occurred, as in this patient with anterior crossbite of both of the maxillary central incisors and the maxillary right cuspid (arrows).
Courtesy Richard Campbell, D.M.D., M.S. & Murray Dock, D.D.S., M.S.D./ Cincinnati Children's Hospital Medical Center & University of Cincinnati College of Medicine

SPEECH NOTES

A crossbite can affect many groups of speech sounds, depending on the severity. There may be obligatory distortions and/or compensatory errors as a result.

If an anterior crossbite causes the maxillary teeth to articulate against the tongue during occlusion, this can cause fronting on sibilants, particularly on s/z. This would be an obligatory distortion. If the tongues moves back to compensate, this causes a lateral distortion.

A complete crossbite (Figure 9–15B), and even a lateral crossbite (particularly if it is bilateral), can cause distorted speech due to oral cavity crowding.

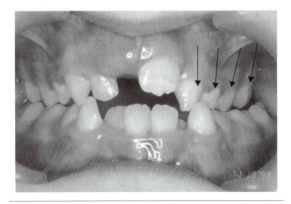

FIGURE 9–14 Unilateral posterior crossbite. The posterior teeth of the patient's maxillary left side are lingual to the mandibular teeth (→). This is referred to as a posterior crossbite. It may also be called a unilateral posterior crossbite.

Courtesy Richard Campbell, D.M.D., M.S. & Murray Dock, D.D.S., M.S.D./ Cincinnati Children's Hospital Medical Center & University of Cincinnati College of Medicine

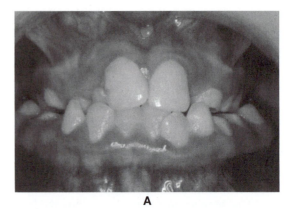

A

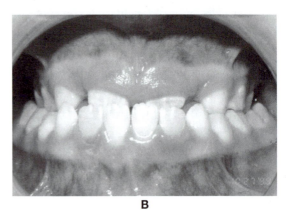

B

FIGURE 9–15 (A and B)   Bilateral crossbite. (A) The maxillary posterior teeth on both sides are lingual to the mandibular teeth. (B) When all the maxillary teeth fit inside the mandibular teeth, a total crossbite exists.

Courtesy Richard Campbell, D.M.D., M.S. & Murray Dock, D.D.S., M.S.D./ Cincinnati Children's Hospital Medical Center & University of Cincinnati College of Medicine

(Figure 9–14), bilateral (Figure 9–15A), or complete (Figure 9–15B). Bilateral posterior crossbites are common in individuals with a history of cleft palate. When mild, a bilateral crossbite may produce a shift of the mandible to one side, which gives the clinical appearance of a unilateral crossbite. A more severe bilateral posterior crossbite rarely produces such a shift of the mandible. Careful examination of the patient's occlusion as the teeth first contact during closure helps to distinguish a bilateral crossbite with mandibular shift from a true unilateral crossbite. Often, a multiple-tooth crossbite involves a combination of anterior as well as posterior teeth.

A *buccal crossbite* occurs when one or more maxillary teeth are positioned buccally such that the maxillary lingual cusps reside buccal to the mandibular cusps. The relatively rare *Brodie crossbite* occurs when the lingual cusps of all the maxillary posterior teeth are buccal to the mandibular teeth. Finally, a *complete crossbite* is when the maxilla is very narrow, and as a result the entire maxillary arch is inside the mandibular arch during occlusion.

Protruding Premaxilla

Infants affected by bilateral complete cleft lip and palate often have a protruding premaxilla at birth. Because the cleft goes through the incisive sutures to the incisive foramen, the premaxilla is untethered by the lateral palatal segments, leaving it in an anterior position. The lateral segments are also displaced medially so that there is no room for the premaxilla to fit in its normal position. Untreated, the

SPEECH NOTES

A protruding premaxilla can affect bilabial competence at rest and also during speech. As a result, bilabial sounds may be produced as labiodental plosives. Although this may be visually distracting, there is usually little speech distortion as a result of this placement.

premaxilla remains protrusive due to lack of space (Figure 9–16A). Past treatment included surgical removal of the premaxilla (Figure 9–16B), but this had major detrimental effects on midfacial growth and, of course, resulted in a lack of maxillary incisors (Proffit, White, & Sarver, 2003). Fortunately, the procedure has been abandoned in the United States and Europe but may still be done in some underdeveloped countries.

OCCLUSION AND ABNORMAL SKELETAL RELATIONSHIPS

Occlusion refers to the way the maxillary and mandibular teeth fit together when the jaws are closed, as when biting. The type of occlusion is determined by the anterior–posterior relationship between the mesiobuccal cusp of the upper molar and the buccal groove of the lower molar. First described by E. H. Angle (1899), the *Angle Classification System* describes normal occlusion and three types of malocclusion. Brilliant in its simplicity, it remains in widespread use today (Table 9–1) (Katz, 1992; Proffit & Fields, 2000). Despite its utility, Angle's classification applies only to the teeth and does not account for the influence of the jaws on tooth position or facial profile.

The way the jaws (not just the teeth) come together is called the *skeletal relationship*. To describe this relationship, contemporary

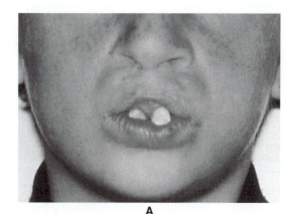

A

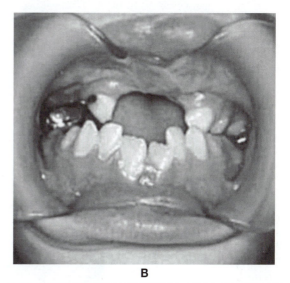

B

FIGURE 9–16 (A and B) (A) Protruding premaxilla. (B) Missing maxillary incisors due to excision of a protruding premaxilla. Fortunately, this procedure is no longer done.

Courtesy Richard Campbell, D.M.D., M.S. & Murray Dock, D.D.S., M.S.D./ Cincinnati Children's Hospital Medical Center & University of Cincinnati College of Medicine

TABLE 9–1 Angle's Classification of Occlusion and Skeletal Relationships

Classification	Example	Skeletal Classification	Diagram
Class I occlusion The *mesiobuccal* cusp of the upper molar occludes in the buccal groove of the lower molar. The remaining teeth are arranged upon a smoothly curving line.	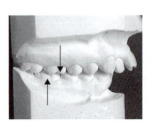 Mesiobuccal Cusp / Mesiobuccal Groove	Class I—Normal	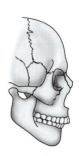
Class I malocclusion The relationship of the molars is normal, but the line of occlusion is incorrect because of malpositioned teeth, rotations, or other causes.		Class I—Normal	(same as above)
Class II malocclusion The lower molar is distally positioned relative to upper molar. The line of occlusion is not specified.	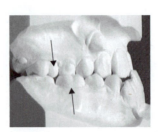	Class II—Mandibular retrusion and/or maxillary protrusion	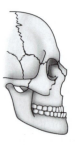
Class III malocclusion The lower molar is mesially positioned relative to upper molar. The line of occlusion is not specified.		Class III—Mandibular protrusion and/or maxillary retrusion	

SPEECH NOTES

Malocclusion of the jaws can have a far more significant effect on speech than the dental anomalies noted above. Depending on the type of malocclusion, the mandible (and thus the tongue) can be positioned too far behind or too far in front of the maxilla, thus affecting the relationship of the tongue tip to the alveolar ridge. The relationship between the upper and lower lip can also be affected.

practitioners have adapted Angle's dental occlusion classification. This is appropriate because in most cases, although not all, the jaw relationship is reflected in the dental relationship. Thus, when the jaws are in normal alignment with each other, practitioners call this a Class I skeletal relationship, even if there are abnormalities in the dentition within the arches. *Malocclusion*, therefore, refers to an abnormal dental or skeletal relationship between the maxillary and mandibular teeth. As a result, the arches do not close together normally during biting.

When the lower jaw is small relative to the upper jaw (retrognathism) or the upper jaw is too far forward (maxillary protrusion), practitioners call it a Class II skeletal relationship.

Again, a Class II dental malocclusion would be expected but does not always occur.

Finally, if the lower jaw is relatively large (prognathism) and/or the upper jaw is relatively small, this is referred to as Class III skeletal relationship and a Class III dental malocclusion would also be likely. Individuals with a history of cleft often have midface deficiency resulting from surgery and scarring, and therefore they commonly have a Class III skeletal occlusion.

The jaw relationship and the soft tissue profile of the forehead, nose, lips, and chin can be measured with a lateral skull X-ray, or *cephalometric radiograph* (also called a *cephalogram*), taken with the patient's head held in a standardized position (Figure 9–17). A cephalometric tracing is done for treatment planning (Figure 9–18).

SPEECH NOTES

When Class II malocclusion (which usually includes micrognathia) is severe, the position of the tongue tip rests under the palate rather than the alveolar ridge. This can cause obligatory distortion of sibilants and even lingual-alveolar phonemes. The individual may compensate by *backing*, which is using the dorsum or the back of the tongue for anterior lingual sounds. In addition to affecting lingual sounds, a Class II malocclusion or protruding premaxilla can interfere with lip closure, causing a lack of bilabial closure at rest and during production of most bilabial sounds (p, b, m). The individual may compensate by producing these with a labiodental placement. This placement causes very little speech distortion, but it can be visually distracting because of abnormal lip placement.

SPEECH NOTES

A Class III malocclusion (which usually includes an anterior crossbite and may include mandibular prognathism) has the most significant effect on speech. In this case, the mandible, along with the tongue, is in an anterior position relative to the alveolar ridge. This causes difficulty with production of sibilant and lingual-alveolar sounds, which require the tongue tip to be under the alveolar ridge. If the tongue remains in the normal position in the mandible while trying to produce these sounds, this will cause the perception of fronting, which is an obligatory distortion (Kummer, Strife, Grau, Creaghead, & Lee, 1989; Moller, 1994; Taher, 1997). If the tongue retracts to compensate for the anterior crowding, this causes the dorsum of the tongue to articulate against the palate, resulting in a lateral distortion (a compensatory error).

Class III malocclusion can also interfere with production of lip sounds. Labiodental (f, v) sounds may be affected due to the difficulty retracting the bottom lip far enough to articulate against the maxillary incisors. To compensate, the individual may use a reverse labiodental placement so that the upper lip articulates with the mandibular incisors (Moller, 1994). Bilabial sounds can also be difficult to produce with this Class III malocclusion. The individual may compensate by using a reverse labiodental production for these sounds as well.

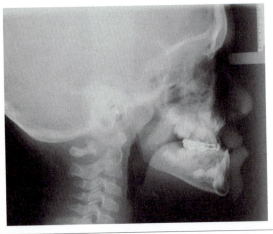

FIGURE 9–17 Cephalometric X-ray. A cephalometric X-ray is a lateral skull film made with a cephalostat, a device with ear rods and a nasal bridge rest to allow reproducible head positioning. This allows comparisons of X-rays of the patient taken at different times for use in longitudinal growth studies.
Courtesy Richard Campbell, D.M.D., M.S. & Murray Dock, D.D.S., M.S.D./ Cincinnati Children's Hospital Medical Center & University of Cincinnati College of Medicine

DENTAL DEVELOPMENT AND STAGES OF TREATMENT

Treatment of dental problems in children with a history of cleft lip and palate is timed to follow the normal stages of dental development. For instance, maxillary expansion to correct a crossbite may be coordinated with the eruption of specific teeth, because this also serves to prepare the patient for secondary alveolar bone grafting. Some interventions may be done to coincide with growth spurts. Others, such as combined orthodontic and orthognathic surgical treatment, may be delayed until the completion of growth (Posnick & Ricalde, 2004).

Infant Stage

Most infants are born without any erupted teeth. The infant stage, therefore, involves the eruption of the primary teeth and lasts until 12 months of age. However, natal or neonatal teeth are common in children with either a

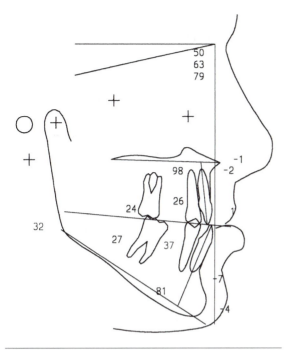

FIGURE 9–18 Cephalometric tracing. A tracing of a cephalometric X-ray is made so that measurement can be drawn without damaging the film. A set of measurements is called an analysis and is frequently named after its founder, for example, the Steiner Analysis or the McNamara Analysis. This particular depiction is the COGS Analysis, or cephalometric analysis for orthognathic surgery, devised by Burstone. The image was generated by Dentofacial Planner.
Courtesy Richard Campbell, D.M.D., M.S. & Murray Dock, D.D.S., M.S.D./ Cincinnati Children's Hospital Medical Center & University of Cincinnati College of Medicine

TABLE 9–2 Tooth Eruption for Primary and Permanent Dentition

Permanent Dentitions

Primary Tooth	Maxillary	Mandibular
Central	10 mo.	8 mo.
Lateral	11 mo.	13 mo.
Canine	19 mo.	20 mo.
1st Molar	16 mo.	16 mo.
2nd Molar	29 mo.	27 mo.
Permanent Tooth		
Central	7.25 yr.	6.25 yr.
Lateral	8.25 yr.	7.5 yr.
Canine	11.5 yr.	10.5 yr.
1st Premolar	10.25 yr.	10.5 yr.
2nd Premolar	11 yr.	11.25 yr.
1st Molar	6.25 yr.	6 yr.
2nd Molar	12.5 yr.	12 yr.
3rd Molar	20 yr.	20 yr.

Data from Proffit and Fields, 2000.

unilateral or a bilateral cleft (Cabete, Gomide, & Costa, 2000). If a tooth is present at birth, a pediatric dentist should examine it to evaluate its stability in the arch. Most often, these teeth are not supernumerary, and every attempt is made to retain them when possible.

The eruption sequence for the primary teeth, as well as for the permanent teeth, is fairly predictable (Table 9–2); however, there is considerable variation from one individual to another with regard to chronological timing. For primary teeth, a variation in eruption of 6 months on either side of the expected eruption

is no cause for alarm. The lower primary incisors are usually the first teeth to erupt, at around 8 months of age. The remaining incisors are close behind, completing their eruption by 10 to 13 months of age. The canines erupt between 19 and 20 months, followed by the first molars at 16 months, and finally the second molars by 27 to 29 months (Proffit & Fields, 2000).

Treatment for an infant with a cleft lip and palate is done in two stages: lip closure at about 12 weeks of age and then palate closure between 9 and 12 months of age. During the first year, clefts of the lip and alveolus, particularly bilateral clefts, require coordinated treatment between the surgeon and the dentist.

Clefts of the lip only, or incomplete clefts of the lip and alveolus, usually don't require

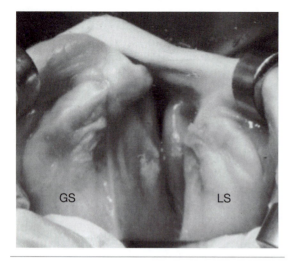

FIGURE 9–19 The occlusal view of the palate of a newborn with unilateral cleft lip and palate. The greater segment (GS) is on the left in the photograph, and the lesser segment (LS) is on the right.

Courtesy Richard Campbell, D.M.D., M.S. & Murray Dock, D.D.S., M.S.D./ Cincinnati Children's Hospital Medical Center & University of Cincinnati College of Medicine

manipulation of the alveolar segment before surgical repair. For a complete or wide unilateral cleft, however (Figure 9–19), many surgeons prefer to have the intra-alveolar gap reduced before surgical closure of the lip. Bilateral clefts of the lip and palate are particularly challenging (Figure 9–20A–C). Not only are there two clefts, but there is often a protruding premaxillary segment (Bartzela et al., 2010; Bitter, 2001). Additionally, the posterior alveolar segments often is narrow. Treatment is usually directed at retracting the protruding premaxillary segment while widening the narrow lateral segments.

There are numerous ways to accomplish alignment of the alveolar segments in both unilateral and bilateral clefts of the palate. Regardless of which technique is chosen, the process is referred to as infant oral *orthopedics* (*premaxillary or palatal orthopedics*) (Figure 9–21A–D). The techniques include, from least invasive to most invasive, taping of the lip (Figure 9–22A–C); elastic straps over the lip and attached to a bonnet; passive molding appliances with or without taping; lip adhesion (temporary surgical closure) before lip repair; and pin retained active intraoral appliances (Cho, 2001; Oosterkamp et al., 2005). Each method has advantages and disadvantages (Table 9–3). The choice of one method over another varies, depending on the individual needs of the patient, the experience of the practitioners, and the overall regard concerning palatal orthopedics at a particular treatment center.

Palatal orthopedic methods are controversial and remain a lively topic of debate among practitioners. Indeed, some authors disparage any repositioning of the palatal segments, believing that these procedures may result in decreased midfacial growth (Berkowitz, Mejia, & Bystrik, 2004; Bongaarts, Kuijpers-Jagtman, van't Hof, & Prahl-Andersen, 2004). Hopefully, further research will clarify the appropriate application of each method (Berkowitz et al., 2005; Braumann, Keilig, Bourauel, & Jager, 2002; Chan, Hayes, Shusterman, Mulliken, & Will, 2003; Millard, Latham, Huifen, Spiro, & Morovic, 1999; Prahl, Kuijpers-Jagtman, van't Hof, & Prahl-Andersen, 2003, 2005).

Because a cleft of the lip and alveolus also affects the nose, *nasal alveolar molding (NAM)* is often done to reposition the deformed nasal cartilage, lengthen the deficient columella, and reposition the alveolar segments (Cutting et al., 1998; Da Silveira et al., 2003). This technique involves applying pressure to the tip of the affected nostril(s) from an intraoral or extraoral approach, using various struts of wire or acrylic (Figure 9–23). Taping of the lip is also frequently done (Grayson & Cutting, 2001; Grayson & Maull, 2004). The molding appliance is worn from early infancy for a period of several months after the lip is closed (Doruk & Kilic, 2005). Proponents of the technique report encouraging results and follow-up

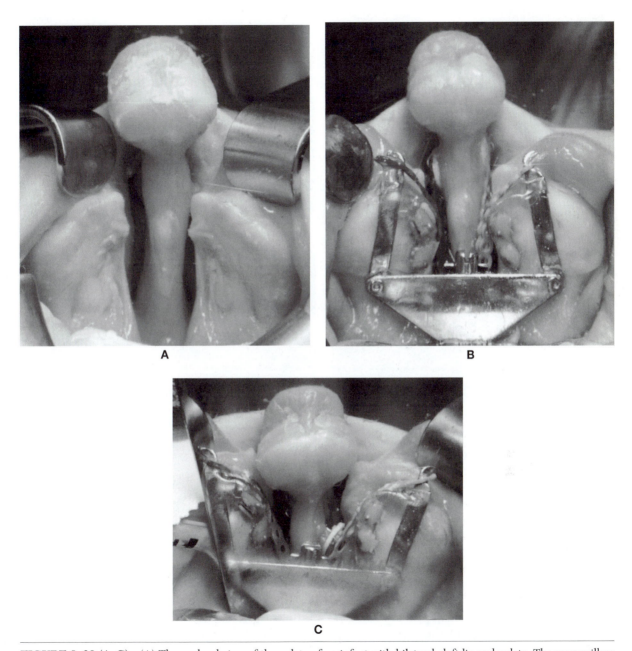

FIGURE 9–20 (A–C) (A) The occlusal view of the palate of an infant with bilateral cleft lip and palate. The premaxillary segment is at the top middle of the photograph, and the two lateral segments are on either side, left or right and posterior to the premaxillary segment in the photograph. (B) A pin-retained appliance used to reposition the segments. (C) The maxillary segment is retracted, and the lateral segment is widened.

Courtesy Richard Campbell, D.M.D., M.S. & Murray Dock, D.D.S., M.S.D./Cincinnati Children's Hospital Medical Center & University of Cincinnati College of Medicine

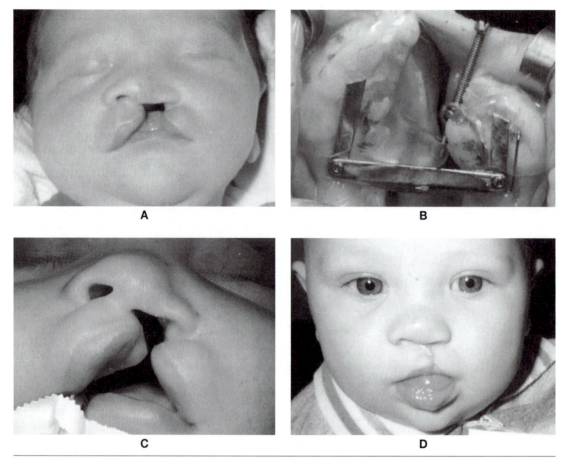

FIGURE 9–21 (A–D) Pin-retained intraoral appliance. (A). A wide unilateral cleft lip and palate. (B) In cases of wide clefts, some surgeons prefer to have the width of the cleft between greater and lesser segments reduced with an appliance. (C) The appliance gives a closer approximation of the lip segments. (D) The close approximation of the segments allows for lip closure with less tension than by other means.

Courtesy Richard Campbell, D.M.D., M.S. & Murray Dock, D.D.S., M.S.D./Cincinnati Children's Hospital Medical Center & University of Cincinnati College of Medicine

findings (Garfinkle, King, Grayson, Brecht & Cutting, 2011; Nazarian Mobin et al., 2011).

Some centers also perform primary alveolar bone grafting in the infant stage, usually with the primary lip repair. An attempt to bridge the gap between the bony segments of the alveolus is made by placing bone formation–inducing material from the rib or the hip into the cleft site (Hathaway, Eppley, Hennon, Nelson, & Sadove, 1999; Hathaway, Eppley, Nelson, & Sadove, 1999). The goal is to unify the alveolar segments into a continuous arch, thus consolidating the maxilla into one piece. Primary grafting is intended to stabilize the arch, thereby preventing future crossbite, and create bone, which provides a path for the eruption of teeth near the cleft (Lee, Grayson, Cutting, Brecht, & Lin, 2004).

Unfortunately, results of primary alveolar bone grafting are mixed. Although some infants gain the desired arch unity and sufficient bone for tooth eruption, many do not. In addition,

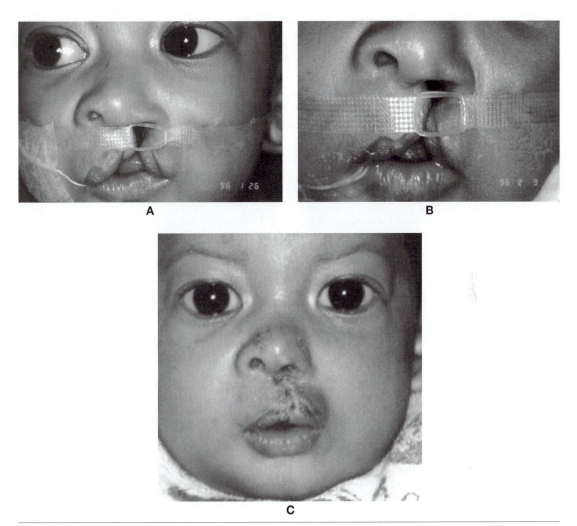

FIGURE 9–22 (A–C)   Taping of the lip. Narrow separations of the lip may be approximated by extraoral taping, in this case with an additional elastic, making surgical closure less difficult. (A) Beginning of taping. This shows separation of lip. (B) After a few weeks, the lip segments are approximated. (C) In this view, taken very shortly after lip closure, one can appreciate that there is little tension across the now joined lip segments.

Courtesy Richard Campbell, D.M.D., M.S. & Murray Dock, D.D.S., M.S.D./Cincinnati Children's Hospital Medical Center & University of Cincinnati College of Medicine

markedly decreased growth of the midface is an undesirable effect that has been associated with primary alveolar bone grafting. Centers debate whether differences in surgical technique and timing relate to success or failure of primary bone grafting (Pfeifer, Grayson, & Cutting, 2002; Sachs, 2002). In particular, much attention has been focused on the amount of gingival,

nasal, and oral mucosa that is manipulated by the surgeon in closing the infant alveolar cleft. This procedure is often called *gingivoperiosteoplasty*, particularly in reference to closing the cleft of the alveolus with raised gingival flaps at the same time that the palatal closure is performed (Millard et al., 1999). Success rates are low, and secondary alveolar bone grafting

TABLE 9–3 Methods of Unilateral Cleft Lip and Palate Closure

Method	Advantages	Disadvantages
Surgical only	Quick; no pre-op manipulations required.	Limited to smaller clefts; no control of segment position post-operatively.
Taping	Noninvasive; no dental impressions required.	Parent cooperation essential; skin irritation common; no control of segments.
Passive molding plates with or without taping	Allows some repositioning of segments; serves as retainers or aids feeding.	Dental impressions required; parents' cooperation is a must; denture adhesives are often used.
Lip adhesion	Decreases size of intra-alveolar gap; allows tension-free closure.	Requires additional surgery; surgeon must perform final closure through scar tissue; no post-op segment control.
Pin-retained active appliance	Greater control of segments; effective at reducing wide clefts; allows tension-free lip closure.	Requires dental impressions or visit for placement; parent cooperation is required; there is surgical placement of the pins; long-term effects on maxillary growth unknown.
Nasal alveolar molding (NAM)	Allows repositioning of the segments; lengthens columella.	Is very labor intensive; periodic dental impressions are required; is uncomfortable for infant; requires significant parent cooperation to learn complex taping techniques; dental adhesives can cause skin irritation.

© Cengage Learing 2014

procedures may be required (Millard et al., 1999; Renkielska, Wojtaszek-Slominska, & Dobke, 2005). After the lip and palate are closed, the infant usually enjoys a reprieve from dental and surgical intervention for a few years until the primary dentition erupts.

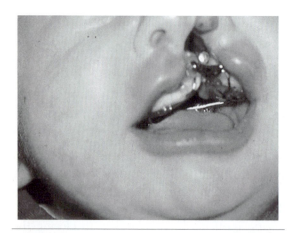

FIGURE 9–23 Extraoral nasal alveolar molding (NAM) appliance in combination with alveolar orthopedics.
Courtesy Richard Campbell, D.M.D., M.S. & Murray Dock, D.D.S., M.S.D./ Cincinnati Children's Hospital Medical Center & University of Cincinnati College of Medicine

Primary Dentition (1–6 Years)

The primary dentition is usually complete by 24 to 30 months of age, with 10 teeth in the upper arch and 10 in the lower arch. Ideally, there should be spacing between all of the primary teeth so that there is room for the larger permanent teeth that will replace them. A child with little or no spacing between the primary teeth is at risk for significant crowding of the permanent teeth (Ngan, Alkire, & Fields, 1999). Children with repaired cleft lip and palate often demonstrate maxillary retrusion, attributed to surgical scarring, as well as a maxilla that is smaller than normal in every dimension due to primary dysplasia of the structures. Therefore, it is not unusual to see crowding of the primary teeth in this population (DiBiase, DiBiase, Hay, & Sommerlad, 2002; Garrahy, Millett, & Ayoub, 2005).

There may be several dental abnormalities in the primary dentition at this stage. The primary lateral incisor and/or the primary canine may be missing because both are in the line of the cleft. Conversely, a supernumerary tooth may be located near the cleft site. They may appear either palatally or labially but are not often directly in the cleft due to its deficit of tissue. Malformations of these teeth are common (Chapple & Nunn, 2001; Maciel, Costa, & Gomide, 2005; Malanczuk, Opitz, & Retzlaff, 1999). Children with clefts are also at risk for periodontal disease localized to teeth near the cleft. Therefore, every effort should be made to establish proper oral hygiene measures at home and early management by a *pedodontist* (pediatric dentist) before age 2 (Chapple & Nunn, 2001; Dewinter et al., 2003; Gaggl, Schultes, Karcher, & Mossbock, 1999; Kirchberg, Treide, &

Hemprich, 2004; Schultes, Gaggl, & Karcher, 1999; Quirynen et al., 2003).

Crossbite in the cleft area is also very common due to the altered anatomy of the palate. The maxilla in unilateral clefts consists of two segments, a *lesser segment* on the cleft side (cleft segment) and a *greater segment* on the noncleft side (noncleft segment) (see Figure 9–19). The greater and lesser segments are not joined at the site of the cleft, and as a result they can be displaced by lip pressure. Therefore, it is common to find crossbite on the affected, lesser segment side. In bilateral clefts, there are three maxillary segments, one premaxillary segment, and two lateral segments. The lateral segments may be displaced medially, which frequently results in a bilateral crossbite. The premaxillary segment may be protrusive (see Figure 9–20).

Children with a repaired cleft lip and palate frequently appear to have a relatively normal upper to lower skeletal (jaw) relationship in the primary dentition (Figure 9–24A).

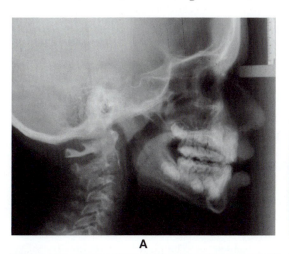 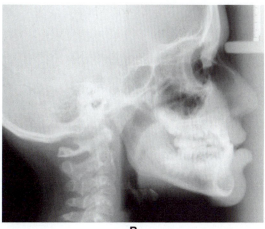

A	B

FIGURE 9–24 (A and B) Normal occlusion in early dentition, which will change in adolescence. (A) The jaw and dental relationships are good in the early mixed dentition cephalogram of a patient with unilateral cleft lip and palate. This patient exhibits a nearly Class I occlusion, and midfacial retrusion is not obvious. (B) Unfortunately, because of the mandibular growth spurt of adolescence, the relationships have changed for the worse. The patient now has a dental and skeletal Class III malocclusion with underbite and underjet, manifestations of the lack of midfacial growth often seen in patients with cleft lip and palate.

Courtesy Richard Campbell, D.M.D., M.S. & Murray Dock, D.D.S., M.S.D./Cincinnati Children's Hospital Medical Center & University of Cincinnati College of Medicine

Unfortunately, this may change with time. The maxilla is smaller in children with a history of cleft than in unaffected children, but the mandible is also normally small at this stage of development. During the adolescent growth spurt, however, the mandible increases to its normal size. As a result, the maxilla appears to become more retrusive relative to the mandible, thereby exposing its deficiency (Figure 9–24B) (Lisson, Hanke, & Trankmann, 2004; Scheuer, Holtje, Hasund, & Pfeifer, 2001; Veleminska, Smahel, & Mullerova, 2003).

Few conditions require orthodontic intervention in the primary dentition. In children with clefts, significant narrowing of the maxillary segments is sometimes addressed in the primary dentition, especially if a crossbite or crowding of the primary teeth occurs. In addition, any crossbite that causes a functional shift of the mandible—that is, a reposturing of the mandible to achieve a more comfortable bite—is addressed as soon as possible. Left untreated, this posturing can cause overgrowth of one *condyle* (jaw joint), resulting in an asymmetry of the mandible so that the chin is deviated to the nonaffected side (Proffit & Fields, 2000).

Treatment for crossbite in the primary dentition involves some form of maxillary expansion. One appliance for maxillary expansion is the *quad helix*. This device consists of orthodontic bands on the most posterior molars and frequently the primary canines as well (Figure 9–25A) (Kirchberg, Treide, & Hemprich, 2004). The bands are connected by a palatal spring that has two posterior loops, each adjacent to a molar, and two anterior loops. These four loops, or helices, give the quad helix its name. Some clinicians prefer to not include the helices, and the resulting W-shaped palatal spring is called a *W-arch*. Another appliance for maxillary expansion to

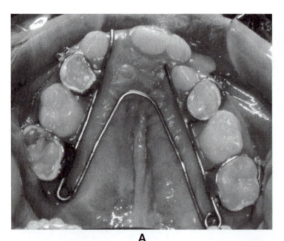
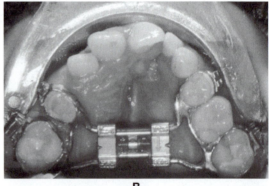

A　　　　　　　　　　　　　　　　　B

FIGURE 9–25 (A and B) Appliances used for maxillary expansion. (A) The quad helix consists of a palatal spring that has four helices. (B) The rapid palatal expander (RPE) consists of a jackscrew mechanism that is activated with a key by the parents. Both appliances are versatile in that they can be modified to fit the individual needs of the patient. For instance, the quad helix actually has only two helices. The anterior helices were not used in this case due to the constricted space of the anterior palate. Both appliances are bulky and may interfere with articulation while in use.

Courtesy Richard Campbell, D.M.D., M.S. & Murray Dock, D.D.S., M.S.D./Cincinnati Children's Hospital Medical Center & University of Cincinnati College of Medicine

correct a crossbite is the *rapid palatal expander* (RPE). This device consists of two or four orthodontic bands connected by a jackscrew in the middle of the palate (Figure 9–25B). Turning the screw creates the necessary force to widen the arch. The rapid palatal expander is capable of delivering very heavy forces, so it is used with caution in the primary dentition. The goal for both of these devices is to create adequate width of the maxilla. Because children with clefts may also have an anterior crossbite, some clinicians may wish to correct incisor position at this time (Sakamoto, Sakamoto, Harazaki, Isshiki, & Yamaguchi, 2002). This is rarely necessary with primary incisors, however, and should be reserved for the permanent incisors, preferably at a stage of nearly completed root development.

Maxillary expansion may be started as early as 4 to 5 years of age in a *cooperative* child, but for most children it's better to wait until the permanent upper first molars erupt. In most cases, expansion and improved access to the cleft area can be accomplished within a few months. Children with repaired palatal clefts must have a fixed lingual upper arch wire to maintain the maxillary expansion. Without proper retention, the scar tissue of the repaired cleft palate exerts a strong tendency toward relapse into crossbite.

In children with repaired cleft palate, maxillary expansion may achieve crossbite correction, but often at the expense of widen-ing a preexisting oronasal fistula. Widening the narrow arch of the cleft palate separates the greater and lesser segments, resulting in tightly stretched tissue over the deficient or absent bone of the palate. Without proper bony support, palatal tissue *necrosis* (death of cellular tissue) may occur, which causes the fistula to manifest. The fistula may be temporarily closed with a removable acrylic obturator. Surgical repair is usually accomplished later with an alveolar bone graft (Proffit et al., 2003).

Early Mixed Dentition (6–9 Years)

Mixed dentition refers to the presence of both primary and secondary teeth. The most noticeable sign that a child with a repaired cleft lip and palate is entering the early mixed dentition stage is the eruption of malpositioned permanent maxillary incisors. The permanent lower central incisors usually erupt first, followed by the upper central incisors, lower lateral incisors, and finally, the upper lateral incisors. The permanent first molars usually erupt shortly after the lower central incisors, but it is not uncommon for them to erupt first.

Figure 9–26A–D shows some examples of misaligned maxillary teeth secondary to a cleft. Although unaesthetic, these crowded incisors should not be corrected with orthodontics at this stage because the root formation remains incomplete. As a general rule, it takes at least

SPEECH NOTES

The quad helix device can interfere with tongue tip movement and thus affect lingual-alveolar sounds temporarily while it is in place. The rapid palatal expander (RPE) goes across the midpart of the palate. As such, it does not interfere with speech production. In fact, it can often be helpful in speech therapy if the goal is to correct palatal-dorsal productions. The child is merely told to elevate the tongue tip in front of the device, while avoiding tongue contact against the device.

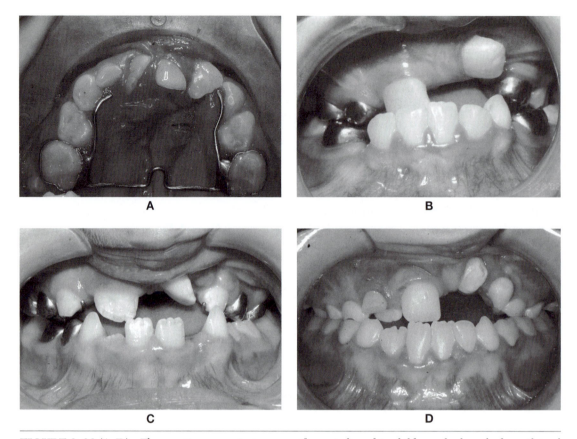

FIGURE 9–26 (A–D)   The erupting upper incisors are often misaligned in children who have had a unilateral or bilateral cleft. Figures A–D show various examples of misaligned maxillary incisors as the result of a cleft.

Courtesy Richard Campbell, D.M.D., M.S. & Murray Dock, D.D.S., M.S.D./Cincinnati Children's Hospital Medical Center & University of Cincinnati College of Medicine

3 years after crown eruption before root formation is complete. The pressure from orthodontic appliances at this stage can damage forming roots, resulting in roots of less than half their normal length. Therefore, correcting anterior misalignment is not advised until after completion of root formation to avoid a poor long-term prognosis for these teeth (Reisberg, 2000; Rivkin, Keith, Crawford, & Hathorn, 2000a, 2000b).

During the mixed dentition stage, the incidence of crossbite increases. This is because the interosseous sutures of the maxilla begin to fuse together, restricting further growth. At the same time, the mandible begins its normal growth spurt. Therefore, the apparent jaw discrepancy increases. If the patient requires maxillary advancement to treat the discrepancy, a *reverse pull headgear (or face mask)* is a nonsurgical option (Figure 9–27A–C). In addition, a face mask can be used to correct a crossbite if it exists. The face mask is attached with labial hooks to a crossbite appliance, such as a quad helix or rapid palatal expander, to provide anchorage (Kawakami, Yagi, & Takada, 2002; Sakamoto et al., 2002). Treatment is usually done before the age of 8, to take advantage of remaining maxillary growth before suture fusion

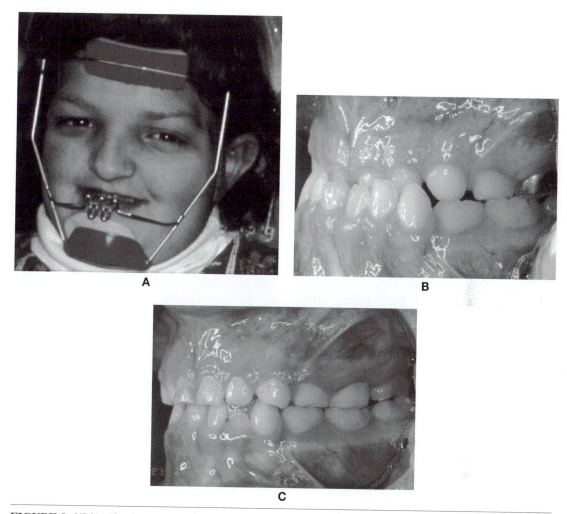

FIGURE 9–27 (A–C) A patient with reverse-pull headgear. (A) Removable reverse-pull headgear, also known as a Delaire facial mask, can be used in cooperative children to correct midfacial retrusion. An appliance attached to the teeth engages the elastic bands on the facemask to generate an anterior force on the teeth that is transmitted to the maxilla and its surrounding interosseous sutures. (B) Underbite due to maxillary deficiency, as shown in this photograph, is an indication for this device before treatment. (C) The correction achievable with the facial mask is readily apparent in this patient.

Courtesy Richard Campbell, D.M.D., M.S. & Murray Dock, D.D.S., M.S.D./Cincinnati Children's Hospital Medical Center & University of Cincinnati College of Medicine

begins. Face-mask treatment requires 12 to 14 hours of wear per day to show midface improvement (Ahn, Figueroa, Braun, & Polley, 1999). Some clinicians report success with the use of a chin cup appliance (Ishikawa, Kitazawa, Iwasaki, & Nakamura, 2000).

Another consideration of the early mixed dentition is the need for an *alveolar bone graft.* This is done to provide bony support for the eruption of the permanent lateral incisor (and later, the canine), as long as the lateral incisor is well formed and suitable for use as a fully functioning tooth (Figure 9–28A–C). Without adequate bone, the erupting tooth will have a periodontal defect, which compromises not only the lateral incisor but other adjacent teeth as well (Shashua & Omnell, 2000; Solis, Figueroa, Cohen, Polley, & Evans, 1998). As with primary bone grafting, a secondary alveolar bone graft is meant to introduce bone matrix–inducing material into the alveolar cleft site. Frequently, bone from the *iliac crest* (part of the greater pelvis) is used, although other sources of bone (e.g., the tibia, cranium, anterior chin, freeze-dried cadaver bone, and artificial substitutes such as hydroxyl apatite) have also been used (Bohman, Yamashita, Baek, & Yen, 2004; Chin, Ng, Tom, & Carstens, 2005; Enemark, Jensen, & Bosch, 2001; Hughes & Revington, 2002; Kalaaji, Lilja, Elander, & Friede, 2001; Nwoku, Al Atel, Al Shlash, Oluyadi, & Ismail, 2005; Sivarajasingam, Peil, Morse, & Shepherd, 2001). When successful, the bone graft stimulates new bone formation in the cleft site to replace the missing segment of the alveolar ridge. This provides bony support for normal eruption of the permanent lateral incisor and later the canine. It also serves to replace the missing part of the nasal floor and piriform (nasal) rim (De Riu, Lai, Congiu, & Tullio, 2004; Hynes & Earley, 2003). Maxillary expansion is usually required, if it hasn't already been accomplished earlier.

Alveolar bone grafting is usually done when the lateral incisor is beginning to reach one-half to two-thirds of normal root length (Hogan, Shand, Heggie, & Kilpatrick, 2003; Matsui, Echigo, Kimizuka, Takahashi, & Chiba, 2005; Murthy & Lehman, 2005). If the maxillary lateral incisor is missing or unusable, the bone grafting can be delayed until the maxillary canine is ready to erupt—usually between ages 11 and 13 (Da Silva Filho, Teles, Ozawa, & Filho, 2000). Some clinicians argue, however, that delaying the bone graft until the time of canine eruption creates a defect around the central incisor. More studies

are needed to evaluate the long-term outcome of periodontal health as it relates to early versus late bone grafting (De Moor, De Vree, Cornelis, & De Boever, 2002; Dempf, Teltzrow, Kramer, & Hausamen, 2002; Kolbenstvedt, Aalokken, Arctander, & Johannessen, 2002; Schultze-Mosgau, Nkenke, Schlegel, Hirschfelder, & Wiltfang, 2003; Witherow, Cox, Jones, Carr, & Waterhouse, 2002).

Secondary alveolar bone grafting is highly predictable in unilateral clefts when the greater and lesser segments are stabilized properly. In these cases, there is close to a 95% success rate (Arctander, Kolbenstvedt, Aalokken, Abyholm, & Froslie, 2005; Bajaj, Wongworawat, & Punjabi, 2003; Hynes & Earley, 2003; Kindelan & Roberts-Harry, 1999; Williams, Semb, Bearn, Shaw, & Sandy, 2003). For bilateral clefts, the success rate approaches 90% when the graft is done on one side at a time (Bohman et al., 2004; Kamakura, Yamaguchi, Kochi, Sato, & Motegi, 2003). When simultaneous grafting of both sides of a bilateral cleft is done, the success rate drops to about 70% (Mao, Ma, & Li, 2000; Shashua & Omnell, 2000).

Late Mixed Dentition (9–12 Years)

Once the permanent incisors and first molars have erupted, visible changes in the dentition are not noticeable for another 2 to 3 years. If there is midface retrusion, however, it may become more noticeable during this stage (see Figure 9–24).

Maxillary expansion for alveolar bone grafting may be done at this stage (if it had not been done before) and is timed around the time of eruption of the maxillary canine. In addition, root formation of the incisors may have progressed to the point that they can be aligned orthodontically, particularly after the alveolar bone graft, which provides sufficient

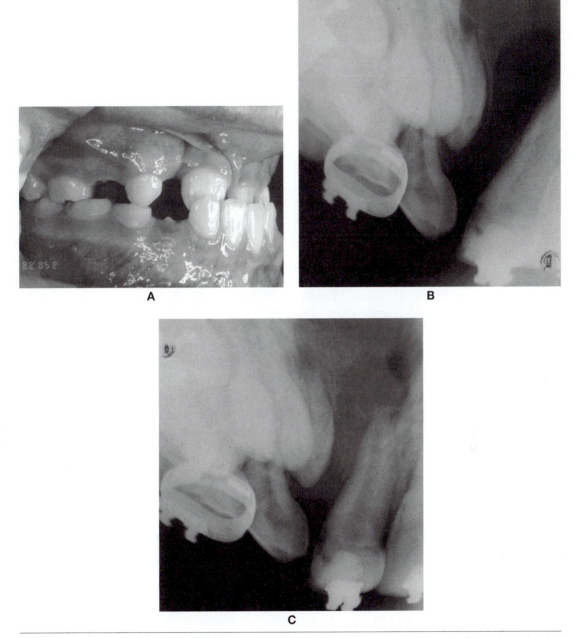

FIGURE 9–28 (A–C)   A patient needing an alveolar bone graft. (A) One can see the notching of the alveolus between the primary canine and the permanent lateral incisor. (B) In the occlusal radiograph, one can see the developing lateral incisor and the deficiency of alveolar bone. This is an indication for alveolar bone grafting. The anterior crossbite and narrowness of the maxilla will be corrected orthodontically prior to the bone graft. This gives the surgeon better access to the cleft and allows the lateral incisor to erupt through normal bone, thereby avoiding periodontal defects. (C) In this example of a larger defect, one can appreciate the deficiency of bone.

Courtesy Richard Campbell, D.M.D., M.S. & Murray Dock, D.D.S., M.S.D./Cincinnati Children's Hospital Medical Center & University of Cincinnati College of Medicine

bone into which to move the incisors, especially in bilateral clefts (Cavassan Ade, de Albuquerque, & Filho, 2004; Semb & Ramstad, 1999). Orthodontics can be started as soon as 1 to 3 months after the bone grafting (Vig, 1999). Missing teeth may be replaced by adding artificial teeth to the orthodontic appliances, at least as a temporary measure.

During the late mixed dentition period, treatment may also be needed for problems common to children without clefts. These problems may include space maintenance for prematurely lost primary teeth, the need to control moderate to severe crowding problems through selective tooth extraction, or correction of jaw position with dentofacial orthopedic measures, such as headgear or functional appliances. The decreased maxillary growth in children with repaired clefts must be considered when prescribing any of these treatment modalities.

A realistic assessment of the risks and benefits of treatment in the late mixed dentition stage has to be done before initiating treatment (Proffit & Fields, 2000). The child with cleft lip and palate is likely to require orthodontic treatment in the permanent dentition, and it is well-known that tooth eruption is frequently delayed in patients with clefts (McNamara, Foley, Garvey, & Kavanagh, 1999). Much of orthodontic treatment depends on the cooperation of the child, and cooperation is not optimal when the child is "burned out" or simply tired of orthodontic treatment (Proffit et al., 2003). Therefore, every attempt should be made to delay or combine treatment whenever possible to avoid "orthodontic fatigue" in the patient (Kapp-Simon, 2004). Most clinicians attempt to accomplish interceptive orthodontic treatment in a short 12- to 18-month period, and then give the child a rest from orthodontics until the permanent dentition completely erupts.

Adolescent Dentition (12–18 Years)

Ideally, by the time of eruption of the permanent dentition, crossbites have been corrected, alveolar bony defects are repaired, the incisors are well aligned, crowding has been managed, and the child has experienced good maxillary growth. Unfortunately, this is not always the case (Veleminska et al., 2003). For many children with clefts, the maxilla remains hypoplastic in all dimensions—vertical, sagittal, and transverse (Gaggl, Schultes, & Karcher, 1999). The adolescent growth spurt may have made these deficits more noticeable because of both the mandible's relatively normal growth and the growth of the nose (Scheuer et al., 2001). The discrepancy due to an underdeveloped maxilla and normal mandible often leads to either a Class III malocclusion with deep underbite or a Class I malocclusion with anterior openbite.

If a severe anterior crossbite persists during growth, the mandibular incisors may overerupt, causing a deep underbite. Because the maxilla is smaller than normal, the middle portion of the face is simply not as long as ideal, and thus the mandible may be overclosed, further contributing to deep underbite. Conversely, in some patients with relatively normal occlusion, mandibular growth may have been directed inferiorly and posteriorly. This allows the teeth to remain in a more normal occlusion but results in a longer facial profile and possible open bite (Lisson, Hanke, & Trankmann, 2004). Fortunately, these two phenomena appear to be occurring less often now because improvements in surgical techniques have led to fewer detrimental effects on maxillary growth. Thus, although percentages vary from one treatment center to another, about 80% of adolescents with a repaired cleft can now be successfully treated with orthodontics alone (Figure 9–29A–D). The remaining 20% or so

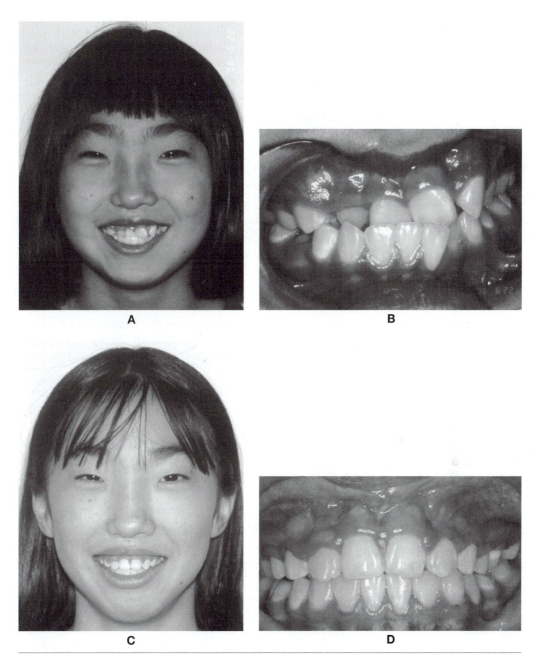

FIGURE 9–29 (A–D) Adolescent treatment with orthodontics only. (A) This patient with right unilateral cleft lip and palate exhibits only mild midfacial retrusion. (B) The anterior crossbite of this patient was judged to be amenable to orthodontic treatment alone. Orthognathic surgery was not considered to be necessary. (C) After adolescent growth and orthodontic treatment, the facial proportions remain well balanced. (D) The post-treatment occlusal result was excellent. One lateral incisor was missing, the remaining lateral incisor was extracted, and the canines were substituted for the lateral incisors.

Courtesy Richard Campbell, D.M.D., M.S. & Murray Dock, D.D.S., M.S.D./Cincinnati Children's Hospital Medical Center & University of Cincinnati College of Medicine

require orthognathic surgery, in addition to orthodontics, to align the dental arches (see Figure 9–21) (Proffit et al., 2003). Of course actual results vary from center to center.

Orthognathic surgery, which is surgery of the bones of the jaws, frequently involves a maxillary Le Fort I osteotomy to reposition the maxilla anteriorly (Figure 9–30A–D and see Figure 19–4) (Heliovaara, Ranta, Hukki, & Rintala, 2002). (See Chapter 19 for more information for the potential effects on speech.) Orthodontic treatment, in preparation for surgery, intentionally worsens the discrepancy between the upper and lower teeth in order to create sufficient space for maximum jaw repositioning.

A recent development in orthognathic surgical treatment is *distraction osteogenesis* (Figure 9–31A–C). This involves making a *corticotomy* (cut in bone) in the middle of a bone, then slowly distracting the cut ends apart with a mechanical device. New osteoid is able to regenerate between the cut ends and, in time, becomes normal bone, obviating the need for bone grafts (Kusnoto, Figueroa, & Polley, 2001). Pioneered in mandibular applications by Molina and Monasterio in Mexico and McCarthy in the United States, this is a very effective treatment option when indicated (Albert, 2000; Kita, Kochi, Imai, Yamada, & Yamaguchi, 2005; McCarthy, Katzen, Hopper, & Grayson, 2002; Molina, 2009). Distraction osteogenesis is espe-cially effective in correcting severe discrepancies that are not amenable to standard surgical techniques. Rigid external distraction osteogenesis for the midface is commonly done (Figueroa & Polley, 1999; Figueroa, Polley, & Ko, 1999; Guyette, Polley, Figueroa, & Smith, 2001; Polley & Figueroa, 2000), although internal appliances are sometimes used as well (Cohen, 1999; Scolozzi, 2008). Orthodontists and surgeons work closely together to determine the final occlusion with these techniques (Motohashi & Kuroda, 1999). The field is rapidly changing; indications and treatment timing are still being developed (Swennen, Figueroa, Schierle, Polley, & Malevez, 2000), and new devices and their variants are being introduced at a rapid pace. At present, distraction osteogenesis is primarily being used to reduce or correct severe facial deformities (Figueroa, Polley, Friede, & Ko, 2004; Liou & Tsai, 2005; Mitsugi, Ito, & Alcalde, 2005; Wang et al., 2005; Yen et al., 2005; Zwahlen & Butow, 2004).

Lastly, an adolescent who has had orthodontics and orthognathic surgery is likely to require prosthodontic replacement of missing teeth. This can be accomplished with removable dental prostheses, such as dentures or partials (see Chapter 20). More commonly, it is corrected with fixed crowns and bridges or dental implants (Moore & McCord, 2004; Reisberg, 2004). *Dental implants* are cylindrical pieces of titanium that can take the place of a

SPEECH NOTES

The effect of distraction on speech as compared to standard surgery has recently been reviewed through a meta-study of the literature (Chanchareonsook, Samman, & Whitehill, 2006). Many studies in the review found that maxillary advancement surgery had no impact on speech or velopharyngeal status. Others reported worsening of speech only in patients with either preexisting velopharyngeal insufficiency or borderline velopharyngeal function before surgery. Although there were very few systematic comparisons between distraction and conventional osteotomy, there seemed to be no clear difference in outcome of one over the other (see Chapter 19 for additional information).

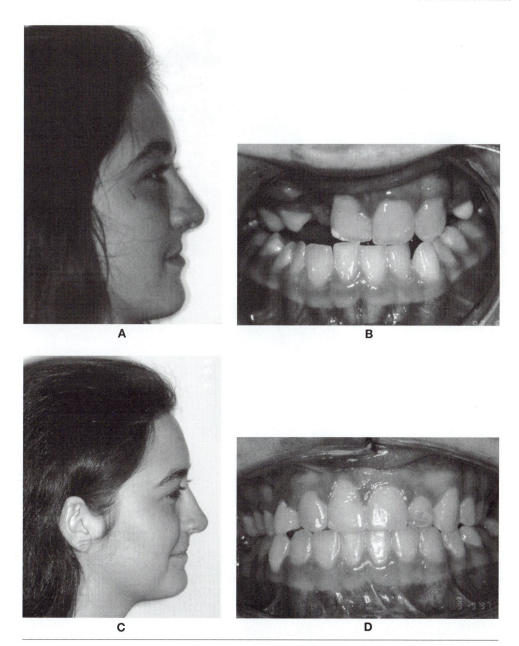

FIGURE 9–30 (A–D) Adolescent dentition treatment orthodontics and orthognathic surgery. (A) This patient with unilateral right cleft lip and palate was judged to need orthodontics and orthognathic surgery to correct her moderate midfacial retrusion. (B) This shows her malocclusion with anterior and posterior crossbite and missing right lateral incisor. (C) After orthodontic preparation, she underwent a Le Fort I maxillary osteotomy to advance the upper jaw and teeth, as well as malar implants to augment the cheeks. As a result, she has an improved profile and upper lip position. (D) Postoperative occlusion is greatly improved as well. Extraction of multiple teeth to correct her malocclusion only (without maxillary advancement surgery) would have lessened her lip support and given her an "aged" or edentulous appearance.

Courtesy Richard Campbell, D.M.D., M.S. & Murray Dock, D.D.S., M.S.D./Cincinnati Children's Hospital Medical Center & University of Cincinnati College of Medicine

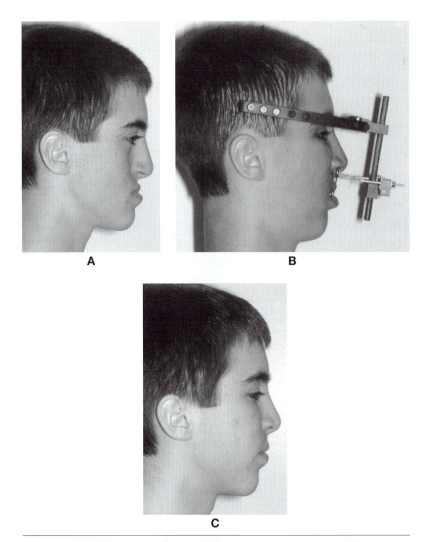

A **B**

C

FIGURE 9–31 (A–C) Rigid external distraction osteogenesis. (A) This patient with bilateral cleft lip and palate exhibits midfacial retrusion that is far outside the limits of conventional orthognathic surgery. (B) He elected to undergo the rigid external distraction procedure of Polley and Figueroa. Following maxillary Le Fort I osteotomy, the rigid framework is attached to the skull with scalp pins, and the maxilla is pulled forward or "distracted" with a screw mechanism over about an 8-week period. (C) Following stabilization, the headframe is removed, and the improvement in facial profile can be readily seen.

Courtesy Richard Campbell, D.M.D., M.S. & Murray Dock, D.D.S., M.S.D./Cincinnati Children's Hospital Medical Center & University of Cincinnati College of Medicine

missing tooth's root and are able to support crowns (Fukuda, Takahashi, & Iino, 2003; Isono et al., 2002). The coordinated involvement of the surgeon, orthodontist, and prosthodontist is required for a successful outcome (Kawakami, Yokozeki, Horiuchi, & Moriyama, 2004; Kearns, Perrott, Sharma, Kaban, & Vargervik, 1997; Kramer et al., 2005; Laine, Vahatalo,

Peltola, Tammisalo, & Happonen, 2002; Sailer, Zembic, Jung, Hammerle, & Mattiola, 2007).

THE ROLE OF SPEECH THERAPY

Speech-language pathologists, dental professionals, and surgeons must work closely together to correct speech problems related to abnormal dentition and/or malocclusion (Pinsky & Goldberg, 1977; Shprintzen et al., 1985; Vallino, Zuker, & Napoli, 2008). The role of the speech-language pathologist is to first determine whether the abnormal speech is related to abnormal structure or abnormal function. If the cause is abnormal structure, it is important to determine whether there are *obligatory distortions* (due to abnormal structure only) or *compensatory productions* (alterations in articulation placement due to abnormal structure). Speech therapy is never appropriate for obligatory distortions (Shprintzen, 1991). Instead, correction of the structural problem (abnormal dentition or malocclusion) corrects the speech without the need for speech therapy (Kummer et al., 1989; Wakumoto et al., 1996). On the other hand, if there are compensatory errors as a result of the structural abnormality, then speech therapy is required for correction, preferably after correction of the abnormal structure. Speech-language pathologists and dentists should coordinate their interventions to coincide with the stages of dental development, as outlined in the preceding sections (Shprintzen, McCall, & Skolnick, 1975). Coordination of treatment timing, sequencing, and follow-up are important for the efficient use of resources and for ensuring the best overall outcome (Shprintzen, 1982).

SUMMARY

Children with clefts or other craniofacial anomalies are at risk for dental and occlusal abnormalities. Most consonants are produced in the anterior portion of the oral cavity. Therefore, dental and occlusal abnormalities often affect speech by interfering with lip and tongue tip placement.

Because so many children with craniofacial anomalies have dental and speech problems, it is important for dental professionals and speech-language pathologists to work closely together. Interdisciplinary communication and coordination will help to determine the appropriate form of treatment needed to achieve a maximal outcome in aesthetics, mastication, and speech.

FOR REVIEW AND DISCUSSION

1. Discuss the number and type of teeth in a normal maxillary and mandibular arch of a 6-year-old. How is adult dentition different?

2. What is the Angle Classification System? Define Class I, Class II, and Class III occlusion. Which type of malocclusion is commonly seen in individuals with a history of cleft lip and palate? What are the factors that can cause that type of malocclusion?

3. What types of dental anomalies have the potential to affect speech? List the category of phonemes that are most likely to be affected by dental anomalies, and list other categories of phonemes that can be affected.

4. What types of compensatory articulation errors might you expect with an anterior crossbite and Class III malocclusion? What is the appropriate treatment?

5. What types of obligatory distortions might you expect with an anterior crossbite and Class III malocclusion? What is the appropriate treatment?

6. Describe the dental concerns and usual dental or orthodontic treatment during the following stages: infant stage, primary dentition (1–6 years), early mixed dentition (6–9 years), late mixed dentition (9–12 years), and adolescent dentition (12–18 years).

REFERENCES

Ahn, J. G., Figueroa, A. A., Braun, S., & Polley, J. W. (1999). Biomechanical considerations in distraction of the osteotomized dentomaxillary complex. *American Journal of Orthodontics & Dentofacial Orthopedics, 116*(3), 264–270.

Akcam, M. O., Evirgen, S., Uslu, O., & Toygar Memikoğlu, U. (2010). "Dental anomalies in individuals with cleft lip and/or palate". European Journal of Orthodontics 32(2), 207–213.

Albert, T. W. (2000). Oral and maxillofacial surgery: Considerations in cleft nasal deformities. *Facial Plastic Surgery, 16*(1), 79–84.

Aljamal, G., Hazza'a, A., & Rawashdeh, M. A. (2010). Prevalence of dental anomalies in a population of cleft lip and palate patients. *Cleft Palate–Craniofacial Journal, 47*(4), 413–420.

Angle, E. H. (1899). Classification of malocclusion. *Dental Cosmos, 41*, 248–264, 350–357.

Arctander, K., Kolbenstvedt, A., Aalokken, T. M., Abyholm, F., & Froslie, K. F. (2005). Computed tomography of alveolar bone grafts 20 years after repair of unilateral cleft lip and palate. *Scandinavian Journal of Plastic & Reconstructive Surgery & Hand Surgery, 39*(1), 11–14.

Bajaj, A. K., Wongworawat, A. A., & Punjabi, A. (2003). Management of alveolar clefts. *Journal of Craniofacial Surgery, 14*(6), 840–846.

Bartzela, T., Katsaros, C., Shaw, W. C., Rønning, E., Rizzell, S., et al. (2010). A longitudinal three-center study of dental arch relationship in patients with bilateral cleft lip and palate. *Cleft Palate–Craniofacial Journal, 47*(2), 167–174.

Berkowitz, S., Duncan, R., Evans, C., Friede, H., Kuijpers-Jagtman, A. M., Prahl-Anderson, B., & Rosenstein, S. (2005). Timing of cleft palate closure should be based on the ratio of the area of the cleft to that of the palatal segments and not on age alone. *Plastic and Reconstructive Surgery, 115*(6), 1483–1499.

Berkowitz, S., Mejia, M., & Bystrik, A. (2004). A comparison of the effects of the Latham-Millard procedure with those of a conservative treatment approach for dental occlusion and facial aesthetics in unilateral and bilateral complete cleft lip and palate: Part I. Dental occlusion. *Plastic and Reconstructive Surgery, 113*(1), 1–18.

Bitter, K. (2001). Repair of bilateral clefts of lip, alveolus and palate. Part 1: A refined method for the lip-adhesion in bilateral cleft lip and palate patients. *Journal of Craniomaxillofacial Surgery, 29*(1), 39–43.

Bohman, P., Yamashita, D. D., Baek, S. H., & Yen, S. L. (2004). Stabilization of an edentulous premaxilla for an alveolar bone graft: Case report. *Cleft Palate–Craniofacial Journal, 41*(2), 214–217.

Bongaarts, C. A., Kuijpers-Jagtman, A. M., van't Hof, M. A., & Prahl-Andersen, B. (2004). The effect of infant orthopedics on the occlusion of the deciduous dentition in children with complete unilateral cleft lip and palate (Dutchcleft). *Cleft Palate–Craniofacial Journal, 41*(6), 633–641.

Braumann, B., Keilig, L., Bourauel, C., & Jager, A. (2002). Three-dimensional analysis of morphological changes in the maxilla of patients with cleft lip and palate. *Cleft Palate–Craniofacial Journal, 39*(1), 1–11.

Cabete, H. F., Gomide, M. R., & Costa, B. (2000). Evaluation of primary dentition in cleft lip and palate children with and without natal/neonatal teeth. *Cleft Palate–Craniofacial Journal, 37*(4), 406–409.

Camporesi, M., Baccetti, T., Marinelli, A., Defraia, E., & Franchi, L. (2010). Maxillary dental anomalies in children with cleft lip and palate: A controlled study. *International Journal of Paediatric Dentistry, 20*(6), 442–450.

Cavassan Ade, O., de Albuquerque, M. D., & Filho, L. C. (2004). Rapid maxillary expansion after secondary alveolar bone graft in a patient with bilateral cleft lip and palate. *Cleft Palate–Craniofacial Journal, 41*(3), 332–339.

Chan, K. T., Hayes, C., Shusterman, S., Mulliken, J. B., & Will, L. A. (2003). The effects of active infant orthopedics on occlusal relationships in unilateral complete cleft lip and palate. *Cleft Palate–Craniofacial Journal, 40*(5), 511–517.

Chanchareonsook, N., Samman, N., & Whitehill, T. L. (2006). The effect of cranio-maxillofacial osteotomies and distraction osteogenesis on speech and velopharyngeal status: A critical review. *Cleft Palate–Craniofacial Journal, 43*(4), 477–487.

Chapple, J. R., & Nunn, J. H. (2001). The oral health of children with clefts of the lip, palate, or both. *Cleft Palate–Craniofacial Journal, 38*(5), 525–528.

Chin, M., Ng, T., Tom, W. K., & Carstens, M. (2005). Repair of alveolar clefts with recombinant human bone morphogenetic protein (rhBMP-2) in patients with clefts. *Journal of Craniofacial Surgery, 16*(5), 778–789.

Cho, B. (2001). Unilateral complete cleft lip and palate repair using lip adhesion and passive alveolar molding appliance. *Journal of Craniofacial Surgery, 12*(2), 148–156.

Cohen, S. R. (1999). Midface distraction. *Seminars in Orthodontics, 5*(1), 52–58.

Cutting, C., Grayson, B., Brecht, L., Santiago, P., Wood, R., & Kwon, S. (1998). Presurgical columellar elongation and primary retrograde nasal reconstruction in one-stage bilateral cleft lip and nose repair. *Plastic and Reconstructive Surgery, 101*(3), 630–639.

Da Silva Filho, O. G., Teles, S. G., Ozawa, T. O., & Filho, L. C. (2000). Secondary bone graft and eruption of the permanent canine in patients with alveolar clefts: Literature review and case report. *Angle Orthodontist, 70*(2), 174–178.

Da Silveira, A. C., Oliveira, N., Gonzalez, S., Shahani, M., Reisberg, D., Daw, J. L., Jr., & Cohen, M. (2003). Modified nasal alveolar molding appliance for management of cleft lip defect. *Journal of Craniofacial Surgery, 14*(5), 700–703.

De Moor, R. J., De Vree, H. M., Cornelis, C., & De Boever, J. A. (2002). Cervical root resorption in two patients with unilateral complete cleft of the lip and palate. *Cleft Palate–Craniofacial Journal, 39*(5), 541–545.

De Riu, G., Lai, V., Congiu, M., & Tullio, A. (2004). Secondary bone grafting of alveolar cleft. *Minerva Stomatologica, 53*(10), 571–579.

Dempf, R., Teltzrow, T., Kramer, F. J., & Hausamen, J. E. (2002). Alveolar bone grafting in patients with complete clefts: A comparative study between secondary and tertiary bone grafting. *Cleft Palate–Craniofacial Journal, 39*(1), 18–25.

Dewinter, G., Quirynen, M., Heidbuchel, K., Verdonck, A., Willems, G., & Carels, C. (2003). Dental abnormalities, bone graft quality, and periodontal conditions in patients with unilateral cleft lip and palate at different phases of orthodontic treatment. *Cleft Palate–Craniofacial Journal, 40*(4), 343–350.

DiBiase, A. T., DiBiase, D. D., Hay, N. J., & Sommerlad, B. C. (2002). The relationship between arch dimensions and the 5-year index in the primary dentition of patients with complete UCLP. *Cleft Palate—Craniofacial Journal, 39*(6), 635–640.

Doruk, C., & Kilic, B. (2005). Extraoral nasal molding in a newborn with unilateral cleft lip and palate: A case report. *Cleft Palate–Craniofacial Journal, 42*(6), 699–702.

Enemark, H., Jensen, J., & Bosch, C. (2001). Mandibular bone graft material for reconstruction of alveolar cleft defects: Long-term results. *Cleft Palate–Craniofacial Journal, 38*(2), 155–163.

Figueroa, A. A., & Polley, J. W. (1999). Management of severe cleft maxillary deficiency with distraction osteogenesis: Procedure and results. *American Journal of Orthodontic and Dentofacial Orthopedics, 115*(1), 1–12.

Figueroa, A. A., Polley, J. W., Friede, H., & Ko, E. W. (2004). Long-term skeletal stability after maxillary advancement with distraction osteogenesis using a rigid external distraction device in cleft maxillary deformities. *Plastic and Reconstructive Surgery, 114*(6), 1382–1392; Discussion 1382–1392.

Figueroa, A. A., Polley, J. W., & Ko, E. W. (1999). Maxillary distraction for the management of cleft maxillary hypoplasia with a rigid external distraction system. *Seminars in Orthodontics, 5*(1), 46–51.

Fukuda, M., Takahashi, T., & Iino, M. (2003). Dentoalveolar reconstruction of a missing premaxilla using bone graft and endosteal implants. *Journal of Oral Rehabilitation, 30*(1), 87–90.

Gable, T. O., Kummer, A. W., Lee, L., Creaghead, N. A., & Moore, L. J. (1995). Premature loss of the maxillary primary incisors: Effect on speech production. *Journal of Dentistry for Children, 62*(3), 173–179.

Gaggl, A., Schultes, G., & Karcher, H. (1999). Aesthetic and functional outcome of surgical and orthodontic correction of bilateral clefts of lip, palate, and alveolus. *Cleft Palate–Craniofacial Journal, 36*(5), 407–412.

Gaggl, A., Schultes, G., Karcher, E. L., & Mossbock, R. (1999). Periodontal disease in patients with cleft palate and patients with unilateral and bilateral clefts of lip, palate, and alveolus. *Journal of Periodontology, 70*(2), 171–178.

Garfinkle, J. S., King, T. W., Grayson, B. H., Brecht, L. E., & Cutting, C. B. (2011). A 12-year anthropometric evaluation of the nose in bilateral cleft lip-cleft palate patients following and cutting bilateral cleft lip and nose reconstruction. *Plastic and Reconstructive Surgery, 127*(4), 1659–1667.

Garrahy, A., Millett, D. T., & Ayoub, A. F. (2005). Early assessment of dental arch development in repaired unilateral cleft lip and unilateral cleft lip and palate versus controls. *Cleft Palate–Craniofacial Journal, 42*(4), 385–391.

Grayson, B., & Cutting, C. B. (2001). Presurgical nasoalveolar orthopedic molding in primary correction of the nose, lip, and alveolus of infants born with unilateral and bilateral clefts. *Cleft Palate–Craniofacial Journal, 38*(3), 193–198.

Grayson, B., & Maull, D. (2004). Nasoalveolar molding for infants born with clefts of the lip, alveolus, and palate. *Clinics in Plastic Surgery, 31*(2), 149–158, vii.

Guyette, T. W., Polley, J. W., Figueroa, A., & Smith, B. E. (2001). Changes in speech following maxillary distraction osteogenesis. *Cleft Palate–Craniofacial Journal, 38*(3), 199–205.

Hathaway, R. R., Eppley, B. L., Hennon, D. K., Nelson, C. L., & Sadove, A. M. (1999). Primary alveolar cleft bone grafting in unilateral cleft lip and palate: Arch dimensions at age 8. *Journal of Craniofacial Surgery, 10*(1), 58–67.

Hathaway, R. R., Eppley, B. L., Nelson, C. L., & Sadove, A. M. (1999). Primary alveolar cleft bone grafting in unilateral cleft lip and palate: Craniofacial form at age 8. *Journal of Craniofacial Surgery, 10*(1), 68–72.

Heliovaara, A., Ranta, R., Hukki, J., & Rintala, A. (2002). Skeletal stability of Le Fort I osteotomy in patients with isolated cleft palate and bilateral cleft lip and palate. *International Journal of Oral & Maxillofacial Surgery, 31*(4), 358–363.

Heliovaara, A., Ranta, R., & Rautio, J. (2004). Dental abnormalities in permanent dentition in children with submucous cleft palate. *Acta Odontologica Scandinavica, 62*(3), 129–131.

Hogan, L., Shand, J. M., Heggie, A. A., & Kilpatrick, N. (2003). Canine eruption into grafted alveolar clefts: A retrospective study. *Australian Dental Journal, 48*(2), 119–124.

Hughes, C. W., & Revington, P. J. (2002). The proximal tibia donor site in cleft alveolar bone grafting: Experience of 75 consecutive cases. *Journal of Craniomaxillofacial Surgery, 30*(1), 12–16; Discussion 17.

Hynes, P. J., & Earley, M. J. (2003). Assessment of secondary alveolar bone grafting using a modification of the Bergland grading system. *British Journal of Plastic Surgery, 56*(7), 630–636.

Ishikawa, H., Kitazawa, S., Iwasaki, H., & Nakamura, S. (2000). Effects of maxillary protraction combined with chin-cap therapy in unilateral cleft lip and palate patients. *Cleft Palate–Craniofacial Journal, 37*(1), 92–97.

Isono, H., Kaida, K., Hamada, Y., Kokubo, Y., Ishihara, M., Hirashita, A., & Kuwahara, Y. (2002). The reconstruction of bilateral clefts using endosseous implants after bone grafting. *American Journal of Orthodontics & Dentofacial Orthopedics, 121*(4), 403–410.

Johnson, N. C. L., & Sandy, J. R. (1999). Tooth position and speech—Is there a relationship? *The Angle Orthodontist, 69*(4), 306–310.

Kalaaji, A., Lilja, J., Elander, A., & Friede, H. (2001). Tibia as donor site for alveolar bone grafting in patients with cleft lip and palate: Long-term experience. *Scandinavian Journal of Plastic & Reconstructive Surgery & Hand Surgery, 35*(1), 35–42.

Kamakura, S., Yamaguchi, T., Kochi, S., Sato, A., & Motegi, K. (2003). Preliminary report of two-stage secondary alveolar bone grafting for patients with bilateral cleft lip and palate. *Cleft Palate–Craniofacial Journal, 40*(5), 449–452.

Kapp-Simon, K. A. (2004). Psychological issues in cleft lip and palate. *Clinics in Plastic Surgery, 31*(2), 347–352.

Katz, M. I. (1992). Angle classification revisited 2: A modified Angle classification *American Journal of Orthodontic and Dentofacial Orthopedics, 102*(3), 277–284.

Kawakami, M., Yagi, T., & Takada, K. (2002). Maxillary expansion and protraction in correction of midface retrusion in a complete unilateral cleft lip and palate patient. *Angle Orthodontist, 72*(4), 355–361.

Kawakami, S., Yokozeki, M., Horiuchi, S., & Moriyama, K. (2004). Oral rehabilitation of an orthodontic patient with cleft lip and palate and hypodontia using secondary bone grafting, osseo-integrated implants, and prosthetic treatment. *Cleft Palate–Craniofacial Journal*, *41*(3), 279–284.

Kearns, G., Perrott, D. H., Sharma, A., Kaban, L. B., & Vargervik, K. (1997). Placement of endosseous implants in grafted alveolar clefts. *Cleft Palate–Craniofacial Journal*, *34*(6), 520–525.

Kindelan, J., & Roberts-Harry, D. (1999). A 5-year post-operative review of secondary alveolar bone grafting in the Yorkshire region. *British Journal of Orthodontics*, *26*(3), 211–217.

Kirchberg, A., Treide, A., & Hemprich, A. (2004). Investigation of caries prevalence in children with cleft lip, alveolus, and palate. *Journal of Craniomaxillofacial Surgery*, *32*(4), 216–219.

Kirschner, R. E., & LaRossa, D. (2000). Cleft lip and palate. *Otolaryngologic Clinics of North America*, *33*(6), 1191–1215, v–vi.

Kita, H., Kochi, S., Imai, Y., Yamada, A., & Yamaguchi, T. (2005). Rigid external distraction using skeletal anchorage to cleft maxilla united with alveolar bone grafting. *Cleft Palate–Craniofacial Journal*, *42*(3), 318–327.

Kolbenstvedt, A., Aalokken, T. M., Arctander, K., & Johannessen, S. (2002). CT appearances of unilateral cleft palate 20 years after bone graft surgery. *Acta Radiologica*, *43*(6), 567–570.

Kramer, F. J., Baethge, C., Swennen, G., Bremer, B., Schwestka-Polly, R., & Dempf, R. (2005). Dental implants in patients with orofacial clefts: A long-term follow-up study. *International Journal of Oral & Maxillofacial Surgery*, *34*(7), 715–721.

Kuijpers-Jagtman, A. M., Borstlap-Engels, V. M., Spauwen, P. H., & Borstlap, W. A. (2000). Team management of orofacial clefts. *Nederlands Tijdschrift voor Tandheelkunde*, *107*(11), 447–451.

Kummer, A. W., Strife, J. L., Grau, W. H., Creaghead, N. A., & Lee, L. (1989). The effects of Le Fort I osteotomy with maxillary movement on articulation, resonance, and velopharyngeal function. *Cleft Palate Journal*, *26*(3), 193–199; Discussion 199–200.

Kusnoto, B., Figueroa, A. A., & Polley, J. W. (2001). Radiographic evaluation of bone formation in the pterygoid region after maxillary distraction with a rigid external distraction (RED) device. *Journal of Craniofacial Surgery*, *12*(2), 109–117; Discussion 118.

Laine, J., Vahatalo, K., Peltola, J., Tammisalo, T., & Happonen, R. P. (2002). Rehabilitation of patients with congenital unrepaired cleft palate defects using free iliac crest bone grafts and dental implants. *International Journal of Oral Maxillofacial Implants*, *17*(4), 573–580.

Lee, C. T., Grayson, B. H., Cutting, C. B., Brecht, L. E., & Lin, W. Y. (2004). Prepubertal midface growth in unilateral cleft lip and palate following alveolar molding and gingivoperiosteoplasty. *Cleft Palate–Craniofacial Journal*, *41*(4), 375–380.

Liou, E. J., & Tsai, W. C. (2005). A new protocol for maxillary protraction in cleft patients: Repetitive weekly protocol of alternate rapid maxillary expansions and constrictions. *Cleft Palate–Craniofacial Journal*, *42*(2), 121–127.

Lisson, J. A., Hanke, L., & Trankmann, J. (2004). Vertical changes in patients with complete unilateral and bilateral cleft lip, alveolus and palate. *Journal of Orofacial Orthopedics*, *65*(3), 246–258.

Maciel, S. P., Costa, B., & Gomide, M. R. (2005). Difference in the prevalence of enamel alterations affecting central incisors of children with complete unilateral cleft lip and palate. *Cleft Palate–Craniofacial Journal, 42*(4), 392–395.

Malanczuk, T., Opitz, C., & Retzlaff, R. (1999). Structural changes of dental enamel in both dentitions of cleft lip and palate patients. *Journal of Orofacial Orthopedics, 60*(4), 259–268.

Mao, C., Ma, L., & Li, X. (2000). A retrospective study of bilateral alveolar bone grafting. *Chinese Medical Sciences Journal, 15*(1), 49–51.

Matsui, K., Echigo, S., Kimizuka, S., Takahashi, M., & Chiba, M. (2005). Clinical study on eruption of permanent canines after secondary alveolar bone grafting. *Cleft Palate–Craniofacial Journal, 42*(3), 309–313.

McCarthy, J. G., Katzen, J. T., Hopper, R., & Grayson, B. H. (2002). The first decade of mandibular distraction: Lessons we have learned. *Plastic and Reconstructive Surgery, 110*(7), 1704–1713.

McNamara, C. M., Foley, T. F., Garvey, M. T., & Kavanagh, P. T. (1999). Premature dental eruption: Report of case. *Journal of Dentistry for Children, 66*(1), 70–72.

Millard, D. R., Latham, R., Huifen, X., Spiro, S., & Morovic, C. (1999). Cleft lip and palate treated by presurgical orthopedics, gingivoperiosteoplasty, and lip adhesion (POPLA) compared with previous lip adhesion method: A preliminary study of serial dental casts. *Plastic and Reconstructive Surgery, 103*(6), 1630–1644.

Mitsugi, M., Ito, O., & Alcalde, R. E. (2005). Maxillary bone transportation in alveolar cleft-transport distraction osteogenesis for treatment of alveolar cleft repair. *British Journal of Plastic Surgery, 58*(5), 619–625.

Molina, F. (2009). Mandibular distraction osteogenesis: A clinical experience of the last 17 years. *Journal of Craniofacial Surgery, 20* (Suppl. 2), 1794–1800.

Moller, K. T. (1994). Dental-occlusal and other oral conditions and speech. In J. E. Bernthal & N. W. Bankson (Eds.), *Child phonology: Characteristics, assessment, and intervention with special populations* (pp. 3–28). New York: Thieme Medical Publishers.

Moore, D., & McCord, J. F. (2004). Prosthetic dentistry and the unilateral cleft lip and palate patient. The last 30 years. A review of the prosthodontic literature in respect of treatment options. *European Journal of Prosthodontics & Restorative Dentistry, 12*(2), 70–74.

Motohashi, N., & Kuroda, T. (1999). A 3-D computer-aided design system applied to diagnosis and treatment planning in orthodontics and orthognathic surgery. *European Journal of Orthodontics, 21*(3), 263–274.

Mouradian, W. E., Omnell, M. L., & Williams, B. (1999). Ethics for orthodontists. *Angle Orthodontist, 69*(4), 295–299.

Murthy, A. S., & Lehman, J. A. (2005). Evaluation of alveolar bone grafting: A survey of ACPA teams. *Cleft Palate–Craniofacial Journal, 42*(1), 99–101.

Nazarian Mobin, S. S., Karatsonyi, A., Vidar, E. N., Gamer, S., Groper, J., Hammoudeh, J. A., & Urata, M. M. (2011). Is presurgical nasoalveolar molding therapy more effective in unilateral or bilateral cleft lip-cleft palate patients? *Plastic and Reconstructive Surgery, 127*(3), 1263–1269.

Ngan, P., Alkire, R. G., & Fields, H., Jr. (1999). Management of space problems in the primary and mixed dentitions. *Journal of the American Dental Association, 130*(9), 1330–1339.

Nwoku, A. L., Al Atel, A., Al Shlash, S., Oluyadi, B. A., & Ismail, S. (2005). Retrospective analysis of secondary alveolar cleft grafts using iliac of chin bone. *Journal of Craniofacial Surgery, 16*(5), 864–868.

Oosterkamp, B. C., Van Oort, R. P., Dijkstra, P. U., Stellingsma, K., Bierman, M. W., &

de Bont, L. G. (2005). Effect of an intraoral retrusion plate on maxillary arch dimensions in complete bilateral cleft lip and palate patients. *Cleft Palate–Craniofacial Journal, 42*(3), 239–244.

Pfeifer, T. M., Grayson, B. H., & Cutting, C. B. (2002). Nasoalveolar molding and gingivoperiosteoplasty versus alveolar bone graft: An outcome analysis of costs in the treatment of unilateral cleft alveolus. *Cleft Palate–Craniofacial Journal, 39*(1), 26–29.

Pinsky, T. M., & Goldberg, H. J. (1977). Potential for clinical cooperation between dentistry and speech pathology. *International Dental Journal, 27*(4), 363–369.

Polley, J., & Figueroa, A. (2000). Re: Maxillary distraction osteogenesis: A method with skeletal anchorage. *Journal of Craniofacial Surgery 11*(3), 295.

Posnick, J. C., & Ricalde, P. (2004). Cleft-orthognathic surgery. *Clinics in Plastic Surgery, 31*(2), 315–330.

Prahl, C., Kuijpers-Jagtman, A. M., van't Hof, M. A., & Prahl-Andersen, B. (2003). A randomized prospective clinical trial of the effect of infant orthopedics in unilateral cleft lip and palate: Prevention of collapse of the alveolar segments (Dutchcleft). *Cleft Palate–Craniofacial Journal, 40*(4), 337–342.

Prahl, C., Kuijpers-Jagtman, A. M., van't Hof, M. A., & Prahl-Andersen, B. (2005). Infant orthopedics in UCLP: Effect on feeding, weight, and length: A randomized clinical trial (Dutchcleft). *Cleft Palate–Craniofacial Journal, 42*(2), 171–177.

Proffit, W. R., & Fields, H. W., Jr. (2000). *Contemporary Orthodontics* (3rd ed.). St. Louis, MO: Mosby.

Proffit, W. R., White, R. P., & Sarver, D. M. (2003). *Contemporary treatment of dentofacial deformity.* St. Louis, MO: Mosby.

Quirynen, M., Dewinter, G., Avontroodt, P., Heidbuchel, K., Verdonck, A., & Carels, C.

(2003). A split-mouth study on periodontal and microbial parameters in children with complete unilateral cleft lip and palate. *Journal of Clinical Periodontology, 30*(1), 49–56.

Reisberg, D. J. (2000). Dental and prosthodontic care for patients with cleft or craniofacial conditions. *Cleft Palate–Craniofacial Journal, 37*(6), 534–537.

Reisberg, D. J. (2004). Prosthetic habilitation of patients with clefts. *Clinics in Plastic Surgery, 31*(2), 353–360.

Renkielska, A., Wojtaszek-Slominska, A., & Dobke, M. (2005). Early cleft lip repair in children with unilateral complete cleft lip and palate: A case against primary alveolar repair. *Annals of Plastic Surgery, 54*(6), 595–597; Discussion 598–599.

Rivkin, C. J., Keith, O., Crawford, P. J., & Hathorn, I. S. (2000a). Dental care for the patient with a cleft lip and palate. Part 1: From birth to the mixed dentition stage. *British Dental Journal, 188*(2), 78–83.

Rivkin, C. J., Keith, O., Crawford, P. J., & Hathorn, I. S. (2000b). Dental care for the patient with a cleft lip and palate. Part 2: The mixed dentition stage through to adolescence and young adulthood. *British Dental Journal, 188*(3), 131–134.

Sachs, S. A. (2002). Nasoalveolar molding and gingivoperiosteoplasty verses alveolar bone graft: An outcome analysis of costs in the treatment of unilateral cleft alveolus. *Cleft Palate–Craniofacial Journal, 39*(5), 570–571.

Sailer, I., Zembic, A., Jung, R. E., Hammerle, C. H., & Mattiola, A. (2007). Single-tooth implant reconstructions: Esthetic factors influencing the decision between titanium and zirconia abutments in anterior regions. *The European Journal of Esthetic Dentistry, 2*(3), 296–310.

Sakamoto, T., Sakamoto, S., Harazaki, M., Isshiki, Y., & Yamaguchi, H. (2002).

Orthodontic treatment for jaw deformities in cleft lip and palate patients with the combined use of an external-expansion arch and a facial mask. *Bulletin of Tokyo Dental College, 43*(4), 223–229.

Scheuer, H. A., Holtje, W. J., Hasund, A., & Pfeifer, G. (2001). Prognosis of facial growth in patients with unilateral complete clefts of the lip, alveolus and palate. *Journal of Craniomaxillofacial Surgery, 29* (4), 198–204.

Schultes, G., Gaggl, A., & Karcher, H. (1999). Comparison of periodontal disease in patients with clefts of palate and patients with unilateral clefts of lip, palate, and alveolus. *Cleft Palate–Craniofacial Journal, 36*(4), 322–327.

Schultze-Mosgau, S., Nkenke, E., Schlegel, A. K., Hirschfelder, U., & Wiltfang, J. (2003). Analysis of bone resorption after secondary alveolar cleft bone grafts before and after canine eruption in connection with orthodontic gap closure or prosthodontic treatment. *Journal of Oral & Maxillofacial Surgery, 61*(11), 1245–1248.

Scolozzi, P. (2008). Distraction osteogenesis in the management of severe maxillary hypoplasia in cleft lip and palate patients. *Journal of Craniofacial Surgery, 19*(5), 1199–1214.

Semb, G., & Ramstad, T. (1999). The influence of alveolar bone grafting on the orthodontic and prosthodontic treatment of patients with cleft lip and palate. *Dental Update, 26*(2), 60–64.

Shashua, D., & Omnell, M. L. (2000). Radiographic determination of the position of the maxillary lateral incisor in the cleft alveolus and parameters for assessing its habilitation prospects. *Cleft Palate– Craniofacial Journal, 37*(1), 21–25.

Shprintzen, R. J. (1982). Palatal and pharyngeal anomalies in craniofacial syndromes. *Birth Defects Original Article Series, 18*(1), 53–78.

Shprintzen, R. J. (1991). Fallibility of clinical research. *Cleft Palate–Craniofacial Journal, 28*(2), 136–140.

Shprintzen, R. J., McCall, G. N., & Skolnick, M. L. (1975). A new therapeutic technique for the treatment of velopharyngeal incompetence. *Journal of Speech and Hearing Disorders, 40*(1), 69–83.

Shprintzen, R. J., Siegel-Sadewitz, V. L., Amato, J., & Goldberg, R. B. (1985). Anomalies associated with cleft lip, cleft palate, or both. *American Journal of Medical Genetics, 20*(4), 585–595.

Sivarajasingam, V., Peil, G., Morse, M., & Shepherd, J. P. (2001). Secondary bone grafting of alveolar clefts: A densitometric comparison of iliac crest and tibial bone grafts. *Cleft Palate–Craniofacial Journal, 38*(1), 11–14.

Solis, A., Figueroa, A. A., Cohen, M., Polley, J. W., & Evans, C. A. (1998). Maxillary dental development in complete unilateral alveolar clefts. *Cleft Palate–Craniofacial Journal, 35*(4), 320–328.

Strauss, R. P. (1998). Cleft palate and craniofacial teams in the United States and Canada: A national survey of team organization and standards of care. The American Cleft Palate–Craniofacial Association (ACPA) Team Standards Committee. *Cleft Palate– Craniofacial Journal, 35*(6), 473–480.

Strauss, R. P. (1999). The organization and delivery of craniofacial health services: The state of the art. *Cleft Palate–Craniofacial Journal, 36*(3), 189–195.

Strong, S. M. (2002). Adolescent dentistry: Multidisciplinary treatment for the cleft lip/palate patient. *Practical Procedures & Aesthetic Dentistry, 14*(4), 333–338; Quiz 340, 342.

Swennen, G., Figueroa, A. A., Schierle, H., Polley, J. W., & Malevez, C. (2000).

Maxillary distraction osteogenesis: A two-dimensional mathematical model. *Journal of Craniofacial Surgery*, *11*(4), 312–317.

Taher, A. (1997). Speech defect associated with Class III jaw relationship. *Plastic and Reconstructive Surgery*, *99*(4), 1200.

Tannure, P. N., Oliveira, C. A., Maia, L. C., Vieira, A. R., Granjeiro, J. M., & de Castro Costa, M. (2012). Prevalence of dental anomalies in nonsyndromic individuals with cleft lip and palate: A systematic review and meta-analysis. *Cleft Palate–Craniofacial Journal*, *49*(2), 194–200.

Trost-Cardamone, J. E. (1997). Diagnosis of specific cleft palate speech error patterns for planning therapy of physical management needs. In K. R. Bzoch (Ed.), *Communicative disorders related to cleft lip and palate* (vol. 4, pp. 313–330). Austin, TX: Pro-Ed.

Turvey, T. A., Vig, K. W. L., & Fonseca, R. J. (1996). *Facial clefts and craniosynostosis, principles and management*. Chapel Hill, NC: W. B. Saunders.

Vallino, L. D., Zuker, R., & Napoli, J. A. (2008). A study of speech, language, hearing, and dentition in children with cleft lip only. *Cleft Palate–Craniofacial Journal*, *45*(5), 485–494.

Vasan, N. (1999). Management of children with clefts of the lip or palate: An overview. *New Zealand Dental Journal*, *95*(419), 14–20.

Veleminska, J., Smahel, Z., & Mullerova, Z. (2003). Facial growth and development during the pubertal period in patients with complete unilateral cleft of lip and palate. *Acta Chirurgiae Plasticae*, *45*(1), 22–31.

Vig, K. W. (1999). Alveolar bone grafts: The surgical/orthodontic management of the cleft maxilla. *Annals of the Academy of Medicine, Singapore*, *28*(5), 721–727.

Wakumoto, M., Isaacson, K. G., Friel, S., Suzuki, N., Gibbon, F., Nixon, F., Hard-castle, W. J., et al. (1996). Preliminary study of the articulatory reorganization of fricative consonants following osteotomy. *Folia Phoniatrica et Logopedica*, *48*(6), 275–289.

Wang, X. X., Wang, X., Yi, B., Li, Z. L., Liang, C., & Lin, Y. (2005). Internal midface distraction in correction of severe maxillary hypoplasia secondary to cleft lip and palate. *Plastic and Reconstructive Surgery*, *116*(1), 51–60.

Wangsrimongkol, T., & Jansawang, W. (2010). The assessment of treatment outcome by evaluation of dental arch relationships in cleft lip/palate. *Journal of the Medical Association of Thailand*, *93*(Suppl. 4), S100–S106.

Williams, A., Semb, G., Bearn, D., Shaw, W., & Sandy, J. (2003). Prediction of outcomes of secondary alveolar bone grafting in children born with unilateral cleft lip and palate. *European Journal of Orthodontics*, *25*(2), 205–211.

Witherow, H., Cox, S., Jones, E., Carr, R., & Waterhouse, N. (2002). A new scale to assess radiographic success of secondary alveolar bone grafts. *Cleft Palate–Craniofacial Journal*, *39*(3), 255–260.

Yen, S. L., Yamashita, D. D., Gross, J., Meara, J. G., Yamazaki, K., Kim, T. H., & Reinisch, J. (2005). Combining orthodontic tooth movement with distraction osteogenesis to close cleft spaces and improve maxillary arch form in cleft lip and palate patients. *American Journal of Orthodontics & Dentofacial Orthopedics*, *127*(2), 224–232.

Zwahlen, R. A., & Butow, K. W. (2004). Maxillary distraction resulting in facial advancement at Le Fort III level in cleft lip and palate patients: A report of two cases. *Oral Surgery, Oral Medicine, Oral Pathology, Oral Radiology & Endodontics*, *98*(5), 541–545.

CHAPTER

10

PSYCHOSOCIAL ASPECTS OF CLEFT LIP/PALATE AND CRANIOFACIAL ANOMALIES

JANET R. SCHULTZ, PH.D., ABPP

CHAPTER OUTLINE

INTRODUCTION

When a baby is born, the infant is not just born to his parents. The child is born into a family, a social network, and society. These layers of context into which the child is born are also forces that impact the child's development. At the same time, the child brings into the world his or her genetic endowment and the characteristics developed during intrauterine life. Among these are temperament, certain instinctual behaviors, and physical appearance. For some children, one characteristic is a cleft lip and/or palate or other craniofacial condition. The child's genetic contribution interacts with the complex context into which he or she is born so that the developing individual is both affected by and affecting that environment.

FAMILY ISSUES

At the birth of any child, the lives of the parents and other family members are changed forever. This is especially true when the child is born with a cleft or other craniofacial condition. There is always an initial shock when parents learn that the child is not what they expected. The parents may struggle with initial issues with attachment. A time of adjustment follows. Finally, the family settles in with the reality of dealing with a child with a chronic medical condition.

Initial Shock and Adjustment

The birth of a child is typically a very happy event. Parents' first questions almost always include "Is the baby alright?" When a baby is born with a cleft lip, there is immediate knowledge of the cleft and, therefore, distress. When an infant is born with a cleft of the velum or a submucous cleft, however, hours (or longer) may elapse before the parents are informed that there is a problem.

For many families, the birth of a child with a cleft is a serious event in their lives. Most have never seen a person with an unrepaired cleft and hence know little about the problem or what can be done about it (Dolger-Hafner, Bartsch, Trimbach, Zobel, & Witt, 1997; Middleton, Lass, Starr, & Pannbacker, 1986). As a result, parents often experience both shock and sadness. There may be a period of mourning for the anticipated child and then adjustment to the child that they actually have (van Staden & Gerhardt, 1995). Strong feelings of love, protectiveness, and excitement often conflict with other feelings of hurt, fear, disappointment, betrayal, resentment, and guilt (Coy, Speltz, & Jones, 2002; Despars et al., 2011). Resolution of these feelings is complicated by a whirlwind of medical concerns that characterize early infancy for children with a cleft.

During the first few weeks of the baby's life, parents of infants with clefts must deal with many challenges. Immediately, they need to learn how to feed the infant. This can be a practical challenge that requires additional time in the already demanding schedule of new parents. Typically, parents mostly lose what would have been restorative time for themselves, such as relaxing, sleeping, and engaging in favorite activities (Winston, Dunbar, Reed, & Francis-Connolly, 2010). There is also the emotional challenge of feeling less than confident and competent about feeding. In most societies, including that of the United States, successful feeding is associated with parental skill and success (Kedesdy & Budd, 1998).

From very early in the child's development, parents also must begin to obtain information about the reason their child has an anomaly as well as about future surgeries and appliances for treatment. During this time, parents may actually find themselves supporting grandparents or other relatives rather than receiving support themselves. Some parents face accusations or perceived accusations about the reason for the cleft from various family members or medical personnel. Additionally, many parents do not remember or do not receive the information they most want to know (Young, O'Riordan, Goldstein, & Robin, 2001).

Parents of infants with visible differences are likely to experience the staring of children, and even other adults, when they take their babies out in public. These experiences may serve to confirm the fears of the child's social rejection, which tend to rise rapidly in the minds of parents at their first contact with the baby (Barr, Thibeault, Muntz, & de Serres, 2007). Therefore, they need to learn how to cope with staring and talk to other people about the baby's cleft. The more visible the anomaly is to the public, the more stressful the situation for parents (Rosenberg, Kapp-Simon, Starr, Cradock, & Speltz, 2011). On the other hand, these challenges may actually help to create strong, protective bonds to the babies. One study found that babies with cleft lip and palate were more securely attached to their parents than those who had cleft palate only (Coy, Speltz, & Jones, 2002).

Mothers of babies with clefts report higher levels of stress than mothers of unaffected babies (Pope, Tilman, & Snyder, 2005; Speltz, Armsden, & Clarren 1990). They may also have more concerns about their competence as parents. There are some mixed findings that mothers may be less responsive to and interactive with infants with clefts than they are with babies without anomalies (Barden, Ford, Jensen, Rogers-Salyer, & Salyer, 1989; Borhini, Habersaat, Muller-Nix, Ansermet, & Hohlfeld, 2001; Field & Vega-Lahr, 1984; Wasserman, Allen, & Solomon, 1986). For example, Barden and colleagues found mothers of children with facial anomalies spent less time in the en face position, provided less physical contact, and smiled and laughed less, compared to mothers of typical children.

Children with any kind of physical anomalies appear to be more at risk of physical abuse than children without anomalies (National Center on Child Abuse and Neglect [NCCAN], 1983). Mothers of children with craniofacial anomalies also reported a higher degree of marital conflict, although there is little evidence that the divorce rate is higher in these families, with mixed findings. About 10% of parents reported that their marriage was adversely affected, whereas a quarter to a third reported that the birth of a child with a cleft brought the parents closer together. Reproductive plans generally were unaltered by the birth of child with a cleft (Andrews-Casal et al., 1998). Regardless, it is known that parents' stress correlates with the child's adjustment later in life (Pope et al., 2005). Therefore, intervening with parents who are experiencing considerable stress may help to prevent adjustment problems for the child.

When the parents have other children, this causes additional challenges during the early adjustment period. Parents may find it difficult to explain to siblings that the baby looks different and has something wrong, while trying to reassure them that the doctors are going to fix the problem. The parents also have to balance the time required for taking care of the baby with the needs of the other children. This can be particularly difficult if the baby requires a long time to feed, has frequent ear infections, is scheduled for many medical visits, or has surgery.

Fortunately, the negative feelings and adjustment problems tend to subside fairly rapidly after the first few weeks, without impairing the parent–child relationship on a long-term basis (Clifford, 1969, 1971) or the quality of life of the parents (Kramer, Baethge, Sinikovic, & Schliephake, 2007). One reason for this relatively rapid resolution is the "fixable" quality of clefts at this point in history. In addition, family support has been found to be a significant factor in the parents' overall adjustment to having a child with a cleft, whereas having a low level of social support is a predictor of depression in mothers of children with clefts (Baker, Owens, Stern, & Willmot, 2009; Bradbury & Hewison, 1994; Sank, Berk, Cooper, & Marazita, 2003). Other factors that affect the parents' adjustment include the extent and visibility of the cleft, and each parent's coping style and level of education (Sank et al., 2003). A study in Germany found that mothers of children with clefts over the age of 1 reported the same levels of quality of life, depression, and anxiety as a normative sample (Weigl, Rudolph, Eysholdt, & Rosanowski, 2005). Overall, negative outcomes are not frequent or severe in most families, especially those who have strong social supports (Baker, Owens, Stern, & Wilmott, 2009).

During the early months, it is very important that parents receive sufficient information and support from health care professionals (generally nurses or pediatricians). New parents need to have someone with whom they can talk who is positive, encouraging, and able to answer their questions. Many parents want contact with other parents who have been through the same experiences (Kerr & McIntosh, 2000; Strauss, Sharp, Lorch, & Kachalia, 1995). Parents seem less afraid to show their vulnerability to sympathetic veterans of the process and may voice more of their fears and questions with them. Many hospitals help parents of newborns with clefts link with other parents so that they can compare experiences and solutions to problems. A common activity is sharing pictures, which the newer parents often use as a peek into the future of their own child. The Internet has also become a resource for medical and parenting information. Some sites specifically focus on cleft palate or other craniofacial conditions. In 1973, the American Cleft Palate–Craniofacial Association launched the Cleft Palate Foundation (CPF) to serve as its public service arm. The CPF website, therefore, is a particularly great source of information for parents of affected children. The website is at http://www.cleftline.org.

Cleft Palate as a Chronic Medical Condition

Parents of a child with a cleft spend a lot of time taking their child to medical appointments, which can pose practical challenges for families. This is especially true for those families with difficulty with transportation, long distances to travel, other preschool children, or particularly limited financial resources. Missing work for appointments may be difficult or employment threatening. The visits may also be stressful as the visits serve to remind them of their baby's "difference." The parents may also be concerned that they will hear more bad news. In some ways, these visits may feel like an evaluation of their efficacy as parents, particularly when feeding has been a major challenge and the physician is charting the infant's growth. It is very important to parents that health care professionals be supportive to them and relate to their child as a person, not as an assortment of physical problems.

The first surgery is a stressful and frightening time for family members. Having a helpless baby taken from their arms for surgery reawakens the sad, frightened, and protective feelings that may have quieted since the birth. For many of the normal challenges of growing up, parents and grandparents have the ability to "make it all better" for their children. When surgery is required, however, the parents and other family members are confronted with their powerlessness to fix the baby's problems. Instead, they have to trust the surgeon and all of the other professionals involved, often leaving them feeling out of control. There is always bit of concern that something might go wrong and that the baby could die as a result of their decision regarding the surgery. The decision as to whether surgery is worth the risk only becomes more complicated as the child grows older and the emphasis of surgery is more on appearance than function.

Children with a history of cleft have been found to exhibit mood and behavior changes following surgery. In a rare longitudinal study of children with a history of cleft, Koomen and Hoeksma (1993) found changes in behavior following surgery that primarily had to do with the infants' apparent increased desire to be in contact with their mothers. They interpreted their findings as suggesting that attachment to parents may be impaired by the cleft repair and the child's subsequent hospitalization. On the other hand, these findings were inconsistent and their significance outside the laboratory of some question.

Parents play a unique role in helping their child through the surgeries that no health professional can assume. It is therefore important that they receive practical advice from

professionals about staying with the infant during the entire hospitalization, preparing siblings for the event and the baby's changed appearance, and caring for the baby after surgery. This advice can increase a parent's sense of being able to contribute to the child's well-being. For the baby, having a parent or other familiar adult available during the entire hospital stay is important for security and comfort (Redsell & Glazebrook, 2010).

Even when there are positive relationships between health care professionals and parents, some aspects of dealing with the medical system can be overwhelming for parents and continue to be problematic for years. For example, dealing with paperwork, insurance authorization and bills can cause frustration and anger with the system. This can lead to misdirected anger toward professionals and even lead to noncompliance to the medical regimen.

The intensity of the family members' negative feelings about the child's cleft and the associated stresses usually diminishes over time, with resurgent peaks at times of surgery, social rejection, or the child's own distress. Parents often experience some fatigue during the whole process and are eager for everything to be done. Disagreement between the parents regarding medical decisions is not unusual. As the child grows older, this disagreement can even be between parents and the child, especially during the teen years. Parental fears may be reawakened when the teenager or adult child moves into a serious relationship where reproductive and hence, genetic issues are important.

When the parent also has a history of cleft, there is an added dimension to the relationship. It usually answers the question of why the child was born with a cleft. Although the parent is in an unusually good position to be knowledgeable about and understanding of the child's situation, there is also the risk that the parent's unresolved negative feelings may color his or her response to the challenges facing the child. Sometimes parents make decisions that reflect an attempt to "get it right this time." It is particularly important to help the parent see differences between his or her situation and that of the child's. An important consideration is the advancement of surgical techniques since the parent's own repair.

Although having a child with a cleft is stressful, there is no evidence that it leads to a higher frequency of psychiatric symptoms in parents (Grollemund et al., 2010). An older study (Goodstein, 1960) compared the personality profiles of parents of children with a history of cleft to those of parents of children with no known abnormalities. Using the *Minnesota Multiphasic Personality Inventory (MMPI)*, the researchers found no significant differences between the groups and no unique patterns emerged. Another study (Baker, Owens, Stern, & Wilmot, 2009) identified parents who make positive meanings out of their parenting situation, particularly those with a strong support system, and those who use coping strategies that involve approaching rather than avoiding the issue (seeking support, problem solving, logical analysis, etc.). However, further research is needed to examine the parents' perspectives about their child's treatment journey (Nelson, Glenny, Kirk, & Caress, 2012).

SCHOOL ISSUES

Once the child enters school, there are additional challenges. Many people, including teachers, underestimate the abilities and intelligence of individuals who have facial anomalies or abnormal speech. Some, but not all, children with clefts or other craniofacial conditions actually do have learning issues, even though they have normal intelligence. Perhaps the greatest concerns for affected children are difficulties with social interactions, periodic teasing, and a relatively negative self-concept.

Knowledge and Expectation of Teachers

Teachers have reported that they do not know much about cleft lip and palate (like most of the population), and what they think they know may be incorrect (Finnegan, 1982). As a group, teachers have also been found to underestimate the intelligence of children with a history of cleft, especially when either appearance or speech is significantly impaired (Richman, 1978). They also may expect less from the children who look different from those who appear normal (Richman & Eliason, 1982). These underestimates shape their expectations of these children and may result in lower performance from these children and less positive evaluations of their academic performance. Several studies have found that children with clefts do not achieve the level that would be predicted by their intelligence alone (Broder, Richman, & Matheson, 1998; Millard & Richman, 2001).

Learning Ability and School Performance

For children and teenagers with a nonsyndromic cleft lip and palate (CLP), intelligence seems to be in the average range, as measured by formal IQ tests (Millard & Richman, 2001; Persson, Becker, & Svenson, 2008). However, these children generally score lower on test sections that require verbal skills, especially oral responses, than on performance-based sections (see Chapter 6 for more information). Children with a CLP who have reading disabilities have been shown to have specific deficits in rapid naming and verbal expression. Their problem does not appear to be phonemic awareness, despite some early attempts to link reading problems to articulation difficulties (Richman & Ryan, 2003). They are also more likely to have serious reading disabilities, often evident in the primary grades (Richman & Millard, 1997).

By contrast, children with cleft palate only (CPO), often associated with various syndromes, tend to score lower on intelligence tests (Persson et al., 2008). Many of these children also have specific learning disabilities (Richman, Ryan, Wilgenbusch, & Millard, 2004). It has been found that over half of children with cleft palate only show significant reading problems in first- and second-grade years, and a full third still show reading problems at age 13. Girls are less often affected than boys (Broder et al., 1998). In addition, children with cleft palate only (CPO) have more speech and language disorders than those with cleft lip and palate or nonaffected peers (Broen, Devers, Doyle, Prouty, & Moller, 1998; Estes & Morris, 1970; Goodstein, 1961; Lamb, Wilson, & Leeper, 1973). Certainly, children who have speech problems often lack self-confidence in reading aloud, which may influence the teachers' evaluation of their abilities. There has been some disagreement in the literature about the intelligence of children, adolescents, and adults with clefts, with some studies suggesting lower scores, but usually still in the average range (McWilliams & Musgrave, 1972). One apparent resolution has been to separate the scores of people with CLP from those with CPO. Studies that separate scores have found that those with CPO score lower on formal intelligence testing than those with CLP (Persson et al., 2008). This finding calls into question older conclusions based on combined groups.

Despite their challenges in school, teenagers with a history of cleft showed only a slightly greater high school dropout rate than their unaffected siblings and those people who went on to college had similar graduation rates (McWilliams & Paradise, 1973). As a group, they attain the same educational levels as other young adults. In fact, one study in Europe found persons with a history of cleft had a lower rate of dropping out than their peers (Ramstad, Ottem, & Shaw, 1995b).

Children with craniofacial anomalies other than CLP and CPO, especially with craniosynostosis, are often found to demonstrate cognitive deficits. For example, a French study found that about a third of children with Apert's syndrome had IQ scores above 70, with a strong affect of timing of surgery (Renier et al., 1996). A later study of children with a craniosynostosis found that as a group the children scored in the average range of intelligence with a mean IQ of 95 (DaCosta et al., 2006). There was, however, a significant difference between those children with a syndromic presentation (mean IQ of 83) and those who were not diagnosed with a syndrome (mean IQ of 104). A 2012 report evaluating factors related to quality of life among children with syndromic craniosynostosis found cognitive functioning to be more problematic for those with Apert, Crouzon and Muenke syndromes, although typically children with Crouzon syndrome have fewer learning problems (deJong, Maliepaard, Bannink, & Mathijssen, 2012).

Syndromes without craniosynostosis, such as Treacher Collins syndrome and hemifacial microsomia, are less frequently associated with problems in cognitive development. A major exception is velocardiofacial syndrome (VCFS). Learning problems have been considered a necessary diagnostic feature when this syndrome was first described (Shprintzen et al., 1978). Later it was suggested that children with VCFS often fit the criteria for non-verbal learning disability (Fuerst, Dool, & Rourke, 1995). Others have found delays that extend into the intellectually impaired range. One study identified significant delays in cognitive development in about half of their sample with VCFS (Swillen et al., 1997). Another study found delays in children younger than 6, with 75% showing at least mild delays (Gerdes et al., 1999).

Other syndromes also include intellectual delay. For example, rates of intellectual delay in Smith-Lemli-Opitz syndrome have been reported to be above 95% (Kelley & Hennekam, 2000). In addition, fetal alcohol syndrome and fetal alcohol spectrum disorder are both associated with high rates of cognitive impairment and learning disabilities (Sokol, Delaney-Black, & Nordstrom, 2003).

Social Interaction

In the early years of a child's life, the negative social implications of the cleft are primarily experienced by the parents. They are the ones who note the stares or answer the questions about the child's condition. By the preschool years, however, the child starts to be asked directly about what happened to his or her lip. Sometimes the question comes from well-meaning adults who believe the child's scar to be from a fall or a minor accident. Other times, it comes from curious peers who notice a difference in the child's appearance. Although preschool children prefer attractive children as friends, they are rarely cruel or tease their peers. They notice differences in appearance, speech, and behavior, but unless the differences interfere, they are not generally important in play relationships. One of the advantages of enrolling the child with a history of cleft in preschool or day care program is the opportunity for the child to build social skills and confidence without parents present at a time when teasing and rudeness is rare.

By school age, a significant number of children with a history of cleft do not have as many friendships as other children their age (Tobiason & Speltz, 1996). This situation appears to be a result of the interaction of several factors. First, children with a history of cleft, especially girls, seem to be more socially inhibited than their peers. They are sometimes reluctant to risk new friendships; other times, they have difficulty in initiating and maintaining new friendships. Second, the lack of friends may relate to the interaction challenges associated with hearing impairment and speech difficulties. Third, concerns about appearance may be a contributor to the lack of friends. To some extent, findings are dependent on who rates the children. For example, one study found that teachers reported lower social competence and less peer acceptance than parents of the same children (Dufton et al., 2011). Parent responses were similar to those of parents of unaffected children. It is not clear whether teachers have a more realistic or negative lens, or perhaps they see a different sample of behavior.

In an experiment, Joyce Tobiasen (1988, 1989) showed pictures of children to second- through fourth-graders. Some of the children in the unretouched photos had no cleft, some had a repaired unilateral cleft, and some had a repaired bilateral cleft. The viewers rated the pictured children on personal qualities. Children rated those with a bilateral cleft as having fewer positive attributes than those with a unilateral cleft, and both cleft groups fared worse than the children without a visible cleft. The younger viewers were harsher in their ratings than the somewhat older ones.

Although the degree of facial impairment is strongly correlated with perceptions of attractiveness and social desirability, the social relationships of an individual child cannot be accurately predicted on the basis of facial attractiveness alone (Feragen, Kvalem, Rumsey, & Borge, 2010; Shute, McCarthy, & Roberts, 2007). The child's temperament, family support, social skills, personal experiences, and coping strategies may also make a difference in that regard.

In most studies, older children and teen-agers reported significant concerns about interpersonal relationships. Sound social relationships can be protective and promote self-esteem in any teen-ager. But for those with craniofacial anomalies, the trend toward over-inhibition and shyness continues into adolescence. Slifer and his colleagues videotaped interactions of 8 to 15-year olds with and without clefts, finding that those with clefts responded less often to questions from peers and made fewer choices during interactions (Slifer et al., 2004). Their parents rated them as less socially competent as well. In addition, those young people with clefts who rated themselves as more socially acceptable were more likely to look their peers in the face. In another study, adult Japanese women with clefts showed fewer physical signs of interest in conversations and smiled less frequently than their counterparts who had no clefts (Adachi, Kochi, & Yamaguchi, 2003).

Problems with social skills may be due to the conversational experiences of those growing up with facial and speech differences (Berger & Dalton, 2011) or these problems may be attributable to neuropsychological differences in individuals with clefts. The latter theory is suggested by the findings of Nopoulos and colleagues (Nopoulos et al., 2005). These researchers found that, as compared to a control group, men with nonsyndromic clefts had morphologic abnormalities in the part of the brain known to govern social functioning,

as noted through MRI imaging. They also reported that the larger the abnormality, the more problems in socializing.

How these differences may relate to romantic outcomes is not yet known. Although the frequency of dating relationships among young people with a history of cleft relative to their peers has not been studied, it appears that teens with a history of cleft show more self-doubts and have lower expectations for relationships than their peers.

Adults with a history of cleft have been found to marry later than their peers and siblings (McWilliams & Paradise, 1973). In studies in other countries, adults have been seen as generally showing good psychological adjustment, but fewer were in long-term relationships or married (Ramstad et al., 1995b). Women, in particular, worried about their appearance (Sinko et al., 2005), but both men and women express concerns about appearance relative to unaffected adults and report that their facial appearance has worked against them socially (Meyer-Marcotty, Gerdes, Stellzig-Eisenhauer, &Alpers, 1999; Sarwer et al., 1999). In the Sarwer and colleagues study, almost 40% of adults felt that their employment and promotion options were affected by their craniofacial anomaly.

In a Danish study, adult women with clefts were likely to have children later than unaffected peers (Yttri, Christensen, Knudsen & Bille, 2011). In contrast, through a meta-analysis of international studies involving three Asian countries and Norway, a study found that psychosocial issues became more important in adulthood than they were in adolescence, especially for men (Hutchinson, Wellman, Noe, & Kahn, 2011). In addition, they found that, overall, individuals with cleft lip and/or palate had responses indicating poorer psychosocial development than non-affected adults.

Teasing

Children with a history of cleft are probably teased more often than their unaffected peers (Broder, Smith, & Strauss, 2001). Teasing seems to be influenced by the child's physical appearance and speech differences, because children tend to report less teasing after surgeries that address those problems. Other factors that affect teasing are the child's personality and social standing and the child's response to teasing. Children who laugh off teasing or respond in kind appear to be teased less than those who respond with distress or helpless anger. The use of humor or attributing teasing to a flaw in the person who does the teasing is protective of the child's self-esteem. It has been found that the experience of being teased affected children more than having a cleft per se (Hunt et al., 2006).

The likelihood of teasing is also affected by the response of adults in the child's environment, especially at school. If the adults help the child to present information to other children about the cleft and the various surgeries, this can reduce teasing and elicit empathy, especially among children in lower grades. Teasing is also reduced when school officials take an active role in demonstrating that respect for all students is expected. On the other hand, when teasing is viewed as an inevitable behavior of children, teasing is more likely to continue or increase.

By high school, teasing tends to diminish or takes on a friendlier tone for children with a history of cleft. There is a greater understanding of clefts and a greater acceptance of differences at this age. When unpleasant teasing continues, however, it can take on a cruel edge and even a group rejection that may result in social withdrawal. Some social scientists see this kind of teasing as having the same power and domination quality as more general "bullying." Hunt and colleagues (2006) found that almost two-thirds of teenagers and young adults reported being teased or bullied, with several reporting physical bullying more frequently than typical peers. Bullying is associated with depression, anxiety, and fear of negative evaluation (Storch et al., 2003).

Self-Perception

Children with a history of cleft have consistently been found to have a more negative self-concept when compared to their unaffected peers (Broder & Strauss, 1989; Kapp-Simon, 1986; Slifer et al., 2003; Sousa, Devare, & Ghanshani, 2009). They see themselves as less acceptable to their peers, less socially competent, less satisfied with their facial appearance, and more often sad or angry than their peers. Children develop a concept of self-worth over time. Broder and Strauss (1989) found that children with both cleft lip and palate scored lower with regard to self-concept than those with an "invisible" cleft palate only, but children with a history of any type of cleft rated themselves less well than unaffected children. Higher levels of acceptance of the cleft were associated with better self-concepts. In school-age children with a history of cleft, greater physical attractiveness correlated with better overall adjustment (Pillemer & Cook, 1989). Similarly, satisfaction with their own appearance was related to the adjustment and older teens and young adults were more satisfied than their younger counterparts (Thomas, Turner, Rumsey, Dowell, & Sandy, 1997). There is some evidence that having appearance-altering surgeries before the teen years contribute to better self-esteem and less social isolation (Pertschuk & Whitaker, 1982).

Generally, teenagers have been found to have more negative feelings about themselves than younger children. Brantley and Clifford

(1979) asked teenagers to report what they thought their parents felt and experienced when they were born. Teens with a history of cleft said that their parents experienced predominantly negative emotions and that their parents did not care to nurture them. Relative to teens with asthma, obesity, or no physical problems, adolescents with a history of cleft reported their parents had higher levels of apprehension about and felt less pride in them. Fortunately, teenagers who view themselves in agreement with their peers and familiar adults tend to be better adjusted.

Physical appearance concerns are consistently greater in persons with a history of cleft across the life span, but in later adolescence and adulthood, women report greater feelings of self-consciousness than their male counterparts and that dissatisfaction with appearance centered on the face, especially the mouth (Clifford, Crocker, & Pope, 1972). Adults with a history of cleft lip were less satisfied with facial appearance than those with a history of cleft palate only, whereas people with a history of cleft palate were more displeased with their speech than those with a history of cleft lip only. More dissatisfaction with their mouth, teeth, lips, voice, and speech was expressed by both cleft groups than by the control group of adults with no history of cleft.

Adults with a history of cleft continue to report some levels of psychological distress. In a study of Norwegian adults, it was found those with a history of cleft had higher levels of anxiety and depression than the unaffected controls (Ramstad, Ottem, & Shaw, 1995a). Their symptoms were strongly associated with more concerns about appearance, dentition, speech, and the possibility of more treatment. The same researchers (1995b) also reported that adults with a history of cleft were less likely to marry than unaffected adults and that when they did marry, it was often later in life. This was particularly true of the group with bilateral cleft lip and palate. Other studies in other countries have found similar results. Although education and employment per se did not differ between those with a history of cleft and the controls, people with a history of cleft appeared to make less money.

CASE REPORT

Andrea's Story

I was born with a severe cleft palate deformity in 1944, a time when no corrective surgery had been done in South Australia. It wasn't until 1958, when a plastic surgeon named Mr. Don Robinson came to the Royal Adelaide Hospital, that I received the operation I needed. I was the first person in the State to have plastic surgery.

In the 1940s, when a mother had an abnormal baby, it was something to be ashamed of and embarrassed about. I was no exception. My early years were spent in the Adelaide Children's Hospital, as I could not feed. This had to be done by gavage method or intravenously. However, as my mother didn't want me, it was convenient for her to have me spend time in hospital. My father was away at the war. When he came home, so did I. He was a loving and caring man.

There were no schools for a child with a speech deformity, so I went to a mainstream school where I was teased relentlessly, every day. I couldn't speak so as to be understood; I just made noises. I struggled with my schooling and was overlooked by the teachers, which left me way behind the other children academically, and

(Continues)

lacking in self-worth. Nothing changed when I went to high school. At home, I wasn't shown love by my mother or siblings.

My father sacrificed the block of land that was to be for the family's dream home to pay for my operation, which cost £500. My mother never forgave me.

Even after my surgery I wasn't accepted at school or at home, but I attended speech therapy three times a week for 4 years and faithfully practised the repetitive exercises.

Following a pharyngoplasty in 1977 and further speech therapy, I now lead a normal life, with only occasional teasing. My wonderful, loving husband gives me constant support (Ogier & Britton, 2013).

By Andrea Ogier

Australia

Printed with permission

SOCIETAL ISSUES

Humans are naturally social beings who require human interaction, communication, and acceptance by others. Individuals with clefts or craniofacial anomalies are often hindered in their communication by speech and hearing difficulties. In addition, they can be viewed more negatively by others because of their appearance and speech.

Physical Attractiveness

One of the forces at work for a child with a cleft is society's response to facial difference. Physical attractiveness, especially facial beauty, is an area that has been well researched, with findings that are among the most reliable and robust in the psychological literature. Some characteristics that people see as attractive or unattractive are cross-cultural; for example, there is no group of people known to find highly blemished skin to be attractive. Other characteristics considered attractive vary considerably between cultures, but even then, attractiveness tends to focus on facial features and body shape. There is some evidence that mouth shape is especially important across cultures, even though the specific standard for

beauty may differ. Dental differences certainly carry meaning for adults, although this is less clear in the case of children.

Within a culture, there is considerable consensus about general characteristics of attractiveness. This consensus develops early. By preschool age, children know the standards of beauty that the adults hold and share those values. In fact, not very long ago, one of the items on a commonly used intelligence test for children asked preschoolers to choose the picture of the "pretty" woman from two choices (Terman & Merrill, 1960, Stanford-Binet Form L-M). This could serve as a developmental test only because the cultural concept of beauty normally is learned before age 4.

More important than the consensual nature of cultural standards of beauty are the meanings associated with being considered either attractive or unattractive. In a nutshell, beauty is equated with goodness. Attractive people are rated as smarter, more friendly, nicer, more likely to be a good friend, and kinder than those who are less attractive. Ethnologists have found that characteristics in babies, such as a round head, large eyes, and short and narrow features are rated as "cute" (witness how most people respond to pandas) and elicit caregiving behaviors from adults. Infants considered to be highly attractive tend to be rated as more likable, smarter, and less problematic. The significance of these ratings and beliefs lie in their power to shape the behavior and attitudes of people, directly and indirectly. These, in turn, become part of the feedback loop that shapes how an individual behaves and views himself or herself.

Physical attractiveness is important across the life span. Cute babies are attributed characteristics that their less attractive peers are not. Preschoolers prefer attractive children as their friends, and the social power of attractiveness continues to increase until the early grade school years and then tends to hold steady until adolescence. Teachers also have more favorable expectations of attractive children than unattractive children (Clifford, 1975). Teachers may respond differentially to more physically attractive children and, as a group, the grades of attractive children are often higher than those of less attractive peers. Attractive teens are more likely to be elected to school office than other youth and, as no surprise to most people, date more frequently and have a higher number of partners. Even being seen with attractive people increases a person's social desirability. Physical attractiveness affects the likelihood of being hired for a job, even when public contact is not a major factor. It may also influence job performance evaluations.

The power of physical attractiveness appears to hold in middle and older age as well, but this is less well established. People sometimes hope that this influence only holds at first impression, but research suggests that this is not the case (Ambady & Rosenthal, 1993; Hosoda, Stone-Romero, & Coats, 2003). Less attractive adults have slower rates of being hired, earning promotions and getting raises (Hosoda et al., 2003). Almost 40% of adults with craniofacial anomalies believe that that happened to them (Sarwer et al., 1999). Although physical attractiveness is only one of many variables contributing to the social responses to a person, it is a powerful force indeed.

Speech Quality

The quality of a person's speech is a factor rather similar to physical attractiveness. First, the quality of speech impacts the social judgments of others, which in turn helps shape behaviors and attitudes. Second, good speech appears to be associated with the assumption that the speaker has positive characteristics. Although children are less likely to initiate conversations with those with impaired speech, adults associate children's speech problems with undesirable personal characteristics. Many adults with dysarthric speech have reported that no matter what they are saying, they feel their comments are discounted or that they are assumed to be retarded or "stupid." This experience has also been noted by adults with acquired speech disorders. Although cultural differences exist in these stereotypes, listeners often believe that people with speech disorders are more likely to be emotionally disturbed (Bebout & Bradford, 1992).

It also appears that speech quality and facial appearance interact with each other in determining how a person is perceived by others. Facial attractiveness may not change ratings of speech quality, but impaired speech seems to lower ratings of physical attractiveness of the speaker. Hypernasality appears to be particularly unattractive to listeners, so that ratings of social desirability of a speaker decrease steadily as nasality increases. Clifford (1987), a well-known psychologist studying effects of cleft lip and palate, concluded that the combination of facial appearance and hypernasality contributed to "a lack of perceived competence" in individuals with a history of cleft.

Hearing Impairment

Having a hearing impairment can add to the social judgments that people make. Many children with a history of cleft have some degree of hearing impairment, which may vary with the frequency of recurrent ear infections. Negative stereotypes exist of people who have hearing impairments, with or without visible hearing aids. More importantly however, hearing is central to many aspects of social interactions among members of the general population (Fujiki, Brinton, & Clark, 2002; Moeller, 2007).

When an individual misunderstands even subtle nuances in a conversation, it shapes the next phase of interaction. If the person is perceived as not understanding some of the communication, he or she can be viewed as annoying or frustrating. With repetition, interactions may be avoided. This is another example of the importance of the social feedback loop.

Stigma

The concept of stigma is a common thread unifying all three areas described above. *Stigma* is the discrediting and objectifying of individuals based on difference from cultural standards. In the case of persons with craniofacial anomalies, they are evaluated in a negative fashion because of their visible difference from the cultural standards of beauty, speech, hearing, and/or social interactions. Stigma diminishes a person's social acceptability, which negatively impacts self-esteem. Another effect is the reduction or blocking of social and economic opportunities. The impact of stigmatization may be felt in the absence of negative intent, as when people stare out of curiosity, ignorance, or sympathy. Essentially,

it is a problem of people being defined by their stigma and coming to anticipate stigmatization as well. They then may behave accordingly, as if stigmatized, regardless of the behavior or attitudes of the other people involved in interactions. People who are disfigured are particularly vulnerable to stigma. In a survey of parents and teens with facial differences, mostly congenital facial anomalies, it was found that stigmatizing experiences occur regularly for at least one-third of them, sometimes on a weekly basis (Strauss et al., 2007).

BEHAVIOR AND PSYCHIATRIC ISSUES

Children with clefts or other craniofacial anomalies are subjected to multiple surgeries and therapies that are not experienced by their unaffected peers. These can cause stress for the child and behavioral issues that require professional intervention. For individuals with certain syndromes, there is also a risk of psychiatric disorders that tend to manifest in adolescence and adulthood.

Behavioral Issues Related to Medical Care

As discussed earlier in this chapter, having to undergo major medical procedures is generally stressful and often difficult for family members and patients. For some, the experience is traumatizing, and for others it is an inevitable event to be faced in a matter-of-fact manner. Multiple surgeries may have a cumulative effect as well.

Psychological interventions can be useful for children with clefts, to help them with concerns related to their treatment. Most children dread even relatively minor procedures, such as injections or having dental caries filled. For a small proportion of children, however, multiple surgeries or medical procedures can contribute to the development of significant anxiety and distress (see Case Report "Brian's Story"). Several studies have demonstrated that teaching children coping skills can help to reduce both the distress associated with a procedure and the time it takes to carry it out (Nocella & Kaplan, 1982; Powers, Blount, Bachanas, & Cotter, 1993). It is also helpful if the psychologist is present for some of the procedures in order to coach the child in coping during the procedure.

When children have to wear devices, such as a distraction device or reverse face mask, the treatment is very visible and can take considerable time. These children and their families often benefit from coaching on how to prepare peers, answer questions, and deal with the inconvenience or discomfort.

Pediatric psychologists can also help children and families with adherence to various treatment recommendations. For example, for children who suck their thumbs past early childhood, a psychologist can help parents develop ways to break this difficult habit through increased awareness and a reward system (Friman & Leibowitz, 1990). Parents are taught to avoid power struggles while focusing on times when the child is not sucking his or her thumb. Similarly, children with clefts often have very poor dental hygiene that prevents needed, and even desired, orthodontia. They avoid brushing because looking in the mirror while brushing teeth forces the child to confront the presence of an undesirable difference in appearance. A psychologist can improve the child's adherence to brushing recommendations, while addressing the underlying concerns expressed through poor hygiene (Dahlquist, 1985; Philippot, Lenoir, D'Hoore, & Bercy, 2005).

Psychiatric Concerns

It should be noted that the rates of diagnosed psychiatric disorders for children and teens with a history of cleft appears no different than that of the population of children as a whole. Studies comparing children with a history of cleft to children with other physical problems and to children with no medical problems have found little difference among the groups. Research to identify a "cleft palate personality" has consistently failed to yield evidence of a consistent type of personality in children, adolescents, or adults with a history of cleft. The biggest risk appears to be for social competence problems, including those relating to development of friendships and participation in organizations (Murray et al., 2010; Richman & Eliason, 1982).

Although overall, there is no known link between nonsyndromic facial anomalies and psychiatric disorders, coping with the added stress and stigmatization may raise the risk of depression or anxiety (Kapp-Simon, Simon, & Kristovich, 1992; Pope & Snyder, 2005). There have been conflicting reports that especially children with craniofacial anomalies are more likely to show symptoms of attention deficit-hyperactivity disorder (ADHD). There have been anecdotal and empirical reports of greater attentional problems (Richman, Ryan, Wilgenbusch, & Millard, 2004), but other research has not supported these findings (Klatt, Schultz, Lee, & Saal, 2002; Speltz, Morton, Goodell, & Clarren 1993). Richman and colleagues (2004) went on to find that only about one-third of the children diagnosed with ADHD actually met the DSM-IV criteria. Statistics have been called into question for ADHD in children with craniofacial anomalies as it has become more evident that airway problems and obstructive sleep apnea (OSA) may manifest as poor attention (Ferini-Strambi et al., 2003; Findley et al., 1986).

More significant psychiatric disorders have been associated with some craniofacial syndromes. The syndrome with the greatest frequency of schizophrenia or mood disorders is velocardiofacial syndrome (VCFS), with some estimates reaching as high as 40% (Papolos, Faedda, & Veit, 1996; Murphy, Jones, & Owen, 1999; Shprintzen, Goldberg, Golding-Kushner, & Marion, 1992). Symptoms typically reach clinical levels in late adolescence or early adulthood. Both Moebius sequence and CHARGE association have been reported to be linked to autism (Miller et al., 2005).

CASE REPORT

Brian's Story

Brian was a 9-year-old boy with a bilateral cleft lip and palate. His surgical repairs had been without complications and he was able to go home at the expected time after each surgery. He was an honor student at a private school considered to be one of the more rigorous in the area. He had friends and had not experienced teasing since second grade. His family was close-knit and generally supportive, except for a typical sibling rivalry with a sister. Brian had interacted well with his physicians and their staff at their offices. His family was careful to adhere to recommendations and reliably attended follow-up appointments.

Unfortunately, Brian became highly anxious at the thought of the hospital after undergoing a bone graft, which he found to be fairly painful at the donor site. The smell of bubble gum, which had been used as a spray on the mask before surgery, brought distress, no matter what the circumstances. A few months later, Brian required PE tube reinsertion. Although this was an uneventful outpatient procedure, Brian's anxiety about the hospital led to nausea and vomiting. He began to have episodes where he felt scared and had cold hands, nausea, and a sensation of salivation.

The usual route from Brian's house to his grandmother's passed near the children's hospital. Brian developed nausea as they neared the hospital, and on several occasions the driver had to pull over to the curb so that he could vomit. They began driving a more convoluted, lengthy route that avoided the hospital area, which eliminated his vomiting. Brian expressed his appreciation for avoiding the hospital but realized it was "stupid" to react so strongly "to nothing." When coming for a craniofacial team appointment at the hospital, he vomited twice, once about four blocks from the hospital and once in the parking lot. Although Brian knew that there was no surgery planned for that day, that fact did nothing to curb his feelings.

Brian was referred to the craniofacial team psychologist to address his symptoms. His family was supportive and hopeful that intervention would lead to greater comfort for Brian and shorter and more pleasant car travel for all. Brian agreed to come to sessions "to get over this," even though the psychologist's office was at the hospital.

At the first visit, the psychologist took a detailed history of Brian's symptoms. She then had Brian monitor his thoughts and feelings throughout the week. From the results, it was evident that Brian had become classically conditioned to this response to the hospital. (He had a similar reaction to patients with cancer who vomit at the sight of the hospital before they receive the chemotherapy that makes them nauseated.) Brian's therapy sessions often included his mother, who enlisted the cooperation of Brian's sister and father to carry out home assignments. Brian was treated with a combination of systematic desensitization and methods to improve and broaden his coping strategies. One of the strategies was for Brian to talk about his fears, concerns, and desires for surgery, and then role-play talking to his surgeon about questions and preferences. Then his mother made an appointment for him to talk to the plastic surgeon with whom the psychologist had previously spoken and prepared. Empowering Brian to be an active participant in his care allowed Brian some sense of control. In three sessions, Brian was able to attend therapy without nausea, and in eight sessions he was able to visit the surgical floors without anxiety. His family resumed more direct driving routes without difficulty, and Brian managed his next surgery 2 years later without relapse.

SUMMARY

A child born with a cleft lip and/or palate does not necessarily develop a major psychopathology as a result (Christensen & Mortensen, 2002). In fact, many individuals with craniofacial conditions are amazingly resilient due to a variety of factors (Mani, Carlsson, & Marcusson, 2010; Strauss, 2001). However, having a facial difference and dealing with speech issues complicates life and presents challenges that children without medical problems generally do not face. These challenges are not restricted to the child, but extend to the family of the child as well. In fact, early in the child's development the majority of the psychological "fallout" of the cleft is on the family, rather than on the child. Later, the challenges to the individual seem most often to be related to school achievement and peer relationships. People with a history of cleft appear to be particularly at risk for diminished social interaction and social competence.

Because of the prevalence of psychological problems in children clefts and in their families, it is strongly recommended that cleft palate and craniofacial teams have a psychologist as a member or at least available on a referral basis. The psychologist can be helpful in addressing the behaviors and attitudes of the child and family that can interfere with an optimal treatment outcome.

FOR REVIEW AND DISCUSSION

1. What are factors that contribute to the shock of having a baby with a cleft? What are some factors that help parents to adjust? What can healthcare professionals do to lessen the immediate shock and distress?

2. Why is cleft palate a "chronic" medical condition? How does this affect the parents? How does it affect the child?

3. What are some issues that a child with a history of cleft lip and palate may experience in school? What are some ways that parents and healthcare providers can lessen these issues? How would you suggest that the child deal with teasing?

4. What are factors that affect self-perception of individuals with a history of cleft lip and palate? How do you explain the fact that some children with significant malformations are better adjusted than other children with minor differences?

5. How does physical attractiveness affect an individual's ability to fit into society? What

is a common perception of that people of individuals with speech problems regarding intelligence? Why do you think this occurs?

6. Describe the role of the psychologist on a craniofacial team and the potential benefit of psychological services to the patient and other team members.

References

Adachi, T., Kochi, S., & Yamaguchi, T. (2003). Characteristics of nonverbal behavior in patients with cleft lip and palate during interpersonal communication. *The Cleft Palate–Craniofacial Journal, 40,* 310–316.

Ambady, N., & Rosenthal, R. (1993). Half a minute: Predicting teacher evaluations from thin slices of nonverbal behavior and physical attractiveness. *Journal of Personality and Social Psychology, 64,* 431–441.

Andrews-Casal, M., Johnston, D., Fletcher, J., Mulliken, J. B., Stal, S., & Hecht, J. T. (1998). Cleft lip with or without cleft palate: Effect of family history on reproductive planning, surgical timing, and parental stress. *Cleft Palate–Craniofacial Journal, 35*(1), 52–57.

Baker, S. R., Owens, J., Stern, M., & Willmot, D. (2009). Coping strategies and social support in the family impact of cleft lip and palate and parents' adjustment and psychological distress. *The Cleft Palate—Craniofacial Journal, 46,* 229–236.

Barden, R. C., Ford, M. E., Jensen, A. G., Rogers-Salyer, M., and Salyer, K. E. (1989). Effects of craniofacial deformity in infancy on the quality of mother-infant interactions. *Child Development, 60,* 819–824.

Barr, L., Thibeault, S. L., Muntz, H., & de Serres, L. (2007). Quality of life in children with velopharyngeal insufficiency. *Archives of Otolaryngology Head and Neck Surgery 133,* 224–229.

Bebout, L., & Bradford, A. (1992). Cross-cultural attitudes toward speech disorders. *Journal of Speech and Hearing Research, 35,* 45–52.

Berger, Z. E., & Dalton, L. J. (2011). Coping with a cleft II: Factors associated with psychosocial adjustment of adolescents with a cleft lip and palate and their parents. *The Cleft Palate–Craniofacial Journal, 48,* 82–90.

Bradbury, E. T., & Hewison, J. (1994). Early parental adjustment to visible congenital disfigurement. *Child Care Health and Development, 20,* 251–266.

Brantley, H. T., & Clifford, E. (1979). Maternal and child locus of control and field dependence in cleft palate children. *Cleft Palate Journal, 16,* 183–187.

Broder, H., Richman, L. C., & Matheson, P. B. (1998). Learning disabilities, school achievement, and grade retention among children with clefts: A two-center study. *Cleft Palate–Craniofacial Journal, 35,* 127–131.

Broder, H., Smith, F. B., & Strauss, R. (2001). Developing a behavior rating scale for comparing teachers' ratings of children with and without craniofacial anomalies. *Cleft Palate–Craniofacial Journal, 38*(6), 560–565.

Broder, H., & Strauss, R. (1989). Self-concept of early primary school-age children with visible or in visible defects. *Cleft Palate Journal, 26*(2), 114–117.

Broen, P. A., Devers, M. C., Doyle, S. S., Prouty, J. M., & Moller, K. T. (1998). Acquisition of linguistic and cognitive skills by children with cleft palate. *Journal of*

Speech, Language, and Hearing Research, 41, 676–687.

Christensen, K., & Mortensen, P. B. (2002). Facial clefting and psychiatric diseases: A follow-up of the Danish 1936–1987 facial cleft cohort. *Cleft Palate–Craniofacial Journal,* 39(4), 392–396.

Clifford, E. (1969). Paternal ratings of cleft palate infants. *Cleft Palate Journal, 6,* 235–243.

Clifford, E. (1971). Cleft palate and the person: Psychological studies of its impact. *Journal of Southern Medical Association, 12,* 1516–1520.

Clifford, E. (1987). *The cleft palate experience: New perspectives on management.* Springfield, IL: Charles C. Thomas.

Clifford, E., Crocker, E. C., & Pope, B. A. (1972). Psychological findings in the adulthood of 98 cleft palate children. *Journal of Plastic and Reconstructive Surgery, 50,* 234.

Clifford, M. M. (1975). Physical attractiveness and academic performance. *Child Study Journal, 5,* 201–209.

Coy, K., Speltz, M. L., & Jones, K. (2002). Facial appearance and attachment in infants with orofacial clefts: A replication. *Cleft Palate–Craniofacial Journal, 39,* 66–72.

DaCosta, A. C., Walters, I., Savarirayan, R., Anderson, V. A., Wrennall, J. A., & Meara, J. G. (2006). Intellectual outcomes in children and adolescents with syndromic and nonsyndromic craniosynostosis. *Plastic & Reconstructive Surgery, 118,* 175–181.

Dahlquist, L. M. (1985). The effects of behavioral intervention on dental flossing skills in children. *Journal of Pediatric Psychology, 10,* 403–412.

deJong, T., Maliepaard, M., Bannink, N., Raat, H., & Mathijssen, I. M. (2012). Health-related problems and quality of life in patients with syndromic and complex craniosynostosis. *Children's Nervous System,* pre-publication, accessed January 15, 2012, from http://www.ncbi.nlm.nih.gov/pubmed/22234545.

Despars, J., Peter, C., Borghini, A., Pierrehumbert, B., Habersaat, S., Muller-Nix, C., Ansermet, F., & Hohlfeld, J. (2011). Impact of a cleft lip and/or palate on maternal stress and attachment representations. *Cleft Palate–Craniofacial Journal, 48,* 419–424.

Dolger-Hafner, M., Bartsch, A., Trimbach, G., Zobel, I., & Witt, E. (1997). Parental reactions following the birth of a cleft child. *Journal of Orofacial Orthopedics, 58,* 124–133.

Dufton, L. M., Speltz, M. L., Kelly, J. P., Leroux, B., Collett, B. R., & Werler, M. M. (2011). Psychosocial outcomes in children with hemifacial microsomia. *Journal of Pediatric psychology, 36,* 794–805.

Estes, R. E., & Morris, H. L. (1970). Relationships among intelligence, speech proficiency, and hearing sensitivity in children with cleft palates. *Cleft Palate Journal, 7,* 763–773.

Feragen, K. B., Kvalem, I. L., Rumsey, N., & Borge, A. I. H. (2010). Adolescents with and without a facial difference: The role of friendships and social acceptance in perceptions of appearance and emotional resilience. *Body Image, 7,* 271–279.

Ferini-Strambi, L., Baietto, C., DiGioia, M. R., Castaldi, P., Castronovo, C., Zucconi, M., & Cappa, S. F. (2003). Cognitive dysfunction in patients with obstructive sleep apnea (OSA): Partial reversibility after continuous positive airway pressure (CPAP). *Brain Research Bulletin, 6,* 87–92.

Field, T. M., & Vega-Lahr, N. (1984). Early interactions between infants with craniofacial anomalies and their mothers. *Infant Behavior & Development, 7,* 527–530.

Findley, L. J., Barth, J. T., Powers, D. C., Wilhoit, S. C., Boyd, D. G. & Surratt, P. M. (1986). Cognitive impairment in patients with obstructive sleep apnea and associated hypoxemia. *Chest, 90,* 686–690.

Finnegan, D. E. (1982). General and special educators' basic information and experience with cleft palate. *Cleft Palate Journal, 19,* 222–229.

Friman, P. C., & Leibowitz, J. M. (1990). An effective and acceptable treatment alternative for chronic thumb- and finger-sucking. *Journal of Pediatric Psychology, 15,* 57–65.

Fuerst, K. B., Dool, C. B., & Rourke, B. P. (1995). Velocardiofacial syndrome. In B. P. Rourke (Ed.), *Syndrome of nonverbal learning disabilities: Neurodevelopmental manifestations* (pp. 119–137), New York: Guilford Press.

Fujiki, M., Brinton, B., & Clarke, D. (2002). Emotion regulation in children with specific language impairment. *Language, Speech, and Hearing Services in Schools, 33,* 102–111.

Gerdes, M., Solot, C., Wang, P. P., Moss, E., LaRossa, D., Randall, P., Goldmuntz, et al. (1999). Cognitive and behavior profile of preschool children with chromosome 22q11.2 deletion, *American Journal of Medical Genetics, 85,* 127–133.

Goodstein, L. D. (1960). MMPI differences between parents of children with cleft palate and parents of physically normal children. *Journal of Speech and Hearing Research, 3,* 31–38.

Goodstein, L. D. (1961). Intellectual impairment in children with cleft palates. *Journal of Speech and Hearing Research, 4,* 287–294.

Grollemund, B., Galliani, E., Soupre, V., Vazquez, M. P., Guedeney, A., & Danion, A. (2010). The impact of cleft lip and palate on the parent-child relationships. *Archives de Pediatric, 17,* 1380–1385.

Hosoda, M., Stone-Romero, E. F., & Coats, G. (2003). The effects of physical attractiveness on job-related outcomes: A meta-analysis of experimental studies. *Personnel Psychology, 56,* 431–462.

Hunt, O., Burden, D., Orth, D., Orth. M., Hepper, P., Stevenson, M., Johnston, C., et al. (2006). Self-reports of psychosocial functioning among children and young adults with cleft lip and palate. *Cleft Palate–Craniofacial Journal, 43,* 598–605.

Hutchinson, K., Wellman, M. A., Noe, D. A., & Kahn, A. (2011). The psychosocial effects of cleft lip and palate in non-Anglo populations: A cross-cultural meta-analysis. *Cleft Palate–Craniofacial Journal, 48,* 497–509.

Kapp-Simon, K. (1986). Self-concept of primary school age children with cleft lip, cleft palate or both. *Cleft Palate Journal, 23,* 24–27.

Kapp-Simon, K. A., Simon, D. J., & Krisovich, S. (1992). Self-perception, social skills, adjustment and inhibition in young adolescents with craniofacial anomalies. *Cleft Palate–Craniofacial Journal, 29,* 352–356.

Kedesdy, J. H., & Budd, K. S. (1998). *Childhood feeding disorders.* Brookes: Baltimore, MD. Kelly, R. I., & Hennekam, R. C. M. (2000). The Smith-Lemli-Opitz syndrome. *Journal of Medical Genetics, 37,* 321–355.

Kerr, S. M., & McIntosh, J. B. (2000). Coping when a child has a disability: Exploring theimpact of parent-to-parent support. *Child: Care, Health and Development, 26,* 309–322.

Klatt, R., Schultz, J., Lee, L., & Saal, H. (2002). Parent and teacher concerns of school age children with isolated cleft lip or cleft palate. Annual Conference of National

Society of Genetics Counselors, Phoenix, Arizona.

Koomen, H., & Hoeksma, J. (1993). Early hospitalization and disturbances of infant behavior and the mother-infant relationship. *Journal of Child Psychology and Psychiatry, 34,* 917–934.

Kramer, F-J., Baethge, C., Sinikovic, H., & Schliephake, H. (2007). An analysis of quality of life in 130 families having small children with cleft lip/palate using the impact on family scale. *International Journal of Oral and Maxillofacial Surgery, 36,* 1146–1152.

Lamb, M., Wilson, F., & Leeper, H. (1973). The intellectual function of cleft palate children compared on the basis of cleft type and sex. *Cleft Palate Journal, 10,* 367.

Mani, M., Carlsson, M., & Marcusson, A. (2010). EDITOR'S CHOICE: Quality of Life Varies with Gender and Age among Adults Treated for Unilateral Cleft Lip and Palate. *Cleft Palate–Craniofacial Journal, 47*(5), 491–498.

McWilliams, B. J., & Musgrave, R. (1972). Psychological implications of articulation disorders in cleft palate children. *Cleft Palate Journal, 9,* 294–303.

McWilliams, B. J., & Paradise, L. P. (1973). Educational, occupational and marital status of cleft palate adults. *Cleft Palate Journal, 10,* 223–229.

Meyer-Marcotty, P., Gerdes, A. B. M., Stellzig-Eisenhauer, A., & Alpers, G. W. (2011). Visual face perception of adults with unilateral cleft lip and palate in comparison to controls—An eye-tracking study. *Cleft Palate–Craniofacial Journal, 48,* 210–217.

Middleton, G. N., Lass, N. J., Starr, P., & Pannbacker, M. (1986). Survey of public awareness and knowledge of cleft palate. *Cleft Palate Journal, 23,* 58–63.

Millard, T., & Richman, L. C. (2001). Different cleft conditions, facial appearance, and speech: Relationship to psychological variables. *Cleft Palate–Craniofacial Journal, 38,* 68–75.

Miller, M. T., Strmland, K., Ventura, L., Johansson, M., Bandim, J. M., & Gilberg, C. (2005). Autism associated with conditions characterized by developmental errors in early embryogenesis: A mini review. *International Journal of Developmental Neuroscience, 23,* 201–219.

Moeller, M. P. (2007). Current state of knowledge: Psychosocial development in children with hearing impairment. *Ear and Hearing, 28,* 729–739.

Murphy, K. C., Jones, L. A., & Owen, M. J. (1999). High rates of schizophrenia in adults with velo-cardio-facial syndrome. *Archives of General Psychiatry, 56,* 940–945.

Murray, L., Arteche, A., Bingley, C., Hentges, F., Bishop, D. V., Dalton, L., Goodacre, T., et al. (2010). The effect of cleft lip on socio-emotional functioning in school-aged children. *Journal of Child Psychology and Psychiatry, and Allied Disciplines, 51,* 94–103.

Nelson, P., Glenny, A. M., Kirk, S., & Caress, A. L. (2012). Parents' experiences of caring for a child with a cleft lip and/or palate: A review of the literature. *Child: Care, Health and Development, 38*(1), 6–20.

Nocella, J., & Kaplan, R. M. (1982). Training children to cope with dental treatment. *Journal of Pediatric Psychology, 7*(2), 175–178.

Nopoulos, P., Choe, L., Berg, S., Van Demark, D., Canady, J., & Richman, L. (2005). Ventral frontal cortex morphology in adult males with isolated orofacial clefts: Relationship to abnormalities in social function.

Cleft Palate–Craniofacial Journal, 42, 138–144.

Ogier, A. & Britton, H. (2013). *Finding My Voice.* Adelaide, Australia: Peacock Publications.

Papolos, D. F., Faedda, G. L., Veit, S., Goldberg, R., Morrow, B., Kucherlapati, R. & Shprintzen, R. J. (1996). Bipolar spectrum disorders in patients diagnosed with velo-cardio-facial syndrome: Does a hemizygous deletion of chromosome 22q11 result in affective disorder? *American Journal of Psychiatry, 153,* 1541–1547.

Persson, M., Becker, M., & Svensson, H. (2008). General intellectual capacity of young men with cleft lip with or without cleft palate and cleft palate alone. *Scandinavian Journal of Plastic and Reconstructive Surgery and Hand Surgery, 42,* 14–16.

Pertschuk, M. J., & Whitaker, L. A. (1982). Social and psychological effects of craniofacial deformity and surgical reconstruction. *Clinical Plastic Surgery, 9,* 297–306.

Pertschuk, M. J., & Whitaker, L. A. (1988). Psychosocial outcome of craniofacial surgery in Children. *Plastic and Reconstructive Surgery, 82,* 741–746.

Philippot, P., Lenoir, N., D'Hoore, W., & Bercy, P. (2005). Improving patients' compliance with the treatment of periodontitis: A controlled study of behavioural intervention. *Journal of Clinical Periodontology, 32,* 653–658.

Pillemer, F. G., & Cook, K. V. (1989). The psychosocial adjustment of pediatric craniofacial patients after surgery. *Cleft Palate Journal, 26,* 201–207.

Pope, A. W., & Snyder, H. T. (2005). Psychosocial adjustment in children and adolescents with a craniofacial anomaly: Age and sex patterns. *Cleft Palate–Craniofacial Journal, 42,* 349–354.

Pope, A. W., Tillman, K., & Snyder, H. T. (2005). Parenting stress in infancy and psychosocial adjustment in toddlerhood: A longitudinal study of children with craniofacial anomalies. *Cleft Palate Craniofacial Journal, 42,* 556–559.

Powers, S. W., Blount, R. L., Bachanas, P. J., & Cotter, M. W. (1993). Helping preschool leukemia patients and their parents cope during injections. *Journal of Pediatric Psychology, 18,* 681–695.

Ramstad, T. E., Ottem, E., & Shaw, W. C. (1995a). Psychosocial adjustment in Norwegian adults who had undergone standardised treatment of complete cleft lip and palate: II. Self-reported problems and concerns with appearance. *Scandinavian Journal of Plastic and Reconstructive Surgery and Hand Surgery, 29,* 329–336.

Ramstad, T. E., Ottem, E., & Shaw, W. C. (1995b). Psychosocial adjustment in Norwegian adults who had undergone standardized treatment of complete cleft lip and palate: I. Education, employment and marriage. *Scandinavian Journal of Plastic and Reconstructive Surgery and Hand Surgery, 29,* 251–257.

Redsell, S., & Glazebrook, C. (2010). Finding a voice: The development of children's healthcare, in S. Redsell & A. Hastings (Eds.), *Listening to children and young people in healthcare consultations.* Abingdon Oxon: Radcliffe Publishing.

Renier, D., Arnaud, E., Cinali, G., Sebag, G., Zerah, M., & Marchac, D. (1996). Prognosis for mental function in Apert's syndrome. *Journal of Neurology, 85,* 66–72.

Richman, L. (1978). Parents and teachers: Differing views of behavior of cleft palate children. *Cleft Palate Journal, 15,* 360–364.

Richman, L. C., & Eliason, M. (1982). Psychological characteristics of children with cleft lip and palate: Intellectual, achievement, behavioral, and personality variables. *Cleft Palate Journal, 19,* 249.

Richman, L. C., & Millard, T. (1997). Brief report: Cleft lip and palate: Longitudinal behavior and relationships of cleft conditions to behavior and achievement. *Journal of Pediatric Psychology, 22,* 487–494.

Richman, L. C., & Ryan, S. M. (2003). Do the reading disabilities of children with cleft fit into current models of developmental dyslexia? *Cleft Palate–Craniofacial Journal, 40,* 154–157.

Richman, L. G., Ryan, S., Wilgenbusch, T., & Millard, T. (2004). Overdiagnosis and medication for attention-deficit hyperactivity disorder in children with cleft: Diagnostic examination and follow-up. *Cleft Palate–Craniofacial Journal, 41,* 351–354.

Rosenberg, J. M., Kapp-Simon, K. A., Starr, J. R., Cradock, M., & Speltz, M. L. (2011). Mothers' and fathers reports of stress in families of infants with and without single-suture craniosynostosis. *Cleft Palate Craniofacial Journal, 48,* 509–518.

Sank, J., Berk, N. W., Cooper, M. E., & Marazita, M. I. (2003). Perceived social support of mothers of children with clefts. *Cleft Palate–Craniofacial Journal, 40*(2), 165–171.

Sarwer, D. B., Bartlett, S. P., Whitaker, L. A., Paige, K. T., Pertschuk, M. J., & Wadden, T. A. (1999). Adult psychological functioning of individuals born with craniofacial anomalies, *Plastic & Reconstructive Surgery, 103,* 412–418.

Shprintzen, R. J., Goldberg, R., Golding-Kushner, K. J., & Marion, R. W. (1992). Late-onset psychosis in the velo-cardio-facial syndrome. *American Journal of Medical Genetics, 42,* 141–142.

Shprintzen, R. J., Goldberg, R. B., Lewin, M. L., Sidoti, E. J., Berkman, M. D., Argamaso, R. V., & Young, D. (1978). A new syndrome involving cleft palate, cardiac anomalies, typical facies, and learning disabilities: Velo-cardio-facial syndrome. *Cleft Palate Journal, 15,* 56–62.

Shute, R., McCarthy, K. R., & Roberts, R. (2007). Predictors of social competence in young adolescents with craniofacial anomalies. *International Journal of Clinical and Health Psychology, 7,* 595–613.

Sinko, K., Jagsch, R., Prechtl, V., Watzinger, F., Hollmann, K., & Baumann, A. (2005). Evaluation of esthetic, functional, and quality-of-life outcome in adult cleft lip and palate patients. *Cleft Palate–Craniofacial Journal, 42,* 355–361.

Slifer, K. J., Beek, M., Amari, A., Diver, T., Hilley, L., Kane, A., & McDonnell, S. (2003). Self-concept and satisfaction with physical appearance in youth with and without oral clefts. *Children's Health Care, 32,* 81–101.

Slifer, K. J., Amari, A., Diver, T., Hilley, L., Beek, M., Kane, A., & McDonnell, S. (2004). Social interaction patterns of children and adolescents with and without oral clefts during a videotaped analogue social encounter. *Cleft Palate–Craniofacial Journal, 41,* 175–184.

Sokol, R. J., Delaney-Black, V., & Nordstrom, B. (2003). Fetal alcohol spectrum disorder. *JAMA, 290*(22), 2996–2999.

Sousa, A. D., Devare, S., & Ghanshani, J. (2009). Psychological issues in cleft lip and palate. *Journal of Indian Association of Pediatric Surgeons, 14,* 55–58.

Speltz, M. L., Morton, K., Goodell, E. W., & Clarren, S. K. (1993). Psychological functioning of children with craniofacial anomalies and their mothers: Follow-up from late infancy to school entry. *Cleft Palate–Craniofacial Journal, 30,* 482–489.

Speltz, M. G., Armsden, G. C., & Clarren, S. S. (1990). Effects of craniofacial birth defects on maternal functioning postinfancy. *Journal of Pediatric Psychology, 15,* 177–196.

Storch, S. A., Bravata, E. A., Storch, J. B., Johnson, J. A., Roth, D. A., & Roberti, J. W.

(2003). Psychosocial adjustment in early adulthood: The role of childhood teasing and father support. *Child Study Journal, 33,* 153–163.

Strauss, R. P. (2001). "Only skin deep": Health, resilience, and craniofacial care. *Cleft Palate–Craniofacial Journal, 38,* 226–230.

Strauss, R. P., & Fenson, C. (2005). Experiencing the "good life": Literary views of craniofacial conditions and quality of life. *Cleft Palate–Craniofacial Journal, 42,* 14–18.

Strauss, R. P., Ramsey, B. L., Edwards, T. C., Topolski, T. D., Kapp-Simon, K. A., Thomas, C. R., Fenson, C., & Patrick, D. L. (2007). Stigma experiences in youth with facial differences: A multi-site study of adolescents and their mothers. *Orthodontics and Craniofacial Research, 10,* 96–103.

Strauss, R. P., Sharp, M. C., Lorch, S. C., & Kachalia, B. (1995). Physicians' communication of "bad news": Parent experiences of being informed of their child's cleft lip/palate. *Pediatrics, 96,* 82–89.

Swillen, A., Devriendt, K., Legius, E., Eyskens, B., Doumoulin, M., Gewillig, M., & Fryns, J. P. (1997). Intelligence and psychosocial adjustment in velocardiofacial syndrome: A study of 37 children and adolescents with VCFS. *Journal of Medical Genetics, 34,* 453–458.

Terman, L. M., & Merrill, M. A. (1960). *Stanford-Binet Intelligence Scale: Manual for the Third Revision, Form L-M.* Oxford, England: Houghton Mifflin.

Thomas, P. S., Turner, S. R., Rumsey, N., Dowell, T., & Sandy, J. R. (1997). Satisfaction with facial appearance among subjects affected by a cleft. *Cleft Palate–Craniofacial Journal, 34,* 226–231.

Tobiasen, J. M. (1988). Psychosocial outcome of craniofacial surgery in children: Discussion. *Plastic and Reconstructive Surgery, 82,* 745–746.

Tobiasen, J. M. (1989). Scaling facial impairment. *Cleft Palate Journal, 26,* 249–254.

Tobiasen, J., & Speltz, M. (1996). Cleft palate: A psychosocial developmental prospective. In S. Berkowitz (Ed.), *Cleft lip and palate: Perspectives in management, vol. II* (15–23). Singular Publishing Group: San Diego.

Van Staden, F., & Gerhardt, C. (1995). Mothers of children with facial cleft deformities: Reactions and effects. *South American Journal of Psychology, 25*(1), 39–46.

Weigl, V., Rudolph, M., Eysholdt, U., & Rosanowski, F. (2005). Anxiety, depression, and quality of life in mothers of children with cleft lip/palate, *Folia Phoniatrica et Logopaedica, 57,* 20–27.

Wasserman, G., Allen, R., & Solomon, C. R. (1986). Limit setting in mothers of toddlers with physical anomalies. *47*(11–12), 290–294.

Winston, K. A., Dunbar, S. B., Reed, C. N., & Francis-Connolly, E. (2010). Mothering occupations when parenting children with feeding concerns: A mixed method study, *Canadian Journal of Occupational Therapy, 77,* 181–189.

Young, J. L., O'Riordan, M., Goldstein, J. A., & Robin, N. H. (2001) What Information Do Parents of Newborns With Cleft Lip, Palate, or Both Want to Know? *Cleft Palate–Craniofacial Journal, 38,* 55–58.

Yttri, J. E., Christensen, K., Knudsen, L. B., & Bille, C. (2011). Reproductive patterns among Danish women with oral clefts. *Cleft Palate–Craniofacial Journal, 48,* 601–608.

ASSESSMENT PROCEDURES: SPEECH, RESONANCE, AND VELOPHARYNGEAL FUNCTION

CHAPTER

11

SPEECH AND RESONANCE ASSESSMENT

CHAPTER OUTLINE

INTRODUCTION

The evaluation of resonance and velopharyngeal function begins with a perceptual speech pathology evaluation. The purpose of this evaluation is to determine whether resonance is normal or abnormal and whether there are any other characteristics of velopharyngeal dysfunction, such as nasal air emission or compensatory articulation productions. A qualified and experienced speech-language pathologist should do the perceptual evaluation of speech and resonance (Smith & Kuehn, 2007).

The goal of the perceptual evaluation is to determine not only whether an abnormality exists but also the type, severity, and possible cause of the disorder. Based on the results of the evaluation, further assessment may be recommended, using instrumental procedures. The ultimate goal of the evaluation is to obtain enough information regarding the disorder to be able to make appropriate recommendations for treatment.

The purpose of this chapter is to review the perceptual evaluation process for individuals who have a history of cleft lip/palate, other craniofacial anomalies, suspected velopharyngeal dysfunction, or a resonance disorder due to other causes. This chapter provides practical suggestions for a thorough assessment of resonance and articulation that correlates to velopharyngeal dysfunction.

TIMETABLE FOR ASSESSMENT

Children with a history of a cleft lip/palate or other craniofacial conditions are at risk for communication disorders. If the child had a cleft of the primary palate, there is a risk of dental or occlusal abnormalities. If the cleft was of the secondary palate, the risk is primarily related to velopharyngeal dysfunction. As noted in Chapter 6, there may also be other problems, such as neurological dysfunction, especially if the child has a craniofacial syndrome. The structural and functional problems that are typical of cleft and craniofacial conditions can cause problems in the areas of articulation, language, phonation, and resonance at different times in development. Therefore, periodic assessments are needed (Smith & Guyette, 2004). The evaluation of velopharyngeal function should be done as soon as it is possible to obtain reliable results.

First Year

The first year of a child's life is usually a time of great joy for the parents. However, when the infant has a congenital anomaly, there is also significant anxiety over what will happen in the future and the ultimate results of treatment. Most people cope best with information rather than with uncertainty. Therefore, the parents should be counseled by various professionals, preferably by members of a cleft palate team, soon after the birth and again early in the first year. These professionals should explain the diagnosis, the effect of the anomalies on function, what might happen in the future, what will be done about it, and the ultimate prognosis.

During the first year, the primary speech-language pathology concerns are feeding, language development, and the development of the physical prerequisites for speech. The family should be assisted with feeding modifications as necessary. In addition, the infant's development should be monitored through parent report, direct observation, or the use of infant scales. If problems in development are noted, further assessment and intervention should be initiated immediately.

During the first year, the speech-language pathologist should counsel the family on methods of speech and language stimulation. It should be emphasized that under the age of 3, language development should be the primary focus. In other words, the quantity of speech is more important than the quality of speech during those early years. However, instructions for stimulating speech sound production after the palate repair are also important to include in this discussion. The speech-language pathologist should reinforce this discussion with a handout that summarizes the information and provides additional suggestions.

Annual Screenings and Periodic Evaluations

The American Cleft Palate–Craniofacial Association has an official publication called the *Parameters for Evaluation and Treatment of Patients with Cleft Lip/Palate or Other Craniofacial Anomalies* (American Cleft Palate–Craniofacial Association, 2009). In this publication, it is recommended that children with a history of cleft lip/palate or craniofacial anomalies receive a screening evaluation of speech and language skills at least twice during the first 2 years of life and at least annually thereafter until the age of 6 years. After the age of 6, screenings should be done annually until after adenoid involution, and at least every 2 years thereafter

until dental and skeletal maturity are reached (American Cleft Palate–Craniofacial Association, 2009). This is often done during the annual visit to the cleft palate or craniofacial team. If problems are suspected during these screening assessments, the child should be scheduled for a more in-depth evaluation.

Around the age of 3, the child should receive a comprehensive evaluation of speech and language. If the child is communicating with connected speech and is able to produce a variety of speech sounds, this is also the appropriate time to evaluate resonance and velopharyngeal function. On the other hand, if the child's speech development and expressive language development are delayed, the assessment of resonance and velopharyngeal function should be done at a later time in order to obtain accurate results.

In addition to the annual evaluations, a perceptual assessment, along with instrumental measures, should be done before any surgery that is designed to improve speech (i.e., pharyngeal flap or sphincter pharyngoplasty) or surgery that might affect speech (i.e., orthognathic surgery) (Pannbacker, & Middleton, 1990). It is very important to document baseline information regarding speech and resonance prior to the surgical procedure. A postoperative assessment should also be done to determine the effect of surgery on speech and whether any further treatment is indicated.

THE DIAGNOSTIC INTERVIEW

Whether a comprehensive evaluation is being done or merely a screening evaluation in a cleft palate clinic, the examiner can obtain valuable information from the family regarding the child's overall communication abilities (Hirschberg & Van Demark, 1997). Therefore, the speech pathology evaluation is usually preceded by an interview with the parent or other family members, as appropriate.

Many clinics send the family a pre-evaluation questionnaire in order to obtain medical and development history, and to determine the current concerns about speech. This information helps the examiner to prepare for the evaluation and can shorten the interview process. However, even if background information was received through a questionnaire or medical record, at least a brief interview should be done before the formal assessment. Examples of interview questions for pediatric patients can be found in Table 11–1.

Parents are usually very good observers of their children and can often effectively compare their child's communication skills with those of siblings or peers. A study by Glascoe (1991) showed that identification of the

parent's concern and skillful observation of the child is often sufficient to identify many speech and language problems. Therefore, a simple rule of thumb is as follows: If the parents are worried about their child's speech, there probably is a good reason.

LANGUAGE SCREENING

Because children with a history of cleft or craniofacial anomalies are at risk for language delay, it is important that their language development be monitored closely throughout the preschool years. This can be done through screening evaluations at the time of the yearly visits to the cleft palate/craniofacial team. If language problems are suspected from the screening evaluation, or if the parents express

---

TABLE 11–1 Sample Questions for Parents: To Be Used When Assessing a Young Child

Current Concern

- What concerns you about your child's speech?
- When did you first become concerned?
- Who referred your child for the evaluation, and what was that person's concern?

Speech Production

- What types of sounds does your child use during vocal play—vowels only or some consonants?
- If the child uses consonants, what are some of the consonants that you hear?
- Are they produced individually or over and over again?
- Does your child "jabber" or use jargon?
- Does your child leave out sounds in words?
- Do you understand your child's speech all of the time, most of the time, some of the time, or hardly at all?
- How well do strangers understand your child's speech?
- Are there any particular speech sounds that are difficult for your child to produce?

Resonance

- Does your child sound nasal? If so, does it sound like your child is talking through her nose, or does it sound like she has a cold?
- Do you ever hear air coming through her nose during speech?
- Do you ever hear a bubbling sound or snorting during speech?
- When did you first notice the problem with nasality?
- If the onset was sudden, what event preceded it?
- Has your child had an adenoidectomy? If so, did it change her speech?
- Does your child's speech vary with the weather, allergies, fatigue, or any other factors?

(Continues)

TABLE 11-1 *(continued)*

Language

- Does your child communicate with gestures, single words, short phrases, incomplete sentences, or complete sentences?
- How many words does your child usually put together in an utterance?
- Does your child leave out the little words (e.g., "of," "to," "the," or "is") in the sentence?
- Is your child communicating as well as other children her age?
- Have you ever had a concern about how well your child understands the speech of others or follows directions?

Medical History

- Was your child born with any congenital problems? If so, what were they? How and when were they treated?
- Does your child have any medical problems, medical diagnoses, or conditions?
- What surgeries has your child undergone?
- Does your child take any medications on a regular basis?
- Does your child hear normally? When was the last hearing test?
- Has your child had many ear infections? If so, how were they treated?
- Does your child have any problems with vision?
- Where is your child on the growth chart?

Developmental History

- Was your child quiet, about average, or very vocal as an infant?
- Did you have any concerns about initial speech development?
- Did your child begin to use words before or after her first birthday?
- When your child was learning to sit up, stand, and walk, did she seem normal or behind other children?
- Did your child walk before or after her first birthday?
- Does your child have any difficulty learning in preschool or school?

Feeding and Oral-Motor Skills

- Does your child have any difficulty chewing, sucking, or swallowing?
- Is there a history of feeding problems?
- Does your child drool or keep her mouth open during the day?

Airway

- Does your child snore at night?
- Does your child ever gasp for breath at night or sleep restlessly?
- Does your child like to breathe through her nose or through her mouth during the day?
- Is your child's breathing ever noisy during the day?
- Does your child have allergies, asthma, or chronic congestion?

Treatment History

- Has your child ever had a speech and/or language evaluation or speech and/or language therapy?
- Is your child currently receiving therapy? If yes, what are the goals?
- Has your child's speech improved in the last 6 months? If so, in what way?

concerns about their child's language development, a comprehensive language evaluation should be done. A comprehensive language evaluation should routinely be done for children who have additional risk factors for language disorders (i.e., hearing loss, developmental delay, or neurological problems). If a language disorder is identified, intervention should be initiated as soon as possible to ensure the best outcome.

The methods for language evaluation are beyond the scope of this text. Instead, the interested reader should consult one of the many books available on this subject. However, a discussion regarding screening methods may be helpful, particularly as it applies to a clinic setting.

One way to screen the language of infants and toddlers is to seek information from the parents through a questionnaire format. The questions must be understandable enough for the parents to answer with confidence and detailed enough to be of value to the examiner. Scherer and D'Antonio (1995) investigated the efficacy of a parent questionnaire as a component of early language screening using the MacArthur Communicative Development Inventory (Fenson et al., 1989). They found that the parent questionnaire can be a valid means of screening language development as compared with other methods.

Although formal screening tests provide structure and a set format, they are not always necessary for language screening. Most experienced examiners can determine whether a child's language is close to age level through the parent interview, observations of the child, and informal testing. An informal screening assessment can be done by these means:

- Observe play behaviors, and the type and complexity of gestures (Scherer & D'Antonio, 1997).

- Ask the child to point to certain objects or follow certain commands.

- Have interesting toys available and observe spontaneous vocalizations and utterances.

- Listen to the child's spontaneous speech while he or she is talking to the parent.

- Ask questions or ask for explanations (see Table 11–2 for examples).

- Have the child repeat sentences, such as those listed in the articulation screening test (see Table 11–3), Even in repeating, the child will usually revert to his or her own form of syntax and morphology, which gives an indication of expressive language abilities.

TABLE 11–2 Sample Questions and Requests for Eliciting Speech

What do you like best ...

- Puppy dogs or kitty cats?
- Baby dolls or teddy bears?
- Cupcakes or cookies?
- Chocolate chip cookies or peanut butter cookies?
- Singing or dancing?
- Baseball or basketball?
- Playing inside or outside?

What do you want to be when you grow up? Why?

What does a fireman do? What does a policeman do? What does a teacher do?

Tell me how you make a peanut butter and jelly sandwich.

Explain the game of baseball to me.

TABLE 11–3 Sample Sentences for Assessment of Articulation Placement and Velopharyngeal Function

Have the child repeat the following sentences:

p	Popeye plays in the pool.
b	Buy baby a bib.
m	My mommy made lemonade.
w	Wade in the water.
j	You have a yellow yo-yo.
h	He has a big horse.
t	Take Teddy to town.
d	Do it for Daddy.
n	Nancy is not here.
k	I like cookies and cake.
g	Go get the wagon.
ŋ	Put the ring on her finger.
f	I have five fingers.
v	Drive a van.
l	I like yellow lollipops.
s	I see the sun in the sky.
z	Zip up your zipper.
ʃ	She went shopping.
ʧ	I ride a choo-choo train.
ʤ	John told a joke to Jim.
r	Randy has a red fire truck.
ɚ	The teacher and doctor are here.
θ	Thank you for the toothbrush.
blends	splash, sprinkle, street

© Cengage Learning 2014

Through these simple methods, the examiner should be able to determine the primary mode of communication (i.e., gestures, signs, single words, short utterances, short sentences, or complete sentences). If the child is communicating with sentences, the examiner should also be able to determine whether the sentences are complete or merely telegraphic; the approximate mean length of utterance (MLU); and whether there are errors of syntax and morphology. Overall, the behaviors of the child, as noted through observation and report, can be compared to norms to estimate the child's developmental level and determine whether formal language testing is necessary.

There are several formal screening tests that allow the examiner to sample the child's communication abilities using a more structured format. Screening tests for children under the age of 3 include the *Receptive-Expressive Emergent Language Scale* (REEL-3), 3rd edition (Bzoch, League, & Brown, 2003); the *Early Language Milestone* (ELM) *Scale*, 2nd edition (Coplan, 1993); and *The Rossetti Infant-Toddler Language Scale* (Rossetti, 2006). These tests are scored through direct observation and parent report. For children between the ages of 2 and 6, the *Fluharty Preschool Speech and Language Screening Test*, 2nd edition (Fluharty, 2000), can be used to screen both articulation and language development. Other preschool language tests include the *Clinical Evaluation of Language Fundamentals® Preschool*, 5th edition (CELF®-5) (Semel, Wiig, & Secord, 2013), and the *Preschool Language Scales*, 5th edition (PLS™-5) (Zimmerman, Steiner, & Pond, 2011).

PERCEPTUAL ASSESSMENT

Although instrumentation is helpful in the assessment of speech, resonance, and velopharyngeal function; the most important tool that we have is the "examiner's ear" (Smith & Kuehn, 2007). In fact, in a survey of speech-language pathologists and cleft palate surgeons in the United States, 99.2% of the 126 respondents who were associated with a cleft palate team reported that they always include a perceptual assessment in the assessment of velopharyngeal insufficiency (Kummer, Clark, Redle, Thomsen, & Billmire, 2011).

In the perceptual evaluation, the ear is used to analyze the acoustic product of velopharyngeal function in order to make inferences about the function of the velopharyngeal mechanism. From a thorough analysis of what is perceived, a determination can be made regarding the status of velopharyngeal function and its potential for change. If there is no abnormality, as judged by a perceptual evaluation, then it does not matter what the instrumental procedures show. It is only when the perceptual evaluation shows an abnormality that treatment is ever initiated (Trindade, Genaro, Yamashita, Miguel, & Fukushiro, 2005).

As part of the perceptual evaluation, the examiner should also determine whether speech sound production is affected by abnormal structure (e.g., velopharyngeal insufficiency or dental malocclusion) versus abnormal function. This determination is particularly important because it impacts the treatment plan (Kummer, 2011). Finally, the perceptual evaluation should include a judgment of phonation.

Some children are naturally loquacious, and little or no effort is needed to elicit spontaneous connected speech. Other children need some prodding. In fact, anyone who works with young children knows that if a child does not want to talk, you can't make that child talk. Instead, you have to find ways to make the child *want* to talk.

To encourage the child to interact and talk during the examination, the following tips may be helpful:

- Be sure to smile and be approachable.
- Don't wear a white coat.
- Talk to the parents first, and only occasionally comment to the child without asking him to talk or respond in any way. Allow him to warm up to the situation.
- Start interacting with the child by making comments about his clothing, a toy, or a picture.
- Ask the child either/or questions, as noted in Table 11–2. Children are much more likely to respond to an either/or question than an open-ended one or a request to repeat.
- Once the child is responding to the either/or questions, then gradually begin asking the child to repeat the test speech samples.
- Once the child is responding, questions that require a longer response can be asked (e.g., "How do you play the game of baseball?").
- If the child still refuses to talk, ask the parent to try to elicit words or conversation while the examiner appears to be not listening.

SPEECH SAMPLES

When assessing speech production, resonance, and velopharyngeal function, it is important to select an appropriate speech sample to obtain the information that is needed for a definitive diagnosis. When testing a child, the speech sample must also be developmentally appropriate in the areas of speech sound production and syntax.

Formal Articulation Tests

The *Iowa Pressure Articulation Test*, a part of the *Templin-Darley Tests of Articulation* (Templin & Darley, 1960), and the *Bzoch Error Pattern Diagnostic Articulation Tests* (Bzoch, 1979) were specifically designed to assess the effects of velopharyngeal insufficiency/incompetence (VPI). However, any formal (or informal) test of speech sound production can also be used for this purpose and provides the information needed.

Although a formal articulation test with single words and single articulatory targets is a standard method to assess speech sound accuracy, it actually provides limited information about the child's actual speech characteristics in normal conversation. Single word production places limited demand on the oral-motor system. In addition, the target phoneme may be affected by the phonemic context. Finally, a single word articulation test that involves naming pictures can be time-consuming to administer. Therefore, an informal test of articulation using repetition and connected speech is often more appropriate and provides better diagnostic information.

Single Sounds

Repetition of single phonemes can be done to estimate a child's phonemic inventory, especially if the child has limited connected speech. Vowels can be repeated in isolation. Some consonants however, especially voiced plosives and affricates, are best evaluated in a consonant-vowel syllable with a low vowel (e.g., /bɑ/, dɑ/, gɑ/, etc.).

Imitation of isolated phonemes can also be used to test resonance and determine whether there is nasal emission. To test for hypernasality, prolongation of a vowel should be used, because vowels are purely resonance sounds. Comparing resonance between a low vowel (e.g., /ɑ/) and a high vowel (e.g., /i/) can be helpful. To test for nasal emission, a pressure-sensitive consonant should be used. The best consonant for this purpose is /s/ because it not only requires oral pressure, but it is also a continuant. Having the child prolong the /s/ further taxes the velopharyngeal mechanism. If hyponasality or cul-de-sac resonance is suspected, prolongation of the /m/ sound is a good test. With the lips totally closed,

the sound has to travel through the pharynx and nasal cavity. If there is obstruction in either cavity, prolongation of the /m/ will be noticeably difficult.

Syllable Repetition

It is often helpful to test phonemes at the syllable level in order to assess one consonant and one vowel at a time. A syllable test eliminates the effects of other contiguous sounds and helps the examiner to determine whether there is phoneme-specific nasal air emission on consonants or phoneme-specific hypernasality on vowels.

The syllable test is done by having the child produce the high-pressure consonants (plosives, fricatives, and affricates) in syllables and in a repetitive manner (e.g., /pɑ, pɑ, pɑ/, /pi, pi, pi/, /tɑ, tɑ, tɑ/, /ti, ti, ti/, etc.). The voiceless phoneme is used rather than its voiced cognate. This is because nasal emission is easier to hear when there is no phonation. In addition, voiceless consonants have a higher degree of air pressure than their voiced cognates, and hence nasal emission is more likely to occur on these consonants.

Each of the pressure-sensitive phonemes should be tested with both a low vowel (such as /ɑ/) and then again with a high vowel (such as /i/). This type of test allows the examiner to assess articulation placement, oral pressure, and the presence of nasal emission on each individual consonant. It also allows the examiner to determine whether hypernasality is vowel specific or occurs only on high vowels (Lee, Wang, & Fu, 2009; Kummer, 2009; Kummer, 2011).

Sentence Repetition

To test speech and resonance in connected speech (and to also obtain some clues regarding expressive language), the examiner should have a battery of sentences for the child to repeat. A sample list of sentences for evaluation of articulation placement, in addition to velopharyngeal function, can be found in Table 11–3.

Each sentence should contain phonemes that are similar in articulatory placement (e.g., "Take Teddy to town"). When evaluating for nasal emission, the sample should contain many pressure-sensitive consonants, particularly those that are voiceless (e.g., "I see the sun in the sky"). When testing for hypernasality, the sample should contain voiced, oral sounds (e.g., "Buy baby a bib"). To separate out the effects of nasal air emission or compensatory errors, the examiner should use a sample of sentences with a large number of low-pressure consonants (e.g., "How are you?"), as can be found in Table 11–4. Finally, to test for hyponasality, the examiner should use sentences with a high frequency of nasal phonemes (e.g., "My mama made lemonade for me"). Sample nasal sentences for assessment of hyponasality can be found in Table 11–5.

By asking the child to repeat these sentences, the examiner can quickly and easily test articulation placement and resonance in a

---

TABLE 11–4 Sample Low-Pressure Sentences for Assessment of Resonance without the Complication of Nasal Air Emission

Have the individual repeat the following sentences:

How are you?

Who are you?

Where are you?

Why are you here?

You are here.

They are here.

Where are they?

They are where you are.

© Cengage Learning 2014

TABLE 11–5 Sample Sentences for Evaluation of Hyponasality

Have the individual repeat the following sentences:

My mama made lemonade for me.

My name is Amy Minor.

My mama takes money to the market.

Many men are at the mine.

Ned made nine points in the game.

My nanny is not mean.

Nan needs a dime to call home.

My mom's home is many miles away.

Many men are needed to move the piano.

© Cengage Learning 2014

---

connected speech environment. The examiner can also determine whether there is consistent or inconsistent nasal emission in connected speech. This is much faster than a single-word articulation test and is actually a more valid test of normal speech production (Hirschberg & Van Demark, 1997).

Counting

Connected speech can often be elicited from a young child by having him count or recite the alphabet. Counting from 60 to 70, or simply repeating "60, 60, 60, 60" can be particularly informative because these numbers contain a combination of a high vowel (/i/), the sibilant /s/, plosives, and even a triple blend (/kst/). As a result, these words require a buildup and continuation of intraoral air pressure, which can particularly tax the velopharyngeal mechanism and may overwhelm a tenuous velopharyngeal valve. Counting from 70 to 79 can be diagnostic as this series contains a nasal phoneme (/n/) followed by an alveolar plosive. (The /t/ in 70 is usually pronounced as /d/ in American English.) Velopharyngeal timing difficulties may become apparent in this speech sample as assimilated hypernasality. If there are concerns regarding possible hyponasality, counting from 90 to 99 allows the examiner to assess the production of the nasal /n/ in connected speech.

Connected Speech

Although a single-word test helps the examiner to isolate the production of individual phonemes, it is important to assess articulation, and particularly resonance, in connected speech. Connected speech increases the demands on the velopharyngeal valving system to achieve and maintain closure. As a result, hypernasality and nasal emission are more apparent in connected speech than in single words. An increase in articulation errors is also common during the production of continuous utterances. Connected speech can be spontaneous, or the examiner can ask the child to repeat syllables or sentences over and over to simulate connected speech.

WHAT TO EVALUATE

Patients with clefts or craniofacial conditions often have disorders of speech sound production, resonance, and voice. Thus, these areas should be the focus of an evaluation. For children under the age of 6, a screening assessment of language should also be done, with further in-depth assessment as needed.

Speech Sound Production

In assessing articulation, it is important to determine whether there are any speech sound errors or distortions. It is also important to identify the type of errors (e.g., placement, phonological, or developmental errors). When there are structural anomalies, the examiner must determine whether there are any

compensatory errors or obligatory distortions. It is necessary to assess the potential cause of the errors (abnormal structure, apraxia or oralmotor dysfunction, phonological disorder, delayed development, or normal developmental error). Finally, the examiner should determine whether there is nasal air emission during the production of pressure-sensitive phonemes, or nasalization of other voiced oral consonants. All of this information is important because it is used as a basis for determining appropriate treatment.

As noted previously, an obligatory error is one where the articulation placement (the function) is normal, but the abnormality of the structure causes distortion of speech. For example, when there is a large velopharyngeal opening, the placement of articulation may be normal, but manner of production is altered from oral to nasal due to the lack of velopharyngeal closure. As a result, voiced plosives may sound closer to their nasal cognates (m/b, n/d, and ŋ/g). These are considered obligatory distortions because articulation placement is normal. Whenever nasal phonemes are primarily heard with connected speech, the examiner should suspect a significant velopharyngeal opening due to these obligatory errors. Another obligatory distortion is nasal emission on consonants, despite normal articulation placement.

Compensatory articulation errors are common in individuals with VPI; therefore, it is important to specifically look for these errors in this population. When compensatory errors occur as a result of VPI, the manner of production may be maintained (e.g., a plosive is substituted with another plosive, and a fricative is substituted with another fricative). However, the placement of production is moved posteriorly to the pharynx, where there is airflow. In other cases, the placement is similar, but the manner is changed to a voiced nasal sound. For example, if the child cannot build up pressure for an /s/ sound or other sibilants, a compensation may be to produce an /n/ (which has a similar placement) instead. A description of various compensatory errors is found in Chapter 7 and therefore will not be repeated here. In addition, Trost-Cardamone (1987) has an instructional videotape in which compensatory productions are nicely demonstrated.

Some compensatory productions can be co-articulated with the normal oral sound. For example, plosives can be produced with normal placement in the oral cavity, but co-articulated with a glottal stop (/ʔ/) for the "plosion." Fricatives and affricates (particularly sibilants) can be co-articulated with a pharyngeal or posterior nasal fricative for the "friction."

To determine the true placement of the sound, the examiner should listen carefully and, if necessary, try to imitate the sound. By imitating the production, the examiner can usually determine the place of production and thus identify the cause of the error. The examiner should also watch the production of each phoneme. Glottal stops, for example, result in visible exaggerated laryngeal movements that can be seen and felt on the patient's neck during articulation.

If the patient is using glottal stops for consonants, without co-articulating the oral placement, this may be confused with a simple consonant omission. To make a distinction between a glottal stop and a true omission, it should be remembered that glottal stops are produced with a rapid voice onset time (like a grunt). If the phoneme is completely omitted, the voice onset is smooth with the initiation of the vowel, and the vowel is longer in duration than if the consonant is substituted by a glottal stop. A final clue to the production of glottal stops is the observation of increased laryngeal activity that can be seen and felt in the throat area.

A pharyngeal fricative can sound similar to a lateral lisp to an inexperienced listener. To make this distinction, the examiner should determine whether the air stream is in the oral or pharyngeal area. If the examiner cannot find the air stream at either side of the dental arch, then the sound is probably produced in the pharynx. See the straw technique below.

The scoring of an articulation test is traditionally done by using phonetic diacritics from the International Phonetic Alphabet (IPA) (Bronsted et al., 1994). However, this system does not include symbols for compensatory productions that are typical of individuals with velopharyngeal dysfunction. Therefore, a set of diacritic symbols for compensatory productions has been proposed by Trost-Cardamone (Trost, 1981; Trost-Cardamone, 1997). The examiner may choose to use these diacritics or to use just the words (e.g., glottal stop, pharyngeal fricative) to describe the errors (which would actually enhance communication with those who are unfamiliar with these symbols).

Stimulability

Stimulability is the ability to correct an abnormal speech sound production when given minimal cues. Stimulability is a good prognostic indicator for whether a speech sound can be corrected with speech therapy and how quickly.

An assessment of stimulability is an important component of the perceptual evaluation of resonance and velopharyngeal function. This is because some compensatory placement errors actually *cause* nasal emission and even hypernasality. For example, the production of a glottal stop, pharyngeal fricative, or nasal fricative is done with the velopharyngeal valve open (Henningsson & Isberg, 1991; Moller, 1991). Therefore, the examiner should determine whether the child is stimulable for elimination of nasal emission or hypernasality with a correction of articulatory placement. If the child is able to produce the sound without nasal air emission or hypernasality merely by changing placement, this suggests that the problem is functional, and hence there is a good prognosis for correction with speech therapy.

Nasal Air Emission

As part of the articulation assessment, the speech-language pathologist should assess for the presence of audible nasal air emission. If it is present, it is important to determine whether the nasal emission is low in intensity, which is usually the result of a larger velopharyngeal opening, or whether it is the "bubbly" nasal rustle (turbulence), which is the result of a small opening (Kummer, Briggs, & Lee, 2003; Kummer, Curtis, Wiggs, Lee, & Strife, 1992). The examiner should also note the occurrence of a nasal snort, which is produced most often with /s/ blends. A nasal grimace commonly accompanies nasal air emission, and this should be reported if it is observed.

The consistency of the nasal air emission should be noted during the articulation test. If nasal emission typically occurs during the production of all pressure-sensitive phonemes, including plosives, then it is considered consistent. If it occurs occasionally on most pressure-sensitive phonemes, then it is inconsistent. If it occurs consistently, but only on specific phonemes, such as sibilants, then it may be phoneme-specific nasal air emission (PSNAE), which is related to faulty articulation rather than VPI. In particular, the production of pharyngeal fricatives or posterior nasal fricatives results in PSNAE because the airflow is in the pharynx and therefore can only be released through the nose.

It is always important to assess for nasal air emission in connected speech. Many patients are able to achieve velopharyngeal closure for short segments and therefore nasal emission may not be noted, even the sentence level. Because connected speech increases the demands on the velopharyngeal mechanism, nasal air emission is more likely to be noted at this level. At times, it is necessary to ask the patient to produce difficult or multisyllabic words (e.g., "60," "basketball") quickly and repetitively to try to tax the velopharyngeal mechanism in order to determine whether there is tenuous closure.

Weak Consonants

The adequacy of intraoral air pressure for the production of pressure-sensitive consonants should be noted. Having the individual repeat sentences loaded with these consonants is a good way to test oral pressure. If these consonants seem to be weak in intensity or pressure, it might be assumed that intraoral air pressure is compromised due to significant nasal air emission (which sometimes is inaudible). Weak consonants are usually associated with both nasal air emission and hypernasality, and are due to a large velopharyngeal opening.

Short Utterance Length

Significant nasal air emission can shorten utterance length. This is because the leak of air through the nose causes the person to have to take more frequent breaths, sometimes even within a sentence, to replenish the airflow. This can be noted by observing the phrasing of utterances in connected speech. In addition, utterance length can be tested by asking the individual to count to 20 and noting when the person takes another breath. Most normal speakers count at least to 15 on one breath.

Oral-Motor Dysfunction

Apraxia of speech can cause inconsistent hypernasality or mixed resonance due to the difficulty in coordinating the movements of the velopharyngeal valve. This can cause errors in closing the valve for oral sounds and opening the valve for nasal sounds. As with placement errors, errors of velopharyngeal closure tend to increase with an increase in utterance length or phonemic complexity. Therefore, the examiner should note the difference in resonance between short, simple utterances and longer, phonemically complex utterances.

Oral-motor dysfunction may be slightly more common in individuals with craniofacial syndromes, particularly those with velocardiofacial syndrome (VCFS), which is a neurodevelopmental disorder (Kummer, Lee, Stutz, Maroney, & Brandt, 2007). When there is hypernasality, particularly in a patient with a syndrome, it is important to determine whether the cause is abnormal structure, abnormal function, or a neuromotor disorder, such as apraxia of speech.

There are several formal tests of apraxia that go from a nonspeech oral level up to the sentence level of production (Hickman, 1997; Kaufman, 1995), but this can also be tested informally. Diadochokinetic exercises can be used to assess the ability to coordinate

---

CASE REPORT

Velocardiofacial Syndrome

Katie, age 2 years 5 months, had a diagnosis of velocardiofacial syndrome. Medical history, which was consistent with this diagnosis, included a submucous cleft, a ventricular septal defect (VSD), and an interrupted aortic valve. Katie was very small for her age, staying consistently under the 10th percentile for both weight and height. She had a history of airway problems as an infant. Early feeding problems were also reported and Katie continued to have difficulty with certain textures. According to the parents, Katie's development of gross motor milestones was essentially within normal limits and her understanding of language seemed normal. However, fine motor skills were abnormal and speech development was delayed.

An assessment revealed that Katie could put words together and even sing nursery rhymes. However, her speech was mostly unintelligible. She communicated primarily with gestures and signs. She had a limited phonemic repertoire consisting of only nasal consonants (/m/, /n/), /h/, glottal stops, and vowels. Occasionally she was able to produce a /d/ approximation. Vowels were on target most, but not all of the time.

Although Katie was able to produce nasal sounds in isolation, she was unable to produce them in certain word positions or with certain vowels. She was also unable to combine them for words such as "mommy," "money," "naming," or "many." When attempting to imitate oral pressure sounds or blow, there was only nasal air emission.

Given all of this information gathered in the evaluation, it was determined that Katie had significant velopharyngeal dysfunction and evidence of significant oral-motor dysfunction.

Recommendations include surgical intervention for correction of the velopharyngeal dysfunction. However, given her age, her size, and her history of airway obstruction, it was decided to delay the surgery for a few months until she was a little bigger. In the meantime, speech therapy, with active involvement of the parents, was recommended to improve articulation placement and ability to combine different articulation positions. This was done with the help of a nose clip both during therapy and at home.

movements for syllables. The individual can be asked to repeat two syllable combinations (e.g., /pʌtʌ, pʌtʌ, pʌtʌ/, etc.) or three syllable combinations (e.g., /pʌtʌkʌ, pʌtʌkʌ, pʌtʌkʌ, pʌtʌkʌ/, etc.). Additionally, the patient can be asked to produce difficult multisyllabic words repetitively (e.g., baseball bat, kitty cat, puppy dog, teddy bear, patty cake, basketball, ice cream cone, etc.). If there is significant hypernasality, the use of words with nasal sounds (e.g., "money," "mommy," "many more," etc.) helps to isolate the oral-motor dysfunction from the VPI.

Resonance

Resonance with connected speech should be judged as either normal or abnormal. If resonance is abnormal, it is very important to determine the type (i.e., hypernasal, hyponasal, cul-de-sac, or mixed) because the type suggests causation and has implications for treatment (Kummer, 2009, 2011). As a general rule, if nasal sounds are heard more frequently than normal or if they are substituted for oral sounds, the resonance is hypernasal. On the other hand, if oral sounds are heard as a substitution for nasal sounds, the resonance is hyponasal. If necessary, the examiner can have the individual repeat sentences loaded with oral sounds and then repeat sentences loaded with nasal sounds if the type of resonance is hard to determine in spontaneous speech. Cul-de-sac resonance sounds as if the voice is muffled and remains in the head. (For comparison, a nasal cul-de-sac resonance can be simulated by imitating hypernasal speech while closing the nose.) Mouth breathing or a history of upper airway obstruction may suggest either hyponasality or cul-de-sac resonance.

Determining the type of resonance is very important, but determining the severity is usually irrelevant. This is because severity of the hypernasality doesn't impact the treatment (Bzoch, 1979). Even if there is mild hypernasality due to VPI, physical management will be required for treatment. Despite this, several authors have suggested the use of an equal-appearing interval scale to rate the severity of deviant resonance with up to seven levels (McWilliams, Morris, & Shelton, 1990; Subtelny, Van Hattum, & Myers, 1972). Although these rating scales have a high degree of face validity, the reliability of these scales is in question. In fact, the more levels on the scale, the less reliable the scale will be. In addition, the severity of hypernasality in a patient who has VPI is usually inconsistent in severity, depending on the utterance length, the speed of production, and effort versus fatigue. If the examiner wants to rate severity, however, it may be best to use a simple four-point scale that includes normal, mild, moderate, and severe as descriptors of severity.

Hypernasality can be phoneme-specific, occurring only on the high vowel /i/. This can be determined by asking the patient to produce syllables with the /i/ vowel and contrasting the resonance with syllables containing the /ɑ/ vowel. In addition, if the patient holds the back of the tongue high during production of other vowels, this will give the perception of hypernasality because it reduces the oral opening and increases transpalatal nasal resonance.

Phonation

Dysphonia is common in individuals with VPI or craniofacial anomalies (McWilliams, Lavorato, & Bluestone, 1973; McWilliams et al., 1990). Therefore, the examiner should listen for characteristics of dysphonia, including hoarseness, breathiness, glottal fry, hard glottal attack, inappropriate pitch level, restricted pitch range, diplophonia, or inappropriate loudness (Kummer & Marsh, 1998). When present, these abnormalities can be rated on a severity scale from mild to severe (Stemple, Glaze, & Gerdeman, 1995; Wilson, 1987). The Consensus Auditory-Perceptual Evaluation of Voice (CAPE-V) is a standardized protocol for evaluation of the auditory perceptual aspects of vocal quality, including roughness, breathiness, strain, pitch and loudness (Kempster et al., 2009). This instrument was developed by a group of experts at a consensus conference and is now what many specialists in voice disorders use today.

In addition to ratings, the ability to sustain phonation for 10 seconds or longer should also be observed. (Dysphonic characteristics may not be noted until the end of the prolonged vowel, as the child begins to run out of air.) Finally, the quality of breath support and the type of breathing pattern should be noted. If the patient has obvious dysphonia, a more comprehensive evaluation of voice should be considered and may include aerodynamic measures, endoscopy, and stroboscopy.

SUPPLEMENTAL EVALUATION PROCEDURES

Experienced clinicians may be able to evaluate all of the above characteristics by merely listening to spontaneous speech or repetition of sounds and sentences. The assessment of experienced evaluators tends to be very reliable (Paal et al., 2005). However, less-experienced clinicians may find it helpful to employ some supplemental tests to more clearly define the speech characteristics and their potential cause. Therefore, the following is a list of simple low-tech and "no-tech" evaluation procedures that may be useful in detecting nasal emission, and in some cases, hypernasality (Kummer, 2009, 2011).

Visual Detection

- ***Mirror Test:*** Some clinicians use the mirror test to determine the presence of nasal emission. For this test, a small mirror (preferably a dental mirror with a narrow rim) is placed under the nares while the patient produces pressure-sensitive sounds (Figure 11–1). If the mirror clouds up with condensation, it indicates nasal emission. This technique can give "false positives" if not done correctly, however. The mirror must be placed under the nares after the patient has already begun talking or it will pick up condensation from normal nasal respiration. In addition, it has to be removed before the patient stops talking because at the end of an utterance, the velum lowers

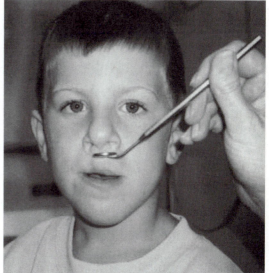

Courtesy Ann W. Kummer, Ph.D./Cincinnati Children's Hospital Medical Center & University of Cincinnati College of Medicine

FIGURE 11–1 A dental mirror for testing nasal air emission. A dental mirror can be held under the nares during speech in order to evaluate nasal air emission. The evaluation is based on the appearance of condensation and should be done carefully to be sure the condensation is not from breathing. Also, this test does not indicate the sound during which the nasal emission occurred.

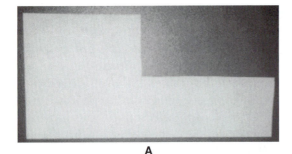

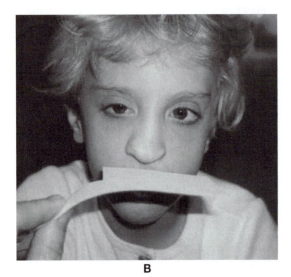

FIGURE 11–2 (A and B) (A) An "air paddle" to be used in testing for nasal air emission. The paddle can be cut (or even torn) from a piece of paper. (B) The paddle is placed underneath the nares during the production of repetitive syllables that have pressure-sensitive consonants. If the paddle moves during speech, this indicates nasal air emission.

Courtesy Ann W. Kummer, Ph.D./Cincinnati Children's Hospital Medical Center & University of Cincinnati College of Medicine

and a puff or air is expelled through the nares. Even when done correctly, this technique does not give information on whether the nasal emission is consistent or just occurred on one phoneme.

- **Air Paddle:** The examiner can actually see nasal emission by using an "air paddle," as first described by Bzoch (1979). An air paddle can be cut (or even torn) from a piece of paper and placed underneath the nares during the production of repetitive syllables with pressure-sensitive consonants (Figure 11–2A and B). It is best to use voiceless consonants because they consist of more air pressure than their voiced cognates and therefore are most likely to show nasal emission. If the paddle moves during the production of these sounds, this indicates that there is nasal air emission. This test is not very sensitive and actually only works when there is a lot of nasal air pressure.

- **See-Scape™:** The See-Scape is a pneumatic device that is sold by several distributors (Pro-Ed; Mayer Johnson; Slosson Educational Publications; AliMed, etc.). A "nasal olive" is placed in the child's nostril. The nasal olive is attached to a flexible tube that is connected to a rigid plastic vertical tube. As the child repeats pressure-sensitive phonemes, a Styrofoam® float will rise in the vertical tube if there is nasal air emission (Figure 11–3). Although this device shows nasal emission when it occurs, it has several disadvantages. First, the retail cost of over $100 is not insignificant. Perhaps the biggest concern, however, relates to infection control. Although this device should be thoroughly cleaned and disinfected between uses, this is not easily done, particularly with the Styrofoam float.

Tactile Detection

- **Feeling the Sides of the Nose:** Vibration from hypernasality can sometimes be felt by placing the fingers lightly on the side of the patient's nose (Figure 11–4). This feeling can be simulated by prolonging an /m/ and feeling the vibration on the nasal cartilage.

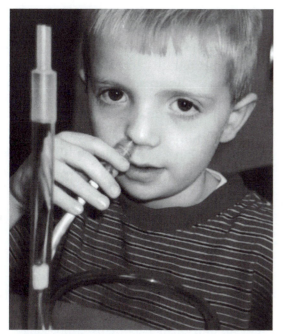

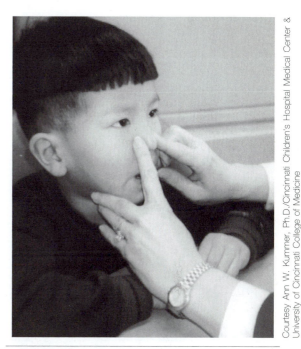

FIGURE 11–3 The use of a See-Scape (Super Duper, Greenville, SC) for testing nasal air emission. The patient places the nasal olive at the entrance to the nostril. If there is nasal air emission during speech production, the Styrofoam stopper will rise in the tube.

FIGURE 11–4 A tactile test of nasal air emission and hypernasality. Nasal air emission or hypernasality can sometimes be felt by placing the index fingers lightly on the individual's nose, in the area of the cartilage that is just below the bone. As the child repeats pressure-sensitive consonants or says "60, 60, 60," the examiner can feel the vibration of nasal air emission or hypernasality.

This is not a very sensitive test, however. Nasal emission from a large velopharyngeal opening cannot be felt on the side of the nose. On the other hand, if there is a nasal rustle (turbulence) due to a small opening, this can easily be felt on the cartilage of the nose due to the turbulence of the airflow.

Auditory Detection

Although visual and tactile detection can be helpful, by far the best evaluation procedures are those that use auditory detection because what is being evaluated is an auditory event (Kummer, 2009, 2001). In addition, the auditory tests are more reliable.

- **Nasal Cul-de-Sac Test:** The nasal cul-de-sac test is done by having the patient

produce an oral speech segment with the nose unoccluded, and then repeat the same speech segment with the nostrils pinched closed (Bzoch, 1979, 1997; Haapanen, 1991) (Figure 11–5). To assess hypernasality with this test, the child is asked to prolong a vowel or repeat a sentence that is devoid of nasal consonants (Kuehn & Henne, 2003). If the velopharyngeal valve is functioning normally and there is no hypernasality, there should be no change in resonance with the closed nose. If there is a dysfunctional velopharyngeal valve causing hypernasality, however, the sound will

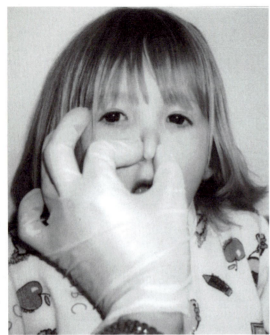

FIGURE 11–5 The nose pinch or "cul-de-sac test." The examiner asks the patient to produce a speech segment and then repeat the segment with the nostrils occluded to determine if there is a difference in resonance.

resonate in the nasal cavity but be blocked by the closed nose, causing cul-de-sac resonance. Therefore, a difference in quality with closure of the nares indicates hypernasality. To assess for nasal air emission, the child is asked to repeat syllables or sentences loaded with pressure-sensitive consonants. If there is an increase in oral pressure with closure of the nose, this is suggestive of significant nasal emission. Finally, to assess hyponasality, the child is asked to produce a nasal sound repetitively (such as /ma, ma, ma/). If there is little or no difference in the quality of the speech with the nose closed, this suggests significant hyponasality.

- **Stethoscope:** A stethoscope can be especially helpful in evaluating the characteristics of velopharyngeal dysfunction. The drum of the stethoscope can be placed on either side of the nose or under the nose. If there is hypernasality or nasal emission during the production of oral sounds, this can be clearly heard through the stethoscope (Figure 11–6). The stethoscope is even more effective if the drum is removed and the tube is placed at the entrance of one nostril. The only disadvantage of this method is that the tubing has to be appropriately disinfected between patients.

- **Listening Tube:** A plastic tube works just like the stethoscope in helping to detect hypernasality and nasal emission. (Suction tubing is readily available in a hospital and can be used for this purpose. It should be cut up into smaller, perhaps 2-foot-long pieces.) When using a tube as part of the evaluation, one end of the tube is placed at the entrance to the child's nostril, and the other end is placed near the examiner's ear as the child produces oral syllables or

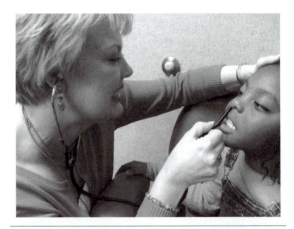

FIGURE 11–6 The use of a stethoscope. The drum is taken off the end so that the tube is placed near the opening of the nostril. This requires disinfection after each use.

sentences (Figure 11–7A). Even a toy whistle can be used for this purpose (Figure 11–7B). The advantage of the tube is that you can make it any length for comfort. The disadvantage is that the examiner needs to be careful to not to forget which end went

in the child's nose and which end went in his or her ear. In addition, the tube needs to be either disinfected or discarded after use.

- ***Straw:*** A straw can be an extremely helpful and reliable tool when making a differential diagnosis about airflow and hypernasality. By placing the short end of a bending straw in the child's nostril and the other end near the examiner's ear, even very slight nasal emission or tenuous velopharyngeal closure can be detected because the sound is amplified in the same way as a stethoscope (Figure 11–8). This technique can be used to identify hypernasality or nasal emission. It can also be used to determine whether an oronasal fistula is symptomatic (see information below). A straw can even be used for the detection of a lateral distortion on sibilants or lingual-alveolar plosives.

It should be noted that of all of these supplemental tests, the straw (or even the listening tube) is the ultimate low-cost, "no-tech" instrument—yet it may be the best way to evaluate hypernasality and nasal emission for several reasons. First, the straw amplifies the sound,

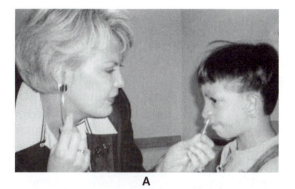

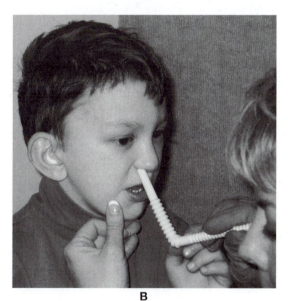

FIGURE 11–7 (A and B) (A) A "listening tube" for a test of nasal air emission and hypernasality. One end of a plastic tube is place in the child's nostril or at the entrance to the nostril, and the other end is placed in the examiner's ear. As the child produces sounds or sentences, the examiner can hear occurrences of nasal air emission or hypernasality. (B) A toy whistle can also be used as a listening tube. Then it can be given to the child to take home as a prize.

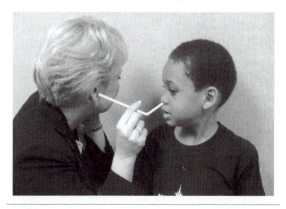

FIGURE 11–8 A straw for a test of nasal air emission and hypernasality. A straw is placed in the child's nostril as he or she produces pressure-sensitive sounds. If there is nasal air emission or hypernasality, this can be heard through the straw.

just like a stethoscope. Therefore, the examiner is able to easily determine whether there is hypernasality, merely by noting whether there is sound through the tube. In addition, the examiner can hear nasal emission clearly, even if it is inaudible in regular speech. Even if the velopharyngeal valve is only slightly inefficient in closing, this inefficiency can be heard as a click, when using a straw. The examiner can hear hypernasality and nasal emission even in a noisy clinic environment because the straw acts almost as a low-tech hearing aid for the examiner. This "equipment" is cheap (less than a penny each) and readily available wherever there is food and drink. The straw is disposable, so it requires no maintenance, and infection control is not an issue. Finally, this method has better validity than visual or tactile detection in that it involves an auditory assessment of an auditory event. Therefore, the straw is highly recommended as a valuable tool for evaluation of resonance, oral and nasal airflow, and velopharyngeal function.

Differential Diagnosis of Cause

Hypernasality and nasal air emission can be caused by VPI, an articulation disorder, or an oronasal fistula. The cause of the problem is important to determine because it has a direct impact on the treatment recommendations (Garrett, Deal, & Prathanee, 2002; Kummer, 2009; Kummer, 2011; Marsh, 2004).

When there is hypernasality or nasal emission, the examiner must first determine whether the cause is structural or functional due to misarticulations (either from mislearning or as compensation for VPI). For example, a nasal rustle commonly occurs with a small velopharyngeal opening due to a structural defect. However, it also occurs in association with the production of a posterior velar fricative, which can be due to mislearning

alone. The differential diagnosis is important because structural defects require surgical intervention, whereas articulation placement errors require speech therapy.

Differential diagnosis is done first by assessing consistency of occurrence. If, for example, the nasal emission is phoneme specific in that it occurs only on certain sounds (particularly sibilants) and never occurs on plosives, this is due to misarticulation. In the same way, if hypernasality only occurs on high vowels (particularly /i/) and never on low vowels, this is also considered phoneme specific and is likely due to faulty articulation. On the other hand, if the nasal emission is inconsistent, but occurs on all pressure sensitive phonemes, the cause is likely to be VPI.

Stimulability testing can also be very helpful in making the correct diagnosis as to cause. If nasal emission or hypernasality are eliminated with a change in articulation placement, this confirms that the cause is faulty articulation and not VPI. For specific suggestions on changing articulatory placement for stimulability testing and for therapy, see Chapter 21.

If the patient has an oronasal fistula and speech is characterized by nasal emission and/or hypernasality, it is important to determine whether these speech characteristics are due to the fistula, to VPI, or to both.

The size of the fistula is one factor that determines its effect on speech. If the fistula is small, it may not be symptomatic for speech because the airflow in the oral cavity is horizontal to the opening. If the fistula is 5 mm or more in diameter, nasal air emission may be noted with the production of some pressure-sensitive consonants. If the fistula is in the area of the incisive foramen (above the tongue tip), it may be symptomatic on anterior sounds (see Figure 2–13). If the fistula is very

CASE REPORT

Phoneme-Specific Nasal Emission

Jeff was a 36-year-old man with a history of "nasality," although he was not born with a cleft palate. When Jeff was a child, his parents were told that he would need surgery to correct the problem. They opted not to have the surgery done. In his early twenties, Jeff sought another opinion and was again told that he would require surgery for correction. Due to his hesitancy to go through with the procedure, the surgery was never done. When he came to our clinic at the age of 36, Jeff reported that his speech had been a barrier in his work and social life and therefore, he was finally ready for the surgery.

Upon examination, the velum appeared to be normal. An assessment of speech revealed the substitution of a pharyngeal fricative for all sibilant sounds (s, z, ʃ, ʒ, ʧ, ʤ), causing nasal emission on those sounds. All other speech sounds were produced correctly with normal air pressure and no evidence of nasal emission. Resonance was normal.

Jeff proved to be stimulable for correct production of all misarticulated sounds when given appropriate cues. (See Chapter 21 for techniques to change articulation placement.) With the change in placement from pharyngeal to oral, there was a total elimination of nasal emission. Given these findings, it was apparent that Jeff had been misdiagnosed with VPI. Instead, he demonstrated phoneme-specific nasal air emission due to mislearning.

Rather than undergoing a surgical procedure, as had been recommended in the past, Jeff was enrolled in speech therapy. Within a few months, he was producing sibilants normally with no nasal air emission and was therefore discharged from therapy.

This case illustrates the importance of a differential diagnosis. In Jeff's case, the nasal emission was due to misarticulation rather than VPI. It is fortunate that he did not follow through with the recommendation for surgery, because that would not have corrected the problem. On the other hand, it is very unfortunate that he was misdiagnosed previously and that the appropriate form of speech therapy was not done when he was a child.

---

large, there may be hypernasality as well (refer to Figure 7–1).

The position of the fistula can also determine its effect on speech. If the fistula is in the area of the incisive foramen, which is common with bilateral clefts, there may be nasal emission during the production of lingual-alveolar sounds if the tongue pushes air into the opening as it elevates for production. On the other hand, if the tongue tip is used to valve the fistula during speech, a lateral distortion will occur. If the fistula is in the midpalatal

area and the tongue is used to valve the fistula, a palatal-dorsal placement with lateral distortion will be noted. A posterior fistula is usually less symptomatic because there are few posterior sounds in speech to force the air stream upward.

To determine whether a fistula is symptomatic, the examiner could temporarily close it with chewing gum (or Fruit Rollups, Janet Middendorf, M.A., personal communication, May 4, 2005). This is time-consuming and messy because the fistula and the gum need to be dried before the gum will stick. Perhaps a better method is for the examiner to compare the occurrence of nasal air emission that occurs on /k/ (which should not be affected by a fistula in the palate) and on anterior sounds, such as /t/ and /p/, using the straw technique for best comparison. If there is no difference in nasal emission, then the source of the nasal air emission is probably the velopharyngeal valve. If there is more nasal emission on anterior sounds than on the sounds that are posterior to the fistula, this suggests that the fistula is symptomatic.

One complicating factor in evaluating VPI in the presence of a fistula is the combined effect of the two. When there is a leak in the system as a result of a fistula, this can cause the velopharyngeal mechanism to function less efficiently (Moller, 1991). Therefore, unless the fistula is closed or obturated, it can be difficult to evaluate the capabilities of velopharyngeal mechanism. It often takes a multidisciplinary approach to determine the symptomatology that is directly due to the fistula, and to formulate the appropriate treatment plan (Sell, Mars, & Worrell, 2006).

An inexperienced examiner may have difficulty discriminating the sound of nasal airflow due to a pharyngeal fricative with the sound of lateral airflow due to a lateral lisp. The examiner should use a straw to first listen for the nasal air emission. Then, the examiner should place the straw at the front of the patient's dental arch during production of a /t/ and then an /s/ sound. If the production is normal, the airstream will be heard through the straw. If the airstream is not heard, the straw should be placed at different positions on the side of the dental arch during the production of the sound. If the air stream is lateralized, it will be heard through the straw at some point on the side of the dental arch rather than in the front.

FOLLOW-UP

The purpose of an evaluation is to determine appropriate treatment recommendations for the patient. In some cases, recommendations may have to be deferred if there is a need for additional testing or consultation from other professionals. The speech-language pathologist should continue to be actively involved with the patient and family until final treatment recommendations are made.

Additional Referrals

Depending on the evaluation results, additional diagnostic procedures may be indicated (e.g., a nasopharyngoscopy evaluation, a videofluoroscopic speech study, a videofluoroscopic swallow study, an ENT evaluation, a sleep study, etc.). Before making referrals for additional evaluations, the speech-language pathologist should always discuss the recommendations with the primary care physician and the referring physician. This is not only common courtesy, but is consistent with the "medical model," where the primary care physician manages the child's overall plan of care.

Recommendations

Based on the particular speech characteristics noted, the examiner will be able to determine whether there is velopharyngeal dysfunction and, if so, the basic cause (structural versus functional). The speech characteristics even allow the examiner to estimate the size of the velopharyngeal gap (see Table 7–1). With this information, the examiner can make appropriate recommendations for treatment. For example, if there is nasal emission and hypernasality, this suggests a large velopharyngeal opening that will require surgical intervention. On the other hand, if there is a nasal rustle that

TABLE 11–6 Recommendations Regarding Treatment Based on Cause of Velopharyngeal Insufficiency (Structural Abnormality)

Velopharyngeal Insufficiency (Structural Abnormality)

- Surgery (postoperative speech therapy as needed)
- Prosthesis—speech bulb
- Speech therapy for articulation and compensatory productions

Velopharyngeal Incompetence (Physiological Abnormality)

- Surgery (postoperative speech therapy as needed)
- Prosthesis—palatal lift
- Speech therapy (particularly if acquired) and therapy for articulation and compensatory productions

Velopharyngeal Mislearning

- Speech therapy only

Symptomatic Palatal Fistula

- Surgery
- Prosthesis—obturator
- Speech therapy for articulation and compensatory production

© Cengage Learning 2014

is phoneme specific or if there are articulation errors that are not obligatory, speech therapy would be appropriate. Speech therapy is appropriate for compensatory productions but should be done after correction of the structure, whenever possible. Table 11–6 has a list of recommendations that can be considered for each cause.

Recommendations should not only be based on the cause and severity of the speech disorder but should also be made considering the potential for improvement, the associated risks, the patient's quality of life, and finally the desires of the patient and family. The examiner must be careful not to impose his or her own value system and personal preferences on the patient and the family. They are the ones who have to live with the consequences of the decision, and therefore they should be the ones

to make informed decisions about the recommended interventions.

Family Counseling

Handouts with labeled drawings are particularly useful in helping the family to understand the anatomy, the problem with speech, and any surgical procedures that are being proposed. Many centers give out their own handouts and brochures that contain specific information regarding their program and facility (see Appendix A). There are handouts in the online materials for this book that can be printed out for families and other professionals. In addition, many informational brochures are available through the Cleft Palate Foundation (CPF) of the American Cleft Palate–Craniofacial Association. These can be accessed at http://www. cleftline.org/.

Evaluation Report

There is a great need for standardization of assessment protocols, and methods of recording and reporting evaluation results (Golding-Kushner et al. 1990; Hirschberg & Van Demark, 1997; Sell, Harding, & Grunwell, 1999). Despite general agreement that standardization is needed, in practice there is still great variability among centers and between providers in the way evaluation results are reported.

The purpose of the evaluation report is to effectively communicate results and recommendations to other professionals and, in some cases, to the family. Therefore, a good evaluation report is one that is clear and concise. Many professionals fail to consider their "customers" when writing the report. Long reports are usually not read and are definitely not appreciated by busy professionals. (Some speech-language pathologists forget that the quality of the evaluation is not judged by the quantity of words in the report.) The report should contain appropriate language and medical terminology but should also be understandable to the readers. (Phonetic symbols are not understood by other professionals and families.) The report should focus on the examiner's impressions (based on the evaluation results) and the recommendations. It is important to be correct and confident in the stated conclusions and recommendations, as they will often result in surgical management.

SUMMARY

A perceptual assessment of speech and resonance gives the examiner information regarding the presence of VPI and its effect on speech production. It is important to assess articulation in order to determine whether there are any obligatory distortions or compensatory errors resulting from VPI. The examiner should determine whether there is nasal emission and whether this is causing weak consonants or short utterance length. If resonance is abnormal, the examiner should determine the type of resonance, but not be particularly concerned about rating the severity. Phonation should also be assessed because dysphonia is common in individuals with VPI.

Although there are instrumental procedures to evaluate velopharyngeal function, the ear remains the best method for judging abnormal speech and resonance. To augment the perceptual assessment, the use of a straw (or other type of tube) is the most appropriate and effective method of assessing the speech correlates of velopharyngeal dysfunction. Finally, differential diagnosis of the cause of hypernasality and/or nasal emission is very important for determination of the appropriate method of treatment.

FOR REVIEW AND DISCUSSION

1. What should be the focus of concern for the speech-language pathologist when the child is a newborn? What should be the focus of concern when the child is a toddler? At what age can velopharyngeal function usually be evaluated? Why can't it be evaluated earlier?

2. What type of information is important to obtain in the diagnostic interview with the parent or guardian?

3. Discuss different types of speech stimuli that can be used in an assessment and the advantages of each type.

4. List the types of errors and distortions that should be identified in the articulation test. Why is it important to identify the type of error?

5. Why is it important to test stimulability? If the child responds well to stimulation, what might that suggest?

6. What sounds would you use to test for hypernasality? What sounds would you use to test for nasal emission? What sounds would you use to test for hyponasality? Explain the reason for each.

7. Describe methods for informally detecting nasality. What is the advantage of auditory detection over visual or tactile detection? What is the advantage of using a straw or listening tube over using a mirror for detection of nasal emission?

8. Your patient has normal resonance but inconsistent nasal emission. He has a small fistula in the middle of the palate. What

would you do to determine whether the nasal emission is due to the fistula or to velopharyngeal insufficiency?

9. Why is a differential diagnosis of the cause of abnormal resonance or nasal emission so important? Discuss possible repercussions of making the wrong diagnosis.

REFERENCES

American Cleft Palate–Craniofacial Association (ACPA). (2009). Parameters for evaluation and treatment of patients with cleft lip/ palate or other craniofacial anomalies. *Cleft Palate–Craniofacial Journal*, *30* (Suppl.), 1–16.

Bronsted, K., Grunwell, P., Henningsson, G., Jansonius, K. J. K., Meijer, M., Ording, U., Sell, K., et al. (1994). A phonetic framework for the cross-linguistic analysis of cleft palate speech. *Clinical Linguistics and Phonetics*, *8*, 109–125.

Bzoch, K. R. (1979). Measurement and assessment of categorical aspects of cleft palate speech. In K. R. Bzoch (Ed.), *Communicative disorders related to cleft lip and palate* (vol. 2, pp. 161–191). Boston: Little, Brown and Company.

Bzoch, K. R. (1997). Clinical assessment, evaluation and management of 11 categorical aspects of cleft palate speech. In K. R. Bzoch (Ed.), *Communicative disorders related to cleft lip and palate* (vol. 4, pp. 261–311). Austin, TX: Pro-Ed.

Bzoch, K. R., League, R., & Brown, V.L. (2003). *Receptive-Expressive Emergent Language Test: A method for assessing the language skills of infants* (3rd ed.). Austin, TX: Pro-Ed.

Coplan, J. (1993). *Early Language Milestone (ELM) Scale* (2nd ed.). Austin, TX: Pro-Ed.

Fenson, L., Dale, P. S., Reznick, J. S., Thai, D., Bates, E., Hartung, P., Pethick, S., et al. (1989). *The MacArthur communicative development inventory*. San Diego, CA: Development Psychology Lab, San Diego State University.

Fluharty, N. B. (2000). *Fluharty Preschool Speech and Language Test* (2nd ed.). Austin, TX: Pro-Ed.

Garrett, J. D., Deal, R. E., & Prathanee, B. (2002). Velopharyngeal assessment procedures for the Thai cleft palate population. *Journal of the Medical Association of Thailand*, *85*(6), 682–692.

Glascoe, F. P. (1991). Can clinical judgment detect children with speech-language problems? *Pediatrics*, *87*(3), 317–322.

Golding-Kushner, K. J., Argamaso, R. V., Cotton, R. T., Grames, L. M., Henningsson, G., Jones, D. L., et al. (1990). Standardization for the reporting of nasopharyngoscopy and multiview videofluoroscopy: A report from an International Working Group. *Cleft Palate Journal*, *27*(4), 337–347; Discussion 347–338.

Haapanen, M. L. (1991). A simple clinical method of evaluating perceived hypernasality. *Folia Phoniatrica*, *43*(3), 122–132. [Published Erratum appears in *Folia Phoniatrica* 1991, *43*(4), 2003.]

Henningsson, G., & Isberg, A. (1991). A cineradiographic study of velopharyngeal movements for deviant versus nondeviant articulation. *Cleft Palate–Craniofacial Journal*, *28*(1), 115–117; Discussion 117–118.

Hickman, L. A. (1997). *Apraxia profile: A descriptive assessment tool for children*. San Antonio, TX: Communication Skill Builders.

Hirschberg, J., & Van Demark, D. R. (1997). A proposal for standardization of speech and hearing evaluations to assess velopharyngeal function. *Folia Phoniatrica et Logopedica*, 49(3/4), 158–167.

Kaufman, N. R. (1995). *Kaufman Speech Praxis Test for Children (KSPT)*. Detroit, MI: Wayne State University Press.

Kempster, B., Gerratt, B., Verdolini Abbott, K., Barkmeier-Kraemer, J., & Hillman, R. E. (2009). Consensus auditory-perceptual evaluation of voice: Development of a standardized clinical protocol, *American Journal of Speech-Language Pathology*, 18, 124–132.

Kuehn, D. P., & Henne, L. J. (2003). Speech evaluation and treatment of patients with cleft palate. *American Journal of Speech-Language Pathology*, 12, 103–109.

Kummer, A. W. (2009). Assessment of velopharyngeal function. In J. E. Lossee & R. E. Kirschner (Eds.), *Comprehensive cleft care* (pp. 589–605). New York: McGraw-Hill.

Kummer, A. W. (2011). Perceptual assessment of resonance and velopharyngeal function. *Seminars in Speech and Language*, 32(2), 159–167.

Kummer, A. W., Briggs, M., & Lee, L. (2003). The relationship between the characteristics of speech and velopharyngeal gap size. *Cleft Palate–Craniofacial Journal*, 40(6), 590–596.

Kummer, A. W., Clark, S. L., Redle, E. E., Thomsen, L. L., & Billmire, D. A. (2011). Current practice in assessing and reporting speech outcomes of cleft palate and velopharyngeal surgery: A survey of cleft palate/craniofacial professionals. *Cleft Palate–Craniofacial Journal*, 49(2), 146–152.

Kummer, A. W., Curtis, C., Wiggs, M., Lee, L., & Strife, J. L. (1992). Comparison of velopharyngeal gap size in patients with hypernasality, hypernasality and nasal emission, or nasal turbulence (rustle) as the primary speech characteristic. *Cleft Palate–Craniofacial Journal*, 29(2), 152–156.

Kummer, A. W., Lee, L., Stutz, L., Maroney, A., & Brandt, J. W. (2007). The prevalence of apraxic characteristics in patients with velocardiofacial syndrome as compared to other populations. *Cleft Palate–Craniofacial Journal*, 44(2), 175–181.

Kummer, A. W., & Marsh, J. H. (1998). Pediatric voice and resonance disorders. In A. F. Johnson & B. H. Jacobson (Eds.), *Medical speech-language pathology: A practitioner's guide*. New York: Thieme.

Lee, G. S., Wang, C. P., & Fu, S. (2009). Evaluation of hypernasality in vowels using voice low tone to high tone ratio. *Cleft Palate–Craniofacial Journal*, 46(1), 47–52.

Marsh, J. L. (2004). The evaluation and management of velopharyngeal dysfunction. *Clinics in Plastic Surgery*, 31(2), 261–269.

McWilliams, B. J., Lavorato, A. S., & Bluestone, C. D. (1973). Vocal cord abnormalities in children with velopharyngeal valving problems. *Laryngoscope*, 83(11), 1745–1753.

McWilliams, B. J., Morris, H. L., & Shelton, R. L. (1990). Diagnosis of phonation and resonance. In B. J. Williams, H. L. Morris, & R. L. Shelton (Eds.), *Cleft palate speech* (pp. 311–319). Philadelphia: B. C. Decker.

Moller, K. T. (1991). An approach to the evaluation of velopharyngeal adequacy for speech. *Clinics in Communication Disorders*, 1(1), 61–65.

Paal, S., Reulbach, U., Strobel-Schwarthoff, K., Nkenke, E., & Schuster, M. (2005). Evaluation of speech disorders in children with cleft lip and palate. *Journal of Orofacial Orthopedics*, 66(4), 270–278.

Pannbacker, M., & Middleton, G. (1990). Integrating perceptual and instrumental procedures in assessment of velopharyngeal insufficiency. *Ear Nose and Throat Journal, 69*(3), 161–175.

Rossetti, L. (2006). *The Rossetti infant-toddler language scale.* East Moline, IL: LinguiSystems.

Scherer, N. J., & D'Antonio, L. L. (1995). Parent questionnaire for screening early language development in children with cleft palate. *Cleft Palate–Craniofacial Journal, 32*(1), 7–13.

Scherer, N. J., & D'Antonio, L. L. (1997). Language and play development in toddlers with cleft lip and/or palate. *American Journal of Speech-Language Pathology, 6* (4), 48–54.

Sell, D., Harding, A., & Grunwell, P. (1999). GOS.SP.ASS/98: An assessment for speech disorders associated with cleft palate and/or velopharyngeal dysfunction (Revised). *International Journal of Language and Communication Disorders, 34*(1), 17–33.

Sell, D., Mars, M., & Worrell, E. (2006). Process and outcome study of multidisciplinary prosthetic treatment for velopharyngeal dysfunction. *International Journal of Language and Communication Disorders, 41*(5), 495–511.

Semel, E., Wiig, E. H., Secord, W. A. (2013). *Clinical evaluation of language fundamentals®—Preschool* (5th ed.). New York, NY: Pearson.

Shprintzen, R. J., & Golding-Kushner, K. J. (1989). Evaluation of velopharyngeal insufficiency. *Otolaryngologic Clinics of North America, 22*(3), 519–536.

Smith, B., & Guyette, T. W. (2004). Evaluation of cleft palate speech. *Clinics in Plastic Surgery, 31*(2), 251–260.

Smith, B. E., & Kuehn, D. P. (2007). Speech evaluation of velopharyngeal dysfunction.

The Journal of Craniofacial Surgery, 18(2), 251–260.

Stemple, J. C., Glaze, L. E., & Gerdeman, B. K. (1995). *Clinical voice pathology: Theory and management.* San Diego, CA: Singular Publishing Group.

Subtelny, J. D., Van Hattum, R. J., & Myers, B. B. (1972). Ratings and measures of cleft palate speech. *Cleft Palate Journal, 9*(1), 18–27.

Templin, M. C., & Darley, F. (1960). *Screening and diagnostic tests of articulation.* Iowa City, IA: Bureau of Educational Research and Service Extension Division, State University of Iowa.

Trindade, I. E., Genaro, K. F., Yamashita, R. P., Miguel, H. C., & Fukushiro, A. P. (2005). Proposal for velopharyngeal function rating in a speech perceptual assessment. *Pro Fono, 17*(2), 259–262.

Trost, J. E. (1981). Articulatory additions to the classical description of the speech of persons with cleft palate. *Cleft Palate Journal, 18*(3), 193–203.

Trost-Cardamone, J. E. (1987). *Cleft palate misarticulations: A teaching tape* [videotape]. Northridge, CA: California State University, Northridge, Instructional Media Center.

Trost-Cardamone, J. E. (1997). Diagnosis of specific cleft palate speech error patterns for planning therapy of physical management needs. In K. R. Bzoch (Ed.), *Communicative disorders related to cleft lip and palate* (vol. 4, pp. 313–330). Austin, TX: Pro-Ed.

Wilson, D. K. (1987). *Voice problems of children* (vol. 3). Baltimore, MD: Williams & Wilkins.

Zimmerman, I. L., Steiner, V. G., & Pond, R. E. (2011). *Preschool Language Scales* (5th ed.). New York, NY: Pearson.

CHAPTER

12

OROFACIAL EXAMINATION

CHAPTER OUTLINE

INTRODUCTION

In speech pathology, an orofacial examination (sometimes called an oral-peripheral examination or perioral examination) involves assessment of oral structures and other facial structures that may be relevant for speech. An intraoral examination (sometimes called an oral mechanism examination) is part of a complete orofacial examination.

An orofacial examination should always be done as part of a speech or resonance evaluation, especially if the individual has a history of cleft or craniofacial anomalies. Unfortunately, many speech-language pathologists have not been taught how to perform a thorough intraoral examination. In fact, research shows that even medical students are not given sufficient instruction or experience in performing oral examinations (Shanks, Walker, McCann, & Kerin, 2011). By performing regular orofacial examinations, speech-language pathologists can increase their familiarity with normal oral structures and will be able to recognize abnormalities more easily (Thomas & Bender, 1993).

Knowledge of the oral structures and their potential effect on speech production and resonance is extremely important in order to make appropriate recommendations for treatment. If there are structural factors that cause or contribute to the deviant speech or resonance, these structural problems should be corrected as soon as possible. When there are obligatory distortions, correcting the structure alone will correct these distortions. In other cases, the compensatory productions need to be corrected with therapy after the structure is normalized.

The examiner should be aware that a judgment regarding velopharyngeal function cannot be made based on an intraoral examination (Smith & Guyette, 2004; Smith & Kuehn, 2007). Velopharyngeal closure occurs behind the velum, usually on the plane of the hard palate. Therefore, it is well above the level that is viewed through the oral cavity. In addition, the examiner cannot see the point of maximum lateral pharyngeal wall movement from an intraoral perspective. In fact, at the oral level, the lateral pharyngeal walls may actually appear to bow outward during phonation. Finally, velopharyngeal function cannot be judged during only a sustained vowel, such as "ah." Instead, the function of the velopharyngeal mechanism must be evaluated based on the movement and closure during connected speech.

Despite these limitations, the examiner can evaluate all of the oral structures that can affect speech and resonance production, including the status of labial competence, dental occlusion, the hard palate, the oral surface of the velum, the uvula, the tonsils, and the tongue (Smith & Kuehn, 2007). As such, an intraoral assessment can provide valuable information that can impact the examiner's overall impressions and recommendations from the assessment.

This chapter describes the methodology for a comprehensive examination of relevant structures and function for the production of normal speech and resonance. In addition, appropriate procedures for infection control are discussed.

General Methodology

An evaluation of the oral cavity is an important part of a speech and resonance evaluation because anomalies of the oral structures can affect both speech production and resonance. It is important to determine whether there are structural anomalies that are affecting speech. If there are such anomalies, the treatment of speech requires physical management in addition to speech therapy. The following sections describe methods for conducting a thorough evaluation of the oral cavity so that appropriate treatment recommendations can be made.

Tools for an Intraoral Examination

An intraoral examination can often be done without special equipment or materials. There are some things that are helpful to have on hand, however, including the following:

- **Gloves:** Used for protection of the patient and the examiner.

- **Flashlight:** Used for illumination of the oral cavity.

- **Tongue blades:** Used to press the back of the tongue down (when necessary) in order to observe the velum and uvula. Also used to inspect the dentition and occlusion by pulling the lips and cheek backward. (Flavored tongue blades should be considered for children.)

- **Dental mirror:** Used like a tongue blade to press the back of the tongue down (when necessary) in order to observe the velum and uvula. Also used to assess the palate for a fistula or for looking up into the pharynx.

- **Alcohol swabs or towelettes:** Used to clean contaminated instruments or surfaces.

- **Sanitizing gel:** Used to sanitize hands, particularly if soap and water are not available.

Examination of the Oral Cavity

If done correctly, a physical examination of the morphology and function of the oral cavity can reveal important information that relates to speech production. Instead of a quick look in the mouth, however, the examiner should carefully inspect the structures and also have a view of some of these structures during function. When conducting an intraoral examination, most healthcare professionals ask the patient to open the mouth and say /ɑ/ (as in "father"). This vowel works well for evaluation of the anterior oral structures, including the hard palate, because it results in a drop of the jaw and anterior part of the tongue. However, the back of the tongue remains high and retracted, thus obstructing the view of the posterior section of the oral cavity and pharynx. In fact, this vowel makes it impossible to bring the back of the tongue down and forward so that the examiner can view the velum, tip of the uvula, tonsils, and pharynx. Because of these problems, a tongue blade is usually required to depress the back of the tongue so that it is low enough for the examiner to view these structures.

If the vowel /æ/ (as in "hat") is used for the examination instead, the patient can be instructed to stick the tongue out and down as far as it will go (Figure 12–1A and B). A young child can be instructed to point his tongue to his shoes or to try to touch his chin with his tongue. This technique brings the back of the tongue down and forward, which opens the view to the back of the oral cavity. It can be argued that this technique alters "typical" velar movement. This may be true, but velopharyngeal function cannot be adequately assessed through an intraoral examination anyway. Regardless, it does provide the examiner with a much better view of the velum, uvula, tonsils, and pharynx. In some young children, the tip of the epiglottis can

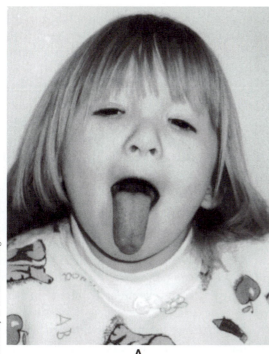

A

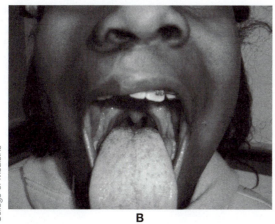

B

FIGURE 12–1 (A and B) The vowel /æ/ (as in "hat") should be used for the examination of the oral cavity. The patient should be instructed to stick the tongue out and down as far as it will go. A young child can be asked to point it to his shoes. Although this does not allow the examiner to see "typical" velar movement, it does provide the examiner with a better view of the velum, uvula, and pharynx as the base of the tongue moves down and forward.

even be seen (Shinohara & Takahashi, 2005). With this vowel, a good examination can usually be done without the use of a tongue blade. Most children, and even many adults, have a strong aversion to the use of tongue blades, for fear of gagging. Therefore, not using a tongue blade is greatly appreciated by these individuals.

If a tongue blade is needed, however, it is important to place it in the proper position. If the blade is placed too far forward, which is a common mistake, pushing downward causes the posterior part of the tongue to mound up so as to further obscure, rather than expose, the back of the oral cavity and the pharynx. If the tongue blade is placed behind the *circumvallate papilla* (a line of prominent taste buds that form an inverted "V" on the posterior tongue), it often elicits the gag reflex. The gag can give the examiner a good view, but it is a quick view and may be the last one that the patient will allow. The correct technique is to place the tongue blade approximately three-quarters of the way back on the tongue. The examiner should then press the tongue downward firmly, while scooping it forward at the same time. The tongue is a strong, muscular organ, so firm pressure is often required to push against resistance.

As the individual phonates, there may be vigorous upward movement of the velum, or very little movement, even in normal speakers. To stimulate movement in order to see the pharynx and the tip of the uvula, the child can be asked to produce the vowel repetitively or to pant ("like a puppy dog"). If this does not stimulate movement, then the examiner can ask the child to do a big yawn with the tongue protruded. This helps to elevate the velum to its fullest extent.

Positioning of the patient is another consideration when performing an intraoral examination. The patient's head should be tilted slightly backward so that the examiner can look directly to the back of the pharynx. The examiner's eye level should be at the level of the patient's oral cavity. For an infant or toddler, it is helpful to place the child on the parent's lap, facing the parent. The child is then laid back so her head is slightly lower than the rest of her body. The examiner should sit opposite the caregiver so that there is a good view of the child's oral cavity from above (albeit upside down). Although this position usually promotes an open mouth posture, the tongue may fall back into the pharynx, requiring the use of a tongue blade. If the child doesn't open mouth enough, the examiner can place a tongue blade between the teeth and apply steady downward pressure on the tongue and mandible. The jaw muscles closing the mouth are powerful but fatigue rapidly, so constant, firm pressure will allow insertion of the tongue blade within a few seconds. When the blade reaches the posterior tongue, the gag reflex causes the mouth to open fully. Alternatively, closing the nose forces the mouth to open for breathing. Finally, crying is not always a bad thing because it does allow the examiner a better intraoral view, especially in this position.

If a submucous cleft is suspected, palatal palpation of the hard palate can be done to determine whether there is a notch in the posterior border. If the examiner is inexperienced or not well trained in this area, palatal palpation can be difficult—not only for the examiner but especially for the patient. The key to successful palpation is to be gentle and slow in feeling the palate. Surprises in the area of the gag reflex are not well received by the child! However, careful palpation of the roof of the mouth with a gloved finger does not cause discomfort. If there is an open cleft or a fistula, it should be remembered that this is a variation in structure—not an open wound.

In preschool and school-aged children, it is best to use the fifth (or little) finger for palpation. This finger is long enough to reach the back of the palate of children in this age group. In addition, this finger is narrow enough to feel a small notch in the palatal bone. For teenagers and adults, the fifth finger is usually not long enough to reach to the back of the hard palate. Therefore, the index finger must be used.

To begin the examination, it is important to wash hands thoroughly and then to don gloves. For a young child, the examiner should begin by merely rubbing or stimulating the outside gums above the maxillary teeth. This helps the patient to become more comfortable and accepting of the examiner's finger in the mouth. The examiner should then stimulate the alveolar ridge behind the teeth by moving the finger from the front of the ridge to the back in the area of the molars. Once the patient is comfortable with that amount of stimulation, the examiner should glide the finger directly behind the last molar, and then slowly move the finger horizontally along the back edge of the hard palate until it reaches the midline (Figure 12–2A and B). This is the point where the notch should be felt if it exists. To feel for the notch, the examiner should try to gently probe the midpoint of the posterior border of the hard palate. With the little finger, the examiner is more likely to feel a small or narrow defect than if the larger index finger is used.

A dental mirror can be especially helpful in visualizing the surface of the palate and a fistula (Figure 12–3). The mirror should be placed under the fistula area, and the light of a flashlight should be directed to the mirror. The light reflects off the mirror to the fistula, which makes it easy to see. If the velum is very short, the dental mirror can also be used to look up into the nasopharynx.

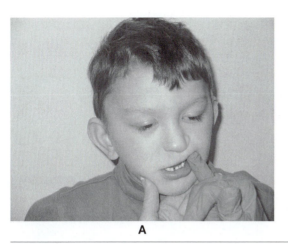
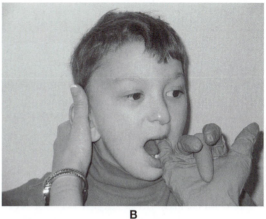

A

B

FIGURE 12–2 (A and B) Method for palpating the hard palate. (A) Using the little finger for children, the examiner can start by putting the finger under the lips and palpating the gum ridge. (B) The finger is then moved between the cheek and gum, around the molars, and then along the back end of the hard palate, until it is in midline.

Courtesy Ann W. Kummer, Ph.D./Cincinnati Children's Hospital Medical Center & University of Cincinnati College of Medicine

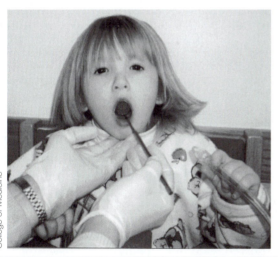

FIGURE 12–3 A dental mirror can be especially helpful in visualizing the palate in order to see a palatal fistula.

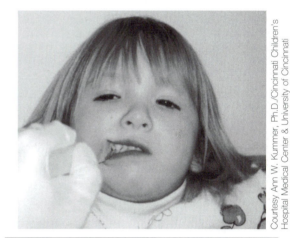

FIGURE 12–4 By inserting a tongue blade between the lateral teeth and the cheeks, the examiner can pull the cheeks away from the teeth to view the occlusal relationships.

Finally, the examiner should assess the skeletal relationship between the maxillary and the mandibular arches during occlusion. As patient "bites down on the back teeth," the examiner should make sure that the bite is with the molars, and not with the incisors. This is done by inserting a tongue blade between the lateral teeth and the cheeks, and then pulling the cheeks away from the teeth to view the occlusal relationships (Figure 12–4).

IMPORTANT OBSERVATIONS

When conducting an orofacial examination, it is important to keep in mind that there are normal variations in structure, which may result in characteristics that are unusual, but not necessarily abnormal or significant. In addition, there may be abnormalities that have no relevance to speech or resonance.

An orofacial examination begins with observation of the external anatomy of the head and face. The facial structures should be observed initially at rest. The examiner should then watch facial gestures, the tongue, and the jaw movement during speech. The examiner should inspect the eyes, ears, nose, mouth, and facial profile for evidence of abnormality or dysmorphology. Most importantly, the examiner should conduct a thorough intraoral examination.

The following describes what should be observed with specific structures.

Eyes

Normally, the eyes should be about one eye's width apart. In certain craniofacial syndromes, however, the spacing between the eyes and the appearance of the eyes is often abnormal (Figure 12–5). There may be excessive spacing between the eyes, called *hypertelorism* (Figure 12–5A), or too little spacing between the eyes, called *hypotelorism*. The opening between the eyelids, called *palpebral fissures*, should also be observed. Narrow palpebral fissures are a phenotypic feature in congenital conditions, such as velocardiofacial syndrome (Figure 12–5B). Finally, the presence of *epicanthal folds* might be noted. These are excess folds of tissue that extend from the upper eyelid to the lower part of the orbit at the inner *canthus* or corner of the eye. This is

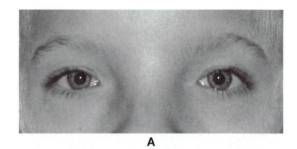

A

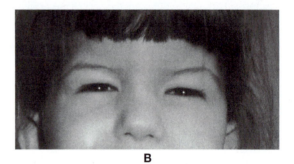

B

FIGURE 12–5 (A and B) Eye anomalies. (A) Hypertelorism (wide-spaced eyes) which is common with several syndromes. (B) Narrow palpebral fissures (eye openings) in a child with velocardiofacial syndrome.
Courtesy Ann W. Kummer, Ph.D./Cincinnati Children's Hospital Medical Center & University of Cincinnati College of Medicine

often seen in Down syndrome and other syndromes, although epicanthal folds are normal in the Asian population.

Ears

The shape and location of the ears should be observed. Many craniofacial syndromes include malformed ears, such as a simplified helix, or *microtia* (Figure 12–6; refer also to Figure 8–1B), which is hypoplasia, or absence of the pinna or auricle of the ear. This is often accompanied by *aural atresia*, which is the congenital absence of the external auditory canal. Aural atresia usually results in a conductive hearing loss, and of course this can have an impact on the quality of speech and

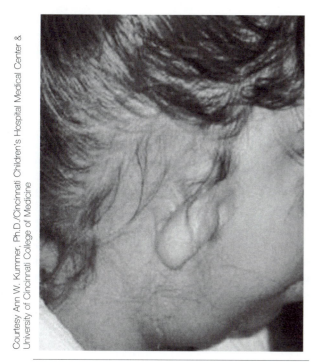

FIGURE 12–6 Microtia in a child with hemifacial microsomia.

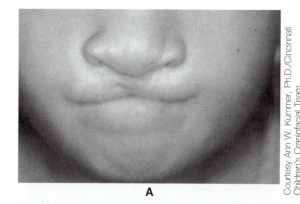

A

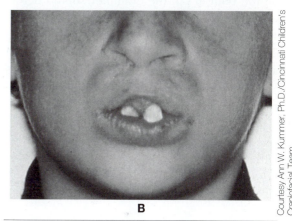

B

possibly resonance when it is bilateral. Ears that are low set (below the level of the eyes), malformed, or bent may also be suggestive of a syndrome.

Lips

The lips should be assessed for *bilabial competence*, which is the ability to achieve bilabial closure at rest and during production of bilabial sounds. When there is bilabial incompetence, the individual may substitute a labiodental placement for bilabial phonemes. This is usually an obligatory distortion and therefore not correctable unless structure is normalized.

There are many causes for bilabial incompetence. For example, if the upper lip is short relative to the vertical length of the maxilla

FIGURE 12–7 (A and B) (A) A short upper lip, making bilabial competence an effort. (B) A protruding premaxilla and short upper lip. Both affect bilabial competence at rest and during speech.

and teeth, bilabial closure may be difficult to achieve and maintain (Figure 12–7A). Sometimes the upper lip is just relatively short because of a skeletal discrepancy, such as a protruding premaxilla (Figure 12–7B) or a Class II malocclusion.

An *open mouth posture* is when the lips are chronically open and the mandible is also involved. A chronic open mouth posture can be due to poor orofacial tone or oral-motor dysfunction. The lack of adequate tone or motor skills also causes drooling. Unfortunately, the chronic open mouth posture can actually increase the production of saliva, which further exacerbates the drooling. An open mouth posture may also be due to upper airway obstruction. Opening the mouth and then moving the mandible and tongue down and forward can help to open the oropharyngeal airway and thus improve nasal and even oral breathing.

The examiner should always look for *lip pits*, which are small depressions in the bottom lip (Figure 12–8A and B). If there is scarring on the bottom lip, the examiner should determine whether there were lip pits that were surgical removed. The finding of lip pits is indicative of Van der Woude syndrome, which also includes cleft palate. This syndrome is autosomal dominant, so it has a 50% recurrence risk for all future pregnancies. Hence,

the finding of lip pits is significant and should be reported.

Uncommonly, there is reduced mobility of the upper lip due to scarring. To assess this, the patient should be asked to sustain exaggerated /i/ (as in "heat") and /u/ (as in "who") sounds. The symmetry and range of lip movement should be noted. Observing the patient produce quick repetitions of the /p/ or /b/ sounds will allow the examiner to assess the ability to make rapid movements with the nose lips.

Finally, when there is a history of cleft lip, there may be excess scarring, the Cupid's bow may be asymmetrical or flat, or the vermilion may extend into the philtral ridges. These are aesthetic issues only and do not affect speech. These types of defects are usually corrected with a later lip revision.

Nose and Airway

The *nasal bridge*, or *nasion*, is the bony structure that is located between the eyes and corresponds to the nasofrontal suture. This structure should be examined, because a flat nasal bridge can affect the nasal airway, causing upper airway obstruction and hyponasality. A bulbous nasal tip is associated with some syndromes (e.g., velocardiofacial syndrome). On the other hand, a flattened nasal tip occurs if the columella is short due to a history of cleft lip. The nares should be inspected for evidence of stenosis that could affect nasal breathing and cause hyponasality or nasal cul-de-sac resonance.

Upper airway obstruction is common in individuals with a history of cleft palate and with other craniofacial anomalies. With a history of unilateral cleft lip and palate, septal deviations often occur. Upper airway obstruction can cause a chronic open mouth posture and anterior tongue position, which can

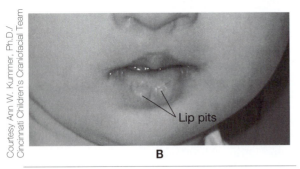

Courtesy Ann W. Kummer, Ph.D./Cincinnati Children's Craniofacial Team

Courtesy Ann W. Kummer, Ph.D./ Cincinnati Children's Craniofacial Team

A

B

FIGURE 12–8 (A and B) Bilateral lip pits, which indicate Van der Woude syndrome. This is an important finding because this syndrome is autosomal dominant.

ultimately result in an anterior open bite. The mandible may be positioned down and forward in order to open the airway further. Additional characteristics of upper airway obstruction include suborbital coloring (darkness under the eyes), which makes the patient appear to be tired; pinched nostrils; and a face that appears elongated and narrow due to the downward position of the mandible. These characteristics have been referred to as the *adenoid facies*, because they are commonly seen in individuals with upper airway obstruction due to adenoid enlargement (Elluru, 2005). Other signs of upper airway obstruction include strident breathing; snoring at night, sleep apnea; and, of course, hyponasality.

To test the nasal airway, the examiner can ask the patient to close the lips and breathe nasally for several minutes. The examiner should observe whether there is any difficulty with nasal breathing. Before opening the mouth, the patient should then inspire deeply through the nose, and then exhale through the nose. Again, the examiner should observe any difficulty, particularly pinching of the nostrils during inspiration. The patency of each nostril can be assessed by having the child close one nostril and then forcibly inspire through the other nostril. If there is obstruction, this will be difficult to do and will result in a high-pitched sound, with the highest sound in the most obstructed nostril. Another test is to ask the patient to prolong an /m/ (which requires the lips to be closed). If there is significant blockage, the patient will be unable to do this easily.

Facial Bones and Profile

The bony structures of the face are important to assess, particularly as they relate to each other. Flattened *zygomas* (cheekbones) are often seen in individuals with a history of cleft

lip and palate or other craniofacial syndromes. The facial profile, which can give an indication of the dysmorphology of the other facial bones, can be evaluated by having the patient turn so that the examiner is viewing the side of the person's face. For a normal profile, imaginary points on the forehead, bridge of the nose, base of the nose, and chin button should all line up in a vertical plane. The examiner should note whether there is maxillary retrusion with midface deficiency. The examiner should also note whether the mandible is either micrognathic or prognathic.

Dentition and Occlusion

Dentition and occlusion should always be assessed because the position of the teeth and the occlusion of the jaws can have a significant effect on articulation. Dental anomalies and malocclusion are common contributors to speech problems in patients with a history of cleft lip and palate or other craniofacial conditions. Missing teeth, rotated teeth, supernumerary teeth, deep bite, overjet, and underjet are all common conditions that can affect speech in this population.

If there are missing teeth, particularly in the maxillary arch, the examiner should determine whether the tongue goes through the created opening during speech. If it does, it is important to observe whether this is due to oral cavity crowding or a tongue thrust, or seems to be merely a misarticulation. If there are rotated or supernumerary teeth, the examiner should determine whether these teeth touch the tongue or interfere with tongue movement during speech, causing a lateral distortion. If there is a deep bite (excessive vertical overlap), the examiner should determine whether it is causing crowding in the oral cavity and restricting tongue movement during speech. If there is an overjet (incisors are labioverted), the examiner should determine whether it affects bilabial competence and bilabial phoneme production. If there is an underjet (incisors are linguoverted), the examiner should determine whether it affects lingual-alveolar sounds and sibilants.

Anterior and lateral crossbites (maxillary teeth are inside the mandibular teeth) are common in the cleft and craniofacial population and can a significant effect on speech (Figure 12–9A–D). There can be an anterior crossbite involving the maxillary incisors, or a lateral crossbite, causing the maxillary arch to be very narrow. In either case, oral cavity crowding during speech is a strong possibility. If the mandible raises or closes normally for speech sound production, the crowding can cause a lateral distortion. On the other hand, the individual may compensate by opening the jaws during speech, resulting in a frontal distortion.

As noted in Chapter 9, a normal occlusal relationship is termed a Class I occlusion according to Angle's (1899) classification (Lin,

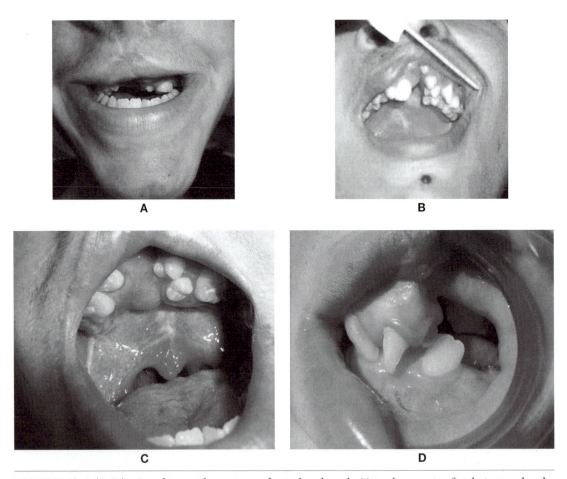

A

B

C

D

FIGURE 12–9 (A–D) Crossbites with missing and misplaced teeth. Note the anterior fistula just under the lip in figure 12–9C.

Courtesy Ann W. Kummer, Ph.D./Cincinnati Children's Hospital Medical Center & University of Cincinnati College of Medicine

Li, Huang, & Wu, 2010). With this type of occlusion, the mandibular molar should line up to be one-half of a tooth in front of the maxillary molar. In addition, the maxillary teeth overlap the mandibular teeth, particularly in the anterior portion of the dental arch. Discrepancy in the relationship between the maxilla and mandible can be particularly problematic for speech. Because the tongue always resides within the mandible, the position of the mandible in relationship to the maxilla can affect tongue tip articulation against the alveolar ridge. Therefore, when malocclusion is noted, the examiner should assess the position of the tongue tip relative to the position of the alveolar ridge. If tongue tip is not under the alveolar ridge, obligatory distortions and/or compensatory productions will be noted.

If the mandible is behind where it should be in relationship to the maxillary arch, this is considered a Class II malocclusion (Figure 12–10). Micrognathia is common with this condition. In severe cases, the tongue tip is under the palate rather than the alveolar ridge. Backing of lingual-alveolar phonemes and labiodental production of bilabials may occur as a result.

On the other hand, if the mandible is forward in relationship to the maxilla, this is considered a Class III malocclusion (Figure 12–11A–C), which can cause a lack of bilabial competence for production of bilabial sounds. It can also result in difficulty producing labiodental sounds, resulting in a reverse labiodental placement (upper lip against mandibular incisors). Lingual-alveolar sounds may be substituted with palatal-dorsal productions.

If the individual had a bilateral cleft of the lip and alveolus, the position of the premaxilla should be assessed. The premaxilla may be positioned in an anterior position, making bilabial closure very difficult, if not impossible. On the other hand, the premaxilla may be

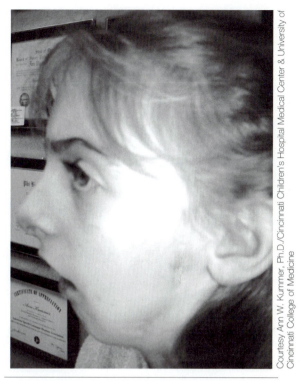

Courtesy Ann W. Kummer, Ph.D./Cincinnati Children's Hospital Medical Center & University of Cincinnati College of Medicine

FIGURE 12–10 Micrognathia and Class II malocclusion. This causes the tongue tip to rest under the hard palate rather than under the alveolar ridge.

retruded so that the teeth are linguoverted. In this case, the examiner should determine whether labiodental, lingual-alveolar, and sibilant phonemes are affected. If there is an open bite (the maxillary teeth do not occlude or overlap the mandibular teeth), the examiner should observer whether the tongue goes through the opening during speech. When there is fronting with an open bite, it is important to determine whether the fronting is due to oral cavity crowding (unlikely in this case), misarticulation, or a tongue thrust (which is often the case). A tongue thrust during swallowing, as well as with speech, can actually be the cause of the open bite.

With all of these dental and occlusal conditions, the examiner should closely

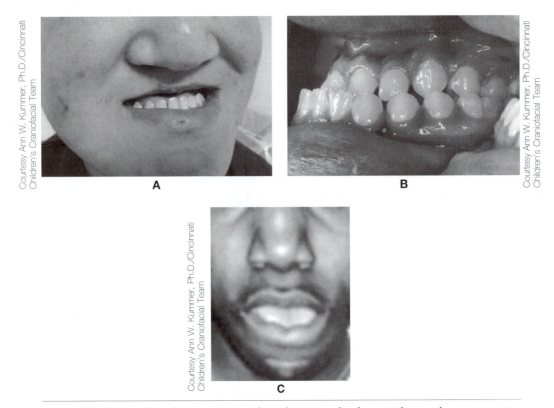

Courtesy Ann W. Kummer, Ph.D./Cincinnati Children's Craniofacial Team

FIGURE 12–11 (A–C)   Three patients with a Class III malocclusion. This results in an anterior tongue position relative to the position of the alveolar ridge.

observe tongue position and movement during speech to note whether there are obligatory distortions due to the abnormal structure, or compensatory misarticulations. This is important to determine because it has an impact on the recommendations for speech therapy versus physical management.

Finally, the status of oral hygiene should be assessed. Poor oral hygiene is common in patients with misaligned teeth because thorough cleaning is much more difficult. In addition, many of these patients are self-conscious about their teeth and simply avoid looking at them. Therefore, they have a particular aversion to brushing. If the examiner observes poor oral hygiene or obvious caries, a referral for dental care should be included in the overall recommendations following the assessment.

Tongue

The function, size, and relative position of the tongue in the oral cavity should be evaluated. The position of the tongue tip relative to the alveolar ridge is particularly important to note. In addition, the size of the tongue relative to the mandibular arch, the palatal arch, and the overall oral cavity space should be assessed. It should be remembered that the infant's tongue is considerably larger relative to the oral cavity space than the tongue of an older child or adult. In addition, the tongue reaches maturation at around the age of 8, whereas the mandible continues to grow for several more years (Arkuszewski, Gaszynska, & Przygonski, 2006). Therefore, at various points during development, the tongue may appear to be relatively large. However, if the tongue is significantly larger than the oral cavity space so that it doesn't fit with attempts to close the teeth, this might indicate a macroglossia (or a narrow mandible), which can affect both dentition and speech (Figure 12–12A). Multiple lobulations of the tongue may be noted in a child with orofaciodigital syndrome (Figure 12–12B). If the patient has had a tongue flap for closure of an oronasal fistula, the scarring and effect on function should be noted. Even with extensive scarring after a tongue flap, there is usually no effect on lingual function with articulation.

Ankyloglossia, commonly called "tongue-tie," is a condition where the person cannot elevate the tongue tip sufficiently to touch the roof of mouth—*with mouth open*, and cannot protrude the tongue tip past the mandibular gingival ridge or mandibular incisors (Figure 12–13A–C). During protrusion, the tongue tip often resembles the top of a heart because the restricted lingual frenulum causes an indentation in midline. If these characteristics are noted, the lingual frenulum under the tongue should be inspected for the location of the attachment and its length.

Although there is a common assumption that ankyloglossia affects speech production, there is actually no evidence in the literature to support this contention (Kummer, 2005). In fact, ankyloglossia usually does not cause abnormal speech—particularly for English speakers. To determine whether the ankyloglossia is affecting articulation, the examiner should assess the individual's ability to elevate the tongue tip for production of /l/ and to protrude the tongue tip

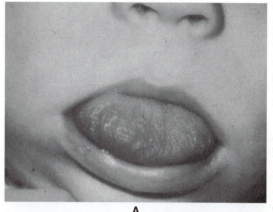

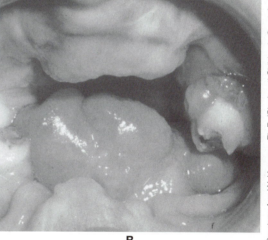

FIGURE 12–12 (A and B) Tongue anomalies. (A) Macroglossia in a patient with Beckwith-Wiedemann syndrome. (B) Lobulated tongue in a patient with orofaciodigital (OFD) syndrome. A lobulated tongue typically does not affect speech.

for production of /θ/. It should be noted that the /l/ sound is produced with the jaw down only slightly, and not with an open mouth position. In addition, /l/ can be produced with the tongue tip down and the dorsum up. The /θ/ sound can be produced with the tongue tip against the back of the incisors or even just under the alveolar ridge, so very little protrusion is actually

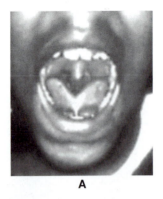

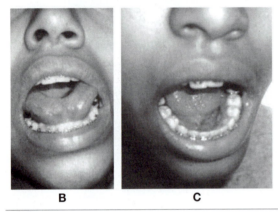

FIGURE 12–13 (A–C) Examples of ankyloglossia (tongue-tie). Note the heart shape at the tip of the tongue in figure 12–13A.

Courtesy Ann W. Kummer, Ph.D./Cincinnati Children's Craniofacial Team

required. There are no other English speech phonemes that are likely to be affected by restriction of the tongue tip. On the other hand, the trilled /r/ sound used in Spanish and some other languages may be difficult to produce with ankyloglossia. In addition, ankyloglossia can be a hindrance for patients with concomitant oral-motor difficulties.

Before recommending a frenulectomy for speech purposes, it is very important to be sure that ankyloglossia is contributing to the speech problem. Of course, frenulectomy can be appropriate for reasons other than speech, including early feeding problems due to difficulty latching on to the nipple, later problems

with bolus manipulation in the oral cavity, and even concerns with the aesthetics of the tongue.

Tonsils

As noted previously, the tonsils are located between the anterior and posterior faucial pillars in the oral cavity. They tend to be largest in the preschool years and then begin to gradually atrophy around age 6. At puberty, there may be a more sudden shrinkage of this lymphoid tissue. Tonsils are virtually nonexistent in most adults.

The presence of tonsils and their relative size can be reported on a 4-point scale. If the tonsils are absent, the rating would be 0. Tonsils that are small and fit within the confines of the faucial pillars are considered to be grade 1 in size. If the tonsils extend to the edge of the faucial pillars, they are rated as grade 2. If they are beyond the pillars, they are rated as grade 3, and if they are very large and meet in midline, they are judged as a grade 4 (refer to Figure 8–8).

When the tonsils are enlarged, they extend toward the midline, extend forward, or extend backward. Regardless, if they extend beyond the faucial pillars, they can have a negative effect on speech. For example, if the tonsils extend in the direction of midline, this can block the transmission of sound into the oral cavity, causing a pharyngeal cul-de-sac resonance. If they extend forward, they can interfere with the production of velar sounds (/k/, /g/). To compensate, the individual is likely to produce these sounds with the dorsum of the tongue (as a palatal-dorsal production) or with the tongue tip (as a lingual-alveolar sound). Finally, if the large tonsils extend backward, they are likely to intrude into the nasopharynx. They can even be positioned between the velum and posterior pharyngeal wall, causing incomplete velopharyngeal closure. When this

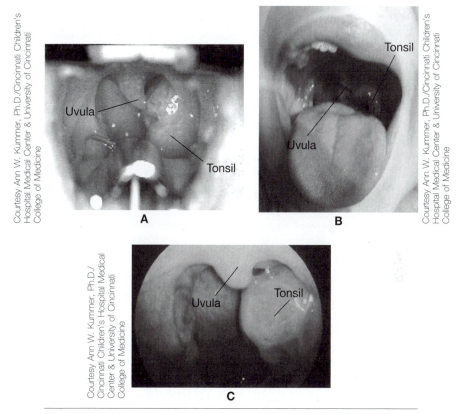

Courtesy Ann W. Kummer, Ph.D./Cincinnati Children's Hospital Medical Center & University of Cincinnati College of Medicine

Courtesy Ann W. Kummer, Ph.D./Cincinnati Children's Hospital Medical Center & University of Cincinnati College of Medicine

Courtesy Ann W. Kummer, Ph.D./ Cincinnati Children's Hospital Medical Center & University of Cincinnati College of Medicine

FIGURE 12–14 (A–C)   Large tonsil on the patient's left side in all three cases. Note the deviation of the uvula. This suggests that the tonsil is intruding into the oropharynx.

occurs, it usually causes a small velopharyngeal gap and thus nasal emission (Kummer, Briggs & Lee, 2003; Kummer, 2011). Resonance is typically mixed with hyponasality and cul-de-sac resonance. If one tonsil is much larger than the other and pushes the velum upward on that side as it intrudes into the pharynx, it will make the uvula point to the side of the large tonsil (Figure 12–14A–C). It should be noted that when the tonsils are markedly asymmetric in size, this may be a sign of malignancy in the larger tonsil, so this observation particularly requires referral to an otolaryngologist.

Alveolus and Hard Palate

As part of the examination, it is very important to note the position of the alveolar ridge as it relates to the position of the tongue tip. If the alveolar ridge is not above the tongue tip, as commonly occurs when there is significant jaw discrepancy, this can cause difficulty with the production of lingual-alveolar sounds and even with other anterior sounds.

Parents of children with a history of cleft may report noticing coloring of food in the child's nostril area after meals. (Chocolate milk, chocolate pudding, and spaghetti sauce seem to be the primary offenders.) This is

Case Report

Oronasal Fistula

Gerald presented as a new patient at the age of 11. He had a history of bilateral complete cleft lip and palate, which were repaired in another state. He had also had a pharyngeal flap for correction of velopharyngeal insufficiency at the age of 4. Gerald received speech therapy for several years in school. The mother reported that her primary concern was Gerald's "nasality."

Upon examination, Gerald's speech was found to be minimally intelligible. His articulation pattern consisted of backing of anterior phonemes. Many compensatory productions were used. Resonance was hyponasal and mouth breathing was noted, suggesting upper airway obstruction. An obstructing pharyngeal flap was suspected.

The surprise came with the intraoral inspection, however. When examining the hard palate, a very large palatal fistula was observed. However, this was packed with food. Gerald was taken to the otolaryngologist, who cleaned out the fistula and the nasal cavity.

Once the fistula was cleaned out and opened, the speech was reevaluated and found to be hypernasal with nasal air emission. The pattern of backing of phonemes was obviously developed as a means to compensate for the position of the open fistula.

Nasopharyngoscopy showed both lateral ports around the flap to be stenosed, which was the cause of the hyponasality and upper airway obstruction when the fistula was impacted. With this information in mind, a fistula repair and lateral port revisions were recommended.

This case study illustrates the importance of an intraoral examination. Although it is not possible to observe velopharyngeal function with an intraoral examination, some observations made in the intraoral examination relate directly to the cause of the speech or resonance disorder.

---

usually an indication of a patent nasolabial fistula, which is under the upper lip and in the line of the cleft. Nasal regurgitation can also be due to a fistula in the area of the incisive foramen but is unlikely to be due to velopharyngeal insufficiency/incompetence (VPI), unless the patient's head is down, as when drinking from a fountain.

To inspect for a nasolabial fistula, the examiner should use a tongue blade or dental mirror to gently raise the upper lip. Using a gloved finger, the fistula usually can be palpated by feeling the top of the gum area just under the buccal sulcus. This type of fistula does not affect speech because it is out of the way of articulation and the airflow.

An examination of the hard palate will reveal the overlying mucosa, which should be uniform in color (Jones, 1989; Schacher et al., 2010). The palatal vault should be evaluated, especially in relationship to the size of the tongue. If the palatal vault is low and flat, or if the maxillary arch is narrow relative to the tongue size, this can reduce the space available for the lingual articulation and can also reduce oral resonance. To compensate for intraoral crowding, the mandible will often lower and the tongue may be forced down and forward during speech. A "V" shape in the hard palate indicates a submucous cleft in the bone. This can extend as far as the position of the

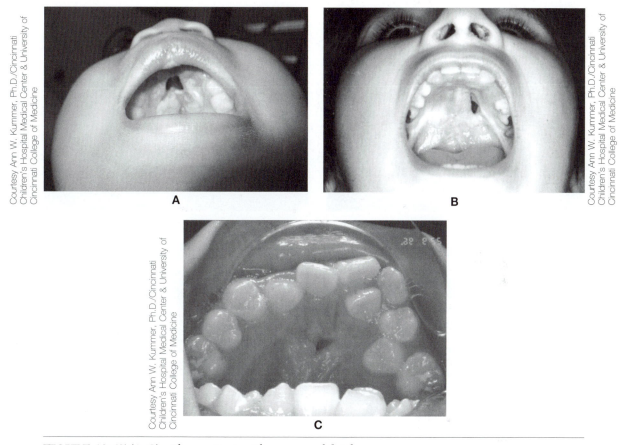

Courtesy Ann W. Kummer, Ph.D./Cincinnati Children's Hospital Medical Center & University of Cincinnati College of Medicine

FIGURE 12–15 (A–C) Three patients with an oronasal fistula.

incisive foramen (just behind the alveolar ridge).

If the patient has a history of cleft palate repair, the examiner should rule out the presence of a palatal (oronasal) fistula in the line of the cleft (Figure 12–15A–C). A tongue flap is often used to close a large fistula (Figure 12–16A–D). If the fistula is small, it may be difficult to see due to the angle of an intraoral view. Despite the use of the mirror, the size of a fistula is often difficult to estimate. It may appear narrow on the oral surface, yet open considerably on the nasal surface. In addition, there may be a furrow or a small depression in the palate that appears

to be a fistula but is actually just a blind pouch that does not go all the way through. If a fistula is identified, its approximate size and location should be noted because these are the determinants as to whether the fistula may be symptomatic for nasal regurgitation or speech.

Occasionally, an examination of the hard palate reveals a palatal torus. A *torus* is a slow-growing nodular protuberance of bone that can occur in either the hard palate or the mandible. There is evidence that both types of tori (plural form of torus) are hereditary. They occur almost twice as often in females than in males (Buddula, 2009; Nortje, 2006;

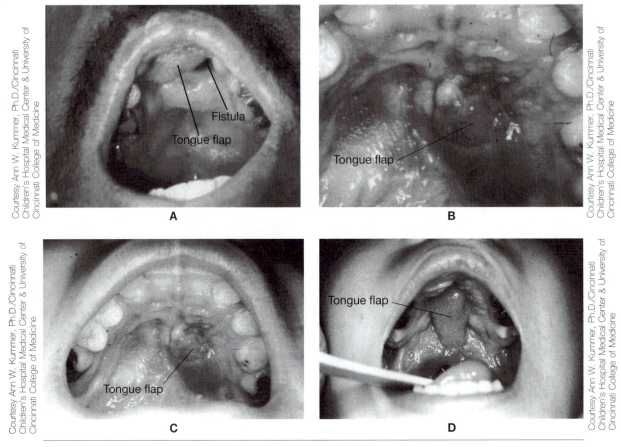

FIGURE 12–16 (A–D)   Tongue flaps. A tongue flap is done to correct a large oronasal fistula. In figure 12–16A, there is still a remaining opening on the right side (patient's left).

Papadopoulos & Lawhorn, 2008; Schwartz, 2005). A *torus palatinus*, also called a *palatal torus*, is a bony protuberance in the midline of the hard palate (Figure 12–17A–D). It has either a flat, spindled, nodular, or a lobular configuration. It is usually asymmetric and is rarely a source of discomfort unless the mucosal surface becomes ulcerated. Therefore, it is of little clinical significance. A torus palatinus does not interfere with speech or any other function unless it is very large.

Velum and Uvula

In an intraoral examination, the clinician should examine velar morphology. A normal velum should be consistent in color and may have a white line down the middle, called the *median palatine raphe*.

If there is a history of cleft palate, it is important to inspect the velum for a fistula, just as is done with the hard palate. If the fistula is anterior to the velar dimple (the point where the velum bends during phonation due to the contraction of the levator muscles), it is likely to be symptomatic, because this location is near the area of maximum air pressure as it enters the oral cavity. On the other hand, a fistula that is posterior to the area of the velar dimple will not affect resonance because it is below the area of velopharyngeal closure and in the area of

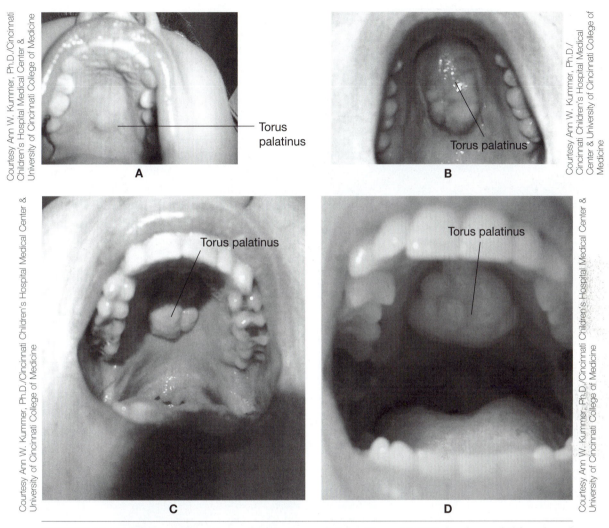

FIGURE 12–17 (A–D)   Different examples of a torus palatinus. Figure 12–17C also shows a bifid uvula and subtle evidence in the velum of a submucous cleft. Figure 12–17D shows a very large torus palatinus that grew to this size following the use of osteoporosis medication. It was interfering with speech and therefore was surgically removed.

velar redundancy (the vertical area of velar contact against the posterior pharyngeal wall).

Although not common, a portion or all of the velum can *dehisce* (pull apart) days or weeks after the palate repair. This may look like an unrepaired incomplete cleft palate (Figure 12–18). In addition, a large velar defect can be noted as a result of previous tumor removal (Figure 12–19A and B).

If there is no history of cleft palate, the examiner should look for characteristics of a submucous cleft (see Figure 2–15A–E in Chapter 2). Signs of a submucous cleft include a zona pellucida, which is a bluish-appearing area in the middle of the velum (Reiter, Brosch, Wefel, Schlomer, & Haase, 2011). This appearance occurs when the velum is thin and hence transparent as a result of the lack of

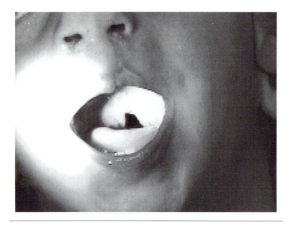

FIGURE 12–18 Velum that has partially dehisced (come apart) after a palate repair.

Courtesy Ann W. Kummer, Ph.D./Cincinnati Children's Hospital Medical Center & University of Cincinnati College of Medicine

muscle in this area. A thin velum is important to note because it can be the cause of nasal resonance, in the absence of VPI, due to transmission of sound energy through it.

If there is a submucous cleft that extends through the velum, the velum may appear to "tent up" in an upside down "V" shape during phonation (Figure 12–20A–C). When this occurs, it is because the levator veli palatini muscles are inserted on the edge of the posterior hard palate rather than in the midline of the velum. The contraction of these muscles results in the "V" shape in the velum. The V-shaped defect may be noted even without phonation, particularly if the submucous cleft extends through velum and the bony hard palate. Even when there is no apparent evidence of a submucous cleft through an intraoral examination, it cannot be ruled out. There may be an occult submucous cleft in the muscles or mucosa on the nasal side of the velum that can only be detected though nasopharyngoscopy (Finkelstein, Hauben, Talmi, Nachmani, & Zohar, 1992). In addition, it should be remembered that even with clear evidence of a submucous cleft, there may be normal resonance and velopharyngeal function.

After examining the basic morphology of the velum, velar function should be observed during phonation. The effective length of the velum is estimated by the position of the velar dimple, which is where the levator veli palatini muscles interdigitate in the velum and pull the velum up and back during

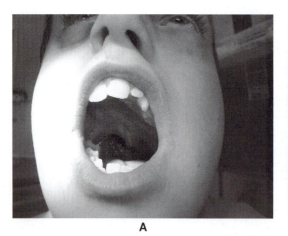

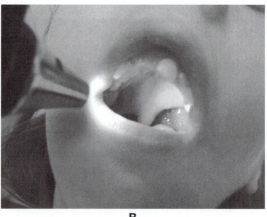

| A | B |

FIGURE 12–19 (A and B)   Velar defect after tumor resection. (A) Defect is on the left in the photo (patient's right side). (B) Defect is on the right in the photo (patient's left side).

Courtesy Ann W. Kummer, Ph.D./Cincinnati Children's Hospital Medical Center & University of Cincinnati College of Medicine

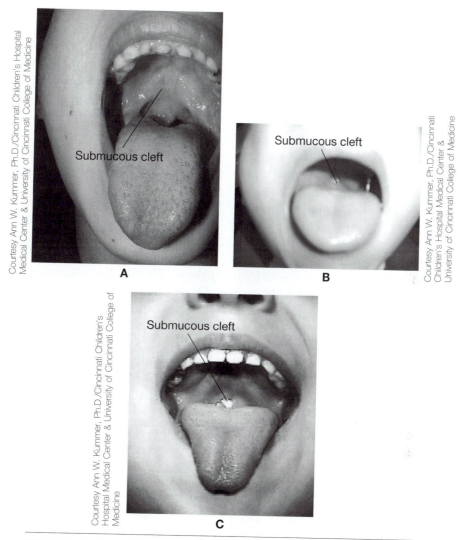

Courtesy Ann W. Kummer, Ph.D./Cincinnati Children's Hospital Medical Center & University of Cincinnati College of Medicine

Submucous cleft

A

Courtesy Ann W. Kummer, Ph.D./Cincinnati Children's Hospital Medical Center & University of Cincinnati College of Medicine

Submucous cleft

B

Courtesy Ann W. Kummer, Ph.D./Cincinnati Children's Hospital Medical Center & University of Cincinnati College of Medicine

Submucous cleft

C

FIGURE 12–20 (A–C)   Examples of a submucous cleft. During phonation, the velum appears to "tent up" in an inverted V-shape, suggesting a submucous cleft.

phonation (Veerapandiyan et al., 2011). The section of the velum that is anterior to the dimple is the effective length because it spans the length of the pharynx that is needed to obturate the nasopharyngeal port during speech. During sustained phonation, the velar dimple should appear to be back approximately 80% of the length of the velum (Mason & Simon, 1977). If the velar dimple is closer to the hard palate than to the uvula, the effective length may be too short, which can cause velopharyngeal insufficiency. On the other hand, the velar dimple may be very close to the uvula, causing the uvula to flip back during phonation. This suggests a short velum with too little vertical surface posterior to the velar dimple to close against the pharyngeal wall.

During phonation, the velum should elevate symmetrically in both a superior and posterior direction, and the velar dimple and uvula should be in midline. If two lateral velar dimples are observed during phonation, this suggests diastasis of the levator veli palatini muscles, which is consistent with a submucous cleft (Boorman & Sommerland, 1985). If there is asymmetrical velar movement, this suggests velopharyngeal incompetence due to unilateral paralysis or *paresis* (weakness) of the velum. In this case, the velar dimple may not be in midline, but instead may be slightly skewed to the better side. In addition, the uvula may point to the better side during phonation. The examiner should particularly look for unilateral velar paralysis or paresis in individuals with hemifacial microsomia. When there is asymmetric velar movement, this usually causes a lateral, rather than central, velopharyngeal gap. This is important to note when making surgical recommendations.

Poor velar movement during phonation in the intraoral exam may suggest velopharyngeal incompetence, but usually it is of no significance because this is common with phonation of a single vowel. Eliciting the gag reflex can confirm the presence of neuromotor function and also show the maximum excursion of the velum. However, this does not correlate well with movement potential for speech. Instead, the examiner can elicit velar movement by asking the patient to produce a vowel (preferably /æ/) repetitively.

In individuals with a history of cleft palate, poor velar movement can be due to abnormal function of the levator veli palatini, despite the palate repair. In other patients, it may be caused by neuromotor dysfunction related to dysarthria, apraxia, or velar paralysis or paresis. Enlarged adenoids can even interfere with the upward movement of the velum during speech.

In addition, there may be an anterior inclination of the pharyngeal wall above the oral level of view, making extensive velar movement unnecessary. Finally, the individual may have a sagittal pattern of closure, making velar movement less important.

During phonation, the velum may appear to be short relative to the position of the posterior pharyngeal wall. This can be deceiving, however, because the oral view is well below the level of velopharyngeal closure. In addition, it is impossible to know the extent of the anterior curvature of the posterior pharyngeal wall toward the velum, which decreases the nasopharyngeal depth at the level of velopharyngeal closure. Finally, the patient's basic pattern of closure cannot be determined from an intraoral perspective. However, if the velum has limited length past the area of the velar dimple, it is very likely to be too short to achieve closure. In this case, the velopharyngeal opening can sometimes be seen by placing a dental mirror just under the nasopharyngeal port.

Inspection of the uvula is important because its appearance may give a clue to a submucous cleft (Finkelstein et al., 1992). Either a bifid uvula (with two separate tags) or a hypoplastic uvula that is short and stubby can suggest a submucous cleft (Figure 12–21A–D; see also Figure 2–15A–C in Chapter 2). In some cases, the uvula may appear to be intact because the saliva helps to "glue" the tags of a bifid uvula together. If the examiner suspects that the uvula is bifid, but is unsure, this can often be determined by placing the tip of a tongue blade just behind the uvula and then flipping it forward (Rivron, 1989; Vilacosta & Canadas Godoy, 2008). If there are two tags, they will separate with this maneuver. (This is not recommended for a young child, however.) It should be remembered that a bifid uvula is a relatively common finding in the general population and does not always indicate a submucous

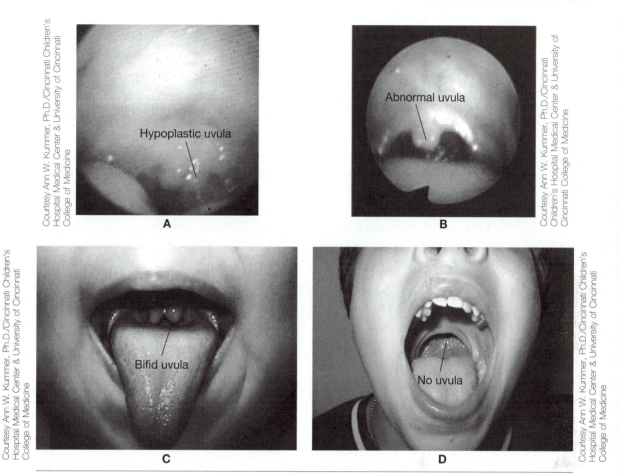

Courtesy Ann W. Kummer, Ph.D./Cincinnati Children's Hospital Medical Center & University of Cincinnati College of Medicine

Hypoplastic uvula

A

Courtesy Ann W. Kummer, Ph.D./Cincinnati Children's Hospital Medical Center & University of Cincinnati College of Medicine

Abnormal uvula

B

Courtesy Ann W. Kummer, Ph.D./Cincinnati Children's Hospital Medical Center & University of Cincinnati College of Medicine

Bifid uvula

C

Courtesy Ann W. Kummer, Ph.D./Cincinnati Children's Hospital Medical Center & University of Cincinnati College of Medicine

No uvula

D

FIGURE 12–21 (A–D) Abnormal uvulae that can suggest a submucous cleft. (A and B) The uvula is hypoplastic with a faint line in the middle. (C) The uvula is clearly bifid. (D) The uvula is absent, which is often the case after a cleft palate repair. This does not affect speech.

cleft (Bagatin, 1985; Saad, 1980; Wharton & Mowrer, 1992). In many cases, the defect includes only the uvula and does not involve the velum. To be safe, however, it is important to counsel individuals with a bifid uvula that they may be at risk for hypernasality following an adenoidectomy.

Posterior and Lateral Pharyngeal Walls

The depth of the posterior pharyngeal wall should be viewed relative to the length of the velum during phonation. When the posterior pharyngeal wall is very deep (and/or the velum is very short), the examiner may be able to look up into the nasopharynx with a dental mirror and flashlight. In most cases, however, the examiner cannot determine whether the pharyngeal wall is too deep or the velum is too short for closure because there is no way to know how the pharynx curves as it courses superiorly and then anteriorly to form the nasal cavity. The pharynx may appear to be very deep at the oral level but may curve sufficiently during the incline so that velopharyngeal closure can be obtained. In addition, the velum may be closing against a large adenoid pad rather than the posterior pharyngeal wall, which cannot be noted with an intraoral examination.

Lateral and posterior pharyngeal wall movement on the oral level can be observed during phonation. There may be very vigorous movement of the pharyngeal walls, which can substantiate that the nervous supply to the pharynx is intact. However, it doesn't necessarily indicate good pharyngeal wall movement in the area of velopharyngeal closure. In addition, poor movement of the lateral pharyngeal walls is not necessarily an indication of a problem. In fact, at the oral level, the lateral pharyngeal walls may actually bow outward during phonation, while bowing inward at a higher plane to assist with closure. Bowing outward at the oral level during phonation is actually a good thing because that opens the oropharynx to facilitate the transmission of airflow and sound into the oral cavity.

If the adenoid pad is very large, the inferior border can occasionally be observed on the posterior pharyngeal wall. It appears as lobulated tissue just behind and under velum during phonation.

Occasionally, the examiner may note a Passavant's ridge during the oral examination. This is a shelf-like ridge that bulges forward from the posterior pharyngeal wall at the oropharyngeal level during phonation and during the gag reflex (Yamawaki, 2003). If a Passavant's ridge is observed from an intraoral view, it is positioned too low to assist with velopharyngeal closure. Therefore, it is no more than an interesting observation.

If the patient has had previous surgery for VPI (velopharyngeal insufficiency or velopharyngeal incompetence), there may be visible evidence of this in the pharynx. For example, a vertical white line on the posterior pharyngeal wall can be a scar from donor site of a pharyngeal flap. In some cases, the actual flaps from the surgery (pharyngeal flap or sphincter pharyngoplasty) can be viewed from an intraoral perspective (see Figure 18–13 and 18–14 in Chapter 18). This usually indicates that the flaps are too low to be maximally effective for speech. In addition, low flaps are more likely to cause sleep apnea (and even swallow problems) because they are near the level of the base of the tongue (see Chapter 18 for more information).

Epiglottis

The epiglottis is located just below the base of the tongue and is relatively high in the hypopharynx in young children. As such, it can sometimes be viewed during an intraoral assessment of a young child, particularly if the child protrudes the tongue to say /æ/ (Shinohara & Takahashi, 2005) (Figure 12–22). As the tongue goes forward, the epiglottis is

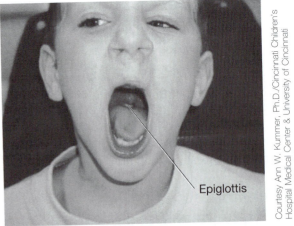

FIGURE 12–22 Epiglottis. Because the epiglottis is closer to the base of the tongue in children than in adults, it can sometimes be seen "popping up" when the child opens his mouth and sticks out his tongue.

pulled upward toward the oropharyngeal isthmus. The epiglottis is not usually seen in adults because the larynx descends in the neck with age, minimizing its ability to be viewed during oral examinations.

Oral-Motor Function

To assess the function of the oral structures, the examiner should request the child to protrude, elevate, depress, and lateralize the tongue tip. The examiner should also ask the patient to purse or smack the lips. What is most important, however, is to evaluate the individual's ability to sequence motor movements for speech. This can be done through the use of diadochokinetic exercises, which require the person to produce a sequence of syllables rapidly. The syllables /p/, /t/, and /k/ have been used for years to assess motor movements for speech. The examiner can use one syllable and have the patient produce it repetitively (e.g., /p, p, p/, etc.) and then the syllables can be combined (e.g., /p, t, k, p, t, k, p, t, k/, etc.). Using meaningless syllables can be difficult for young children, however. Therefore, it may be more effective to have the child produce common multisyllabic words repetitively (e.g., "patty cake," "puppy dog," "baby doll," "bubble gum," "peanut butter," "teddy bear," "kitty cat," "basketball," "baseball bat," etc.).

In diadochokinetic testing, it is more important to look at the accuracy of production than the number of repetitions. If consonants are omitted, substituted, or reversed, and errors increase with utterance length or phonemic complexity, the possibility of *childhood apraxia of speech (CAS)*, also called "verbal apraxia," or just "apraxia" should be considered.

The examiner should also look for characteristics of dysarthria and more subtle signs of oral-motor dysfunction, including a chronic open mouth posture in the absence of upper airway obstruction, and an anterior tongue position. With the open mouth and anterior tongue position, drooling commonly occurs. This can be subtle, with just a little moisture on the chin, or it can be copious so that the child wears a bib or carries a cloth. If the child has feeding difficulties by history or by observation, this could also be an indication of oral-motor dysfunction.

If there is an anterior open bite, the possibility of a tongue thrust should also be considered. This can be determined by gently scratching the tip of the tongue with a tongue blade to provide a tingling sensation, and then having the child take a drink of water. After the swallow, the examiner asks the child to report whether the tongue tip went up (against the alveolar ridge), forward (against or between the incisors), or down (against the mandibular incisors). If the child consistently reports that the tongue goes forward or down with the swallow, a tongue thrust should be suspected (Dahan, Lelong, Celant, & Leysen, 2000; Eslamian & Leilazpour, 2006; Fraser, 2006; Peng, Jost-Brinkmann, Yoshida, Chou, & Lin, 2004; Piyapattamin, Soma, & Hisano, 2002). If the child is unable to report the direction of the tongue movement, this can be observed by asking the child to swallow while the lips are held open with a tongue blade. If there is an anterior open bite, observing the tongue movement during swallowing is usually easy.

Putting It All Together

During the orofacial examination, the examiner should determine the physical factors that appear to be interfering with articulation and/or resonance. Although the examiner should focus on assessing anomalies that can contribute to a speech or resonance disorder, other anomalies should also be noted. This is particularly important if these abnormalities require additional referral or follow-up (e.g., dental caries) or they provide evidence of a syndrome (e.g., hypertelorism). Even non-orofacial features, such as short stature or long and slender digits (Figure 12–23), should be noted by the examiner, as these can provide clues to a syndrome. (These particular features are suggestive of velocardiofacial syndrome.) Some relevant anomalies or medical conditions that are not readily seen, such as heart or kidney anomalies, may be recorded in the medical record or reported by the parents. When anomalies are noted that require additional evaluation or follow-up, the speech-language pathologist should discuss the findings with the primary care physician and referring physician, and suggest referrals to other specialists, as appropriate.

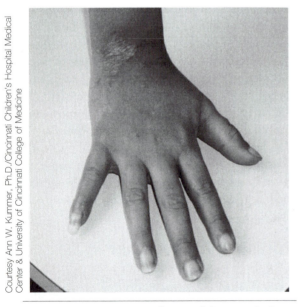

FIGURE 12–23 Long and tapered fingers, which are often found with velocardiofacial syndrome.

INFECTION CONTROL DURING THE EXAMINATION

A discussion of the intraoral examination would not be complete without a section on infection control. Knowledge of infection control is important to protect the healthcare provider and prevent the spread of infection to those individuals who are being served. Speech-language pathologists should practice good infection control procedures because they are in close physical contact with the individuals in their care, and they are often working around and even in the mouth. Unfortunately, most speech-language pathologists have had little training on appropriate infection control procedures unless they have obtained it from on-the-job experience (Bankaitis, Kemp, Krival, & Bandaranayake, 2006; Mosheim, 2005).

The most common causes of communicable diseases in healthcare environments are the human immunodeficiency virus (HIV), hepatitis B virus (HBV), cytomegalovirus I (CMV), methicillin-resistant staphylococcus aureus (MRSA) bacteria, clostridium difficile (C-diff) bacteria, and the tuberculosis bacteria. Professionals must also be concerned about the transmission of minor diseases, such as the common cold and influenza. Pediatric settings are a particular concern because children generally have poor personal hygiene habits and hence are very susceptible to infection (Krewedl, 1999).

In 1988, the Centers for Disease Control and Prevention (CDC) in Atlanta published guidelines for infection control called Universal Blood and Body Fluid Precautions (UBBFP). They have since been revised and are now called *Standard Precautions* (CDC, 2005). Standard precautions contain recommended procedures that are designed to protect the patient, the professional, and all others in a healthcare environment from the spread of infection. These procedures are based on the assumption that every patient and healthcare provider is a potential carrier of an infectious disease and that any body fluid may contain contagious microorganisms. The American Speech-Language-Association Hearing Association (ASHA) adopted these guidelines and recommended them to its membership in 1990. There are now documents and links on the ASHA website related to standard precautions and infection control (ASHA, 2012). Despite the fact that standard precautions have been recommended for more than two decades, there is evidence to suggest that they are not consistently or appropriately used by many healthcare professionals (Aultman & Borges, 2011).

Handwashing

The role of the human hands in the transmission of infection was recognized even before the establishment of microbiology as a science (Kerr, 1998). For many years, handwashing has been considered the single most important means of preventing the spread of infection in a healthcare setting (Akyol, Ulusoy, & Ozen, 2006; CDC, 2005; CDC, 2013; World Health Organization, 2009; Gallagher, 1999; Ginsberg & Clarke, 1972; Horton, 1995; Kiernan, 1999). Handwashing reduces the number of potential pathogens on the hands and interrupts the opportunity of transferring organisms to patients and others.

Unfortunately, healthcare workers are not always compliant in washing their hands as often as they should (Aultman & Borges, 2011). As a result, *nosocomial* (hospital-acquired) *infections* continue to be a principal cause of morbidity and even mortality in healthcare settings (Brunetti et al., 2006; Kennedy, Elward, & Fraser, 2004; Picheansathian, Pearson, & Suchaxaya, 2008). It is widely believed that if all healthcare providers used the proper technique for handwashing and this became a habit, infection rates in healthcare facilities would drop dramatically (Brown & Persivale, 1995). Certainly, greater awareness of this problem may help to generate improvement.

Hands should be washed before and after every patient contact and especially before and after an intraoral examination. It is best if hands are washed in front of the parents and child. This models appropriate hygienic behavior (Bellet, 1996). The use of examination gloves does not eliminate the need for handwashing (Bowman & Nicholas, 1990; Hopkins, 1989; Ripper, 1988; Shogren, 1988). It is important to wash hands before putting on gloves because there can be a perforation in the glove that is not readily visible. It is also necessary to wash hands after glove removal, because the warm, moist environment in the glove is conducive to rapid bacterial multiplication (Mayone-Ziomek, 1998). Finally, hands should be washed after contact with potentially contaminated surfaces.

Both the CDC and the World Health Organization (WHO) have published guidelines on appropriate handwashing in a hospital environment (CDC, 2005; CDC, 2013; & WHO, 2009). The WHO recommendations for proper handwashing with soap and water are stated as follows:

- Wet hands with water.

- Apply enough soap to cover all hand surfaces.

- Rub hands palm to palm, right palm over left dorsum with interlaced fingers and vice versa;

- Rub hands palm to palm with fingers interlaced.

- Rub backs of fingers to opposing palms with fingers interlocked.

- Rub rotationally, left thumb clasped in right palm and vice versa.

- Rub rotationally backward and forward, with clasped fingers of right hand in left palm and vice versa.

- Rinse hands with water.

- Dry hands thoroughly with a single use towel.

- Use towel to turn off faucet.

For more information or to see illustrations, go to the WHO Web site at http://whqlibdoc.who .int/publications/2009/9789241597906_eng.pdf.

If soap and water are not immediately available, or if hands are not visibly dirty or contaminated, antimicrobial handwipes or gels can be used for antisepsis. Antimicrobial handwashing products (e.g., 2% chlorhexidine gluconate, triclosan) should be used before contact with newborns, immunocompromised patients, and patients on high-risk units, and before an invasive procedure. Recommendations for hand hygiene using an alcohol-based gel are published on the WHO site noted on page 155.

Gloves

With the standard precautions approach to infection control, the examiner should assume that all human secretions, including saliva, could be infectious or contain bloodborne pathogens. Therefore, the examiner must wear personal protective equipment (PPE) when performing any task that has the risk of contact with the patient's secretions or when the professional is engaged in any type of evaluation or treatment that requires physical contact with the patient's mouth or nose. Gloves are the best form of protection for an intraoral examination.

Until recently, latex gloves were used in most healthcare settings. However, latex allergies have become very common. To minimize sensitization of healthcare workers and exposure to latex-sensitive patients, most institutions have now eliminated the use of latex gloves. Hospital gloves are now made of vinyl, nitrile, or a synthetic material.

Gloves should always be worn during an intraoral examination, during a feeding evaluation or therapy, and also while performing a nasopharyngoscopy exam. They should fit tightly because loosely fitted gloves interfere with the manipulation of objects. Gloves should be changed immediately if holes, rips, or tears are visible, and as needed during the patient's care. When removing gloves, they should be pulled off so that they are inside out, and then immediately discarded (Figure 12–24A–C). This prevents physical contact with the contaminated surface of the gloves. Because all gloves are designed for single-patient use, they are discarded in the waste can after each patient.

Patient Equipment and Supplies

Tongue blades, dental mirrors, and other tools for an intraoral assessment should not be placed directly on a desk or table after use. Instead, these tools should be placed on a clean paper towel or tissue until they can be cleaned or discarded.

Disposable items should be used for intraoral examinations or manipulation whenever possible. It is easier to dispose of an item and use a new one for the next person than to have to wash and disinfect the item between uses. Items that are manufactured to be

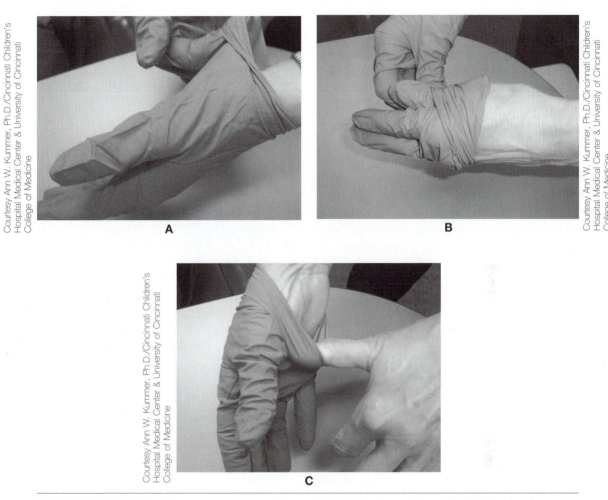

Courtesy Ann W. Kummer, Ph.D./Cincinnati Children's Hospital Medical Center & University of Cincinnati College of Medicine

A

Courtesy Ann W. Kummer, Ph.D./Cincinnati Children's Hospital Medical Center & University of Cincinnati College of Medicine

B

Courtesy Ann W. Kummer, Ph.D./Cincinnati Children's Hospital Medical Center & University of Cincinnati College of Medicine

C

FIGURE 12–24 (A–C)   Proper way to remove gloves. (A) Grab the glove at the wrist. (B) Pull the glove off so that it is inside out. (C) Put thumb under the wrist of the second glove and pull it off inside out.

disposable can usually not be adequately washed or disinfected. Therefore, all disposable items should be discarded immediately after use.

Items that are not disposable, such as a dental mirror, should be cleaned and sanitized in a dishwasher if possible. Alternatively, the item can be thoroughly cleansed with hot soapy water and then wiped down with alcohol. Both ethyl alcohol and isopropyl alcohol have a broad spectrum of antimicrobial activity that counteracts vegetative bacteria, fungi, and viruses (including HIV) (Widmer & Frei, 1999). In addition, alcohol has many qualities that make it suitable for low-level and intermediate-level disinfection, including the fact that it is fast acting (15–30 seconds), and it readily evaporates. Sterilization, as opposed to disinfection, is required to destroy bacterial spores, however. Items contaminated with saliva only and intact mucous membranes are resistant to bacterial spores. Therefore, sterilization is usually not necessary unless the instruments have the potential for exposure to blood. On the other hand, C-diff bacteria are not killed with alcohol, so if this disease is a concern, chlorine bleach wipes should be used.

All patient equipment and supplies should be stored in a clean and safe manner that protects the items from exposure or contamination to body fluids, known soiled items, dust, particulate matter, and moisture. Supplies should always be stored at a minimum of 4–6 inches off the floor to enable floor cleaning and to protect from accidental damage or contamination with floor cleaning solutions.

Surface Disinfection

All therapy or patient care rooms should be equipped with spray disinfectant products and disinfectant towelettes (Bankaitis et al., 2006).

Flat surfaces, such as tables and armchairs, can be contaminated with saliva or mucous during a session. Therefore, they should be cleaned and disinfected with a disinfecting agent between patients.

SUMMARY

The structure and function of the oral articulators and the structures of the oral cavity have a direct impact on the quality and intelligibility of speech. Therefore, when speech or resonance problems are noted, a thorough intraoral orofacial examination must be done. The examiner must rule out structural abnormalities that may require surgical or orthodontic treatment prior to the initiation of speech therapy. In addition, a keen eye and a thorough examination can help to detect previously undiagnosed conditions.

FOR REVIEW AND DISCUSSION

1. Describe the best method for viewing the intraoral structures with the least amount of stress or discomfort for the patient.

2. What are the particular anomalies that can be observed of the eyes, ears, nose, lips, and facial bones? Why are these observations an important part of a speech pathology examination?

3. What is the purpose of palatal palpation? Describe how this is done and what should be felt.

4. What observations of the velopharyngeal mechanism can be made through an

intraoral examination? Why can't velopharyngeal function be viewed by looking in the mouth?

5. Describe a method for evaluating dental occlusion. Why is it important to assess occlusion? What are the implications for treatment recommendations?

6. Discuss the evaluation of the structure and function of the tongue and what should be considered. What are some techniques that could be used to evaluate tongue function?

7. Describe methods of infection control when performing an intraoral examination.

REFERENCES

Akyol, A., Ulusoy, H., & Ozen, I. (2006). Handwashing: A simple, economical and effective method for preventing nosocomial infections in intensive care units. *Journal of Hospital Infection*, 62(4), 395–405.

American Speech-Language-Hearing Association (ASHA). (2012). Infection control in speech-language pathology. Accessed January 11, 2013, from http://www.asha.org/slp/infectioncontrol.htm.

Angle, E. H. (1899). Classification of malocclusion. *Dental Cosmos, 41*, 248–264, 350–357.

Arkuszewski, P., Gaszynska, E., & Przygonski, A. (2006). A method for determination of tongue size in patients with mandibular prognathism. *Annales Academiae Medicae Stetinensis*, 52(Suppl. 3), 125–129.

Aultman, J. M., & Borges, N. J. (2011). The ethical and pedagogical effects of modeling "not-so-universal" precautions. *Medical Teacher*, 33(1), e43–49.

Bagatin, M. (1985). Submucous cleft palate. *Journal of Maxillofacial Surgery, 13*(1), 37–38.

Bankaitis, A. U., Kemp, R. J., Krival, K., & Bandaranayake, D. (2006). *Infection control for speech-language pathology*. St. Louis, MO: Auban.

Bellet, P. S. (1996). Physical examination. In R. C. Baker (Ed.), *Pediatric primary care*. Philadelphia: Lippincott Williams & Wilkins.

Boorman, J. G., & Sommerland, B. C. (1985). Levator veli palati and palatal dimples: Their anatomy, relationship, and clinical significance. *British Journal of Plastic Surgery, 38*, 326–332.

Bowman, A. M., & Nicholas, T. J. (1990). Improving compliance with universal blood and body fluid precautions in a rural medical center. *Journal of Nursing Quality Assurance, 5*(1), 73–81.

Brown, J. W., & Persivale, E. J. (1995). Managing the front line of infection control: Handwashing. *Director, 3*(1), 36–37.

Brunetti, L., Santoro, E., De Caro, F., Cavallo, P., Boccia, G., Capunzo, M., & Motta, O. (2006). Surveillance of nosocomial infections: A preliminary study on hand hygiene compliance of healthcare workers. *Journal of Preventive Medicine and Hygiene, 47*(2), 64–68.

Buddula, A. (2009). Staining of palatal torus secondary to long term minocycline therapy. *Journal of Indian Society of Periodontology, 13*(1), 48–49.

Centers for Disease Control and Prevention (CDC). (2013). Handwashing: Clean hands save lives. Accessed January 11, 2013, from http://www.cdc.gov/handwashing/

Centers for Disease Control and Prevention (CDC). (2005). Appendix 11: Recommendations for application of standard precautions for the care of all patients in all healthcare settings. Accessed January 11, 2013, from http://www.cdc.gov/sars/guidance/I-infection/app1.html.

Cook, S., Rieger, M., Donlan, C., & Howell, P. (2011). Testing orofacial abilities of children who stutter: The Movement, Articulation, Mandibular and Sensory awareness (MAMS) assessment procedure. *Journal of Fluency Disorders*, 36(1), 27–40.

Dahan, J. S., Lelong, O., Celant, S., & Leysen, V. (2000). Oral perception in tongue thrust and other oral habits. *American Journal of*

Orthodontics and Dentofacial Orthopedics, 118(4), 385–391.

Elluru, R. G. (2005). Adenoid facies and nasal airway obstruction: Cause and effect? *Archives of Otolaryngology-Head & Neck Surgery, 131*(10), 919–920.

Eslamian, L., & Leilazpour, A. P. (2006). Tongue to palate contact during speech in subjects with and without a tongue thrust. *European Journal of Orthodontics, 28*(5), 475–479.

Finkelstein, Y., Hauben, D. J., Talmi, Y. P., Nachmani, A., & Zohar, Y. (1992). Occult and overt submucous cleft palate: From peroral examination to nasendoscopy and back again. *International Journal of Pediatric Otorhinolaryngology, 23*(1), 25–34.

Fraser, C. (2006). Tongue thrust and its influence in orthodontics. *International Journal of Orthodontics Milwaukee, 17*(1), 9–18.

Gallagher, R. (1999). This is the way we wash our hands. *Nursing Times, 95*(10), 62–65.

Ginsberg, F., & Clarke, B. (1972). Handwashing is simple, effective infection control, so why won't people wash their hands? *Modern Hospital, 119*(4), 132.

Hopkins, C. C. (1989). AIDS. Implementation of universal blood and body fluid precautions. *Infectious Disease Clinics of North America, 3*(4), 747–762.

Horton, R. (1995). Handwashing: The fundamental infection control principle. *British Journal of Nursing, 4*(16), 926, 928, 930–933.

Jones, J. A. (1989, October 30). Integrating the oral examination into clinical practice. *Hospital Practice, 24*(10A), 23–27, 30, 39.

Kennedy, A. M., Elward, A. M., & Fraser, V. J. (2004). Survey of knowledge, beliefs, and practices of neonatal intensive care unit healthcare workers regarding nosocomial infections, central venous catheter care, and hand hygiene. *Infection Control and Hospital Epidemiology, 25*(9), 747–752.

Kerr, J. (1998). Handwashing. *Nursing Standards, 12*(51), 35–39; Quiz 41–42.

Kiernan, M. (1999). Handwashing in infection control. *Community Nurse, 5*(7), 19–20.

Krewedl, A. (1999, August 23). Infection control in pediatric settings. *Advance*, pp. 26–27.

Kummer, A. W. (2005, December 27). To clip or not to clip? That's the question. *The ASHA Leader, 10*(17), 6–7, 30.

Kummer, A. W. (2011). Types and causes of velopharyngeal dysfunction. *Seminars in Speech and Language, 32*(2), 150–158.

Kummer, A. W., Briggs, M., & Lee, L. (2003). The relationship between the characteristics of speech and velopharyngeal gap size. *Cleft Palate—Craniofacial Journal, 40*(6), 590–596.

Lin, X. F., Li, S. H., Huang, Z. S., & Wu, X. Y. (2010). [Relationship between occlusal plane and masticatory path in youth with individual normal occlusion.] *Zhonghua Kou Qiang Yi Xue Za Zhi, 45*(6), 370–375.

Mason, R. M., & Simon, C. (1977). An orofacial examination checklist. *Language, Speech, and Hearing Services in the Schools, 8*(3), 155–163.

Mayone-Ziomek, J. M. (1998). Handwashing in healthcare. *Dermatological Nursing, 10*(3), 183–188.

Mosheim, J. (2005, October 24). Infection control: Protocols protect the clinician and patient. *Advance for Speech-Language Pathologists & Audiologists*, PP. 7–9.

Nortje, C. J. (2006). General Practitioners radiology. Case 39. Diagnosis. Palatal torus. *SADJ Journal of the South African Dental Association, 61*(2), 081.

Papadopoulos, H., & Lawhorn, T. (2008). Use of a palatal flap for torus reduction. *Journal of Oral and Maxillofacial Surgery*, *66*(9), 1969–1970.

Peng, C. L., Jost-Brinkmann, P. G., Yoshida, N., Chou, H. H., & Lin, C. T. (2004). Comparison of tongue functions between mature and tongue-thrust swallowing—An ultrasound investigation. *American Journal of Orthodontics and Dentofacial Orthopedics*, *125*(5), 562–570.

Picheansathian, W., Pearson, A., & Suchaxaya, P. (2008). The effectiveness of a promotion programme on hand hygiene compliance and nosocomial infections in a neonatal intensive care unit. *International Journal of Nursing Practice*, *14*(4), 315–321.

Piyapattamin, T., Soma, K., & Hisano, M. (2002). Temporary tongue thrust: Failure during orthodontic treatment. *Australian Orthodontic Journal*, *18*(1), 39–46.

Reiter, R., Brosch, S., Wefel, H., Schlomer, G., & Haase, S. (2011). The submucous cleft palate: diagnosis and therapy. *International Journal of Pediatric Otorhinolaryngology*, *75*(1), 85–88.

Ripper, M. (1988). Universal blood and body fluid precautions. *Journal of Advances in Medical Surgical Nursing*, *1*(1), 21–25.

Rivron, R. P. (1989). Bifid uvula: Prevalence and association in otitis media with effusion in children admitted for routine otolaryngological operations. *Journal of Laryngology & Otology*, *103*(3), 249–252.

Saad, E. F. (1980). The underdeveloped palate in ear, nose and throat practice. *Laryngoscope*, *90*(8, Pt. 1), 1371–1377.

Schacher, B., Burklin, T., Horodko, M., Raetzke, P., Ratka-Kruger, P., & Eickholz, P. (2010). Direct thickness measurements of the hard palate mucosa. *Quintessence International*, *41*(8), e149–156.

Schwartz, A. J. (2005). Insertion of a folded laryngeal mask airway around a palatal torus. *American Association of Nurse Anesthetics Journal*, *73*(3), 211–216.

Shanks, L. A., Walker, T. W., McCann, P. J., & Kerin, M. J. (2011). Oral cavity examination: Beyond the core curriculum? *British Journal of Oral and Maxillofacial Surgery*, *49*(8), 640–642.

Shinohara, E. H., & Takahashi, A. (2005). View of the epiglottis during examination of the oral cavity. *British Journal of Oral and Maxillofacial Surgery*, *43*(3), 264.

Shogren, E. (1988). An ounce of prevention is worth a pound of cure: Using universal blood and body fluid precautions in your work setting. *MNA Accent*, *60*(2), 35–36.

Smith, B., & Guyette, T. W. (2004). Evaluation of cleft palate speech. *Clinics in Plastic Surgery*, *31*(2), 251–260.

Smith, B. E., & Kuehn, D. P. (2007). Speech evaluation of velopharyngeal dysfunction. *The Journal of Craniofacial Surgery*, *18*(2), 251–260.

Thomas, J. E., & Bender, B. S. (1993). What to look for after you say "Open wide." *Postgraduate Medicine*, *93*(7), 109–110.

Veerapandiyan, A., Blalock, D., Ghosh, S., Ip, E., Barnes, C., & Shashi, V. (2011). The role of cephalometry in assessing velopharyngeal dysfunction in velocardiofacial syndrome. *Laryngoscope*, *121*(4), 732–737.

Vilacosta, I., & Canadas Godoy, V. (2008). Images in clinical medicine. Bifid uvula and aortic aneurysm. *The New England Journal of Medicine*, *359*(2), e2.

Wharton, P., & Mowrer, D. E. (1992). Prevalence of cleft uvula among school children in kindergarten through grade five. *Cleft Palate–Craniofacial Journal*, *29*(1), 10–12; Discussion 13–14.

Widmer, A. F., & Frei, R. (1999). Decontamination, disinfection, and sterilization. In P. R. Murray, E. J. Baron, M. A. Pfaller, F. C. Tenover, & R. H. Yolken, (Eds.), *Manual of clinical microbiology* (pp. 138–164). Washington, DC: ASM Press.

World Health Organization. (2009). *WHO guidelines on hand hygiene in health care*. Geneva, Switzerland: WHO Press . Accessed January 11, 2013, from http://whqlibdoc.who.int/publications/ 2009/9789241597906_eng.pdf.

Yamawaki, Y. (2003). Forward movement of posterior pharyngeal wall on phonation. *American Journal of Otolaryngology,* 24(6), 400–404.

CHAPTER

13

OVERVIEW OF INSTRUMENTAL PROCEDURES*

CHAPTER OUTLINE

*This chapter may be all that is needed for graduate students and general practitioners regarding instrumentation. Chapters 14 through 17 are designed to help practicing speech-language pathologists learn how to actually perform these procedures and interpret the results.

INTRODUCTION

Velopharyngeal insufficiency/incompetence (VPI) can be diagnosed by an experienced and knowledgeable speech-language pathologist based on the characteristics of the speech, as determined through a perceptual speech evaluation (Hinton, 2009). However, instrumental assessment of the velopharyngeal valve can provide important additional information. In some cases, this information can be used to help determine the surgical procedure for the patient. It can also help in measuring change as a result of surgery or therapeutic intervention (Karnell, 2011).

There are two basic categories of instrumental procedures for evaluation of velopharyngeal function—those that give indirect yet objective information and those that give direct yet subjective information. Indirect instrumental procedures include the use of nasometry and aerodynamic instrumentation. The advantage of these procedures is that they provide objective data regarding the results of velopharyngeal function, such as acoustic output or airflow and air pressure. They are considered indirect measures because they do not allow visualization of the structures. Direct instrumental procedures include videofluoroscopy and nasopharyngoscopy. The advantage of these procedures is that they allow the examiner to directly visualize the structures of the velopharyngeal valve during speech (and swallowing). However, these procedures require interpretation of the examiner, and therefore they are somewhat subjective.

The purpose of this chapter is to provide an overview of the types of instrumentation that are available for evaluation of velopharyngeal function. The uses and relative advantages and disadvantages of each procedure are discussed.

INDIRECT MEASURES

Indirect instrumental procedures (nasometry and speech aerodynamics) give objective data regarding the physical correlates of velopharyngeal function, such as acoustic output, airflow, and air pressure. The advantage of objective data is that they can be compared to standardized norms for interpretation. In addition, data from these instruments can be used for determination and comparison of treatment outcomes. For example, such data can be used to determine the outcome of surgery or therapy, or they can be used to compare treatment outcomes between professionals and centers.

The disadvantage of indirect procedures is that they do not allow visualization of the structures.

In late 2009, a survey was sent to plastic surgeons, otolaryngologists, and speech-language pathologists who are members of the American Cleft Palate–Craniofacial Association (ACPA) and work with patients with VPI. Of the 126 respondents, more participants reported using nasometry (28.9%) than aerodynamic measures (4.3%) (Kummer, Clark, Redle, Thomsen, & Billmire, 2012). Still, less than a third of respondents reported using instrumentation to obtain objective measures. For a comparison of advantages of each direct procedure, see Table 13–1.

TABLE 13-1 The Relative Advantages (+) of Nasometry (NS) over Aerodynamic (AD) Procedures and Vice Versa

Advantages	NS	AD
Can obtain an accurate estimate of the size of the VP opening	−	+
Results not affected by articulation errors or mixed resonance	−	+
Provides information on the patency of the nasal airway during breathing	−	+
Measures resonance in addition to audible nasal emission	+	−
Can be used to determine phoneme-specific nasal emission	+	−
Can determine the effect of a fistula versus VPI	+	
Can assess VP function in connected speech	+	−
Can be used for speech biofeedback	+	−

© Cengage Learning 2014

Nasometry

Nasometry is a method of measuring the acoustic correlates of resonance, audible nasal emission, and velopharyngeal function through a computer-based instrument. The Nasometer II (KayPENTAX, Montvale, N.J.) includes a Nasometer Headset (Figure 13–1A) or a Hand-Held Separator (Figure 13–1B), each of which has two directional microphones on either side of a sound separator plate. The sound separator plate is placed between the child's upper lip and nose (Figure 13–2A and B).

The speech sample for nasometry usually consists of standardized passages where normative data are available. The Zoo passage and Nasal passage were the first to have normative data. Later, the MacKay-Kummer Simplified Nasometric Assessment Procedures-Revised (SNAP-R) (Kummer, 2005) was developed to provide more diagnostic value and also to make it easier for evaluation of children. When an individual's score is compared to normative data for that passage, a judgment can be made regarding the normalcy of resonance. High scores, in comparison to normative data, suggest hypernasality; low scores, in comparison, suggest hyponasality.

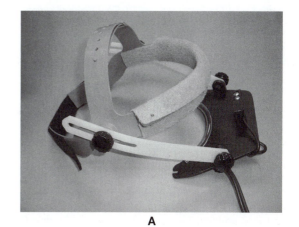

A

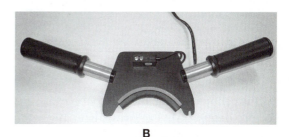

B

FIGURE 13–1 (A and B) (A) The Nasometer II Headset. (B) The Nasometer II Hand-Held Separator.

Courtesy of Kay PENTAX/Montvale, NJ and Ann W. Kummer, Ph.D./Cincinnati Children's Hospital Medical Center & University of Cincinnati College of Medicine

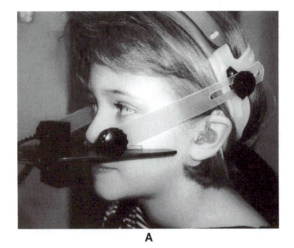

A

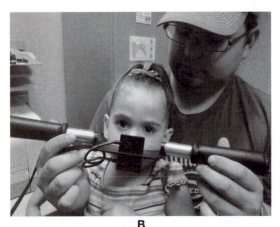

B

FIGURE 13–2 (A and B) (A) Placement of the Nasometer II Headset on a patient. The sound separator plate should be perpendicular to the face or in a horizontal position. The microphones should be directly in front of the mouth and the nose. (B) Placement of the Hand-Held Separator. The separator plate should be placed in the same position as with the Headset.

Courtesy of Kay PENTAX/Montvale, NJ and Ann W. Kummer, Ph.D./ Cincinnati Children's Hospital Medical Center & University of Cincinnati College of Medicine

During production of the speech passage, the Nasometer II captures data regarding acoustic energy from both the nasal (N) cavity and the oral (O) cavity in real time. The Nasometer II then calculates the average ratio of nasal over total (nasal plus oral) acoustic energy and converts this to a percentage value

called the *nasalance score*. This gives the examiner information about the percentage of nasality in speech. The nasalance score can be depicted, therefore, as follows:

$$\text{Nasalance} = N \div (N + O) \times 100.$$

Nasometry is useful in that it supplements what is heard through the perceptual evaluation and what is seen through direct instrumental measures (Karnell, 2011; Sweeney & Sell, 2008). In addition to evaluating characteristics of velopharyngeal dysfunction, nasometry can also be used to assess upper airway obstruction and hyponasality through their acoustic correlates during speech. It has even been used to evaluate and treat resonance of children with hearing impairment. Nasometry can be used effectively for pre- and post-surgical comparisons. Finally, it can provide visual feedback for the patient during therapy.

Speech Aerodynamics

Speech aerodynamics is a procedure to measure the mechanical properties of airflow and air pressure during speech production (Figure 13–3). Because speech production requires a buildup and release of air pressure during consonant production, aerodynamic procedures are ideal to assess air pressure and airflow during speech. The aerodynamic procedure involves the use of oral and nasal catheters, which are connected to pressure transducers. There is also a flow tube that is connected to a heated pneumotachograph. The *transducers* convert the detected air pressure or flow into electrical signals. The *pneumotachograph* determines the rate of airflow.

Aerodynamic instrumentation can be used in the evaluation of VPI because it can provide objective documentation of intraoral air pressure levels and the amount of nasal air emission. The data collected allow the examiner to calculate an estimate of velopharyngeal

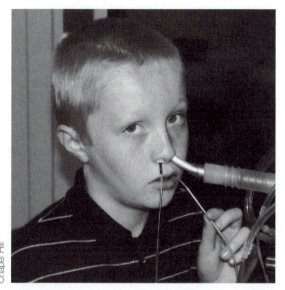

FIGURE 13–3 The pressure-flow technique to estimate velopharyngeal orifice areas during speech production. A flow tube is placed in the nose, and pressure catheters are placed in the mouth and nostril.

orifice size during consonant production. Aerodynamic methods can be used to provide information on the timing aspects of velopharyngeal function during certain phonetic contexts and the patency of the nasal airway during breathing (Smith & Kuehn, 2007; Zajac & Mayo, 1996). This information can be used as a basis for making diagnostic decisions that impact the recommendations for treatment of VPI. Aerodynamic instrumentation can also provide evidence of airway obstruction through measurements of nasal airway resistance.

Although aerodynamic instrumentation is used in some clinics, it is not widely used at this time. Only 4.3% of respondents to the 2009 survey reported using it clinically (Kummer et al., 2012). Perhaps this is because it is technically complex and is typically limited to stop-plosive sounds, especially bilabials, due to practical constraints on placement of the oral pressure-sensing tube. However, pressure-flow measures can be useful in research (Karnell, 2011).

DIRECT MEASURES

Direct instrumental procedures (videofluoroscopy and nasopharyngoscopy) allow the examiner to visualize aspects of the velopharyngeal valve during speech. These procedures allow the examiner to look for the cause of velopharyngeal dysfunction and also to determine the location of a velopharyngeal gap. This information is important for surgical planning.

Through direct procedures, the examiner can view both the anatomy of the velopharyngeal structures and the physiology during function (e.g., speech and swallowing). The examiner can also directly observe defects that cause VPI. Because there is a wide spectrum of anatomic and physiologic causes for VPI, this information is important to obtain so that the appropriate and most effective treatment can be determined. Finally, direct procedures can be helpful in assessing the placement of a prosthetic device or evaluating the results of surgical procedures for correction of VPI (e.g., pharyngeal flap, sphincter pharyngoplasty, etc.). (See Chapter 18 for additional information about surgical procedures.)

Videofluoroscopy was the gold standard for evaluation of velopharyngeal function in the 1970s. In the 1980s, flexible nasopharyngoscopy became an option. In the same survey noted above, more respondents reported using nasopharyngoscopy routinely (59.3%) than videofluoroscopy (19.2%) (Kummer et al., 2012). For a comparison of advantages of each direct procedure, see Table 13–2.

Although the structures and function of the velopharyngeal valve can be seen through these measures, the evaluation of what is seen is still subjective and open to examiner judgment and interpretation. Therefore, the usefulness of these procedures depends greatly on the experience of the examiner(s).

TABLE 13–2   Videofluoroscopy (VF) versus Nasopharyngoscopy (NP). Yes (+), No (–)

Advantages	VF	NP
Can see tongue movement during speech	+	–
Can see the entire posterior pharyngeal wall during speech	+	–
Can see the point on the posterior pharyngeal wall of VP contact*	+	–
Has the best resolution and is in natural color	–	+
Can see morphology of the nasal surface of the velum and identify an occult submucous cleft	–	+
Can see entire adenoid, including irregularities in the surface that can affect the velopharyngeal seal	–	+
Can see pulsations of medially displaced carotid arteries in patients with velocardiofacial syndrome	–	+
Can see tonsils intruding into the pharynx, which can affect resonance and VP function	–	+
Can view the vocal folds and determine the presence of vocal nodules	–	+
Can see most of the valve at once, including the lateral walls moving against the velum	–	+
Can see even very small VP gaps	–	+
Can determine the pattern of closure and the exact location of the opening which is important for surgical planning		+
Can see ports after a pharyngeal flap or sphincter pharyngoplasty		+
Does not require radiation and injection of barium (which is noxious) in the nasopharynx	–	+
Parent can hold the child in his or her lap during the procedure	–	+
Can give the parents the results and recommendations immediately after the procedure	–	+
Can be used for speech biofeedback	–	+

*Some surgeons want this information to know where to position a flap or sphincter in the pharynx. Others argue that you should just place it as high in the pharynx as possible so that this view is not needed.
© Cengage Learning 2014

Videofluoroscopy

Videofluoroscopy is a radiological technique used to obtain real-time moving images of internal structures. This is done through the use of a fluoroscope, which consists of an X-ray source and fluorescent screen. A *videofluoroscopic speech study* provides visualization of the velopharyngeal valve during speech, along with simultaneous audio recording. Therefore, this procedure is useful in the evaluation of velopharyngeal dysfunction (Dudas, Deleyiannis, Ford, Jiang, & Losee, 2006) (Figures 13–4, 13–5, 13–6, and 13–7). Videofluoroscopy is also used to assess swallowing and is called either a *modified barium swallow (MBS)* or a *video-fluoroscopic swallowing study*. Videofluoroscopy requires fluoroscopy equipment and a video capture system. This is usually available in radiology departments.

Because videofluoroscopy involves two-dimensional imaging, a videofluoroscopic speech study requires several views in order to see all aspects of the velopharyngeal port (Dudas, et al., 2006; Lam, Starr, Perkins, Lewis, Eblen, Dunlap, & Sie, 2006; Smith & Kuehn, 2007; Ysunza, Pamplona, & Morales, 2011; Ysunza, Pamplona, Ortega, & Prado, 2008). On the lateral (sagittal) view, where the beam goes through the side of the head from ear to ear, the examiner can see the occlusion of the jaws, the hard palate, tongue, velum,

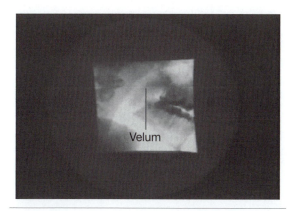

FIGURE 13–4 Lateral view showing a short velum relative to the posterior pharyngeal wall, which results in velopharyngeal insufficiency.
Courtesy Ann W. Kummer, Ph.D./Cincinnati Children's Hospital Medical Center & University of Cincinnati College of Medicine

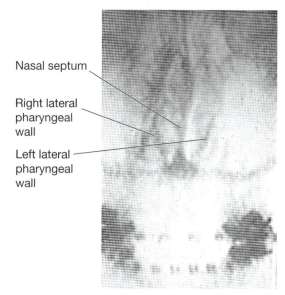

FIGURE 13–6 Frontal view showing the nasal septum in midline. The lateral pharyngeal walls are well coated with barium and bow outward during nasal breathing, as noted in the frame.
Courtesy Ann W. Kummer, Ph.D./Cincinnati Children's Hospital Medical Center & University of Cincinnati College of Medicine

posterior pharyngeal wall, adenoids, and larynx. During speech, the movement of the tongue can also be observed. On the frontal view, also called the anterior–posterior (AP) view because the beam goes from the front of the face to the back, the examiner can see the septum and lateral pharyngeal walls. Finally, on the base view, where the beam goes from under the chin up through the port, the examiner can see the

outline of the lateral and posterior pharyngeal walls, and to some extent the velum. There are

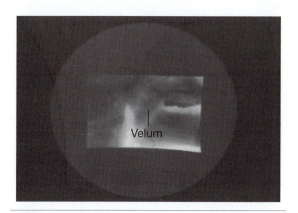

FIGURE 13–5 Lateral view showing a velum of normal length but poor movement during speech, which results in velopharyngeal incompetence.
Courtesy Ann W. Kummer, Ph.D./Cincinnati Children's Hospital Medical Center & University of Cincinnati College of Medicine

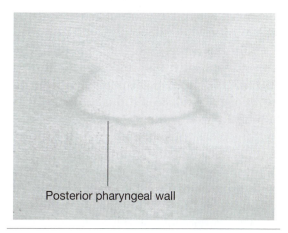

FIGURE 13–7 Base view with the posterior pharyngeal wall at the bottom of the screen. The open port can be clearly seen.
Courtesy Ann W. Kummer, Ph.D./Cincinnati Children's Hospital Medical Center & University of Cincinnati College of Medicine

other supplementary views that can be used as needed. To obtain an impression of the function of the entire velopharyngeal valve, all views must be considered together. To be able to see the pharyngeal walls, a coating of barium is usually required. This is usually introduced into the pharynx by a rubber catheter that goes through the nose.

Videofluoroscopy for speech is done in a radiology department by a radiologist and/or a radiology technician. However, these studies should always be interpreted by both a radiologist and a speech-language pathologist.

Nasopharyngoscopy

Nasopharyngoscopy (also called *nasendoscopy* or *videonasendoscopy*) is a minimally invasive nasal endoscopic procedure that allows direct visual observation and analysis of the velopharyngeal mechanism during speech (Karnell, 2011; Ramamurthy, Wyatt, Whitby, Martin, & Davenport, 1997; Shetty, Frampton, & Patel, 2009; Smith & Kuehn, 2007; Strauss, 2007). The required equipment includes a flexible fiberoptic nasopharyngoscope and a cold light source. It is preferable to also have a monitor and recording system.

With this procedure, the nasopharyngoscope is inserted into the nose and then directed back to the pharynx where the tip "periscopes" down to see the nasopharyngeal structures from above (Figure 13–8). Nasopharyngoscopy allows the examiner to view the nasal surface of the velum (Figure 13–9). Various other nasopharyngeal structures can be viewed, including the nasal cavity and turbinates, the posterior choana an each side, the nasal surface of the velum, the velopharyngeal valve, the Eustachian tube orifices, the nasopharynx, adenoids, base of the tongue, pharyngeal and lingual tonsils, vallecula and pyriform spaces, epiglottis, glottis, and vocal

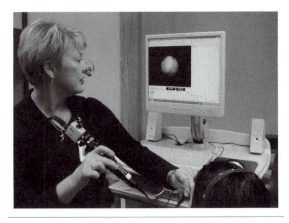

FIGURE 13–8 The nasopharyngoscopy procedure with the patient positioned to see the monitor.
Courtesy of Kay PENTAX/Montvale, NJ and Ann W. Kummer, Ph.D./ Cincinnati Children's Hospital Medical Center & University of Cincinnati College of Medicine

folds. Nasopharyngoscopy is used to assess the results of surgery for velopharyngeal insufficiency/incompetence (e.g., pharyngeal flap or sphincter pharyngoplasty). Nasopharyngoscopy

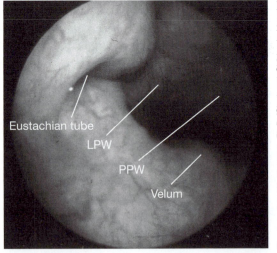

Courtesy Ann W. Kummer, Ph.D./Cincinnati Children's Hospital Medical Center & University of Cincinnati College of Medicine

FIGURE 13–9 A nasopharyngoscopy view of normal velopharyngeal structures. The nasal surface of the velum is always at the bottom of the screen, and the posterior pharyngeal wall is always at the top of the screen. The opening to the Eustachian tube can be seen on the left side of the view.

is not only a powerful tool in the evaluation of velopharyngeal function, but it is also commonly used in the evaluation of swallowing, upper airway obstruction, and the structure and function of the larynx and vocal cords.

Nasopharyngoscopy can be done by a physician. However, it is also in the scope of practice for specially trained speech-language pathologists. Regardless, the recorded study should be reviewed by both the speech-language pathologist and the surgeon to determine the appropriate course of treatment.

Speech Sample for Videofluoroscopy/ Nasopharyngoscopy

With either videofluoroscopy or nasopharyngoscopy, the composition of the speech sample used with the patient is very important. This is because if the speech sample does not adequately tax the velopharyngeal mechanism, the study may not identify mild or inconsistent VPI. In addition, the speech sample for each patient should be designed to test the patient's specific speech errors based on the observations from the speech assessment.

In general, the speech sample for both videofluoroscopy and nasopharyngoscopy should include a combination of repetition of syllables, counting, and repetition of sentences loaded with pressure-sensitive phonemes.

It is helpful to have the patient repeat certain syllables with pressure-sensitive phonemes and high and low vowels (e.g., /pɑ, pa, pɑ/; /pi, pi, pi/; /ta, ta, tɑ/; /ti, ti, ti/; /kɑ, ka, kɑ/; /ki, ki, ki/; /sɑ, sa, sɑ/; /si, si, si/; etc.). This helps to illustrate phoneme-specific openings that are due to misarticulation. To test the effect of the fistula on the velopharyngeal valve, the examiner should compare velopharyngeal function on repeated velar syllables (e.g., /kɑ/ and /ki/), which would be produced behind the

fistula, and repeated syllables with anterior sounds (e.g., /tɑ/, /ti/, /sɑ/, /si/, /pɑ/, /pi/). Having the individual prolong an /s/ can be informative, as in some cases the velopharyngeal closure that is initially achieved may break down with this task.

Having the patient count from 60 to 70 or repeat "60, 60, 60, 60" is particularly helpful because the combination of plosives, the sibilant /s/, a high vowel (/i/), and even a triple blend (/kst/) is particularly taxing on the velopharyngeal mechanism (Kummer, 2011).

The examiner should have the patient repeat some sentences loaded with pressure-sensitive consonants (see Table 11–3). Because the /s/ sound is most often affected by VPI, the sample should include at least one sentence with a frequent occurrence of this sound. The sentence "Sissy sees the sun in the sky" is particularly good because it not only contains many /s/ sounds, but it also contains an /s/ blend and a high vowel (/i/), which further challenge the velopharyngeal mechanism. In addition, this sentence has some nasal sounds in the middle, so the velum has to go up and down for the sentence.

If apraxia of speech is suspected as a cause of velopharyngeal dysfunction, having the child repeat multisyllabic words with a combination of placement points can be helpful (e.g., "baseball bat," "kitty cat," "puppy dog," "teddy bear," "patty cake," "basketball," "ice cream cone," etc.) (Kummer, 2011).

Reporting the Results of Videofluoroscopy/ Nasopharyngoscopy

Some centers report results of nasopharyngoscopy and videofluoroscopy with a purely narrative report. Others use a numeric scale or a checklist format to rate various parameters of structure and function. In 1990, a multidisciplinary group proposed a system for reporting direct observations of the movement of the velopharyngeal structures from their resting position to the opposing structure, using a ratio scale (Golding-Kushner et al., 1990). It is not known how often this scale is used today. Regardless of the method used, what is most important is that there is consistency in the observations that are made in each study and in the way that the studies are reported. Fortunately, precise measurements are not necessary for determination of treatment. Instead, documentation of the size, location, and cause of the opening are what is most important (Karnell, 2011).

Although the results are used to make treatment recommendations and also to report to other professionals, they should also be shared with the family. It is important that the person who counsels the family uses clear, easy-to-understand language. After the initial explanation, it may also be helpful to play the videotape of the procedure and point out the structures and their function. All medical terms should be clearly defined. When discussing the function of the velopharyngeal mechanism, supplementary pictures and diagrams should be used.

Magnetic Resonance Imaging (MRI)

Magnetic resonance imaging (MRI) is a non-invasive method to produce a very clear and detailed view of internal body structures, using a magnetic field and radio waves. It has only recently been used to evaluate the structures of the velopharyngeal valve. MRI can provide high-resolution images of the soft tissues of the velopharyngeal sphincter in all planes. Therefore, MRI has been used successfully for the evaluation of obstructive sleep apnea in pediatric patients (Barrera, Holbrook, Santos, &

Popelka, 2009; Donnelly, Shott, LaRose, Chini, & Amin, 2004; Zhang, Ma, Li, Wang, & Wang, 2011). It has also proved to be an effective method of imaging and examining the morphology of the levator veli palatini muscle and related structures (Perry, Kuehn, Sutton, Goldwasser, & Jerez, 2010) or for diagnosing an occult submucous cleft palate (Kuehn, Ettema, Goldwasser, Barkmeier, & Wachtel, 2001).

Some authors have suggested the use of MRI as a means for evaluating velopharyngeal function in addition to velopharyngeal structure (Atik et al. 2008; Drissi et al. 2011). However, a primary disadvantage of MRI is the static nature of the imaging. To view velopharyngeal closure, an image is typically taken during production of a vowel or sustained /s/. Therefore, movement of the structures during speech cannot be appreciated. In addition, MRI only shows a two-dimensional view, although the use of serial images and computer modeling to obtain 3D images has been suggested (Serrurier, 2008). Other disadvantages include noise in the scanner, the potential for claustrophobia during the exam, and current expense. Because of these disadvantages, MRI is not currently a standard procedure for clinical evaluation of velopharyngeal function. However, it is providing information that is very valuable for research.

SUMMARY

The best way to evaluate resonance disorders and velopharyngeal dysfunction is an experienced examiner's ear. Despite that, instrumental procedures can provide very valuable additional information to augment the perceptual evaluation results. Indirect procedures (e.g., aerodynamic instrumentation and nasometry) provide objective data relative to the function of the velopharyngeal valve. Objective data allow for better comparison of treatment results between professionals and centers. Direct procedures (e.g., videofluoroscopy and nasopharyngoscopy) provide visual information about the structures and function of the velopharyngeal valve. This information is important for finding the cause of the velopharyngeal dysfunction and the location of the velopharyngeal gap.

Because instrumentation is expensive and it requires specialty training for use, these procedures are usually done in a medical center, particularly one that has a craniofacial program. There are low-tech instruments (including a straw) that can be used effectively in other clinical settings (see Chapter 11).

For Review and Discussion

1. If the perceptual assessment is sufficient in diagnosing VPI, what are the reasons for using instrumentation?

2. What is the difference between direct measures and indirect measures? What are the advantages of each type of measure? What are the disadvantages?

3. What are the primary advantages of nasopharyngoscopy over videofluoroscopy?

What are the primary advantages of videofluoroscopy over nasopharyngoscopy?

4. What would be the advantages and disadvantages of using MRI for a clinical assessment?

5. What type of speech sample could you use with each type of instrumentation?

6. Why is instrumentation typically available only in certain specialty centers?

References

Atik, B., Bekerecioglu, M., Tan, O., Etlik, O., Davran, R., & Arslan, H. (2008). Evaluation of dynamic magnetic resonance imaging in assessing velopharyngeal insufficiency during phonation. *Journal of Craniofacial Surgery*, *19*(3), 566–572.

Barrera, J. E., Holbrook, A. B., Santos, J., & Popelka, G. R. (2009). Sleep MRI: Novel technique to identify airway obstruction in obstructive sleep apnea. *Otolaryngology—Head and Neck Surgery*, *140*(3), 423–425.

Donnelly, L. F., Shott, S. R., LaRose, C. R., Chini, B. A., & Amin, R. S. (2004). Causes of persistent obstructive sleep apnea despite previous tonsillectomy and adenoidectomy in children with down syndrome as depicted on static and dynamic cine MRI. *American Journal of Roentgenology*, *183*(1), 175–181.

Drissi, C., Mitrofanoff, M., Talandier, C., Falip, C., Le Couls, V., & Adamsbaum, C. (2011). Feasibility of dynamic MRI for evaluating velopharyngeal insufficiency in children. *European Radiology*, *21*(7), 1462–1469.

Dudas, J. R., Deleyiannis, F. W., Ford, M. D., Jiang, S., & Losee, J. E. (2006). Diagnosis and treatment of velopharyngeal insufficiency: Clinical utility of speech evaluation and videofluoroscopy. *Annuals of Plastic Surgery*, *56*(5), 511–517; Discussion 517.

Golding-Kushner, K. J., Argamaso, R. V., Cotton, R. T., Grames, L. M., Henningsson, G., Jones, D. L., et al. (1990). Standardization for the reporting of nasopharyngoscopy and multiview videofluoroscopy: a report from an International Working Group. *Cleft Palate Journal*, 27(4), 337–347; Discussion 347–348.

Hinton, V. A. (2009). Instrumental measures of velopharyngeal function. In J. E. Lossee & R. E. Kirschner (Eds.), *Comprehensive Cleft Care* (pp. 607–617). New York: McGraw-Hill.

Karnell, M. P. (2011). Instrumental assessment of velopharyngeal closure for speech. *Seminars in Speech and Language*, 32(2), 168–178.

Kuehn, D. P., Ettema, S. L., Goldwasser, M. S., Barkmeier, J. C., & Wachtel, J. M. (2001). Magnetic resonance imaging in the evaluation of occult submucous cleft palate. *Cleft Palate–Craniofacial Journal*, 38(5), 421–431.

Kummer, A. W. (2011). Perceptual assessment of resonance and velopharyngeal function. *Seminars in Speech and Language*, 32(2), 159–167.

Kummer, A. W., Clark, S. L., Redle, E. E., Thomsen, L. L., & Billmire, D. A. (2012). Current practice in assessing and reporting speech outcomes of cleft palate and velopharyngeal surgery: a survey of cleft palate/craniofacial professionals. *Cleft Palate–Craniofacial Journal*, 49(2), 146–152.

Lam, D. J., Starr, J. R., Perkins, J. A., Lewis, C. W., Eblen, L. E., Dunlap, J., & Sie, K. C. (2006). A comparison of nasendoscopy and multiview videofluoroscopy in assessing velopharyngeal insufficiency. *Otolaryngology-Head and Neck Surgery*, 134(3), 394–402.

Perry, J., Kuehn, D., Sutton, B., Goldwasser, M., & Jerez, A. (2010, Feb. 17). MRI and 3D computer modeling of the levator veli palatini muscle before and after primary palatoplasty. *Cleft Palate–Craniofacial Journal*. Epub ahead of print.

Ramamurthy, L., Wyatt, R. A., Whitby, D., Martin, D., & Davenport, P. (1997). The evaluation of velopharyngeal function using flexible nasendoscopy. *Journal of Laryngology & Otology*, 111(8), 739–745.

Serrurier, A., & Badin, P. (2008). A three-dimensional articulatory model of the velum and nasopharyngeal wall based on MRI and CT data. *Journal of the Acoustic Society of America*, 123(4), 2335–2355.

Shetty, S., Frampton, S., & Patel, N. (2009). Flexible nasendoscopy. *Clinical Otolaryngology*, 34(2), 169–171.

Smith, B. E., & Kuehn, D. P. (2007). Speech evaluation of velopharyngeal dysfunction. *Journal of Craniofacial Surgery*, 18(2), 251–261; Quiz 266–257.

Strauss, R. A. (2007). Flexible endoscopic nasopharyngoscopy. *Atlas of the Oral and Maxillofacial Surgery Clinics of North America*, 15(2), 111–128.

Sweeney, T., & Sell, D. (2008). Relationship between perceptual ratings of nasality and nasometry in children/adolescents with cleft palate and/or velopharyngeal dysfunction. *International Journal of Language & Communication Disorders*, 43(3), 265–282.

Ysunza, A., Carmen Pamplona, M., & Santiago Morales, M. A. (2011). Velopharyngeal valving during speech, in patients with velocardiofacial syndrome and patients with non-syndromic palatal clefts after surgical and speech pathology management. *International Journal of Pediatric Otorhinolaryngology*, 75(10), 1255–1259.

Ysunza, A., Pamplona, M. C., Ortega, J. M., & Prado, H. (2008). Video fluoroscopy for evaluating adenoid hypertrophy in children. *International Journal of Pediatric Otorhinolaryngology*, 72(8), 1159–1165.

Zajac, D. J., & Mayo, R. (1996). Aerodynamic and temporal aspects of velopharyngeal function in normal speakers. *Journal of Speech, Language and Hearing Research*, 39(6), 1199–1207.

Zhang, X., Ma, L., Li, S., Wang, Y., & Wang, L. (2011). A functional MRI evaluation of frontal dysfunction in patients with severe obstructive sleep apnea. *Sleep Medicine*, 12(4), 335–340.

C H A P T E R

14

NASOMETRY

CHAPTER OUTLINE

INTRODUCTION

Nasometry is a method of measuring the acoustic correlates of resonance and velopharyngeal function through a computer-based instrument. Nasometry testing gives the examiner a *nasalance score*, which is the percentage of nasal acoustic energy of the total (nasal plus oral) energy. Because nasometry does not include visualization of the velopharyngeal structures, it is considered an *indirect measure*. The advantage of the nasometry is that it provides objective data that can be compared to standardized norms for interpretation. Nasometry is useful in the evaluation of resonance because it supplements what is heard through the perceptual evaluation and what is seen through direct instrumental measures (Sweeney & Sell, 2008). It can also be a valuable treatment tool because it provides visual feedback for the patient. Finally, it can be used effectively for pre- and post-treatment comparisons.

The purpose of this chapter is to describe nasometry and its use in the evaluation and treatment of individuals with resonance disorders.

NASOMETRY AND ITS CLINICAL USES

Nasometry was developed as a means to quantify the acoustic correlates of velopharyngeal function during speech. Nasometry supplements the perceptual assessment of resonance, which by its nature, is subjective.

Development of Nasometry

The first instrument to measure nasal and oral acoustic energy was developed by Samuel Fletcher in 1970. This instrument was called TONAR, which is an acronym for The Oral-Nasal Acoustic Ratio (Fletcher & Bishop, 1970). The TONAR was later updated, revised, and then renamed the TONAR II (Fletcher, 1976a; Fletcher, 1976b). Although the TONAR instruments provided objective data regarding the acoustic product of speech, the data acquisition was somewhat unreliable (Dalston, 1997). Samuel Fletcher, along with colleagues

Larry Adams and Martin McCutcheon at the University of Alabama, Birmingham, developed the Nasometer based on Fletcher's early work. It was then introduced by Kay Elemetrics Corp. in 1986 (Fletcher, 1970; Fletcher, Adams, & McCutcheon, 1989).

In 2002, a second version of the Nasometer was released as Nasomete™ II, Model 6400 (KayPENTAX, n.d.[b]). Although the Nasometer II is fundamentally the same as the original version, it captures data through analog and digital circuitry, rather than just analog circuitry. Additionally, Nasometer II captures the speech signal, which can be played back.

The latest hardware/software version is the Nasometer™ II, Model 6450. With this version, there is a built-in sound chip installed in the hardware. The hardware connects to the host computer via a USB interface. This design allows the Nasometer II to be used with laptops as well as desktop computers.

Two other instruments have been developed to measure nasalance: the NasalView

(Tiger Electronics, Seattle, Wash.) and the OroNasal System (Glottal Enterprises, Syracuse, N.Y.). These instruments are not as widely used, perhaps because there are no published normative studies for their use. In addition, it has been shown that there are significant differences in the nasalance scores of these instruments, so norms established for the Nasometer cannot be used with them (Bressmann, 2005; Lewis & Watterson, 2003). Because of these findings and the fact that the Nasometer is widely used internationally, the remainder of this chapter focuses on nasometry using Nasometer II, Model 6450 (Kay-PENTAX, n.d.[b]).

What Is a Nasometer?

A *Nasometer* is a computer-assisted instrument that measures the relative amount of nasal acoustic energy in an individual's speech. The Nasometer provides an easy, noninvasive method for obtaining objective data regarding resonance during speech by analyzing the acoustic energy from both the oral and nasal cavities in real time. As such, it can be a valuable tool in both the evaluation of resonance disorders and in treatment of functional resonance problems.

The Nasometer provides data of the relative amount of nasal resonance in speech for a passage. This is done by capturing data regarding acoustic energy in both the nasal (N) cavity and the oral (O) cavity during speech and in real time. The Nasometer software then calculates the average ratio of nasal over total (nasal plus oral) acoustic energy. This ratio is converted to a percentage value called the *nasalance score*. The nasalance score can be depicted, therefore, as follows:

$$\text{Nasalance} = N \div (N + O) \times 100.$$

When an individual's score is compared to normative data, a judgment can be made regarding the normalcy of resonance. High scores, in comparison to normative data, suggest hypernasality; low scores, in comparison, suggest hyponasality.

Purpose and Clinical Uses

Since its introduction, the Nasometer has been a useful tool in the evaluation of resonance and velopharyngeal function of patients with a history of cleft palate (Dalston, 1991b; Dalston, 1991c; Dalston, 1997; Hardin, Van Demark, Morris, & Payne, 1992; Karnell, 1995; Karnell, 2011; van der Heijden, Hobbel, van der Laan, Korsten-Meijer, & Goorhuis-Brouwer, 2011). It has even been used to evaluate and treat resonance of children with hearing impairment (Hassan et al., 2011; Tatchell, Stewart, & Lapine, 1991). Nasometry is used to assess upper airway obstruction and hyponasality through their acoustic correlates during speech (Dalston et al., 1991a; Dalston et al., 1991b; Hardin et al., 1992; Hong, Kwon, & Jung, 1997; Nieminen, Lopponen, Vayrynen, Tervonen, & Tolonen, 2000; Parker, Clarke, Dawes, & Maw, 1990). It has even been suggested as a means of selecting at-risk individuals for adenoidectomy (Kummer, Myer, Smith, & Shott, 1993; Parker, Maw, & Szallasi, 1989; Williams, Eccles, & Hutchings, 1990; Williams, Preece, Rhys, & Eccles, 1992).

Very often, nasometry is used to measure changes in resonance following surgical procedures (Dejonckere & van Wijngaarden, 2001; Eckardt, Teltzrow, Schulze, Hoppe, & Kuettner, 2007; Mueller, Neuber, Schelhorn-Niese, & Schumann, 2007; Soneghet et al., 2002; Van Lierde, De Bodt, Baetens, Schrauwen, & Van Cauwenberge, 2003; Van Lierde, Monstrey, Bonte, Van Cauwenberge, & Vinck, 2004). It is also used to show the effects of various forms of treatment, including CPAP (Sweeney, Sell, & O'Regan, 2004), prosthetic management

(Rieger, Wolfaardt, Seikaly, & Jha, 2002), and speech therapy. Finally, nasometry can be used as part of singing pedagogy.

EQUIPMENT

The Nasometer requires a host computer, specialized software, an external module, a headset, and a means for calibration. These components are described here.

Hardware and Software

The Nasometer II requires the use of a host computer and specialized software. The system components include a Nasometer II external module (Figure 14–1) and either a Nasometer Headset (Figure 14–2A) or a Hand-Held Separator (Figure 14–2B), each of which has

two directional microphones on either side of a sound separator plate. The equipment connection and software installation instructions can be found in the *Nasometer II, Model 6450 Installation, Operations and Maintenance Manual* (KayPENTAX, [a]).

Calibration

Prior to its first use and at periodic intervals, the Nasometer should be calibrated according to the manufacturer's instructions. This is necessary to be sure that the data collection and analyses are accurate. The Nasometer comes with a calibration stand. The sound separator plate is placed in the calibration stand located on the top of the Nasometer II external hardware module. The provided calibration slot ensures that both microphones are equidistant from the calibration speaker (approximately 6 inches

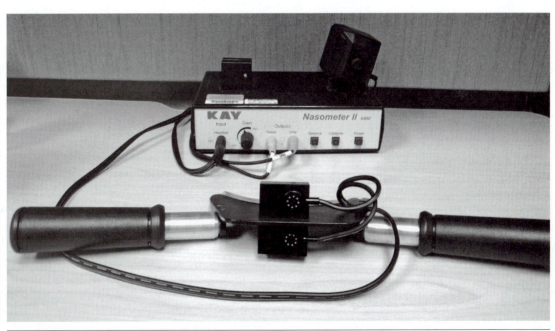

FIGURE 14–1 Basic Nasometer equipment. The Nasometer requires the use of an IBM-compatible or Apple computer, a Nasometer box, which is connected by a cable to an interface printed circuit board in the computer, and a Nasometer Headset or Hand-Held Separator that is used for data collection. Nasometer software is installed on the computer's hard drive.

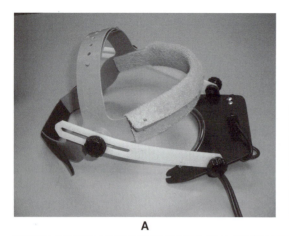
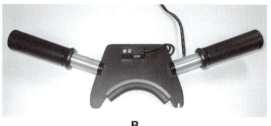

A **B**

FIGURE 14–2 (A and B)   (A) The Nasometer II Headset. (B) The Nasometer II Hand-Held Separator.
Courtesy of Kay PENTAX/Montvale, NJ and Ann W. Kummer, Ph.D./Cincinnati Children's Hospital Medical Center & University of Cincinnati College of Medicine

[15 cm]) (Figure 14–3). When a tone from the external module is presented to the microphones, both the nasal and oral microphones register the tone equally. If the two microphones are not balanced so that the tone registers above or below the 50% mark, calibration adjustments are made in the Nasometer II software to balance any detected sensitivity differences between the two microphones.

NASOMETRIC PROCEDURES

For comprehensive information about nasometric procedures, the reader should consult the Nasometer II Manual that comes with the equipment. Although extensive instruction regarding nasometry procedures is beyond the scope of this text, some basic information is important to cover.

Placing the Headset/Hand-Held Separator

Either the Nasometer II Headset or the Hand-Held Separator can be used for data collection. Before use (and also after use), the examiner

should wipe the sound separator plate and plastic guard with a chlorine wipe in order to disinfect and sanitize it. The device is then plugged into the external module.

The Nasometer II Headset is placed on the individual's head and secured using the top adjustment band and the Velcro® strip in the back. When in place, the sound separator plate should fit snugly between the child's upper lip and nose. The microphones should be directly in front of the mouth and the nose, and the plate should be perpendicular to the face (or in a horizontal position). An angle in excess of 15 degrees in either direction can affect the integrity of the data (KayPENTAX, n.d.[a]). Once the plate is in proper position, the top and then the bottom adjustment knobs are tightened to keep the plate in place and add further stability. The plastic tubing along the plate promotes a tight seal while softening the force against the face. The proper placement of the Nasometer II Headset is seen in (Figure 14–4A and B).

Positioning the Nasometer II Headset on young children can be a challenge. Despite the examiner's best efforts, there are times when

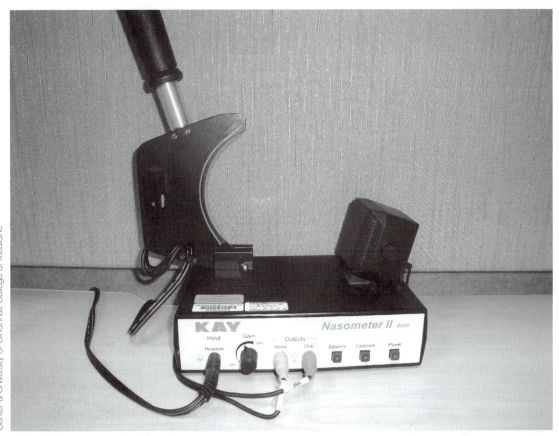

Courtesy of Kay PENTAX/Montvale, NJ and Ann W. Kummer, Ph.D./Cincinnati Children's Hospital Medical Center & University of Cincinnati College of Medicine

FIGURE 14–3 Calibration. During calibration, the separator plate should be placed so that both microphones are equidistant from the Nasometer box and about 12 inches in front of the calibration speaker.

the child simply refuses to put it on. In addition, young children are often not tolerant of keeping it on during the time that the examiner is recording the data in between passages. The Nasometer II Headset has another disadvantage that the headgear must be sanitized between uses.

Because of the challenges in using the Headset and problem with disinfection, many examiners will prefer to use the newer Hand-Held Separator (Figure 14–4C and D). This device has two handles to hold the separator plate in place so there is no need for the headgear. In some cases, the Hand-Held

Separator can be held in place by the child. For young children, however, it is preferable to have the child sit in the parent's lap and then have the parent hold the device in place from behind. The device can be set down in between passages, and it is easier to clean than the original Headset.

Preparing the Child for the Exam

Most young children cooperate very well with Nasometry (van der Heijden et al., 2011). To ensure best cooperation, the child should be told what to expect, even before the day of

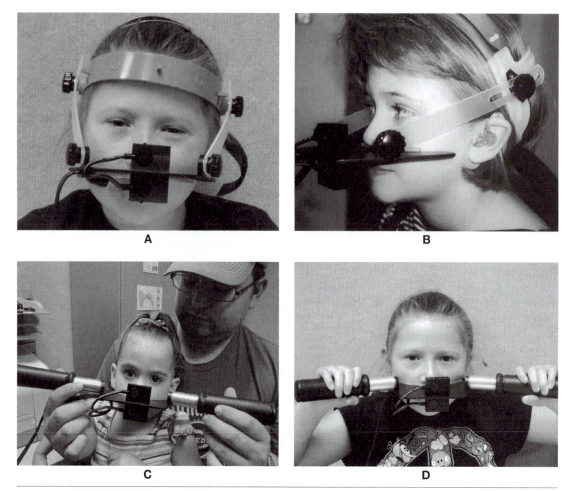

FIGURE 14–4 (A–D)   (A and B) Placement of the Nasometer II Headset on a patient. The sound separator plate should be perpendicular to the face or in a horizontal position. The microphones should be directly in front of the mouth and the nose. (C and D) Placement of the Hand-Held Separator. The separator plate should be placed in the same position as with the Headset.

Courtesy of Kay PENTAX/Montvale, NJ and Ann W. Kummer, Ph.D./Cincinnati Children's Hospital Medical Center & University of Cincinnati College of Medicine

the appointment. This can be done by sending parents information describing the exam and a picture or drawing of the Nasometer. The sentences or speech samples that will be used in the exam should be included so that the child can practice repeating them at home. At Cincinnati Children's Hospital Medical Center, we send the child a coloring book prior to an evaluation. In the book,

one page explains the nasometry procedure (Figure 14–5).

To ease the child's fears and promote cooperation for the evaluation, the examiner should make the procedure as nonthreatening as possible. For example, at Cincinnati Children's we may tell the child that he will be playing a computer game and wearing a "superhero" mask. He will talk to the computer through the

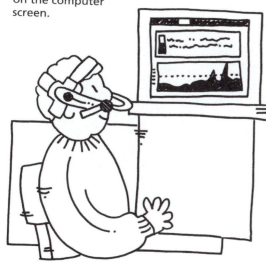

Do you like computer games?

We hope so because the speech pathologist has one for you to play. With this game, you get to wear a super hero mask that fits around your face.

When you talk into microphones on the mask, you will see funny blue lines on the computer screen.

FIGURE 14–5 Page out of a coloring book used to prepare the patient for the examination.

microphones because "computers don't have ears." When the computer can hear him talk, it will make lots of blue "mountains." It helps to have the child feel the plate and the plastic tubing that will come in contact with his face. The examiner can explain that the separator plate will "hug" around his face during data collection. Even if the child is not fully cooperative, a few syllables or short utterances usually result in the collection of data that can be useful.

Data Collection

Once the separator plate is in place, the child is asked to read or repeat standardized speech passages (Figure 14–6). To start data collection, the examiner presses the F12 key, and to stop data collection the examiner presses the space bar. The microphones pick up acoustic energy from the oral cavity and the nasal cavity simultaneously. The sound separator plate provides sufficient separation between the oral and the nasal signals (about 25 dB of separation), but there may be some spillover.

In order to compare the individual's performance with normative data, a standardized speech segment must be used. There are several standardized passages in English that can be displayed on the screen with the Nasometer software.

Normed Passages in English

The first nasometric norms were established for the following three passages: the Zoo Passage (Fletcher, 1972), the Rainbow Passage (Fairbanks, 1960), and Nasal Sentences (Fletcher, 1978). These passages for Nasometer II and their norms (mean scores and standard deviations) can be found in Appendix 14–1.

The Zoo Passage consists of sentences that are devoid of nasal phonemes. Therefore, this passage allows the examiner to determine whether velopharyngeal closure can be achieved and maintained throughout connected speech. Of course, without nasal consonants, this passage does not test the effects of the timing of closure with the transitions between nasal and oral phonemes (Sweeney & Sell, 2008). If there are problems with velopharyngeal timing or movement, this is more likely to be demonstrated with the Rainbow Passage. In this passage, 11.5% of the consonants are nasal consonants, which is representative of the percentage of nasal consonants in normal Standard American English. If hyponasality is suspected, the Nasal Sentences passage is used. In this passage, 35% of the phonemes are nasal consonants, which is more than three times

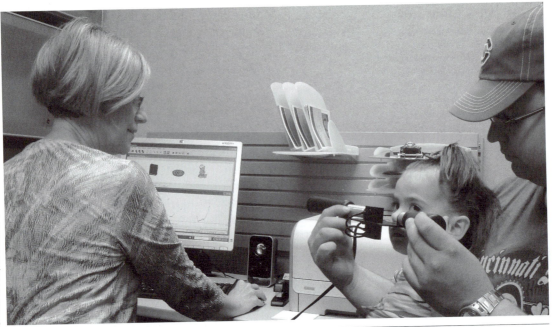

FIGURE 14–6 Nasometer procedure for data collection. The individual is asked to read or repeat certain speech passages for data collection.

as many nasal sounds as would normally occur in Standard American English. This passage allows the examiner to test the individual's ability to open the velopharyngeal port for normal nasal resonance. The results can also provide evidence for nasal obstruction.

Although the original passages are still commonly used, particularly with adults, they have certain disadvantages. They are hard to use with individuals who cannot read, have a limited attention span, or have limited compliance. The Zoo and Rainbow Passages are long and awkward, and some of the sentences are semantically and syntactically complex. Some of the words are difficult to pronounce, especially for children who have incomplete phonological acquisition. This increases the possibility of production errors. When the passage is produced with articulation substitutions or deletions, the nasalance score associated with it loses some validity. A pause with

the use of "um" is particularly problematic. The phonetic heterogeneity of these passages also limits their diagnostic use. It makes it impossible to isolate the effects of phoneme-specific nasal emission, phoneme-specific hypernasality, or a fistula versus the effects of velopharyngeal insufficiency/incompetence (VPI) on the nasalance score because the score is computed based on the average from a variety of consonants and vowels.

In an effort to determine the best and most efficient way to collect nasometric data while avoiding the pitfalls of the original passages, some investigators have found that reliable measures of nasalance can be obtained using much shorter passages (Kummer, 2005; MacKay & Kummer, 1994; Watterson, Lewis, & Foley-Homan, 1999; Wozny, Kuehn, Oishi, & Arthur, 1994). In addition, it has been reported that the clinically relevant information provided in the Rainbow Passage can be obtained using the other speech samples (Dalston & Seaver, 1992), so this passage can be deleted from the test battery in most cases.

Given the limitations of the first three standardized passages, the *Simplified Nasometric Assessment Procedures (SNAP Test)* (Kummer, 2005; MacKay & Kummer, 1994) was developed at Cincinnati Children's Hospital Medical Center for the purpose of providing more appropriate standardized passages for children. It was also designed to enhance the diagnostic value of nasometry by allowing the examiner to determine nasalance on specific phonemes, thus avoiding the problem of phonetic heterogeneity. Normative data was first obtained using the Nasometer I Model 6200. With the introduction of Nasometer II, another normative study was conducted, and the test form was revised. The SNAP Test-R (Kummer, 2005) with normative data for Nasometer II can be found in Appendix 14–2.

The SNAP Test-R consists of a battery of passages divided into three subtests. Any or all of these subtests can be used by the examiner, but they are usually selected based on the age of the child; the anticipated level of cooperation; the child's level of literacy; and, most importantly, on the specific characteristics or etiologies that need to be evaluated.

Subtest I, the *Syllable Repetition/Prolonged Sounds Subtest*, includes 14 consonant-vowel (CV) syllables of pressure-sensitive consonants (plosives and fricatives) and nasal sounds (/m/ and /n/) combined with either the low vowel /ɑ/ (as in "father") or the high vowel /i/ (as in "tea"). Subtest I also includes two prolonged vowels /ɑ/ and /i/, and two prolonged consonants /s/ and /m/. To administer the syllables part of this subtest, the individual is asked to repeat the syllables at a normal rate until the screen is full of relatively even peaks. Approximately six to eight syllables should be produced during the 2-second period. The prolonged sounds should be produced until the screen is full.

The oral consonants of this subtest are used to evaluate velopharyngeal function. An abnormally high score on these passages suggests VPI with hypernasality and/or nasal emission. The nasal phonemes subtest is used to evaluate the patency of the nasopharynx and nasal cavity for normal nasal resonance. An abnormally low score on these passages suggests a nasopharyngeal blockage and hyponasality. The nasal syllables or another nasal passage should always be used following surgery to correct VPI (e.g., pharyngeal flap or sphincter pharyngoplasty) because these procedures have the potential side effect of upper airway obstruction.

There are several advantages of Subtest I. Most importantly, it has better diagnostic value than longer passages that contain a mixture of consonants and vowel types. With a single consonant and single vowel per passage, it is easier for the examiner to determine the effects of type of phoneme on velopharyngeal function. For example, the examiner can identify phoneme-specific nasal emission by comparing the relative nasalance on sibilant phonemes (particularly /s/) versus plosives sounds. The examiner may determine that there is abnormally high nasalance on high vowels as compared to low vowels, suggesting either a high tongue position or a thin velum as possible causes. Finally, higher nasalance scores on anterior sounds (/tɑ/ or /sɑ/) versus posterior sounds (/kɑ/) suggest that there is a fistula that is symptomatic for speech.

In addition to isolating phonemes for an in-depth analysis, Subtest I is particularly appropriate for children who have a short attention span, poor cooperation, or a limited phonemic repertoire. For example, if the child cannot produce velar sounds (/k/, /g/) then the velar passage would not be used.

Subtest II, the *Picture-Cued Subtest*, contains passages that are essentially phonetically homogeneous. For each passage, one carrier phrase (e.g., "Pick up the …") is used with three pictures to complete three sentences (e.g., "Pick up the book." "Pick up the pie." "Pick up the baby.") In this subtest, there is a passage that focuses on each of the following: bilabial plosives, lingual-alveolar plosives, velar plosives, sibilant fricatives, and nasals.

To administer this subtest, the examiner should model the three sentences of the passage for the child and then ask the child to say the sentences with the pictures used as cues. The examiner may use the images displayed on the computer screen (Figure 14–7A–D). The sentences alone could also be printed and used for older patients (including adults) who are able to read. Ideally, the individual should say the set of three sentences twice so that there are a total of six sentences produced for each passage.

The advantage of Subtest II is that it allows the examiner to elicit a form of connected speech, yet each passage is loaded with similar consonants, thus enhancing its diagnostic value. The same carrier phrase is used for each set in order to increase the subtest's simplicity while reducing the chance of production errors.

Subtest III, the *Paragraph Subtest*, consists of two short, easy-to-read passages (Figure 14–8A and B). These passages can be either read or repeated after the examiner. The first passage contains primarily plosive phonemes, whereas the second passage is loaded with phonemes. The examiner can select either or both passages, depending on the articulation ability of the individual and the diagnostic goals of the examiner. These passages are more phonetically heterogeneous than the other two subtests and include some nasals but are still more homogeneous than the Zoo and Rainbow passages.

Normative Studies for Other Languages

Normative data for Nasometer I and Nasometer II has been gathered from thousands of normal English-speaking speakers using standardized passages (e.g., Zoo, Rainbow, Nasal Sentences, and passages from the SNAP Test-R). Similarly, passages with normative data have also been developed and normed in other English dialects and many other languages around the world.

Some authors suggest that nasalance scores can vary with language (Anderson, 1996; Leeper, Rochet, & MacKay, 1992; Nichols, 1999; Santos-Terron, Gonzalez-Landa, & Sanchez-Ruiz, 1990; van Doorn & Purcell, 1998). This may be true, depending on the balance of high vowels versus low vowels in the language. However, the nasalance score for a passage is dependent on its particular phonemic composition, regardless of the language. Passages with more high vowels have higher average nasalance scores in comparison to passages with more low vowels, regardless of language (Awan, Omlor, & Watts, 2011; Kummer, 2005; Lewis, Watterson, & Blanton, 2008; Mandulak & Zajac, 2009). Therefore, different passages in the same language will have different normative nasalance scores. The relative nasalance between languages cannot be directly compared unless the passages have the same high vowel/low vowel composition.

Some normative studies have suggested that nasalance scores vary with dialect when the same passage is used (Leeper et al., 1992; Seaver, Dalston, Leeper, & Adams, 1991), and even with racial group or culture (Mayo, Floyd, Warren, Dalston, & Mayo, 1996). Because consonants are produced essentially the same, regardless of dialect, these differences must be in the production of the vowels. Nasalized vowels are presumably the cause of a *nasal*

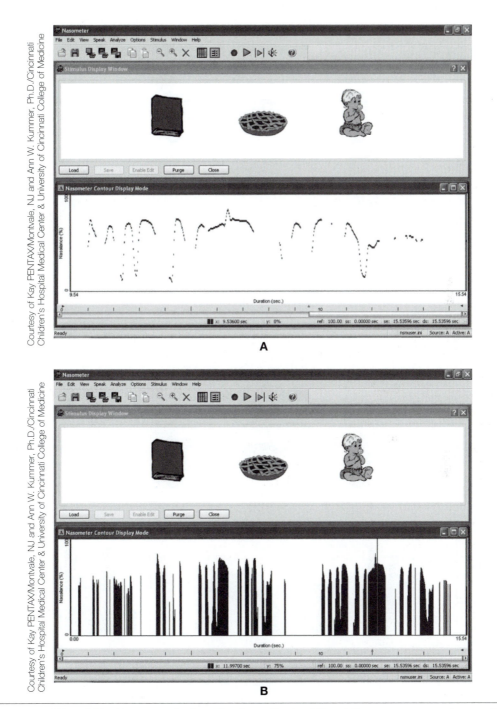

A

B

FIGURE 14–7 (A and B) Nasometer displays after data collection. The nasalance percentage points are displayed on the computer screen in real time as the individual is speaking. For normal speech and the production of only oral sounds, the data points are usually between the 10 to 20 percentage points above the baseline. (A) A contour display of data from the Bilabials Passage of the SNAP Test. The pictures are displayed on the screen. (B) A filled contour display of the same data.

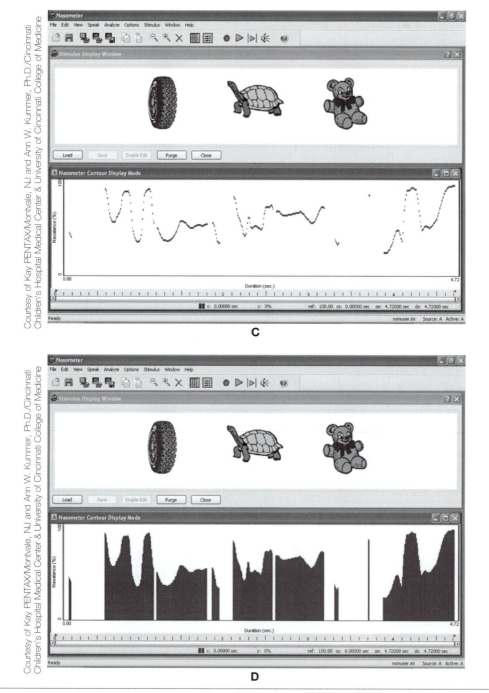

FIGURE 14–7 (C and D) (C) A contour display of data from the Lingual-Alveolars Passage of the SNAP Test. (The pictures are displayed on the screen.) (D) A filled contour display of the same data.

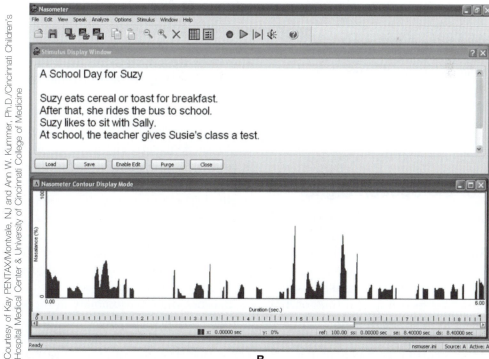

FIGURE 14–8 (A and B) (A) A contour display of data from the Paragraph Subtest of the SNAP Test. (B) A filled contour display of the same data.

twang, which is exaggerated nasality as noted in some dialects (perhaps the southern dialect in American English, because this dialect seems to use more high vowels than other English dialects). It might be assumed that dialects, accents, or even languages that use more high vowels or a higher tongue position might be expected to have slightly higher nasalance scores as compared to those with a greater incidence of low vowels or a lower tongue position (Lewis & Watterson, 2003). There may also be a difference in dialects between the timing of closure when transitions are made between nasal consonants and vowels (Mayo et al., 1996).

With the introduction of the Nasometer II, normative studies were repeated. These studies found slight differences that are not clinically significant between the two versions (Kummer, 2005; Watterson, Lewis, & Foley-Homan, 1999). However, the new norms should be used with Nasometer II.

NASOMETRIC RESULTS

As data is collected during the speech segment, a visual depiction of the relative amount of nasal acoustic energy in the speech is displayed in real time on the screen. Once the speech segment is completed, summary descriptive statistics can be obtained and saved.

Display of the Speech Signal

As the individual is speaking, the speech signal enters the microphones and the software computes the nasalance score which, as noted previously, is the percentage of nasal acoustic energy of the total energy. This nasalance value is displayed during speech in real time on the bottom of the screen as a nasogram.

A *nasogram* is a contour display of the individual data points in sequence as they are collected in real time during the production of a passage. The nasogram is recorded and can be saved for later review along with the auditory playback feature. The contour display can be changed to a bar graph, which is helpful in therapy. For young children, there are also games and animated graphics to help keep the child engaged.

The default is the Contour Display mode (Nasogram) (Figures 14–7A 14–7C and 14–8A), where the percentage nasalance is displayed on the vertical (x) axis and the time is displayed on the horizontal (y) axis. The contour can be filled in as an option (Figures 14–7B, 14–7D, and 14–8B). The Bar Display mode also shows nasalance on the horizontal axis in real time, but only one frame of data shows at a time (Figure 14–9).

Result Statistics

Once the passage has been read or repeated, the examiner can obtain descriptive statistics for that segment of speech. This is done by clicking **Analyze** from the menu, and then **Compute Result Statistics**, which brings up a statistics box (Figure 14–10). Table 14–1 shows definitions of each value.

For evaluation, the most important statistic is the *mean nasalance score*, which is the mean of all the single means. The mean nasalance score is compared to normative data to determine if there is an abnormality and if so, the approximate degree of severity. The minimum and maximum percent nasalance scores give the range of nasalance and can help the examiner to judge the variability during speech. For treatment, the threshold can be useful in setting a target for the individual to achieve.

Because there is variability in the scores of normal speakers and the scores do not always match perceptual impressions, Bressmann and colleagues (Bressmann et al., 2000) suggested

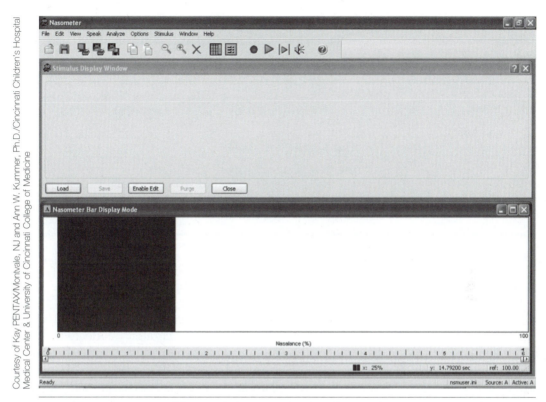

Courtesy of Kay PENTAX/Montvale, NJ and Ann W. Kummer, Ph.D./Cincinnati Children's Hospital Medical Center & University of Cincinnati College of Medicine

FIGURE 14–9 Horizontal bar graph shows nasalance results in real time. It can be used to provide feedback in therapy.

TABLE 14–1 Important Nasometry Statistics

- Mean (%)—the mean nasalance percentage points for the entire passage
- Min (%)—the lowest nasalance value in the data, excluding zero values (important when assessing hyponasality)
- Max (%)—the highest nasalance value in the data (important when assessing hypernasality)
- Threshold (%)—An assigned target nasalance value that is indicated by the placement of the reference cursor
- Above (%)—the percentage of the nasalance trace that is greater than the ratio value set by the location of the reference cursor
- Below (%)—the percentage of the nasalance trace that is less than the ratio value set by the location of the reference cursor

© Cengage Learning 2014

---

adding two new measures to the nasometric evaluations: the *nasalance distance*, which they define as the range between maximum and minimum nasalance; and the *nasalance ratio*, which is the minimum nasalance divided by maximum nasalance. These numbers give an indication of the variability of nasalance within a passage.

Sensitivity and Specificity of the Nasalance Score

There have been several studies to evaluate the sensitivity and specificity of the nasalance score as it is correlated to another measure. The *sensitivity* refers to the extent to which the score is able to correctly identify individuals

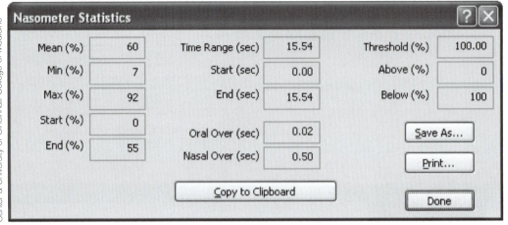

FIGURE 14–10 Summary statistics of these results. The statistic that is listed as the "mean" is actually the mean of all of the percentage points for the entire passage.

with abnormal resonance. The *specificity* refers to the extent to which the score correctly excludes individuals with normal speech from the abnormal group.

Dalston and colleagues (Dalston et al., 1991c) conducted a study to determine the extent to which nasometric results using Nasometer I corresponded with aerodynamic estimates of velopharyngeal orifice area. Using an oral speech passage and a cutoff nasalance score of 32, the sensitivity of the Nasometer scores in correctly identifying the presence or absence of velopharyngeal areas in excess of 0.10 cm was 0.78 and 0.79, respectively. As a second part of the study, the nasalance results were compared to clinical judgments of hypernasality. Again, using the score of 32 as the threshold of abnormality, the sensitivity and specificity of nasometry in correctly identifying subjects with more than mild hypernasality in their speech was 0.89 while the specificity was 0.95. Hardin and others (1992) conducted a similar study, but used a cutoff score of 26. In this study, a sensitivity coefficient of 0.87 and a specificity coefficient of 0.93 were obtained.

Ninety-one percent of the nasometry-based classifications accurately reflected listener judgments of hypernasality. Watterson, McFarlane, and Wright (1993) also found a significant correlation between nasalance and judgments of hypernasality on an oral speech passage. These results suggest that the Nasometer is an appropriate instrument that can be of value in assessing individuals suspected of having velopharyngeal impairment.

Dalston and associates (Dalston et al., 1991b) conducted a complementary study to determine the extent to which nasometric scores corresponded with clinical judgments of hyponasality and aerodynamic measurements of nasal cross-sectional area. Among the 38 adult subjects with moderate to severe nasal airway impairment as identified with aerodynamic studies, the sensitivity of the nasalance scores in correctly identifying these individuals was 0.38, whereas the specificity was 0.92. Among a group of 76 individuals, the sensitivity and specificity of nasometry in correctly identifying the presence or absence of hyponasality, as determined by perceptual assessment, was 0.48 and 0.79 respectively. However, when individuals with audible nasal emission were eliminated from analysis, the sensitivity rose to 1.0 and the specificity rose to 0.85. This study suggests that the sensitivity of nasometry in the identification of hyponasality with nasal air emission is not as strong as the sensitivity for identification of hypernasality or hyponasality alone.

Karnell (1995) suggested that one reason for a lack of agreement between perceptual measures and the nasalance results is that nasometry does not permit discrimination between nasal acoustic energy due to hypernasality and nasal acoustic energy due to audible nasal airflow. Hypernasal resonance occurs on vowels and nasal air emission occurs during the production of consonants. However, the presence of either can give the impression of "hypernasality," as judged by the listener. To test resonance, without the effect of nasal air emission, Karnell used a "low-pressure" speech sample that contained only consonants that do not require intraoral air pressure. The nasalance results from this sample were compared to the results of the "high pressure" sentences from the Zoo Passage. He found that the scores for some individuals were significantly different in the two passages. From this study, he suggested that those individuals with hypernasal resonance obtain elevated nasalance scores on the low-pressure and high-pressure speech samples, because the resonance occurs primarily on the vowels. In contrast, those individuals with normal resonance but with nasal air emission, especially the turbulent nasal rustle, will have low scores or normal scores on the low-pressure sample, but will have higher nasalance scores on the speech sample with high-pressure consonants. This observation seems true in our clinical experience and is another reason to consider the nasalance score based on what is heard perceptually.

INTERPRETATION OF NASOMETRIC RESULTS

There are many factors that can affect the nasalance score. First, the expected nasalance score for a given passage is dependent on the vowel composition of that passage. This is why the normative score is not exactly the same for all oral passages in the same language. In addition, the score must be interpreted with knowledge of patient's speech sound production during the passage. This is because the use of glottal stops or pharyngeal sounds elevates the score, even in the presence of a normally functioning velopharyngeal valve. Finally, the examiner should interpret the score based on information obtained from the intraoral examination.

Expected Nasalance Results

The degree of nasalance in normal speech is dependent on the type of sounds produced. For example, voiceless oral consonants in normal speech actually have no nasalance. This is because there is no phonated sound (and therefore no nasal resonance) and there is no nasal emission of the airstream. Therefore, when producing a sustained /s/, for example, the nasalance score is 0, and there is no tracing on the screen. In contrast, all voiced consonants have some nasal resonance. This can be demonstrated by producing a sustained /z/ and contrasting it with the voiceless cognate /s/. Although the nasalance score varies according to voicing, it does not seem to vary between the low-pressure and high-pressure consonants (Watterson, Lewis, & Deutsch, 1998).

Because all vowels are voiced, they all have some degree of nasal resonance. This can be seen on the screen when prolonging a vowel.

The degree of nasalance varies, depending on the type of vowel produced (Lewis & Watterson, 2003). There is more nasalance on high vowels than on low vowels, as can be noted on the SNAP Test-R (Kummer, 2005). In fact, the nasalance for /i/ is usually at least 10 percentage points higher than that for the low vowel /ɑ/.

One might question how it is possible to have nasal resonance, as represented by nasalance, on oral consonant syllables when the velopharyngeal valve is completely closed. There are actually two reasons for nasalance on voiced oral consonants. One is that the sound separator plate cannot totally block reception of the signal from one side of the plate to the other side. Therefore, there may be some spillover between the microphones during the production of voiced phonemes, particularly vowels (KayPENTAX, n.d.[a]). The other reason is that there seems to be a transpalatal transmission of sound during production of voiced phonemes, particularly vowels (Awan et al., 2011; Gildersleeve-Neumann & Dalston, 2001). It can be assumed that the hard palate is like a brick wall and allows little sound to go through it. On the other hand, the soft palate is more like a heavy curtain—allowing some sound to pass through into the nasal cavity.

High vowels have more nasal resonance than low vowels because the high tongue position results in a smaller oral passage and hence increased impedance to the oral cavity. At the same time, there is increased sound pressure against the soft tissues of the velum (S. G. Fletcher, personal communication, May 12, 1999). In contrast, low vowels result in a larger oral cavity size and less impedance. Therefore, oral resonance is more pronounced on low vowels. Overall, a normal nasalance score for a passage with all oral sounds is usually under 20%.

In evaluating nasal resonance, a prolonged nasal sound often results in scores that are in the 90s. However, when nasal consonants are combined with oral consonants in connected speech, the resulting nasalance score is between 50% and 70%.

Interpretation of the Nasalance Score

When various phonemes are combined together for connected speech, the resultant average nasalance score for speakers with normal resonance depends on the passage and its phonemic content of voiced versus voiceless consonants and high versus low vowels. Passages with more voiced consonants and/or high vowels have a higher average nasalance than those with more voiceless consonants and/or low vowels. Therefore, it is difficult to compare norms for different passages, even in the same language. When one of the standardized passages is used, however, the nasalance score of the individual can be compared to normative data for that particular passage.

Because nasalance and resonance are on a continuum, there is a borderline area between clearly normal and clearly abnormal. Therefore, there is no single score that serves as an absolute or definitive cutoff point between normal and abnormal resonance. Despite this fact, Dalston, Neiman, and Gonzalez-Landa (1993) suggested the score of 28 as the threshold between normal and abnormal for the Zoo Passage, using Nasometer I. In addition, suggested thresholds (based on about two standard deviations from the mean) are given for the various passages of the SNAP-R, which was normed on Nasometer II. In looking at all the norms for a passage devoid of nasal phonemes, it can be said that in general, a score under about 20% suggests no hypernasality, scores between 30% and 40% are in the mild range, and scores over 40% can be considered clearly hypernasal (Smith & Kuehn, 2007).

Given the large borderline range and the variability of scores based on phonemic content of the passage, the results of nasometric testing must always be interpreted by the speech pathologist in the context of the perceptual assessment. This is important because many factors can affect the nasalance score. For example, an individual's nasalance score can be in the normal range if there is normal resonance, even in the presence of audible nasal air emission. On the other hand, the nasalance score may be as much as two standard deviations above the normative mean, yet the person may still have very acceptable speech.

If there is obstruction in the vocal tract causing cul-de-sac resonance, the obstruction may impede the transmission of resonance in both the oral and the nasal cavities, resulting in an essentially normal nasalance score, because the nasalance score is a ratio of the two. In the same way, if there is a combination of hyponasality and hypernasality, both aspects are combined for the average nasalance score (Dalston et al., 1991a). If there is nasal turbulence (or a nasal rustle), this may result in a high nasalance score due to the degree of nasal distortion, even though it may be due to a small velopharyngeal opening. On the other hand, a large velopharyngeal opening may give a moderate nasalance score due to the lack of intensity of both oral and nasal acoustic energy. A breathy vocal quality or low volume can even influence the nasalance score to some degree.

Articulation errors can also affect the nasalance score. If pharyngeal fricatives or posterior nasal fricatives are substituted for sibilant phonemes, the nasal emission associated with these articulation productions will produce an elevated nasalance score, particularly on passages that contain a large number of sibilants. The same is true if nasal sounds are substituted for oral sounds (for example, the substitution of /ŋ/ for /l/). Although these errors are due to faulty articulation placement rather than true velopharyngeal dysfunction, this cannot always be distinguished by the Nasometer if heterogeneous passages are used. Because there are so many factors that can affect the nasalance score, nasometry should always serve as a supplement to clinical judgment, but not as a substitute for it.

With prior information from the perceptual and oral examination, the examiner can interpret the nasalance scores with more confidence. In addition, certain patterns of scores can be diagnostic, as can be seen through the following case studies:

CASE REPORTS

Case 1

Oral Passages	Nasalance Score
Bilabial Plosives	11
Lingual-Alveolar Plosives	11
Velar Plosives	13
Sibilant Fricatives	46

Analysis: All passages are within the normal range, with the exception of the sibilants. This suggests phoneme specific nasal emission on sibilants, which can be corrected with speech therapy.

(continues)

(continued)

Case 2

Oral Passages	Nasalance Score
Bilabial Plosives	15
Lingual-Alveolar Plosives	48
Velar Plosives	13
Sibilant Fricatives	43

Analysis: Velar phonemes are normal, but anterior phonemes show high nasalance scores. This indicates normal velopharyngeal function but a symptomatic fistula that is just above the tongue tip.

Case 3

Oral + /ɑ/ Syllables	Nasalance Score
pɑ, pɑ, pɑ,...	5
tɑ, tɑ, tɑ...	8
kɑ, kɑ, kɑ...	8
sɑ, sɑ, sɑ,...	7
ɑ, ɑ, ɑ...	7

Oral + /i/ (as in "tea") Syllables	Nasalance Score
pi, pi, pi...	38
ti, ti, ti...	37
ki, ki, ki...	37
si, si, si...	39
i, i, i...	37

Analysis: Low vowel syllables are normal, but high vowel syllables are abnormally high. This suggests phoneme-specific hypernasality on high vowels due to an abnormally high tongue position. Another possibility is a thin velum.

Interpretation of the Nasogram

The configuration of the nasogram can be useful when the results of the entire passage are displayed on the screen. Some general guidelines in interpretation are as follows:

During production of an oral passage with no nasals:

- Normal oral resonance is typically between 10 to 15 percentage points.

- The expected difference between vowels /ɑ/ and /i/ is about 10 percentage points when combined with oral consonants and about 20 percentage points when combined with nasal consonants.

- The higher the contour is on the screen, the more hypernasality to expect.

- If most of the data points appear normal (and the nasalance score is normal), but there are occasional high peaks, this suggests normal resonance but inconsistent nasal emission.

- A gradual rise in the curve throughout the passage suggests muscle fatigue, which could indicate neuromotor problems.

- There should be no data points during production of a prolonged /s/ or /ʃ/. If there is a break in velopharyngeal closure, this will be seen on the screen.

- If either /s/ or /ʃ/ in isolation or in syllables is high and all other phonemes others are normal, consider phoneme-specific nasal emission due to the substitution of a pharyngeal fricative or posterior nasal fricative.

- If lingual-alveolars and bilabials are significantly higher than velars, this could be due to a symptomatic fistula.

- If vowels are high, but prolonged /s/ is zero, this could be due to a thin velum, high tongue position, or vowel-specific nasality.

During production of a nasal passage:

- If the data points are low and remain toward the bottom of the screen, this indicates hyponasality and also suggests upper airway obstruction.

The nasogram can be particularly helpful in counseling individuals and their families. With the visual display, it is easier for the examiner to explain what is happening during speech as well as the relative severity of the problem.

USE IN TREATMENT

In addition to its utility as diagnostic tool, nasometry can be useful in treatment by providing the individual with real-time visual feedback regarding nasality and tangible goals. This is useful in eliminating nasal emission or hypernasality that is functional or phoneme specific. It is also helpful following VPI surgery because it helps the patient to learn to use the new velopharyngeal mechanism. As a form of biofeedback, it can even be used to modify resonance in certain cases of velopharyngeal incompetence (Heppt, Westrich, Strate, & Mohring, 1991).

Although the Nasometer is a great tool for providing biofeedback in therapy, it should be noted that *biofeedback is only effective if the individual's velopharyngeal mechanism is anatomically and physiologically capable of achieving and maintaining normal velopharyngeal closure during connected speech*. If there is velopharyngeal insufficiency or incompetence, physical management (a prosthetic device or surgery) is needed for improvement or correction of speech.

Games are provided as part of the software to help to motivate young patients (Figure 14–11A and B). The options on the Nasometer games can be changed to access different display formats, including the filled contour display, bar display, or inverted contour display, depending on the therapy task (Figure 14–12). The green reference cursor line can be placed on the nasogram according to the needs of the patient and the therapy goals. The patient works with a goal of keeping the nasalance trace below the reference line level during speech. After the speech task has been completed, the clinician can open the statistics box to obtain the percentage above and below the threshold. This can serve as a basis for charting progress.

To address specific errors, such as a phoneme-specific nasal emission on /s/, the child is instructed to eliminate the tracings on the nasogram that occur when he produces the

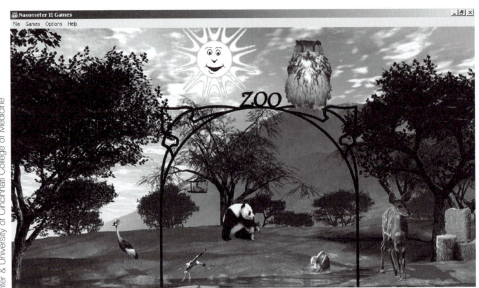

Look at this book with us. It's a story about a zoo. That is where bears go. Today it's very cold out of doors, but we see a cloud overhead that's a pretty white fluffy shape. We hear that straw covers the floor of cages to keep the chill away; yet a deer walks through the trees with her head high. They feed seeds to birds so they're able to fly.

PLAY Click PLAY or press Space Bar to start game.   48.93 %   11 sec.

A

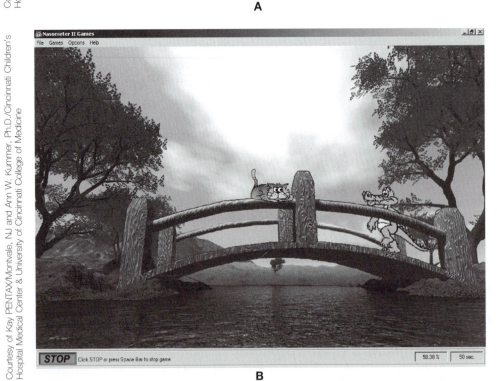

STOP Click STOP or press Space Bar to stop game   58.38 %   50 sec.

B

FIGURE 14–11 (A and B) Nasometer games. All games provide biofeedback, with the ability to set a nasalance threshold. When achieving the desired threshold, the child is rewarded with an emerging picture.

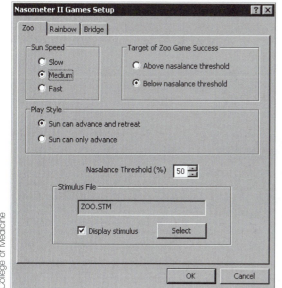

/s/ phoneme. It may be helpful to contrast minimal paired words with and without the /s/ phoneme. For example, because the /s/ phoneme should not be visible on the nasogram, words such as "mile" and "smile" should look similar, as noted in Figure 14–13A. When there is a phoneme-specific nasal rustle, an obvious difference can be noted in the tracings, as can be seen in Figure 14–13B.

One big advantage of the Nasometer is that the tracing with the audio can be replayed for the child again and again. This allows the child to see and hear the nasal emission. For more information regarding the use of nasometry in treatment, please refer to Chapter 21.

FIGURE 14–12   The options on the Nasometer games can be changed to meet the needs of each therapy session.

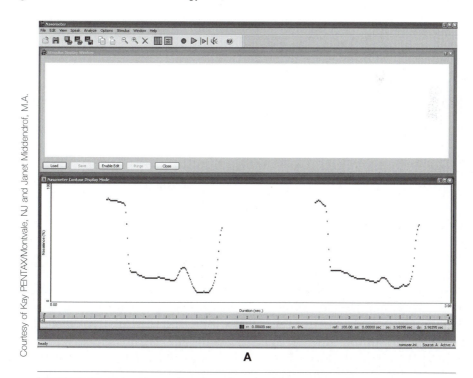

A

FIGURE 14–13A   The words "mile" and "smile." (A) Normal speech production of the word "mile" and then "smile." Note that the two tracings are very similar in appearance due to the fact that there is no nasalance on the /s/ sound.

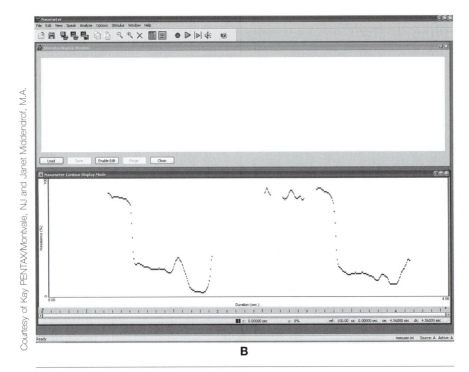

Courtesy of Kay PENTAX/Montvale, NJ and Janet Middendrof, M.A.

B

FIGURE 14–13B (B) Production of the word "mile" and then "smile" with a nasal rustle on /s/. Note that in this case, there is a high squiggly line at the beginning of the word "smile" due to the nasal rustle on /s/.

Summary

Nasometric testing is an easy, noninvasive procedure used to obtain objective data regarding the results of velopharyngeal function (Hirschberg et. al., 2006). The nasalance score can be compared to normative data in order to gauge the type and degree of abnormality. Nasometry is an excellent means of substantiating the subjective findings of the speech pathologist. In addition, the Nasometer provides a visual display that is helpful in counseling individuals and families. Finally, nasometry is an excellent means for providing visual biofeedback regarding the results of velopharyngeal function during speech, and therefore it can be very useful during treatment.

Although nasometry can be a very valuable part of an evaluation of resonance and velopharyngeal function, it should not be viewed as an independent diagnostic measure. Because the nasalance score can be affected by articulation errors, production errors, mixed nasality, and other factors, the objective measurements provided by nasometry should be interpreted based on an accompanying perceptual evaluation by a qualified speech pathologist. In addition, just like with aerodynamic instrumentation, nasometry can give objective scores, but cannot show the cause of velopharyngeal dysfunction or the location and size of the defect in the same manner that the direct measures can do. Therefore, the results of the nasometry testing must be integrated into a test battery for a complete evaluation of velopharyngeal function.

FOR REVIEW AND DISCUSSION

1. What is the Nasometer, and what are the equipment components?

2. What does the nasalance score measure? How is it calculated?

3. What are the standardized tests for use with nasometry? What type of passage should be used for testing hyponasality? What type of passage would be appropriate for testing hypernasality?

4. If the child has only plosives in his phonemic repertoire, what passages could be used?

5. Why is the nasalance score not 0 with normal speech and normal velopharyngeal closure?

6. If the child has a high nasalance score on the sibilants passage, but other scores are normal, what might you conclude? What would you recommend?

7. If a child with a history of cleft palate has a high nasalance score on plosives and lingual-alveolars but a normal score on velars, what might you suspect to be the cause? What would you do next? What would you recommend?

8. Why is the nasalance score 0 during prolongation of the /s/ sound?

9. Which passage would have the highest nasalance score in normal speech: repetitive /pi/ or repetitive /pɑ/? Why?

REFERENCES

Anderson, R. T. (1996). Nasometric values for normal Spanish-speaking females: A preliminary report. *Cleft Palate–Craniofacial Journal, 33*(4), 333–336.

Awan, S. N., Omlor, K., & Watts, C. R. (2011). Effects of computer system and vowel loading on measures of nasalance. *Journal of Speech, Language and Hearing Research, 54*(5), 1284–1294.

Bressmann, T. (2005). Comparison of nasalance scores obtained with the Nasometer, the Nasal View, and the OroNasal System. *Cleft Palate–Craniofacial Journal, 42*(4), 423–433.

Bressmann, T., Sader, R., Whitehill, T. L., Awan, S. N., Zeilhofer, H. F., & Horch, H. H. (2000). Nasalance distance and ratio: Two new measures. *Cleft Palate–Craniofacial Journal, 37*(3), 248–256.

Dalston, R. M. (1997) The use of nasometry in the assessment and remediation of velopharyngeal inadequacy. In K. R. Bzoch (Ed.), *Communicative disorders related to cleft lip and palate* (vol. 4, pp. 331–346). Austin: Pro-Ed.

Dalston, R. M., Neiman, G. S., & Gonzalez-Landa, G. (1993). Nasometric sensitivity and specificity: A cross-dialect and cross-culture study. *Cleft Palate–Craniofacial Journal, 30*(3), 285–291.

Dalston, R. M., & Seaver, E. J. (1992). Relative values of various standardized passages in the nasometric assessment of patients with velopharyngeal impairment. *Cleft Palate–Craniofacial Journal, 29*(1), 17–21.

Dalston, R. M., Warren, D. W., & Dalston, E. T. (1991a). The identification of nasal obstruction through clinical judgments of hyponasality and nasometric assessment of speech acoustics. *American Journal of Orthodontics and Dentofacial Orthopedics, 100*(1), 59–65.

Dalston, R. M., Warren, D. W., & Dalston, E. T. (1991b). A preliminary investigation concerning the use of nasometry in identifying patients with hyponasality and/or nasal airway impairment. *Journal of Speech and Hearing Research*, *34(1)*, 11–18.

Dalston, R. M., Warren, D. W., & Dalston, E. T. (1991c). Use of nasometry as a diagnostic tool for identifying patients with velopharyngeal impairment. *Cleft Palate–Craniofacial Journal*, *28(2)*, 184–188; Discussion 188–189. [Published Erratum appears in *Cleft Palate–Craniofacial Journal*, 1991, 28(4), 446.]

Dejonckere, P. H., & van Wijngaarden, H. A. (2001). Retropharyngeal autologous fat transplantation for congenital short palate: A nasometric assessment of functional results. *Annals of Otology, Rhinology, & Laryngology*, *110(2)*, 168–172.

Eckardt, A., Teltzrow, T., Schulze, A., Hoppe, M., & Kuettner, C. (2007). Nasalance in patients with maxillary defects—Reconstruction versus obturation. *Journal of Craniomaxillofacial Surgery*, *35(4–5)*, 241–245.

Fairbanks, D. (1960). *Voice and articulation drill book* (pp. 127–127). New York, NY: Harper and Row.

Fletcher, S. G. (1970). Theory and instrumentation for quantitative measurement of nasality. *Cleft Palate Journal*, *7*, 601–609.

Fletcher, S. G. (1972). Contingencies for bioelectronic modification of nasality. *Journal of Speech and Hearing Disorders*, *37*, 329–346.

Fletcher, S. G. (1976a). "Nasalance" vs. listener judgments of nasality. *Cleft Palate Journal*, *13*, 31–44.

Fletcher, S. G. (1976b). Theory and use of Tonar II: A status report. *Biocommunications Research Reports*, *1*, 1–38.

Fletcher, S. G. (1978). *Diagnosing speech disorders from cleft palate*. New York: Grune & Statton.

Fletcher, S. G., Adams, L., & McCutcheon. (1989). Cleft palate speech assessment through oral-nasal acoustic measures. In K. R. Bzoch (Ed.), *Communicative disorders related to cleft lip and palate* (pp. 246–257). Boston: College Hill Press.

Fletcher, S. G., & Bishop, M. E. (1970). Measurement of nasality with Tonar. *Cleft Palate Journal*, *7*, 610–621.

Gildersleeve-Neumann, C. E., & Dalston, R. M. (2001). Nasalance scores in noncleft individuals: Why not zero? *Cleft Palate–Craniofacial Journal*, *38(2)*, 106–111.

Hardin, M. A., Van Demark, D. R., Morris, H. L., & Payne, M. M. (1992). Correspondence between nasalance scores and listener judgments of hypernasality and hyponasality. *Cleft Palate–Craniofacial Journal*, *29(4)*, 346–351.

Hassan, S. M., Malki, K. H., Mesallam, T. A., Farahat, M., Bukhari, M., & Murry, T. (2012). The effect of cochlear implantation on nasalance of speech in postlingually hearing-impaired adults. *Journal of Voice*, *26(5)*, 669.e17–22.

Heppt, W., Westrich, M., Strate, B., & Mohring, L. (1991). [Nasalance: A new concept for objective analysis of nasality]. *Laryngorhinootologic*, *70(4)*, 208–213.

Hirschberg, J., Bok, S., Juhasz, M., Trenovszki, Z., Votisky, P., & Hirschberg, A. (2005). Adaptation of nasometry to Hungarian language and experiences with its clinical application. *International Journal of Pediatric Otorhinolaryngology*, *70(5)*, 785–798.

Hong, K. H., Kwon, S. H., & Jung, S. S. (1997). The assessment of nasality with a Nasometer and sound spectrography in patients with nasal polyposis. *Otolaryngology–Head & Neck Surgery*, *117(4)*, 343–348.

Karnell, M. P. (1995). Nasometric discrimination of hypernasality and turbulent nasal airflow. *Cleft Palate–Craniofacial Journal*, 32(2), 145–148.

Karnell, M. P. (2011). Instrumental assessment of velopharyngeal closure for speech. *Seminars in Speech and Language*, 32(2), 168–178.

KayPENTAX (n.d.[a]). Installation, operations, and maintenance manual: Nasometer II, Model 6450. Lincoln Park, NJ: KayPENTAX.

KayPENTAX. (n.d.[b]). Accessed January 15, 2013, from http://www.kayelemetrics.com/index.php?option=com_product&controller=product&Itemid=3&cid%5B%5D=78&task=pro_details.

Kummer, A. W. (2005). The MacKay-Kummer SNAP Test-R: Simplified nasometric assessment procedures. KayPENTAX. Accessed January 15, 2013, from http://www.kayelemetrics.com/index.php?option=com_product&controller=product&Itemid=3&cid%5B%5D=78&task=pro_details.

Kummer, A. W., Myer, C. M. L, Smith, M. E., & Shott, S. R. (1993). Changes in nasal resonance secondary to adenotonsillectomy. *American Journal of Otolaryngology*, 14(4), 285–290.

Leeper, H. A., Rochet, A. P., & MacKay, I. R. A. (1992). Characteristics of nasalance in Canadian speakers of English and French. *Proceedings of the International Conference on Spoken and Language Processes*, 5, 49–52.

Lewis, K. E., & Watterson, T. (2003). Comparison of nasalance scores obtained from the Nasometer and the NasalView. *Cleft Palate–Craniofacial Journal*, 40(1), 40–45.

MacKay, I.R.A., & Kummer, A. W. (1994). Simplified nasometric assessment proce-

dures. In Kay Elemetrics Corp. (Ed.), *Instruction manual: Nasometer model 6200-3* (pp. 123–142). Lincoln Park, NJ: Kay Elemetrics Corp.

Mandulak, K. C., & Zajac, D. J. (2009). Effects of altered fundamental frequency on nasalance during vowel production by adult speakers at targeted sound pressure levels. *Cleft Palate–Craniofacial Journal*, 46(1), 39–46.

Mayo, R., Floyd, L. A., Warren, D. W., Dalston, R. M., & Mayo, C. M. (1996). Nasalance and nasal area values: Cross-racial study. *Cleft Palate–Craniofacial Journal*, 33(2), 143–149.

Mueller, K., Neuber, B., Schelhorn-Niese, P., & Schumann, D. (2007). Diagnostic value of nasometry – representative study of patients with cleft palate and normal subjects. *Folia Phoniatrica et Logopaedica*, 59(5), 219–226.

Nieminen, P., Lopponen, H., Vayrynen, M., Tervonen, A., & Tolonen, U. (2000). Nasalance scores in snoring children with obstructive symptoms. *International Journal of Pediatric Otorhinolaryngology*, 52(1), 53–60.

Parker, A. J., Clarke, P. M., Dawes, P. J., & Maw, A. R. (1990). A comparison of active anterior rhinomanometry and nasometry in the objective assessment of nasal obstruction. *Rhinology*, 28(1), 47–53.

Parker, A. J., Maw, A. R., & Szallasi, F. (1989). An objective method of assessing nasality: A possible aid in the selection of patients for adenoidectomy. *Clinical Otolaryngology*, 14(2), 161–166.

Rieger, J., Wolfaardt, J., Seikaly, H., & Jha, N. (2002). Speech outcomes in patients rehabilitated with maxillary obturator prostheses after maxillectomy: A prospective study. *International Journal of Prosthodontics*, 15(2), 139–144.

Santos-Terron, M. J., Gonzalez-Landa, G., & Sanchez-Ruiz, I. (1990). Nasometric patterns in the speech of normal child speakers of Castilian Spanish. *Revista Espanola de Foniatrica, 4,* 71–75.

Seaver, E. J., Dalston, R. M., Leeper, H. A., & Adams, L. E. (1991). A study of nasometric values for normal nasal resonance. *Journal of Speech and Hearing Research, 34*(4), 715–721.

Smith, B. E., & Kuehn, D. P. (2007). Speech evaluation of velopharyngeal dysfunction. *The Journal of Craniofacial Surgery, 18*(2), 251–261.

Soneghet, R., Santos, R. P., Behlau, M., Habermann, W., Friedrich, G., & Stammberger, H. (2002). Nasalance changes after functional endoscopic sinus surgery. *Journal of Voice, 16*(3), 392–397.

Sweeney, T., & Sell, D. (2008). Relationship between perceptual ratings of nasality and nasometry in children/adolescents with cleft palate and/or velopharyngeal dysfunction. *International Journal of Language and Communication Disorders, 43*(3), 265–282.

Sweeney, T., Sell, D., & O'Regan, M. (2004). Nasalance scores for normal-speaking Irish children. *Cleft Palate–Craniofacial Journal, 41*(2), 168–174.

Tatchell, J. A., Stewart, M., & Lapine, P. R. (1991). Nasalance measurements in hearing-impaired children. *Journal of Communication Disorders, 24*(4), 275–285.

van der Heijden, P., Hobbel, H. H., van der Laan, B. F., Korsten-Meijer, A. G., & Goorhuis Brouwer, S. M. (2011). Nasometry cooperation in children 4–6 years. *International Journal of Pediatric Otorhinolaryngology, 75*(3), 420–424.

van Doorn, J., & Purcell, A. (1998). Nasalance levels in the speech of normal Australian children. *Cleft Palate Craniofacial Journal, 35*(4), 287–92.

Van Lierde, K. M., De Bodt, M., Baetens, L, Schrauwen, V., & Van Cauwenberge, P. (2003). Outcome of treatment regarding articulation, resonance, and voice in Flemish adults with unilateral and bilateral cleft palate. *Folia Phoniatrica et Logopedica, 55*(2), 80–90.

Van Lierde, K. M., Monstrey, S., Bonte, K., Van Cauwenberge, P., & Vinck, B. (2004). The long-term speech outcome in Flemish young adults after two different types of palatoplasty. *International Journal of Pediatric Otorhinolaryngology, 68*(7), 865–875.

Watterson, T., Lewis, K. E., & Deutsch, C. (1998). Nasalance and nasality in low-pressure and high-pressure speech. *Cleft Palate–Craniofacial Journal, 35*(4), 293–298.

Watterson, T., Lewis, K. E., & Foley-Homan, N. (1999). Effect of stimulus length on nasalance scores. *Cleft Palate–Craniofacial Journal, 36*(3), 243–247.

Watterson, T., McFarlane, S. C, & Wright, D. S. (1993). The relationship between nasalance and nasality in children with cleft palate. *Journal of Communication Disorders, 26*(1), 13–28.

Williams, R. G., Eccles, R., & Hutchings, H. (1990). The relationship between nasalance and nasal resistance to airflow. *Acta Otolaryngology (Stockholm), 110*(5/6), 443–449.

Williams, R. G., Preece, M., Rhys, R., & Eccles, R. (1992). The effect of adenoid and tonsil surgery on nasalance. *Clinical Otolaryngology & Allied Sciences, 17*(2), 136–140.

Wozny, C. G., Kuehn, D. P., Oishi, J. T., & Arthur, J. L. (1994, November). *Effect of passage length on nasalance values in normal adults.* Paper presented at the American Speech-Language-Hearing Association, New Orleans, LA.

STANDARD NASOMETRIC PASSAGES SUPPLIED BY KAYPENTAX

ZOO PASSAGE[*]

Look at the book with us. It's a story about a zoo. That is where bears go. Today it's very cold out of doors, but we see a cloud overhead that's a pretty, white, fluffy shape. We hear that straw covers the floor of cages to keep the chili away; yet a deer walks through the trees with her head high. They feed seeds to birds so they're able to fly.

[*]The Zoo Passage excludes nasal consonants.

RAINBOW PASSAGE[**]

When the sunlight strikes raindrops in the air, they act like a prism and form a rainbow. The rainbow is a division of white light into many beautiful colors. These take the shape of a long round arch, with its path high above, and its two ends apparently beyond the horizon.

There is, according to legend, a boiling pot of gold at one end. People look, but no one ever finds it. When a man looks for something beyond his reach, his friends say he is looking for the pot of gold at the end of the rainbow.

[**]In the Rainbow passage, 11.5% of the consonants are nasal consonants.

NASAL SENTENCES[***]

Mama made some lemon jam.

Ten men came in when Jane rang.

Dan's gang changed my mind.

Ben can't plan on a lengthy rain.

Amanda came from Bounding, Maine.

[***]The Nasal Sentences Passage is loaded with nasal phonemes so that 35% of the total phonemes in these sentences are nasal consonants. This is more than three times as many as would be expected in Standard American English sentences.

Normative data for standardized passages collected on 40 adult subjects using Nasometer II (KayPENTAX, n.d.[b]):

Test Passage	Mean Nasalance	SD of Mean
Zoo Passage	11.25	5.63
Rainbow Passage	31.47	6.65
Nasal Sentences	59.55	7.96

© Cengage Learning 2014

Score Sheet for the SNAP Test-Revised

The Mackay-Kummer SNAP Test-R
Simplified Nasometric Assessment Procedures
Revised 2005

Name:	Date:
Age:	Examiner:

Subtest I: Syllable Repetition/Prolonged Sounds Subtest

Instructions: Repeat or prolong until the screen is full.

Oral + /ɑ/ Syllables	Norms	SD	Score (Threshold: ≥15)
pɑ, pɑ, pɑ,...	6	3	
tɑ, tɑ, tɑ,...	7	4	
kɑ, kɑ, kɑ,...	7	4	
sɑ, sɑ, sɑ,...	7	5	
ʃɑ, ʃɑ, ʃɑ...	7	4	

Oral + /i/ Syllables	Norms	SD	Score (Threshold: ≥35)
pi, pi, pi...	17	7	
ti, ti, ti...	17	7	
ki, ki, ki...	18	8	
si, si, si...	17	8	
ʃi, ʃi, ʃi...	16	8	

Nasal + /a/ Syllables	Norms	SD	Score (Threshold: ≤40)
ma, ma, ma,...	53	13	
na, na, na,...	53	11	

Nasal + /i/ Syllables	Norms	SD	Score (Threshold: ≤60)
mi, mi, mi...	72	13	
ni, ni, ni...	74	11	

Prolonged Sounds	Norms	SD	Score (Threshold: +/–2 SDs)
Prolonged /a/	6	3	
Prolonged /i/	19	9	
Prolonged /s/	0	0	
Prolonged /m/	93	3	

SNAP Test-Revised, page 2.
Name:_____

Subtest II: Picture Cued Subtest

Instructions: Produce a sentence with the carrier phrase and picture. Do each twice.

Oral Passages	Norms	SD	Score (Threshold: ≥22)
Bilabial Plosives	11	5	
Lingual-Alveolar Plosives	11	5	
Velar Plosives	13	6	
Sibilant Fricatives	12	5	
Nasal Passage	Norms	SD	Score (Threshold: ≤45)
Nasals	54	9	

Subtest III: Paragraph Subtest

Instructions: Read or repeat each passage

Passages (Reading)	Norms	SD	Score (Threshold: >25)
Bilabial Plosives (w/nasals)	16	5	
Passages (Reading)	Norms	SD	Score (Threshold: >20)
Sibilant Fricatives (w/o nasals)	10	4	

Notes:

_____

_____

_____

Important: The threshold value for each test is an approximation of the beginning of a borderline range of abnormal resonance. These values were estimated based on Standard deviations (about two higher for orals, about one lower for nasals) and clinical experience. It should be noted that a small number of normal speakers will score outside two Standard deviations of the mean for both orals and nasals. Therefore, the suggested threshold values should be used as general guidelines and not as absolute markers between normal and abnormal resonance. The scores on nasometry should always be used as a means to support clinical judgment but never to replace it.

Pick up the . . .

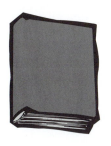
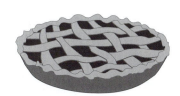
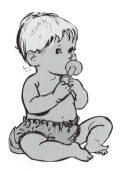

Take a . . .

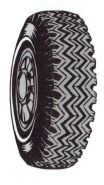
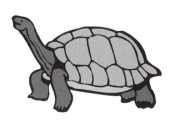
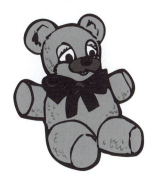

Go get a . . .

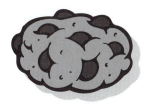
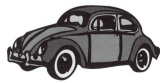
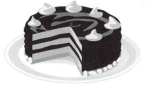

Suzy sees the . . .

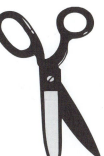
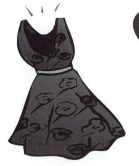
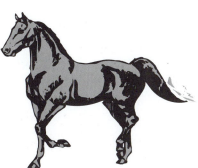

Mama made some . . .

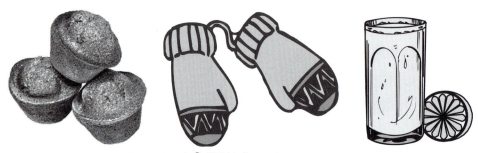

CHAPTER

15

SPEECH AERODYNAMICS

DAVID J. ZAJAC, PH.D.

CHAPTER OUTLINE

INTRODUCTION

Aerodynamics is the branch of physics that deals with the mechanical properties of air and other gases in motion. Because speech production requires a buildup and release of air pressure at the various valving points in the vocal tract, aerodynamic principles can be used to study the speech process. Aerodynamic procedures are especially well suited to study velopharyngeal function given that two of the primary symptoms of velopharyngeal dysfunction—loss of oral air pressure and nasal air emission—are aerodynamic in nature. Although aerodynamic assessment is typically done with older children because of the need for their cooperation, some new modifications have extended its use to toddlers and even infants.

The purpose of this chapter is to describe the principles and practice of aerodynamic assessment of the velopharyngeal mechanism and nasal passages of individuals with resonance disorders.

WHY AERODYNAMIC ASSESSMENT?

Aerodynamic processes are indeed responsible for all acoustic aspects of speech production. Beginning with inspiration, air enters the lungs due to the expansion of the thorax and the generation of negative air pressure relative to the atmosphere. During expiration, positive subglottal pressure (Ps) is generated due to passive relaxation of the thorax and, if needed, active contraction of the muscles of respiration. Positive Ps is responsible for the rapid displacement of the vocal folds that results in the quasiperiodic release of air for all voiced speech sounds. The articulators of the upper vocal tract further modify airflow for sound production. During production of the stop-plosive /p/, for example, the lips momentarily impede airflow resulting in a buildup and release of air pressure. The air bursts resulting from the release of the articulators provide important acoustic cues to the place of articulation of stop consonants. In addition, the

articulators create relatively prolonged noise by constricting the size of the upper vocal tract. During production of the fricative /s/, for example, the tongue approximates the alveolar ridge, resulting in a reduction of cross-sectional area and the generation of turbulent airflow.

Adequate production of speech requires an effective velopharyngeal (VP) mechanism. During production of oral pressure consonants, the VP mechanism must separate the oral and nasal cavities. Conversely, during production of nasal consonants the VP mechanism must allow some degree of oral-nasal coupling. As indicated by Sussman (1992) and others, the following perceptual speech symptoms commonly occur in individuals with cleft palate due to VP dysfunction and/or other structural defects: (1) weak pressure consonants, (2) nasal air emission, (3) hypernasality, (4) hyponasality, and (5) compensatory articulation (p. 211–212). Although the first two symptoms have clear aerodynamic foundations, perceptual descriptions vary and are not well defined. Sussman (1992) described weak pressure consonants as sounds that "appear muffled and lack clarity." As indicated by Peterson-Falzone, Hardin-Jones, and Karnell (2001), nasal air emission may or may not be audible depending on the status of the nasal passages. Audible nasal air emission may also be masked by or attributed to acoustic deviations resulting from faulty oral articulation, especially those related to sibilant production. Clearly, aerodynamics should be considered an essential assessment method to determine the extent of weak pressure consonants and nasal air emission. Although hypernasality and hyponasality are complex acoustic-perceptual phenomena associated with vowels and nasal consonants, respectively, they too may have identifiable aerodynamic substrates.

Because of these factors, aerodynamic techniques should form an important part of the diagnostic procedures for individuals when VP dysfunction is suspected. Indeed, a comprehensive evaluation of VP function must include both perceptual and instrumental techniques (Peterson-Falzone et al., 2001). When aerodynamic techniques are appropriately employed, they provide objective documentation of intraoral air-pressure levels, rates of nasal air emission, and estimates of VP orifice size during consonant production (Smith & Kuehn, 2007). In addition, aerodynamic methods can be used to provide information on the timing aspects of VP function during certain phonetic contexts and the patency of the nasal airways during breathing (Smith & Kuehn, 2007). Such information can provide a firm basis for diagnostic decisions and/or post-management evaluation of individuals with cleft palate and/or VP dysfunction.

The following sections describe (a) basic principles of the pressure-flow technique, (b) instrumentation and calibration of equipment, (c) aerodynamic assessment of nasal respiration, and (d) aerodynamic assessment and characteristics of speech production in cleft palate. The first two sections lay the groundwork and theory of aerodynamic assessment techniques. The third section is included because, as indicated, the nasal airway impacts the perceptual aspects of speech production. The final section provides a detailed examination of aerodynamic characteristics of normal and cleft palate speech.

BASIC PRINCIPLES OF THE PRESSURE-FLOW TECHNIQUE

Warren and DuBois (1964) were the first to describe the use of aerodynamic principles to study the dynamics of the VP mechanism during speech. Their procedure has often been referred to as the *pressure-flow technique*. By placing catheters with small openings in the oral cavity and in one nostril, and inserting a flow tube into the other nostril, estimation can be made of the cross-sectional area of the VP port. The technique thus provides an indirect method of determining the presence and extent of VP dysfunction.

Derivation of the "Orifice Equation"

As described by Warren and DuBois (1964), the cross-sectional area of a constriction or an orifice can be calculated if the differential pressure across the orifice and rate of airflow are measured simultaneously. In an ideal situation (see Figure 15–1), the static pressures (e.g., pressures associated with the moving airstream) are determined before the orifice (Point A) and at a point near the constriction (Point B). The difference between these

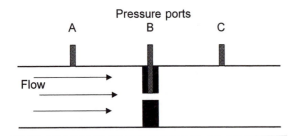

FIGURE 15–1 The area of a constriction can be calculated if the rate of airflow and the pressure loss across the constriction are measured. Either the dynamic pressure loss (from A to B) or the stagnation pressure loss (from A to C) is measured.

Courtesy David J. Zajac, Ph.D./University of North Carolina at Chapel Hill

pressures is the dynamic pressure loss. Assuming that airflow is steady or nonturbulent, the area of the orifice can be calculated using the dynamic pressure loss and a modification of Bernoulli's equation as follows:

$$A = \hat{V}/k[2(p_1 - p_2)/D]^{1/2}$$

where A is orifice area in cm^2, $\hat{V}$ is airflow in ml/s, p_1 is static pressure in dynes/cm before the orifice, p_2 is static pressure in dynes/cm at the orifice, and D is the density of air (0.001 gm/cm). As indicated by Warren and DuBois (1964), however, ideal or "theoretical" conditions do not exist in the human anatomy. In addition, because of practical limitations involving the placement of pressure probes, the static pressure at the constriction cannot be measured. Therefore, the pressure-flow technique uses a stagnation pressure (e.g., pressure associated with a low-velocity or nonmoving airstream) detected at Point C in Figure 15–1 to determine the pressure loss. As noted by Yates, McWilliams, and Vallino (1990), the pressure loss created by the orifice is nearly equal to the dynamic pressure at the orifice if the flow velocities before and after the orifice are small. Because these conditions are

assumed in the human anatomy, and indirectly confirmed by Zajac and Yates (1991), the substitution of a stagnation pressure for a dynamic pressure is used in the pressure-flow technique.

As further noted by Warren and DuBois (1964), the substitution of a pressure measured downstream of the orifice is valid if the kinetic energy of the gas passing through the orifice is lost due to turbulence on the nasal side of the orifice. Because the "theoretical" equation does not take turbulence into account, the calculated area differs from the actual area. To overcome this problem, Warren and DuBois (1964) introduced a "correction factor k." This was a dimensionless coefficient, 0.65, derived from model tests of the upper vocal tract. Using short tubes that varied in area from 2.4 to 120.4 mm^2, they determined that an average value of 0.65 would suffice for the range of areas typically encountered in speakers with inadequate VP structures.

Based on their model tests, Warren and DuBois (1964) modified the theoretical equation as follows:

$$A = \hat{V}/k[2(p_1 - p_2)/D]^{1/2}$$

where k is 0.65. Although Warren and DuBois (1964) referred to this as a "working equation," it has subsequently become known as the *orifice equation*, which is now defined as the formula to calculate the minimal cross-sectional area of the VP valve by measuring the differential pressure across the orifice and rate of airflow simultaneously.

Application of the Pressure-Flow Technique

Air pressures during consonant production can be associated with a moving airstream (e.g., the fricative /s/) or a nonmoving air volume (e.g., the stop-plosive /p/). To detect these air pressures, catheters with small openings must be positioned behind the articulators of interest. To detect static pressures associated with fricative sounds, care must be taken to ensure that the opening of the catheter is positioned perpendicular to the direction of airflow. To detect stagnation pressures associated with stop consonants, the orientation of the catheter within the vocal tract is inconsequential—as long as it is behind the articulator of interest—due to equal pressure being exerted in all directions (Baken & Orlikoff, 2000). Practical placement of the catheters, therefore, is an important issue that will be addressed below.

Warren and DuBois (1964) originally used a balloon-tipped catheter placed in the posterior oropharynx (see Figure 15–2A and B). The catheter was passed through a nostril and secured by a cork at a level just below the resting velum. The catheter was then connected to a calibrated differential air pressure transducer referenced to atmospheric pressure. A larger plastic tube was fitted to the

speaker's other nostril and connected to a calibrated flowmeter. Because the balloon-tipped catheter was positioned behind the tongue, stagnation pressures associated with the place of articulation of all stop sounds (e.g., bilabials, lingual-alveolars, and velars) could easily be detected. These pressures reflected the driving pressure before the VP orifice, corresponding to Point A in Figure 15–1. Warren and DuBois (1964) noted that the use of a thin-walled balloon reduced pressure measurements by approximately 3% as compared to an open-tip catheter. The balloon was used, however, to eliminate the possibility of saliva occluding the catheter. An additional advantage of using a transnasal placement of a catheter is that it does not interfere with tongue movements during articulation.

A disadvantage of the pressure-flow technique, as illustrated in Figure 15–2, is that the differential pressure recorded during speech also includes a nasal pressure component when the VP portal is open. To overcome this problem, Warren and DuBois (1964) first instructed the speaker to breathe lightly

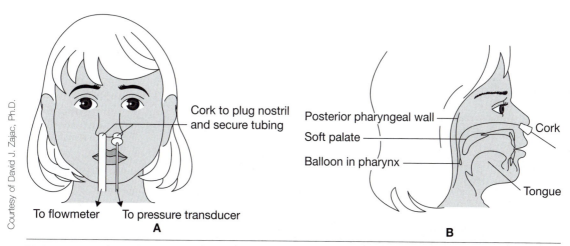

FIGURE 15–2 (A and B) The pressure-flow method as originally described by Warren and Dubois (1964). (A) Front view. (B) Side View. A balloon-tipped catheter is placed in the oropharnyx.

through the nose with the lips closed. The differential pressure and nasal airflow values obtained during breathing were then plotted as x and y coordinates. As noted by Warren and DuBois (1964), although the differential pressure in theory also contains a VP orifice component during breathing, at low rates of nasal airflow typical of speech, this component is too small to be recorded. During speech, the measured flow rate for a specific segment is used to determine the nasal pressure component from the breathing plot. This pressure is then subtracted from the differential pressure obtained during speech.

In a subsequent report by Warren (1964), the pressure-flow technique was modified to permit direct estimation of the differential pressure across the VP orifice during speech production. As illustrated in Figure 15–3, a catheter was placed in the oral cavity to detect oral-pharyngeal pressure below the VP orifice and another catheter was placed in one of the nostrils. The latter catheter was held by a cork stopper that also served to occlude the nostril and create a stagnation pressure downstream

of (i.e., beyond) the VP orifice. The oral and nasal catheters were connected to a calibrated differential pressure transducer. The remaining nostril was used to detect nasal airflow as described above. These modifications, especially the elimination of a balloon passed through the VP port, greatly facilitated clinical application of the pressure-flow technique.

A final modification of the pressure-flow technique was described by Warren, Dalston, Trier, and Holder (1985). Instead of recording differential oral-nasal pressure by means of a single transducer, they recorded oral and nasal pressures separately by using two pressure transducers—each referenced to atmospheric pressure. The differential pressure needed for the orifice equation was then calculated from the oral and nasal pressure values. An advantage of this modification was that true oral air pressure was obtained that could be compared to normative data. An estimate of subglottal pressure, therefore, could also be inferred from the oral pressure value during production of voiceless stop consonants.

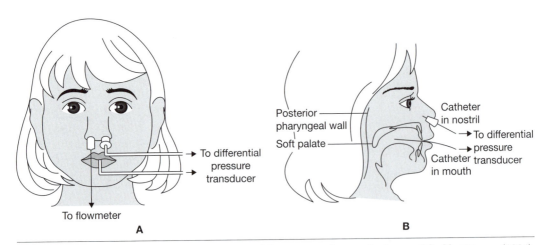

Courtesy of David J. Zajac, Ph.D.

A

To differential pressure transducer

To flowmeter

B

Posterior pharyngeal wall

Soft palate

Catheter in nostril

To differential pressure transducer

Catheter in mouth

FIGURE 15–3 (A and B) Front and side views of the pressure-flow method as modified by Warren (1964). Open-end catheters are placed in the nostril and the oropharnyx.

INSTRUMENTATION AND CALIBRATION

The basic equipment for speech aerodynamics includes catheters, a flow tube, transducers, and a heated pneumotachograph. Calibration equipment is also required. These instruments are described in the following sections.

Equipment

The speech aerodynamic procedure involves the use of a nasal catheter, an oral catheter with small opening into the oral cavity, and a flow tube for the other nostril. *Transducers* then convert the detected air pressure or flow into electrical signals for further processing. Transducers vary in construction, design, and performance characteristics. Figure 15–4 illustrates two types of differential air pressure transducers useful for speech work. A variable *capacitance* (ability to store energy) transducer (Figure 15–4A) consists of a diaphragm and an insulated electrode that forms a variable capacitor. As pressure is applied to the high (center) port relative to the low (or atmospheric) port, capacitance increases in proportion. Two of the transducers shown in Figure 15–4A have a pressure range of 0–15 inches (~0–38 cm) of water, useful for recording most pressures associated with speech activities. The upper limit of these transducers, for example, is approximately twice as high as pressures associated with even loud speech. The other two transducers shown have a pressure range of 0–0.5 inches (0–1.27 cm) of water, useful for recording the typically low airflow rates associated with speech. Solid state transducers are illustrated in Figure 15–4B. Again, two of the transducers have relatively high ranges required for speech pressures, whereas two have lower ranges appropriate for recording speech airflow. Both types of transducers have good response times (especially the solid state) and exhibit little drift (especially the variable capacitance).

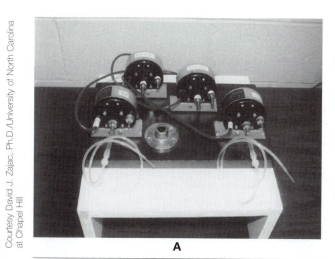

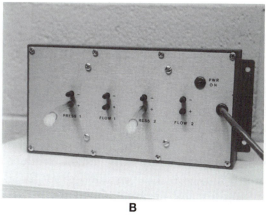

A   **B**

FIGURE 15–4 (A and B) (A) Four variable-capacitance differential pressure transducers. The two in the foreground are used to measure air pressures. The two in the background are used to measure airflows. (B) Four solid-state differential pressure transducers. Two are used to measured air pressures and two are used to measure airflows.

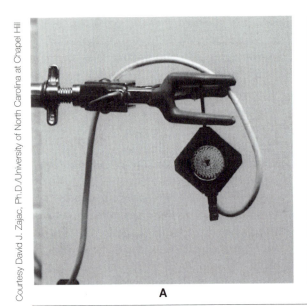
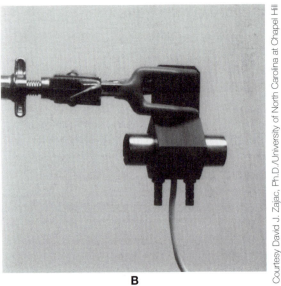

Courtesy David J. Zajac, Ph.D./University of North Carolina at Chapel Hill

A

B

Courtesy David J. Zajac, Ph.D./University of North Carolina at Chapel Hill

FIGURE 15–5 (A and B) (A) Front view of a bidirectional pneumotachograph showing resistive channels. (B) Side view of pneumotachograph showing static pressure ports.

The recording of speech airflow also requires the use of a heated *pneumotachograph*, which is a device that determines the rate of airflow. This device, illustrated in Figure 15–5, provides a resistance by channeling airflow through a bundle of small-diameter tubes housed within a larger conduit. The two pressure taps are connected to the ports of a differential pressure transducer. As indicated above, because the pressure drops associated with rates of airflow during speech are relatively low, a pressure transducer with a range of 0–0.5 or 0–1.0 inches (1.27–2.54 cm) of water is appropriate. The rate of airflow through the pneumotachograph is determined by measuring the differential pressure drop. Higher rates of airflow produce a proportionally higher pressure drop for the given resistance. Pneumotachographs are available in different sizes for different applications. As indicated by Baken and Orlikoff (2000), the Fleisch 1 pneumotachograph (Figure 15–5) is appropriate for many speech applications. It has a maximum useful flow rate of 1.0 L/s, a resistance of 1.5 cm H_2O/L/s, and a dead space of 15 ml.

Calibration

Calibration of pressure-flow instrumentation is required to ensure that the output of the transducers is consistent with a known input. Calibration of pressure transducers is typically done using a *manometer*, which is a device that usually consists of a liquid column to measure pressures.

The U-tube water manometer consists of a U-shaped glass tube partially filled with water. A scale—usually in centimeters of water (cm H_2O)—is positioned so that zero aligns with the meniscus (curve) of the water column. When a pressure is applied to one leg of the manometer, it depresses the column of water in that leg while elevating the column of water in the other leg. The amount of applied pressure is determined by summing the magnitude of displacement in both legs of the manometer. If the first column was depressed by 3 cm, for example, and the second column was elevated by 3 cm, then a total pressure of 6 cm H_2O would be applied.

A well-type manometer (Figure 15–6) is similar to a U-tube, but it provides direct reading of applied pressures. This type of manometer has a calibrated reservoir (the left leg in Figure 15–6) filled with gauge oil of a specific gravity. Zero on a centimeter scale is aligned with the meniscus of the reservoir. When pressure is applied to the reservoir, it causes the fluid to rise in a connected column. The height of the column of fluid indicates the applied pressure. Although a well-type manometer is easier to use than a U-tube, it has the disadvantage that specific gauge oil must be used to ensure accurate calibration. Digital manometers are also available that eliminate the need for any type of fluid-filled device.

Calibration of the pneumotachograph is typically accomplished by using a compressed air supply and *rotameter*, a device to measure rate of airflow, as illustrated in Figure 15–7. A float or ball in the rotameter rises in proportion to the applied rate of airflow. A Gilmont rotameter is shown in Figure 15–7. This rotameter is calibrated in arbitrary units from 0 to 100. The units must be converted to ml/s (or L/s) by means of a calibration curve provided by the manufacturer. Other types of rotameters are available that are calibrated in units such as ml/s. A large volume syringe (e.g., 1–3 liters) may also be used to apply a known quantity of air across the pneumotachograph for calibration purposes. The advantage of this approach is that it eliminates the need for a compressed air supply that may not be available in all test settings.

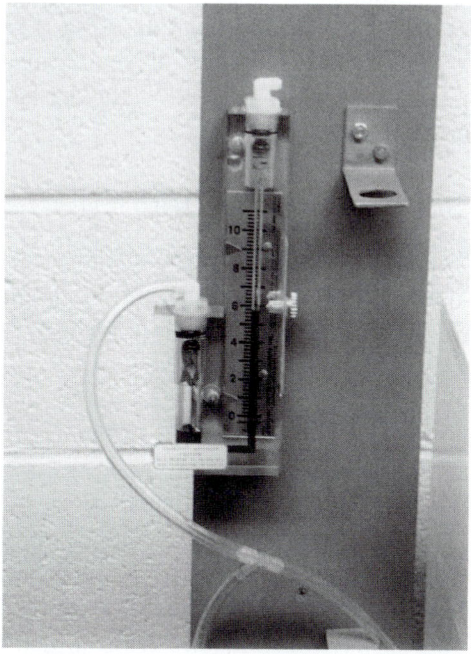

FIGURE 15–6 Well-type manometer. Applied pressure to the reservoir (left side) displaces the column of fluid on the right.

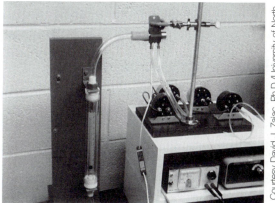

FIGURE 15–7 Calibration of pneumotachograph. A compressed air supply (not shown) delivers a known flow rate to a rotameter (left side in figure) that is coupled to a pneumotachograph and differential pressure transducer.

Calibration of computer-based aerodynamic systems also involves the use of software programs that determine and store calibration (or scale) factors for the various pressure transducers. The numerical scale factors indicate the relationship between the electrical voltage output of the transducer and the known input (i.e., the applied air pressure or flow).

Currently, there are several manufacturers of speech aerodynamic equipment. They typically provide the basic components for complete assessment of patients, including calibration devices and software programs. If clinicians are not familiar with calibration procedures, it is suggested that they seek assistance from someone with the requisite background (e.g., electrical technician, mechanical engineer) to set up and calibrate the instrumentation.

ASSESSMENT OF THE NASAL AIRWAY

Aerodynamic instrumentation can be used to evaluate nasal respiration and to quantify upper airway obstruction. Because nasal respiration involves resistance to airflow by both the nasal cavity and the velopharynx, obstruction may occur at either or both of these sites.

Nasal Airway Obstruction

Nasal airway obstruction is common in individuals with a history of cleft lip/palate or other craniofacial anomalies. This can be caused by maxillary retrusion, cranial base anomalies, a narrow hypopharynx, or enlarged adenoids—all of which restrict the nasopharyngeal airway. Other conditions such as a septal deviation, choanal atresia, or a stenotic naris can also restrict the size and patency of the nasal cavity. Even acute conditions, such as congestion or mucosal hypertrophy, can reduce nasal airway

size. Any condition that obstructs and therefore attenuates the airflow through the nasopharynx or nasal cavity is a cause of nasal airway obstruction. Such obstruction may cause hyponasal resonance.

Individuals with cleft lip/palate are also susceptible to nasal airway obstruction as a consequence of the surgical procedures used to repair the defects. Indeed, work by Warren and colleagues indicated that children with repaired unilateral cleft lip and palate have significantly reduced nasal airway size as compared to noncleft children (Warren, Hairfield, Dalston, Sidman, & Pillsbury, 1988). Individuals with a cleft of the soft palate who undergo secondary surgical procedures for residual velopharyngeal insufficiency are also at risk for posterior nasal airway obstruction. Such obstruction may not only result in hyponasal resonance, it may also interfere with health and daily living activities if severe enough to cause obstructive sleep apnea. Therefore, the evaluation of nasal resistance during respiration is of significance to both the speech-language pathologist and otolaryngologist.

Nasal Resistance and Rhinomanometry

Traditionally, measurements of nasal airway resistance have been obtained by using the techniques of anterior and posterior rhinomanometry (Smith & Kuehn, 2007). These techniques involve the measurement of the pressure encountered by air passing through the nasal cavity (Clement, 1984). With posterior rhinomanometry (Figure 15–8), the differential pressure between the oropharynx and the external nostrils, along with the simultaneous rate of nasal airflow, are determined. The resulting nasal airway resistance measure, therefore, includes components of both the velopharynx and the nasal cavities. As

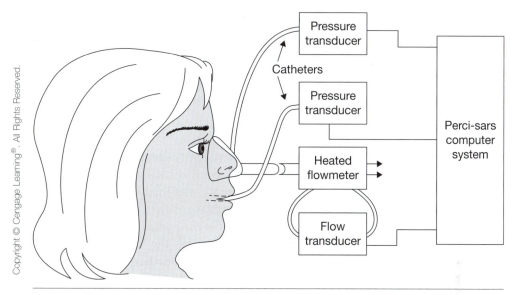

FIGURE 15–8 Posterior rhinomanometry. Both nostrils are evaluated simultaneously.

previously indicated, however, the relaxed velum typically produces a negligible pressure drop during quiet breathing. With anterior rhinomanometry (Figure 15–9), the differential pressure is obtained between the exit of the nose and the atmosphere. This is achieved by occluding one of the nostrils with a cork/ catheter assembly. As previously described, this condition creates a stagnation pressure downstream of the velopharynx. This pressure serves as the upstream (or driving) pressure to atmosphere. Because of the need to occlude a nostril, anterior rhinomanometry measures the resistance of the unoccluded nostril only. To

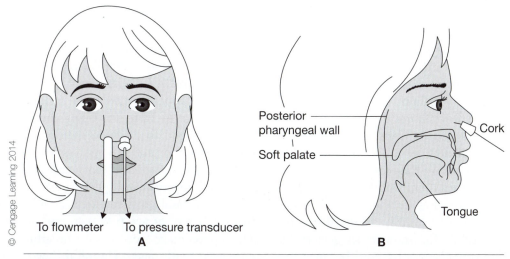

FIGURE 15–9 (A and B) (A) Front view of anterior rhinomanometry. Each nostril is evaluated separately. (B) Side view.

obtain resistance of the other nostril, the cork/catheter assembly and the nasal flow tube are reversed, and the measurement is repeated. With either anterior or posterior rhinomanometry, it is important that the individual maintain lip closure while breathing in order to obtain valid results.

Once differential air pressure and nasal airflow measures are obtained by either anterior or posterior rhinomanometry, nasal resistance (R_n) may be calculated as follows:

$$R_n = P/\hat{V}_n$$

where P is differential pressure in cm H_2O and $\hat{V}_n$ is nasal airflow in L/s. Nasal resistance, therefore, is expressed in units of cm H_2O/L/S. Although this formula is universally accepted for the calculation of nasal resistance, it is valid only when turbulent flow conditions are not present during nasal respiration (Clement, 1984). Depending on the degree of respiratory effort (i.e., the driving pressure provided by the lungs), airflow through the nasal cavity may be laminar or turbulent. *Laminar airflow* is steady and smooth due to the lack of significant resistance. When airflow is laminar in nature, the relationship between pressure and flow is linear, and the above equation for nasal resistance is valid. Convolutions and irregularities in the passages of the nasal cavities may cause *turbulent airflow*, which is chaotic and irregular. When airflow becomes turbulent, the pressure-flow relationship is quadratic and the resistance equation must be modified accordingly. To overcome this problem, many clinicians measure nasal resistance at relatively low rates of airflow to avoid turbulent conditions and to ensure that comparisons among individuals are valid (Allison & Leeper, 1990; Berkinshaw, Spalding, & Vig, 1987; Warren, Duany, & Fischer, 1969). Berkinshaw and colleagues (1987), for example, suggested that a flow rate of 0.250 L/s be used because it is

laminar in nature and can easily be achieved by individuals even with nasal obstruction.

Estimation of Nasal Cross-Sectional Area

Warren (1984) demonstrated that the "orifice equation" could also be applied to pressure-flow measurements obtained during rhinomanometry to estimate nasal cross-sectional area. The use of an area measure effectively circumvents the problem of calculating nasal resistance when airflow is turbulent. This approach permits the calculation of the *nasal valve*, which is the smallest cross-sectional area of the nasal cavity. The nasal valve is located approximately 1 cm posterior to the entrance of the nose from the pharynx and is bordered by the septal wall medially, the alar cartilage laterally, and the anterior portion of the inferior turbinate (Bridger, 1970). There is a nonlinear relationship between nasal cross-sectional area and nasal airflow in adults with varying degrees of nasal obstruction (Warren, Hairfield, Seaton, & Hinton, 1987). Warren and colleagues showed that the rate of nasal airflow was controlled by nasal cross-sectional area only when the nasal airway size was less than 0.40 cm^2.

Subsequent studies have indicated that the size of the nasal airway is age-dependent (Smith, Patil, Guyette, Brannan, & Cohen, 2004; Warren et al., 1988; Warren, Hairfield, & Dalston, 1990). As with facial growth, nasal airway size appears to continue to increase up until the age of 16 to 18. Using the pressure-flow technique to evaluate children between the ages of 6 and 15 years, Warren and colleagues (1990) found that nasal airway size increased approximately 0.032 cm^2 each year, and mean nasal cross-sectional area increased from 0.21 cm^2 at age 6 to 0.46 cm^2 at age 14. The percentage of nasal breathing also increased with age. Therefore, age should always be considered when assessing the status of the nasal airway in children and adolescents.

Clinical Procedures: Posterior Rhinomanometry

The specific procedures of posterior rhinomanometry (Figure 15–8) are summarized as follows:

1. Nasal resistance and area are measured for both nostrils during inhalation and exhalation of quiet respiration.

2. A heated pneumotachograph is connected to a nasal mask, which is fitted snugly over the patient's nose. The rate of nasal airflow is measured in L/s and recorded by a computer.

3. A catheter connected to a pressure transducer is placed in the patient's mouth. This catheter detects oropharyngeal air pressure. Pressure is measured in cm H_2O and recorded by the computer.

4. A second catheter connected to a pressure transducer is inserted through the wall of the nasal mask. This catheter detects mask pressure—or the pressure external to the nostrils.

5. During the examination, the patient breathes quietly through the nose while maintaining lip closure. Simultaneous recordings are made of the rate of nasal airflow, oropharyngeal pressure, and mask pressure.

The pressure-flow breathing records from an adult without nasal obstruction are illustrated in Figure 15–10. The figure shows oropharyngeal pressure, nasal (i.e., mask) pressure, nasal airflow, and calculated differential pressure from top to bottom, respectively. The three cursors labeled "I" indicate peak flow points during inspiration where measurements of nasal resistance and area were calculated. The three cursors labeled "E" show corresponding measurements made during expiration. All measurements and means are printed at the bottom of the figure. In addition, the rectangular boxes labeled "E Means" and "I Means" on the left of the figure provide a summary of the mean measurements for each parameter except nasal resistance. The mean nasal areas of the individual were 62.2 and 67.5 mm^2 during expiration and inspiration, respectively. As indicated by Warren (1984), a mean nasal area of approximately 60 mm^2 is typical of adults without nasal impairment.

Clinical Procedures: Anterior Rhinomanometry

The specific procedures of anterior rhinomanometry (Figure 15–9) are summarized as follows:

1. Nasal resistance and area are measured for each nostril separately during both inhalation and exhalation of quiet respiration.

2. A nasal flow tube connected to a heated pneumotachograph is placed snugly in one nostril of the patient. The rate of nasal airflow is measured in L/s and recorded by a computer.

3. A cork/catheter assembly connected to a pressure transducer is placed in the patient's other nostril. This catheter detects nasal cavity air pressure. Pressure is measured in cm H_2O and recorded by the computer.

4. During the examination, the patient breathes quietly through the nose while maintaining lip closure. Simultaneous recordings are made of the rate of nasal airflow and nasal cavity pressures. The

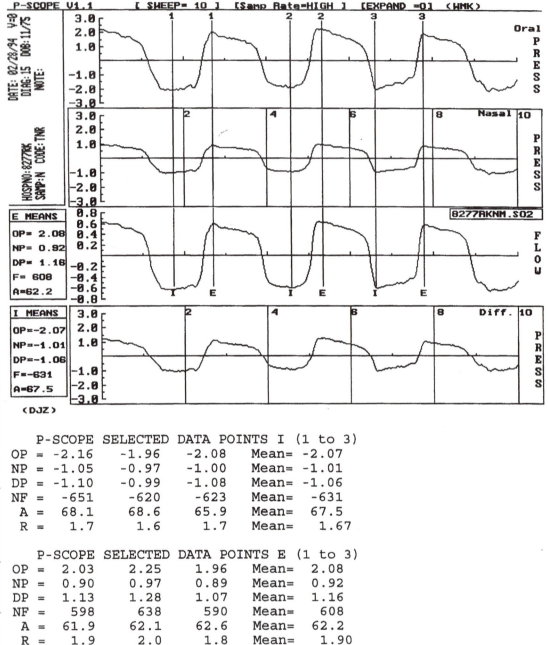

```
        P-SCOPE SELECTED DATA POINTS I (1 to 3)
OP =  -2.16    -1.96    -2.08    Mean=  -2.07
NP =  -1.05    -0.97    -1.00    Mean=  -1.01
DP =  -1.10    -0.99    -1.08    Mean=  -1.06
NF =   -651     -620     -623    Mean=   -631
 A =   68.1     68.6     65.9    Mean=   67.5
 R =    1.7      1.6      1.7    Mean=   1.67

        P-SCOPE SELECTED DATA POINTS E (1 to 3)
OP =   2.03     2.25     1.96    Mean=   2.08
NP =   0.90     0.97     0.89    Mean=   0.92
DP =   1.13     1.28     1.07    Mean=   1.16
NF =    598      638      590    Mean=    608
 A =   61.9     62.1     62.6    Mean=   62.2
 R =    1.9      2.0      1.8    Mean=   1.90
```

FIGURE 15–10 Pressure-flow recordings of breathing from an adult without nasal obstruction during posterior rhinomanometry. Calculated nasal area (a) is expressed in mm; calculated nasal resistance (R) is expressed in cm $H_2O/L/s$.

nasal flow tube and cork/catheter assembly are then reversed and the procedures repeated. As noted by Riski (1988), care must be taken when using anterior rhinomanometry to ensure that an airtight seal is obtained with the nasal flow tube and that the cork/catheter assembly does not deform the nasal valve area of the unoccluded nostril.

Using the above procedures, left and right nasal areas during inspiration for the individual illustrated in Figure 15–10 were 43.8 and 17.9 mm^2, respectively. Because the individual did not have posterior nasal airway obstruction, the summation of the left and right nasal areas (61.7 mm^2) approximates the total nasal area (67.5 mm^2) obtained by posterior rhinomanometry.

It must be noted that if an individual has significant posterior nasal obstruction, then the two techniques will not correspond. The use of both anterior and posterior rhinomanometry therefore has the potential to identify the site of nasal obstruction in patients with clefts of either the primary and/or secondary palates. Although it is beyond the intended scope of this chapter, some clinicians have discussed the use of rhinomanometric techniques to partition the VP and nasal components of measured nasal resistance. The interested reader is referred to Smith, Fiala, and Guyette (1989).

SPEECH AERODYNAMICS AND VELOPHARYNGEAL FUNCTION

The pressure-flow technique is ideally suited to determine the magnitude of intraoral air pressure levels and the rates of nasal air emission during consonant production, which are inversely related. It is important to realize, however, that intraoral air pressures vary somewhat with the type of consonant and phonetic context. Voiceless sounds are known to have greater intraoral pressure than voiced sounds due to the open glottis. In addition, intraoral air pressures tend to remain relatively constant at approximately 3.0 cm H_2O or higher, even in individuals with severe velopharyngeal dysfunction (Dalston, Warren, Morr, & Smith, 1988). This can be partly explained by the effects of increased nasal airway resistance, which is common in patients with a history of clefting as indicated above. Individuals with inadequate VP closure may also compensate for the oral pressure loss by increasing respiratory effort (Warren, Dalston, Morr, & Hairfield, 1989). Intraoral air pressures, therefore, may be affected by both increased nasal resistance and respiratory effort. Similarly, the rate of nasal airflow may be affected by increased nasal resistance. Measures of oral air pressure and/or nasal airflow, therefore, should be used with caution as indicators of VP function. The pressure-flow technique, however, which uses differential oral-nasal pressure, circumvents these limitations by providing estimates of the size of the VP orifice that are, in theory, unaffected by changes in either respiratory effort and/or nasal resistance.

Clinical Procedures

The pressure-flow technique is noninvasive and involves minimal risk to the patient. However, there is always the inherent risk that patients, especially children, may accidentally harm themselves around pressure-flow (or any laboratory) equipment. Standard safety precautions, therefore, should be followed. Care should also be taken to ensure that flow tubing and/or corks do not have sharp edges that may irritate or cut the nasal skin and/or mucosa.

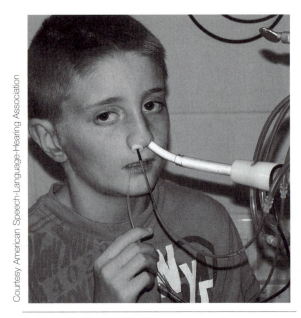

FIGURE 15–11 The pressure-flow technique to esti-mate velopharyngeal orifice areas during speech production. A flow tube is placed in the nose and pressure catheters are placed in the mouth and nostril.

The pressure-flow technique requires a certain level of cooperation in that the patient must place a flow tube in the nose and pressure catheters in the mouth and nostril. Figure 15–11 illustrates application of the pressure-flow technique with a school-age child. The specific procedures for estimating VP orifice size are as follows:

1. A plastic flow tube is inserted into the patient's more patent nostril. If anterior rhinomanometry has previously been performed, then the nostril with the larger area is selected. Otherwise, indirect estimation of the more patent nostril can be made using a mirror or detail reflector during quiet breathing with the mouth closed (Kuehn & Henne, 2003). The flow tube is connected to a heated pneumotachograph. The rate of nasal airflow is measured in L/s and recorded by a computer.

2. A cork/catheter assembly connected to a pressure transducer is placed in the patient's other nostril. This catheter detects a stagnation pressure downstream of the VP orifice. Pressure is measured in cm H_2O and recorded by the computer.

3. A catheter connected to a pressure transducer is placed in the patient's mouth. This catheter detects oral air pressure. Pressure is measured in cm H_2O and recorded by the computer.

As previously indicated, placement of the pressure catheter must be behind the articu-lator of interest in order to record a valid pressure. Also, if the target consonant is associated with a moving airstream (e.g., /s/), then the open end of the catheter must be positioned perpendicular to the direction of airflow. Because of these requirements, clini-cians most often evaluate VP function during production of the bilabial stop consonants. To evaluate the alveolar /s/ sound, the oral cath-eter can be occluded at the distal end, side holes placed in the catheter wall, and the catheter inserted to an area behind the alveolar ridge. Inserting the catheter from the side of the mouth during /s/ production often reduces interference with articulation. To detect stag-nation pressures associated with velar stops, a buccogingival catheter placement may be used. This approach permits valid detection of pressures associated with all oral consonants.

During the examination, simultaneous recordings are made of oral air pressure, nasal air pressure, and the rate of nasal airflow as the patient produces a series of speech samples designed to evaluate the VP mecha-nism. The speech samples typically employed by this author include the syllables /pi/, /pa/, /mi/, /si/; the word "hamper"; and the sentence "Peep into the hamper." The oral syllables are used because the VP mechanism must maintain closure during their repetition. The word "hamper" is tested because it contains the /mp/ sequence, which requires the speaker to rapidly adjust the VP mechanism from an open to closed configuration, thus allowing assessment of the dynamic aspects of VP closure (Smith & Kuehn, 2007). The sentence is included to embed the word "hamper" in an utterance and thus approximate the conditions associated with continuous speech. The fricative /s/ is tested because this sound is often associated with nasal air emission in speakers with VP function. In addition, learned phoneme-specific nasal air emission (PSNAE) is often associated with /s/ production. (This latter phenomenon is described in the following sections.) Overall, the pressure-flow technique can provide valuable information regarding intraoral pressure levels, the rates of nasal air emission, and estimates of velopharyngeal orifice size during consonant production.

The following sections present actual pressure-flow recordings of speakers with adequate VP function and with varying degrees of velopharyngeal dysfunction. The pressure-flow data were collected using the PERCI P-SCOPE system (MicroTronics, Chapel Hill, N.C.). In the recordings, oral pressure, nasal pressure, and nasal airflow are illustrated from top to bottom, respectively. In some recordings, calculated differential oral-nasal pressure is displayed. The pressures are shown in units of cm H_2O; airflow is expressed in L/s. Estimated VP areas are expressed in mm^2. Measurements were made at peak oral pressures for all oral consonants and at peak nasal flow for all nasal consonants. The locations of measurements are indicated by numbered cursors in the recordings. Estimated VP areas are most accurate when the measurements are taken at the point of peak flow, where the rate of flow change is zero (Warren, 1997). Peak pressures were used for oral consonants because (1) there is typically no nasal airflow for speakers with adequate VP function, and (2) peak nasal airflow typically coincides with peak pressure for speakers with inadequate velopharyngeal function. If peak nasal airflow does not coincide with peak oral air pressure, then measurements should be made at the flow peak. Care should be taken, however, to ensure that oral air pressure is not less than nasal air pressure as this invalidates area calculations. This situation often occurs in speakers with significant VP dysfunction.

Speech Aerodynamics of Normal Velopharyngeal Function

The following case history shows the typical pressure-flow results of an adult male speaker with normal velopharyngeal function.

CASE REPORT

Pressure-Flow Recordings from an Adult Male Speaker with Normal VP Function

Figures 15–12 through 15–14 illustrate the pressure-flow recordings from an adult male speaker with normal VP function saying the syllable /pi/, the word "hamper," and the sentence "Put the baby in the buggy," respectively. In Figure 15–12, the syllable is repeated eight times on a single breath, with relatively equal stress placed on each syllable. The magnitude and shape of the oral air-pressure pulses are strikingly consistent across the repeated productions. Typically, if equal stress is not maintained throughout an utterance, the first

(Continues)

(Continued)

pulse may have greater magnitude than the following pulses due to higher relaxation pressure available at the beginning of a breath group. The rise in slope of the first pressure pulse may also be steeper due to the lack of voicing from a preceding vowel. As indicated above, voicing tends to reduce the magnitude of air pressure available to the oral cavity.

Figure 15–12 also illustrates that nasal air pressure and nasal airflow are present and in synchrony during respiration before and after the utterance. This confirms the patency of both nostrils required for valid estimation of the VP orifice area. Normal onset and offset nasal air emissions are evident at the beginning and end of the utterance. Onset nasal emission reflects the transition of the VP mechanism from an open configuration during breathing to a closed configuration during speech. Offset nasal emission reflects the converse transition from speech to breathing. Close examination of the nasal airflow signal reveals that the speaker exhibited approximately 40–50 ml/s of airflow during the beginning of the second pressure pulse. This type of inconsistent nasal airflow may have occurred due to several reasons. First, even in the presence of airtight VP closure, muscular contractions of the velum may displace the nasal volume of air (Lubker & Moll, 1965). This phenomenon, however, is typically characterized by both positive and negative flows with rates less than ±10 ml/s (Thompson and Hixon, 1979; Hoit, Watson, Hixon, McMahon, & Johnson, 1994). Second, the nasal airflow may have occurred due to inadvertent movement of the flow tube. Artifact airflow resulting from compression of the flow tube, however, would also be bidirectional and relatively small in magnitude. Third, the VP mechanism of the speaker may have actually opened momentarily. Indeed, VP closure may not be complete for vowels as compared to consonants, especially low vowels (Bell-Berti & Krakow, 1990; Moll, 1962). Although the speaker produced the high vowel /i/, VP closure may still have been incomplete, giving rise to nasal emission when oral pressure increased to a level that was sufficient to overcome the resistance of the nasal cavity. This last explanation may be most likely because the nasal airflow occurred following the initial vowel and did not reoccur during any of the subsequent syllables. One may speculate, therefore, that the speaker was able to implement an adjustment that was facilitated by auditory feedback, aerodynamic feedback, or a combination of both.

Figure 15–13A illustrates the same speaker saying the word "hamper" five times. Nasal air pressure and airflow are evident throughout the nasalized segments of each word. P-SCOPE software (MiroTronics, Chapel Hill, N.C.) was used to measure oral air pressure, nasal air pressure, nasal airflow, and to calculate VP orifice areas of the /m/ and /p/ segments. The three vertical cursors labeled "M" indicate peak nasal flow where measurements were made for the /m/ segments. The three vertical cursors labeled "P" indicate peak oral pressure where measurements were made for the /p/ segments. As expected, peak nasal airflow associated with /m/ occurred before peak oral pressure for /p/. In addition, anticipatory nasal airflow occurred during the phonetic segments preceding peak nasal flow for /m/.

Figure 15–13B illustrates a single production of "hamper" with accompanying notation to indicate the phonetic segments. As illustrated, nasal airflow was higher during the voiceless /h/ than during the vowel immediately preceding the nasal consonant. This was expected due to increased resistance provided by the vocal folds during voicing. Nasal airflow reached its peak during the /m/ segment when lip closure occurred. Although not shown in the illustration, the simultaneous acquisition of the speech audio signal facilitated the identification of phonetic segments. This capability is available in a newer version of the software (PERCI-SARS, MicroTronics, Chapel Hill, N.C.).

As indicated in the measurements of Figure 15–13A, mean oral pressure of the speaker during /p/ averaged approximately 5–6 cm H_2O. This value is typical of normal adult speakers saying "hamper" (Zajac & Mayo, 1996). Children typically average higher oral pressures (7–8 cm H_2O) than adults, depending on their specific age (Zajac, 2000). The reason for higher pressures is most likely due to the tendency of children to speak louder than adults. Nasal airflow of the speaker during the /p/ segments in Figure 15-13 averaged 26 ml/s and the estimated VP area was 1.2 mm^2. Although these values are typical of both children and adults (Zajac, 2000), children tend to exhibit even lower rates of nasal airflow and smaller VP areas. This may be due to the fact that children typically possess greater amounts of adenoid tissue and smaller nasal and pharyngeal cross-sectional areas than adults. Nasal airflow of the speaker during the /m/ segments averaged 191 ml/s and the estimated VP area was 24.4 mm^2.

Finally, Figure 15–14 shows an example of continuous speech. The sentence "Put the baby in the buggy" was produced by the previous speaker. To record the oral pressures associated with the various consonants, a polyethylene catheter was heated and then molded so that its distal end approximated a 90-degree angle. The catheter was placed along the buccogingival sulcus with its angled end around the last mandibular molar, approximating the midline of the posterior oropharynx behind the tongue. This placement and orientation of the catheter permitted the valid recording of pressures associated with all consonants regardless of place of articulation. As illustrated in Figure 15–14, the voiceless consonants were associated with higher oral pressures than voiced consonants. This effect was most evident during production of /p/ and /b/, sounds that differ only in voicing. Consistent with normal VP function, Figure 15–14 also reveals the absence of nasal air pressure and flow during the utterance except for the nasal segment.

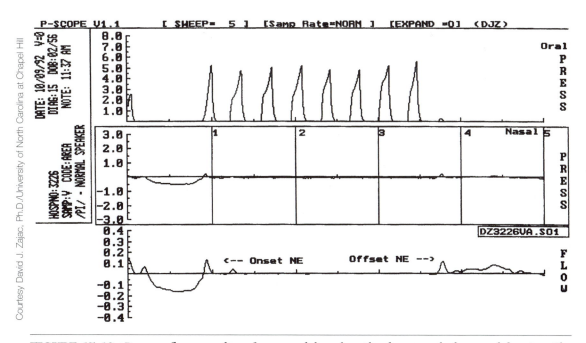

FIGURE 15–12 Pressure-flow recordings from an adult male with adequate velopharyngeal function. The syllable /pi/ was repeated eight times. Onset and offset nasal emission (NE) are evident at the beginning and end of the utterance.

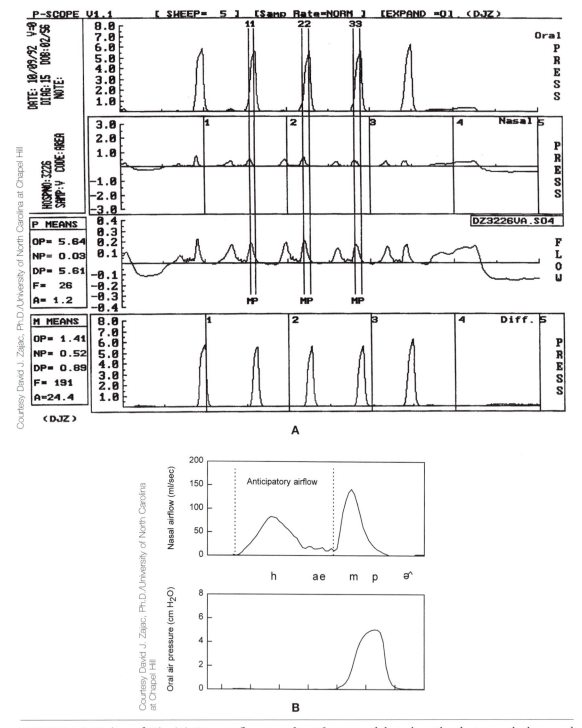

Courtesy David J. Zajac, Ph.D./University of North Carolina at Chapel Hill

Courtesy David J. Zajac, Ph.D./University of North Carolina at Chapel Hill

FIGURE 15–13 (A and B) (A) Pressure-flow recordings from an adult male with adequate velopharyngeal function. The word "hamper" was repeated five times. (B) Pressure-flow recordings of a single production of "hamper" with phonetic notation.

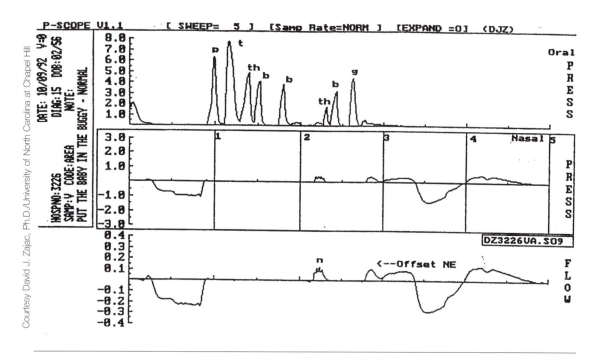

FIGURE 15–14 Pressure-flow recordings from an adult male with adequate velopharyngeal function. The sentence, "Put the baby in the buggy," was produced.

Speech Aerodynamics of Velopharyngeal Dysfunction

The following case histories show the pressure-flow results of various speakers with velopharyngeal dysfunction function.

Modifications for Young Children

The standard approach to pressure-flow testing (Figure 15–11) requires some degree of cooperation from the child and patency of both nostrils. If either or both of these conditions are lacking, the clinician may still gain valuable aerodynamic information by modifying the approach.

CASE REPORT

Pressure-Flow Recordings from a 12-Year-Old Boy with a Repaired Bilateral Cleft Lip and Palate

Figure 15–15 illustrates the pressure-flow recordings from a 12-year-old boy with a repaired bilateral cleft lip and palate while he repeated the syllable /pi/. Perceptually, the boy's speech was characterized by consistent but mild hypernasality, suggesting marginal VP function. Oral air pressures were somewhat reduced and variable during the utterance, ranging from approximately 2.5 to 5.5 cm H_2O. Consistent nasal airflow occurred during the /p/ and vowel segments, averaging approximately 75 and 40 ml/s, respectively. In Figure 15–15, nasal airflow

(Continues)

(Continued)

during /p/ segments is reflected by the flow peaks and numbered vertical cursors. Nasal airflow during vowels is reflected by the variable flow occurring between the flow peaks.

It must be noted that nasal airflow during vowel segments may not be readily detected by the pressure-flow method. This occurs because oral resistance to airflow is generally less than nasal resistance. Most of the airflow, therefore, will be shunted through the oral cavity even in the presence of a VP gap. The appearance of consistent nasal airflow during vowels in the speaker suggests the use of increased respiratory effort, altered lingual articulation as compensatory behaviors, and/or relatively reduced nasal airway resistance. Because of the consistent nasal air loss during /p/ production, however, the oral pressure measures may not be good indicators of overall respiratory effort.

The estimated size of this boy's VP gap was approximately 6 mm^2 during production of the /p/ segments. Based on this VP area, the boy's VP function would be categorized as "borderline adequate" according to criteria proposed by Warren and colleagues (1989). They suggested that VP areas under 5.0 mm^2 reflected adequate VP function, 5.0–9.9 mm^2 was borderline adequate, 10.0–19.9 mm^2 was borderline inadequate, and greater than 20 mm^2 was inadequate. It must be emphasized that these categories refer to the "respiratory requirements" of speech production, not perceptual aspects. The boy, whose recordings are illustrated in Figure 15–15, was capable of generating borderline-adequate oral air pressures for speech while clearly sounding hypernasal. This is an important distinction that clinicians must bear in mind when interpreting the VP area categories suggested by Warren and colleagues (1989). Overall, the pressure-flow records of the boy clearly indicate the marginal nature of his VP function. Borrowing a diagnostic term from Morris (1984), the boy, whose recordings are illustrated in Figure 15–15, may be considered to exhibit VP function that is "almost but not quite" adequate.

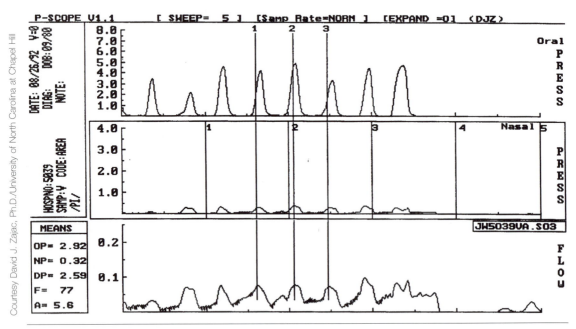

Courtesy David J. Zajac, Ph.D./University of North Carolina at Chapel Hill

FIGURE 15–15 Pressure-flow recordings from a 12-year-old boy with repaired cleft lip and palate. The syllable /pi/ was repeated eight times. Estimates of velopharyngeal area were calculated at peak nasal airflow associated with the /p/ segments.

Case Report

Pressure-Flow Recordings from a 7-Year-Old Girl with a Repaired Bilateral Cleft Lip and Palate

Figure 15–16 illustrates another example of a speaker with marginal VP function. The pressure-flow records are from a 7-year-old girl with a repaired bilateral cleft lip and palate while repeating the syllable /pi/. Perceptually, she exhibited inconsistent hypernasality and moderate hoarseness. The girl repeated the syllable eight times. Because the P-SCOPE software was set to trigger automatically on a positive oral air-pressure value, only partial pressure-flow data were recorded for the first syllable. The seven numbered cursors in the figure, therefore, indicate pressure-flow measurements that were made for the last seven syllables. These measurements are listed at the bottom of the figure.

Initially, the girl exhibited relatively low rates of nasal airflow during both consonant and vowel segments of the syllables. Estimated VP orifice areas during /p/ production were well under 5 mm^2 for the second (cursor 1) and third (cursor 2) syllables. During production of the fifth syllable (cursor 4), however, VP orifice size increased dramatically to almost 40 mm^2, causing a drop in oral pressure to 1.42 cm H$_2$O. Beginning with the next syllable (cursor 5), the girl appeared to use a compensatory strategy as evidenced by a rise in oral pressure with concomitant decreases in both nasal airflow and estimated orifice size. By production of the seventh syllable (cursor 6), she had achieved essentially airtight VP closure. It should be noted that the duration of her oral air-pressure pulses increased during this process. Warren and colleagues (1989) have suggested that increased respiratory effort is a compensatory strategy employed by speakers with inadequate VP function. The increased duration of the oral air-pressure pulses suggests that some type of respiratory strategy occurred. Such a strategy, however, may also result in laryngeal hyperfunction and perceived dysphonia. Indeed, as previously noted, the girl exhibited vocal hoarseness. Again, using the diagnostic terms of Morris (1984), the VP function of this speaker may be categorized as "sometimes but not always" adequate.

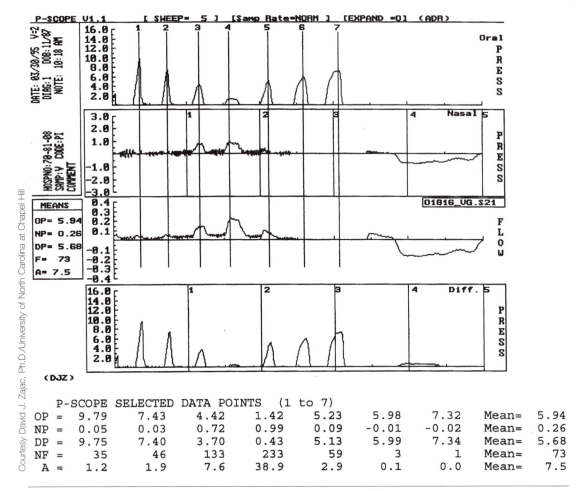

Courtesy David J. Zajac, Ph.D./University of North Carolina at Chapel Hill

```
P-SCOPE SELECTED DATA POINTS   (1 to 7)
OP =  9.79    7.43    4.42    1.42    5.23    5.98    7.32   Mean=  5.94
NP =  0.05    0.03    0.72    0.99    0.09   -0.01   -0.02   Mean=  0.26
DP =  9.75    7.40    3.70    0.43    5.13    5.99    7.34   Mean=  5.68
NF =    35      46     133     233      59       3       1   Mean=    73
 A =   1.2     1.9     7.6    38.9     2.9     0.1     0.0   Mean=   7.5
```

FIGURE 15–16 Pressure-flow recordings from a 7-year-old girl with repaired cleft lip and palate. The syllable /pi/ was repeated eight times.

CASE REPORT

Pressure-Flow Recordings from a 5-Year-Old Girl with an Unrepaired Submucous Cleft Palate and Hypernasal Speech

The pressure-flow characteristics of a speaker with severe VP dysfunction are presented in Figure 15–17 and Figure 15–18. The speaker was an almost 5-year-old girl with an unrepaired submucous cleft palate and hypernasal speech. Videofluoroscopy confirmed VP dysfunction. In Figure 15–17, she repeated the syllable /p/ four times. Because of the extent of her VP dysfunction, nasal air pressures (2.86 cm H_2O) were slightly but consistently higher on average than oral air pressures (2.84 cm H_2O). This finding—relatively rare except in cases of severe dysfunction—invalidates the estimated VP orifice area shown in the figure. Nasal airflow during

/p/production was 181 ml/s on average. It should also be noted, however, that relatively little nasal airflow was evident during vowel productions, as seen by the essentially baseline levels between the flow peaks.

In Figure 15–18, the same speaker repeated the word "hamper" five times. Because P-SCOPE software was set to an automatic trigger mode, pressure-flow data associated with the initial syllable in the first "hamper" were not recorded. The most striking feature of Figure 15–18 is the complete overlap of oral pressure, nasal pressure, and nasal airflow during the /mp/ segments as indicated by the numbered vertical cursors. In essence, oral-nasal coupling was so complete that the speaker was unable to aerodynamically distinguish the /m/ from the /p/ segments in the words. Warren and colleagues (1989) showed that this overlap of pressure and airflow is a distinctive feature of inadequate VP function when orifice areas exceed 20 mm^2. Zajac and Mayo (1996) provided normative pressure-flow and timing data for the /mp/ segment in adult speakers. They reported a mean temporal separation of the nasal airflow and oral pressure pulse of approximately 70–75 ms. Also demonstrated in Figure 15–18 is the speaker's inability to generate adequate oral air pressures. This is especially apparent after the initial productions of "hamper" when oral pressures dropped from approximately 2.5 cm H_2O (cursor 1) to 1.0 cm H_2O (cursor 2).

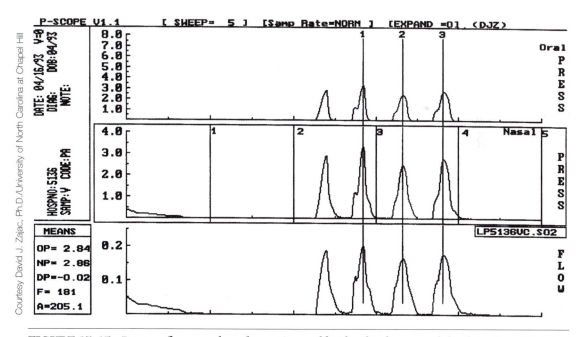

FIGURE 15–17 Pressure-flow recordings from a 5-year-old girl with submucous cleft palate. The syllable /pa/ was repeated four times. Note: Because differential pressure was slightly negative (see Means box), the area calculation is invalid as discussed in the text.

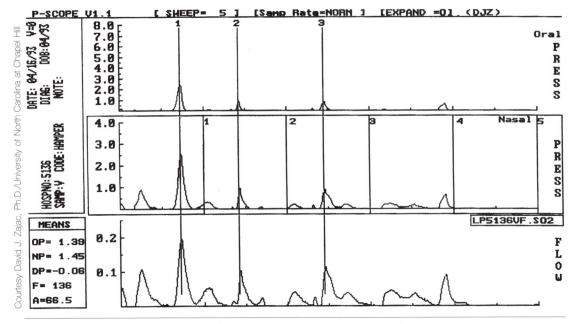

Courtesy David J. Zajac, Ph.D./University of North Carolina at Chapel Hill

FIGURE 15–18 Pressure-flow recordings from a 5-year-old girl with submucous cleft palate. The word "hamper" was repeated five times.

CASE REPORT

Pressure-Flow Recordings from a 10-Year-Old Girl with a Repaired Cleft Palate and a Superior-Based Pharyngeal Flap

The pressure-flow recordings of "hamper" from a 10-year-old girl with a repaired cleft palate and a superior-based pharyngeal flap are illustrated in Figure 15–19. Perceptually, the girl's speech was characterized by hyponasality, suggesting an obstructive pharyngeal flap. The aerodynamic correlate is clearly seen as a severe reduction in nasal airflow associated with the /m/ segments. In addition, expected anticipatory nasal airflow was entirely absent. Because rhinomanometric testing indicated normal nasal airway size prior to the secondary palatal surgery, these findings confirmed the suggestion of an obstructive pharyngeal flap.

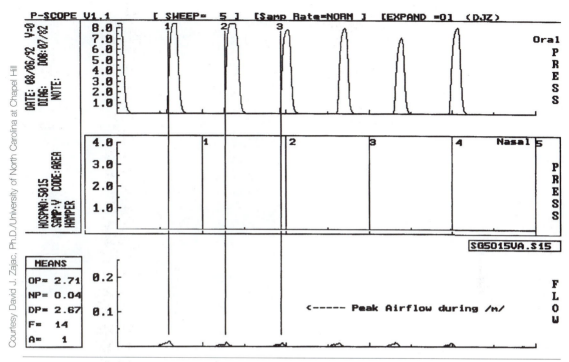

FIGURE 15–19   Pressure-flow recordings from a 10-year-old girl with a repaired cleft palate and a superior-based pharyngeal flap. The word "hamper" was repeated seven times.

CASE REPORT

Pressure-Flow Recordings from a 6-Year-Old Boy without a History of Cleft Palate Who Exhibited a Pattern of Phoneme-Specific Nasal Emission (PSNE)

Figure 15–20 illustrates the pressure-flow recordings of a 6-year-old boy without a history of cleft palate who exhibited a pattern of Phoneme-Specific Nasal Emission (PSNE). Although the boy exhibited adequate VP function, his findings are presented because they have differential diagnostic value. The boy's speech was characterized by audible nasal air emission associated with all sibilant speech sounds. Trost (1981) has described this type of articulation as a "posterior nasal fricative." All stop-plosive sounds and the /f/ and /v/ fricative sounds, however, were produced orally, indicating a learned articulatory pattern for the posterior nasal fricatives. The pressure-flow recordings in Figure 15–20 illustrate production of the target syllable /si/. Nasal airflow was evident during all expected /s/ segments (nasal pressure is not shown in the figure). More interesting, however, was the virtual lack of oral air pressures. As previously noted, oral air pressure is typically maintained at some minimal level even in the presence of severe VP dysfunction. The boy, however, had learned a pattern of phoneme-specific nasal emission that included the simultaneous articulation of a middorsum palatal stop during the posterior nasal fricative. This pattern of oral stopping was confirmed by subsequent perceptual and acoustic analyses of the separate oral and nasal audio signals obtained from the microphones of a Nasometer. In essence, the oral air pressure recordings were nearly atmospheric because the oral catheter was positioned at the alveolar ridge in anticipation of /s/. This anterior placement of the catheter did not detect the pressure buildup at the palatal location of stop articulation.

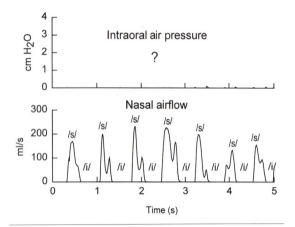

FIGURE 15–20 Pressure-flow recordings from a 6-year-old boy who exhibited a pattern of Phoneme-Specific Nasal Emission (PSNE). The syllable /si/ was repeated seven times. Oral air pressures were not detected due to deviant articulation.

Courtesy David J. Zajac, Ph.D./University of North Carolina at Chapel Hill

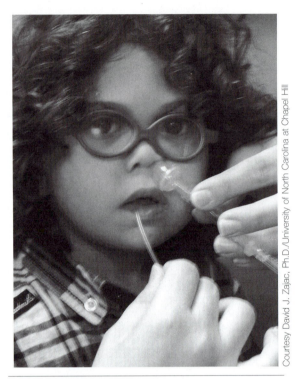

FIGURE 15–21 Determination of differential oral-nasal pressure of a young child.

One modification involves the acquisition of only differential oral-nasal air pressure data. As illustrated in Figure 15–21, the nasal pressure catheter is inserted into the nose while the clinician holds the oral pressure catheter behind the lips of the child. Because nasal airflow is not obtained, VP orifice area cannot be calculated. Adequacy of VP closure, however, can be inferred from differential pressure. According to Warren, Putnam Rochet, and Hinton (1997), VP closure is adequate if differential pressure is greater than 3.0 cm H_2O during production of /p/ in the word "hamper"; VP closure is borderline if differential pressure is between 1.0 and 2.9 cm H_2O; and closure is inadequate if differential pressure is below 1.0 cm H_2O. Similar to VP orifice area, differential oral-nasal pressure is relatively unaffected by changes in respiratory effort. Thus, this approach yields valid results even with young children who typically tend to speak louder than older children and adults.

A second modification of the pressure-flow technique involves the use of a mask to obtain both nasal airflow and nasal air pressure during speech. This approach is often necessary if a child is hesitant to insert tubes/catheters in the nose, and/or has a unilateral nasal obstruction. The equipment configuration for this approach is the same as for posterior rhinomanometry (refer to Figure 15–8). Although an estimate of VP orifice area can be obtained, it requires a differential pressure correction because the differential pressure recorded also includes a nasal pressure component. This is similar to the original method described by Warren and DuBois (1964). The differential pressure correction can be readily obtained by simply having the child breathe through the nasal mask with the lips closed around the oral pressure catheter.

Recently, Hoit and colleagues (Bunton, Hoit, & Keegan Gallagher, 2011; Thom, Hoit,

Hixon, & Smith, 2006) described a relatively simple aerodynamic technique to determine VP closure in infants and toddlers. The technique involves detection of nasal ram air pressure by means of a double-pronged cannula inserted into the nostrils. The end of the cannula is attached to a differential pressure transducer. As seen in Figure 15–22, the cannula does not occlude the nostrils of the child. Rather, the prongs of the cannula function as a *pitot tube*, a device used to determine airflow velocity, to detect nasal airflow emitted around the cannula. Because it is not part of a closed system, the cannula is relatively unaffected by movement artifacts. During utterances that are produced with VP closure, output of the pressure transducer shows a flat (atmospheric) trace. Conversely, during utterances that are produced with an open VP port, output of the pressure transducer shows a positive trace, as seen in Figure 15–23. Most young children readily adapt to wearing the cannula, or "nose microphone." A regular lapel microphone is used to record voice. A disadvantage of this technique is that information is limited to knowing whether the VP port is open or closed. Estimates of relative VP port size cannot be calculated.

Precautions and Limitations of the Pressure-Flow Technique

There are several factors of which the clinician must be aware during the acquisition and interpretation of pressure-flow measures. First, as previously indicated, to obtain accurate measures, the equipment must be properly calibrated. During an examination, all tubing, masks, corks, and catheters must be intact, snugly fitted to the patient (except the infant nasal cannula), and securely connected to other instrumental components. Tubing must be free of kinks, and nasal masks must not be

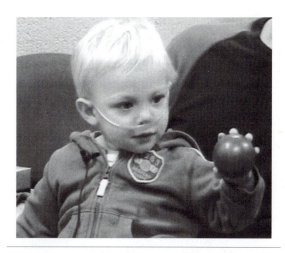

FIGURE 15–22 Double-pronged cannula used to record nasal air pressure during speech of young children and vocalizations of infants.
Courtesy David J. Zajac, Ph.D./University of North Carolina at Chapel Hill

so tight that they distort the nasal valve (Warren, 1997). To estimate VP orifice size, both nostrils of the patient must be patent if the standard pressure-flow configuration (Figure 15–11) is used.

One concern is that the accuracy of VP orifice size estimations decreases significantly with openings that are 80 mm^2 or above (Warren, 1997). This occurs due to the limits of the pressure transducers in detecting small pressure changes. As previously indicated, however, most perceptual characteristics of VP dysfunction are clearly evident when orifice size exceeds 20 mm^2.

There is also debate in the literature about the appropriate value of the correction factor k to be used in the orifice equation (Muller & Brown, 1981; Pelorson, 2001; Yates et al., 1990). As noted by Yates and colleagues (1990), 0.65 may not be the most appropriate value for the geometry of the human VP orifice. Because of this uncertainty, it should be emphasized that VP area estimates are only relative measures. That is, as long as

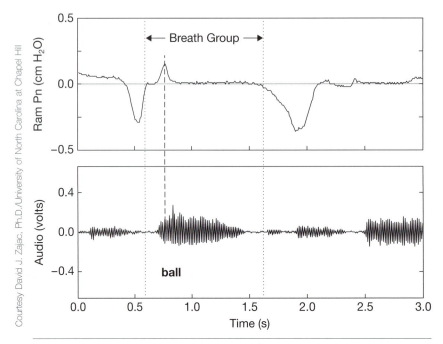

FIGURE 15–23 Nasal air pressure (top) and audio signal (bottom) during production of "ball" by a 2 year-old with repaired cleft lip and palate. Dashed vertical line shows positive nasal air pressure associated with the /b/ segment indicating an open velopharyngeal port. Nasal air pressure was obtained as illustrated in Figure 15–22.

speakers exhibit similar VP orifice geometries, a relative comparison among individuals is possible using any value of k. Indeed, Hixon (1966) omitted the k value entirely when estimating oral port sizes during fricative production.

Last, it must be reemphasized that, although the pressure-flow technique has the advantage of providing objective data relative to VP closure, it does not provide information about resonance of the sound during speech. Therefore, clinical evaluation of resonance should be done by perceptual assessment and/or the use of other instrumental techniques, such as nasometry.

SUMMARY

Since the original report by Warren and DuBois (1964), aerodynamic measures have been used by many researchers and clinicians to study the function of the velopharyngeal mechanism. The pressure-flow technique can give the examiner objective information regarding the approximate size of a velopharyngeal opening during speech, the extent of nasal emission and the presence of airway obstruction. Because of this, it should be considered an invaluable tool in the assessment of patients with cleft palate and/or suspected velopharyngeal dysfunction.

For Review and Discussion

1. What is meant by speech aerodynamics? Why is it relevant to evaluate this in an individual with questionable velopharyngeal closure?

2. What is the pressure-flow technique? What does it measure? What information can be obtained from a pressure-flow evaluation?

3. Describe the equipment necessary for a pressure-flow examination. Where are the catheters and flow tube placed?

4. What does the orifice equation measure when there is velopharyngeal insufficiency? What does it measure when assessing upper airway obstruction?

5. Which consonant would be expected to have a higher degree of intraoral pressure—a /p/ or a /b/? Why?

6. What types of speech utterances are typically used in a pressure-flow evaluation? Why do you think that short speech segments are used instead of longer segments?

7. What is the diagnostic significance of nasal airflow measures? What is the diagnostic significance of orifice size estimates? What does a VP orifice size of 40 mm^2 suggest?

8. What are the advantages of the pressure-flow technique? What are the disadvantages?

References

Allison, D. L., & Leeper, H. A. (1990). A comparison of noninvasive procedures to assess nasal airway resistance. *Cleft Palate Journal, 27,* 40–44.

Baken, R. J., & Orlikoff, R. F. (2000). *Clinical measurement of speech and voice* (2nd ed.). San Diego, CA: Singular.

Bell-Berti, F., & Krakow, R. A. (1990). Anticipatory velar lowering: A coproduction account. *Haskins Laboratories Status Report on Speech Research, SR-103/104,* 21–38.

Berkinshaw, E. R., Spalding, P. M., & Vig, P. S. (1987). The effect of methodology on the determination of nasal resistance. *American Journal of Orthodontic Dentofacial Orthopedics, 92,* 196–198.

Bridger, G. P. (1970). Physiology of the nasal valve. *Archives of Otolaryngology—Head & Neck Surgery, 92,* 543–553.

Bunton, K., Hoit, J. D., & Gallagher, K. (2011). A simple technique for determining velopharyngeal status during speech production. *Seminars in Speech and Language, 32*(1), 69–80.

Clement, P. A. R. (1984). Committee report on standardization of rhinomanometry. *Rhinology, 22,* 151–155.

Dalston, R. M., Warren, D. W., Morr, K. E., & Smith, L. R. (1988). Intraoral pressure and its relationship to velopharyngeal inadequacy. *Cleft Palate Journal, 25,* 210–219.

Hixon, T. J. (1966). Turbulent noise sources for speech. *Folia Phoniatrica, 18,* 168–182.

Hoit, J. D., Watson, P. J., Hixon, K. E., McMahon, P., & Johnson, C. L. (1994). Age and velopharyngeal function. *Journal of Speech and Hearing Research, 37,* 295–302.

Kuehn, D. P., & Henne, L. J. (2003). Speech evaluation and treatment of patients with cleft palate. *American Journal of Speech-Language Pathology, 12,* 103–109.

Lubker, J., & Moll, K. (1965). Simultaneous oral-nasal airflow measurements and cine-fluorographic observations during speech production. *Cleft Palate Journal*, 2, 257–272.

Moll, K. L. (1962). Velopharyngeal closure on vowels. *Journal of Speech and Hearing Research*, 17, 30–77.

Morris, H. L. (1984). Marginal velopharyngeal incompetence. In H. Winitz (Ed.), *Treating articulation disorders: For clinicians by clinicians*. Baltimore, MD: University Park Press.

Muller, E. M., & Brown, W. S. (1981). Variations in the supraglottal air pressure waveform and their articulatory interpretation. In N. Lass (Ed.), *Speech and language: Advances in basic research and practice* (vol. 4, pp. 317–389). New York, NY: Academic Press.

Pelorson, X. (2001). On the meaning and accuracy of the pressure-flow technique to determine constriction areas within the vocal tract. *Speech Communication*, 35, 179–190.

Peterson-Falzone, S., Hardin-Jones, M., & Karnell, M. (2001). *Cleft Palate Speech* (3rd ed.). St Louis, MO: Mosby.

Riski, J. E. (1988). Nasal airway interference: Consideration for evaluation. *International Journal of Orofacial Myology*, 14, 11–21.

Smith, B. E., Fiala, K. J., & Guyette, T. W. (1989). Partitioning model nasal airway resistance into its nasal cavity and velopharyngeal orifice areas during steady flow conditions and during aerodynamic simulation of voiceless stop consonants. *Cleft Palate Journal*, 21, 18–21.

Smith, B. E., & Kuehn, D. P. (2007). Speech evaluation of velopharyngeal dysfunction. *The Journal of Craniofacial Surgery*, 18(2), 251–261.

Smith, B. E., Patil, Y., Guyette, T. W., Brannan, T. S., & Cohen, M. (2004). Pressure-flow measurements for selected oral sound segments produced by normal children and adolescents: A basis for clinical testing. *Journal of Craniofacial Surgery*, 15(2), 247–254.

Sussman, J. E. (1992). Perceptual evaluation of speech production. In L. Brodsky, L. Holt, & D. H. Ritter-Schmidt (Eds.), *Craniofacial anomalies: An interdisciplinary approach*. St. Louis, MO: Mosby Yearbook.

Thom, S. A., Hoit, J. D., Hixon, T. J., & Smith, A. E. (2006). Velopharyngeal function during vocalization in infants. *Cleft Palate Craniofacial Journal*, 43(5), 539–546.

Thompson, A. E., & Hixon, T. J. (1979). Nasal airflow during normal speech production. *Cleft Palate Journal*, 16, 412–420.

Trost, J. E. (1981). Articulatory additions to the classical description of the speech of persons with cleft palate. *Cleft Palate Journal*, 18, 193–203.

Warren, D. W. (1984). A quantitative technique for assessing nasal airway impairment. *American Journal of Orthodontics*, 86, 306–314.

Warren, D. W. (1997). Aerodynamic assessments and procedures to determine extent of velopharyngeal inadequacy. In K. R. Bzoch (Ed.), *Communicative disorders related to cleft lip and palate* (4th ed.). Austin TX: Pro-Ed.

Warren, D. W., Dalston, R. M., Morr, K., & Hairfield, W. (1989). The speech regulating system: Temporal and aerodynamic responses to velopharyngeal inadequacy. *Journal of Speech and Hearing Research*, 32, 566–575.

Warren D. W., Dalston, R. M., Trier, W. C, & Holder, M. B. (1985). A pressure-flow technique for quantifying temporal patterns of palatopharyngeal closure. *Cleft Palate Journal*, 22, 11–19.

Warren, D. W., Duany, L. F., & Fischer, N. D. (1969). Nasal pathway resistance in normal and cleft lip and palate subjects. *Cleft Palate Journal, 6,* 134–140.

Warren, D. W., & DuBois, A. (1964). A pressure-flow technique for measuring velopharyngeal orifice area during continuous speech. *Cleft Palate Journal, 1,* 52–71.

Warren, D. W., Hairfield, W. M., & Dalston, E. T. (1990). Effect of age on nasal cross-sectional area and respiratory mode in children. *Laryngoscope, 100,* 89–93.

Warren, D. W., Hairfield, W. M., Dalston, E. T., Sidman, J. D., & Pillsbury, H. C. (1988). Effects of cleft lip and palate on the nasal airway in children. *Archives of Otolaryngology—Head & Neck Surgery, 114,* 987–992.

Warren, D. W., Hairfield, W. M., Seaton, D. L., & Hinton, V. A. (1987). The relationship between nasal airway cross-sectional area and nasal resistance. *American Journal of Orthodontic Dentofacial Orthopedics, 92,* 390–395.

Warren, D. W., Putnam Rochet, A., & Hinton V. (1997). Aerodynamics. In M. McNeil (Ed.), *Clinical management of sensorimotor speech disorders.* New York, NY: Thieme Medical Publisher.

Yates, C. C, McWilliams, B. J., & Vallino, L. D. (1990). The pressure-flow method: Some fundamental concepts. *Cleft Palate Journal, 27,* 193–198.

Zajac, D. J. (2000). Pressure-flow characteristics of /m/ and /p/ production in speakers without cleft palate: Developmental findings. *Cleft Palate–Craniofacial Journal, 37*(5), 468–477.

Zajac, D. J., & Mayo, R. (1996). Aerodynamic and temporal aspects of velopharyngeal function in normal speakers. *Journal of Speech and Hearing Research, 39,* 1199–1207.

Zajac, D. J., & Yates, C. C. (1991). Accuracy of the pressure-flow method in estimating induced velopharyngeal orifice area: Effects of the flow coefficient. *Journal of Speech and Hearing Research, 34,* 1073–1078.

ENDNOTE

[1]Although Yates and colleagues (1990) inferred that Warren and DuBois (1964) used "rectangular, thin plate orifices," Warren has clarified that the original model actually used short tubes to derive the k coefficient (personal communication, March 27, 2000).

CHAPTER

16

VIDEOFLUOROSCOPY

INTRODUCTION

Velopharyngeal insufficiency/incompetence (VPI) can be diagnosed based on the characteristics of the speech as determined through a perceptual speech evaluation alone. However, instrumental assessment of the velopharyngeal valve, as can be done through videofluoroscopy, is usually indicated to determine the cause, the approximate size, and particularly the location of the velopharyngeal opening. This information is important to obtain so that the best form of surgical intervention can be determined.

Videofluoroscopy is an imaging technique used to obtain real-time moving images of internal structures. This is done through the use of a fluoroscope, which consists of an X-ray source and fluorescent screen. A *videofluoroscopic speech study* is the use of moving images of the velopharyngeal valve, along with simultaneous audio recordings, for the evaluation of velopharyngeal function during speech (Dudas, Deleyiannis, Ford, Jiang, & Losee, 2006; Lam et al., 2006; Rowe & D'Antonio, 2005; Shprintzen, 1995; Smith & Kuehn, 2007; Ysunza, Pamplona, Ortega, & Prado, 2008, 2011). Videofluoroscopy can help the examiner assess both the anatomical and physiological abnormalities that are causing VPI. This information is important so that the optimal surgical or prosthetic treatment for the patient can be determined. Videofluoroscopy is also used to assess swallowing and is called either a *modified barium swallow (MBS)* or a *videofluoroscopic swallowing study*.

Videofluoroscopy was first used for direct visualization of velopharyngeal function in the late 1960s and early 1970s, and it has been used ever since. With the advent of nasopharyngoscopy, however, it is not used as extensively as it once was, although it is still used by many centers, at least occasionally. Therefore, the professionals who treat patients with velopharyngeal dysfunction should be knowledgeable of its uses, advantages, and disadvantages. In addition, videofluoroscopy continues to be a powerful tool in the evaluation of swallowing disorders.

The purpose of this chapter is to explain how videofluoroscopy is used in evaluating velopharyngeal function. The specific procedures for a videofluoroscopic speech study are reviewed, and the interpretation of images is discussed as it relates to the diagnosis of VPI and recommendations for treatment.

HISTORY OF RADIOGRAPHY FOR VPI

Radiography refers to the use of the roentgen ray (X-ray) to image internal body parts. As the ray goes through the body, it creates an image on the other side. The image then shows structures as light images and air space as a dark image. Because the beam goes entirely through a structure, it projects the summation of all of the parts of that structure through which the beam passes. In other words, it shows whether the matter is consistent throughout or only occurs in a small portion of the line of the beam.

Conventional radiography depends on the natural attenuation of the different tissues. *Attenuation* is the combined absorption and scattering of radiation proton particles by the tissues. When there is greater attenuation, as in bone, fewer radiation particles reach the image, resulting in less exposure and hence an image that is near the white end of the spectrum. When there is less attenuation (as in air), more radiation particles reach the film, resulting in more exposure, so the image is near the black end of the spectrum.

Traditionally, radiographic images were recorded on film or videotape. Most systems now use high-resolution digital imaging. The many advantages of digital radiographs include the fact that they can be viewed on a computer, are of greater resolution, and can be stored electronically.

Most radiographic images are planar, or two-dimensional, in nature. To image a three-dimensional volume structure adequately, it must be examined in three mutually perpendicular planes to fully appreciate that structure (Pelo, Tassiello, Boniello, Gasparini, & Longobardi, 2006; Skolnick & Cohn, 1989; Skolnick, McCall, & Barnes, 1973). Of course, the velopharyngeal port is a three-dimensional volume structure.

Lateral Cephalometric X-rays

Lateral cephalometric X-rays are still radiographic images of the midsagittal plane of the head. They are typically taken in a dental professional's office, using a standard head holder. Through a process called *laminography*, which involves careful measurement of the distances and angles between particular landmarks on the image, orthodontists and oral surgeons use lateral cephalometric images to study and measure the craniofacial bones and parameters of growth.

The lateral "ceph" is a still picture that can be taken during phonation of a vowel or production of a prolonged /s/. It shows the hard palate, the velum at rest, velar length and height during phonation, and the posterior pharyngeal wall. The lateral ceph illustrates the cervical spine, angle of the cranial base, and the morphologic features of the facial skeleton. Cervical spine and cranial base anomalies that affect the position of the pharyngeal wall for velopharyngeal closure can be identified through this procedure. In the 1950s, lateral cephalometric X-rays were used extensively in cleft palate research. In fact, the role of adenoid tissue in velopharyngeal closure was better understood with the use of this procedure (Smith & Kuehn, 2007).

Despite its value in certain circumstances, cephalometric images are no longer used for routine assessment of velopharyngeal function for several reasons. First, the lateral ceph shows only the midsagittal section of the velopharyngeal portal. The lateral pharyngeal walls cannot be viewed. As a result, the examiner is likely to misdiagnose the presence or absence of velopharyngeal insufficiency about 30% of the time, as compared with the use of a multiview technique (Major, Flores-Mir, & Major, 2006; Williams & Eisenbach, 1981). Another problem is that the lateral ceph is a still image that can only show structure, but speech is dynamic with continual movement. Therefore, the ceph is not a good representation of true speech because the movement of the velopharyngeal structures cannot be evaluated (Kuehn & Henne, 2003). Finally, the image is a summation of all of the parts through which the beam travels. If the velum is touching on just one part of the posterior pharyngeal wall, it looks like complete closure on the lateral view because of this summation effect. Therefore, small openings are not easy to detect.

Cineradiography

The use of *cineradiography* as a method for evaluating velopharyngeal function was first introduced in the early 1950s. Often referred to as a *cine study*, this technique involved taking a series of 16 to 24 frames of radiographs per second, which were recorded on motion picture film. Multiple views were taken for appreciation of all aspects of the velopharyngeal valve. Although this procedure was far better than a lateral ceph, which showed only one view and no movement, there was no way to simultaneously record sound, and thus the speech, so correlating movement patterns with speech phonemes was not possible (Shprintzen, 1995). Another major disadvantage of this procedure was the relatively high dosage of radiation per study.

Videofluoroscopy

A significant methodological advancement was made with the introduction of radiographic procedure using videofluoroscopy (Skolnick, 1969, 1970; Skolnick & McCall, 1971). Through the use of multiple views, videofluoroscopy allows the examiner to visualize the structures and function of the velopharyngeal mechanism (Skolnick & Cohn, 1989). Unlike cineradiography, it allows simultaneous audio recording of the speech.

Multiview videofluoroscopy can be used to confirm the presence of a velopharyngeal opening and estimate the size of that opening (Lam et al., 2006). The cause of VPI can be differentiated between a short velum and a poor velar movement. Videofluoroscopy is not as helpful in assessing the extent and symmetry of lateral pharyngeal wall motion. In comparison with nasopharyngoscopy, videofluoroscopy is superior in showing the vertical movement of the velum during speech. It also provides a view of the entire length of the posterior pharyngeal wall during closure, which cannot be seen with nasopharyngoscopy.

Videofluoroscopy can help the examiner in determining surgical and prosthetic options for the treatment of VPI. It can also be helpful in assessing the placement of a prosthetic device, particularly a palatal lift. Finally, it can be used to evaluate the effects of surgical procedures, such as adenoidectomy, maxillary advancement, and a retropharyngeal implant (Havstam et al., 2005; Kendall, Leonard, & McKenzie, 2004).

Videofluoroscopy is not a good method for a postoperative evaluation of a pharyngeal flap or sphincter pharyngoplasty because the lateral ports after a pharyngeal flap and the central port after a sphincter pharyngoplasty cannot be easily visualized with videofluoroscopy. Therefore, if surgical revision may be needed for port insufficiency or for port obstruction, nasopharyngoscopy is a much better procedure.

Before using videofluoroscopy for evaluation of velopharyngeal function, the speech-language pathologist should refer to the practice document regarding videofluoroscopy, published by the American Speech-Language-Hearing Association (ASHA, 2004).

PREPARATION OF THE PATIENT

Most patients who require an evaluation of velopharyngeal function are children. For best results, it helps to prepare the patient and the family for the procedure before the day of the exam. Many centers send information to the family regarding the videofluoroscopy procedure at the time that the appointment is scheduled. Information about what to expect should also be sent to the child, preferably in the form of a storybook or coloring book. The child can even be given a list of the standard phrases and sentences to practice at home. When the patient and family receive information before the examination, the child is more likely to be cooperative during the procedure.

Regardless of prior preparation, the child may be nervous during the examination. Therefore, it is important that the speech-language pathologist and/or X-ray technologist speak calmly and softly to the child. It is best to tell the child exactly what will be done before it is done. The parents can help by encouraging the child and offering the child a reward for completing the study.

VIDEOFLUOROSCOPY PROCEDURE

The velopharyngeal port is a three-dimensional structure that operates as a sphincter, with movement from all sides of the port. With fluoroscopic imaging, however, only two-dimensional views can be obtained (Shprintzen, 1995; Shprintzen, Rakof, Skolnick, & Lavorato, 1977; Skolnick, 1975; Skolnick, McCall, & Barnes, 1973). Therefore, in order to fully evaluate all sides of the velopharyngeal port with fluoroscopy or any other form of radiography, it is necessary to obtain three mutually perpendicular planes (Kane, Butman, Mullick, Skopec, & Choyke, 2002; Skolnick & Cohn, 1989; Skolnick & McCall, 1971).

The views most commonly used with videofluoroscopy include the lateral view, the frontal view, and the base view. The name of the view (e.g., lateral view) denotes the direction in which the radiation beam passes through the body. In addition to the standard views, there are some supplemental views (Towne's view and oblique view) that can also be used for certain diagnostic circumstances. When multiple views are used, the examiner is able to evaluate the motion of all structures of the velopharyngeal valve.

Lateral View

For the *lateral view*, the beam enters the side of the head. As such, it shows the velum and posterior pharyngeal wall in a midsagittal plane. The examiner is able to view the effective length of the velum, velar movement and height during speech, the entire posterior pharyngeal wall, tongue movement, and the patency of an oronasal fistula when barium is injected in the nasal cavity.

For the lateral view, the patient is ideally placed in an upright position. The fluoroscopic table is vertically positioned, and the patient stands or sits between the table and the fluoroscopic screen (Figure 16–1). The head remains in a neutral position with the patient looking straight ahead.

For a young child who has difficulty holding still, the child can lie on the table on his or her side (Figure 16–2). A special pillow is used to support and stabilize the head. The disadvantage of this position is the potential effect of gravity on velar movement, although this effect may be negligible (Perry, 2010). In order to be sure that the head is not rotated or tilted during the study, the X-ray technician should always be sure that the ramus on both sides of the mandible are superimposed on the view. This is very important because if a true lateral view is not obtained, the beam will not go straight through the port. Therefore, it may appear that there is closure when there is not.

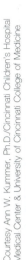

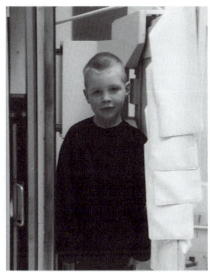

FIGURE 16–1 Patient position for the lateral view. The fluoroscopic table is vertically positioned and the patient stands or sits between the table and the fluoroscopic screen. The head remains in a neutral position with the patient looking straight ahead.

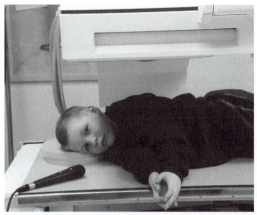

FIGURE 16–2 Alternate patient position for the lateral view. This is used if the patient needs more head support. For a young child who has difficulty holding still, the child can lie on the table on his or her side. A special pillow is used to support and stabilize the head. The disadvantage of this position is the potential effect of gravity on velar movement, although this effect may be negligible.

Frontal View

For the *frontal view* (also called the *anterior–posterior* or simply the *AP view*), the X-ray beam is directed through the nose so that it is tangential to the plane of the velar eminence, which is usually appreciated as an arc between the lateral pharyngeal walls. This allows the examiner to visualize the lateral pharyngeal walls at rest and during speech.

For the frontal view, the patient is positioned to face forward so that the beam is directed straight through the front of the nose. The patient can be upright or placed in a supine position (Figure 16–3). It is very important that the head is centered for the frontal projection and is not rotated. This can be determined by observing the nasal septum and making sure that it appears to be in midline. The septum should be equidistant from the lateral margins of the maxillary cavity, and the incisor teeth should appear to be on either side of the nasal septum, allowing for deviations in structures. During nasal breathing, the lateral pharyngeal

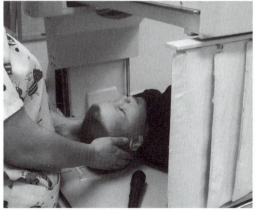

FIGURE 16–3 Patient position for the frontal or AP (anterior–posterior) view. The patient is placed in a supine position and the head is centered. This can be determined by observing the nasal septum through the fluoroscope and making sure that it appears to be in midline.

walls can be seen to bow outward on either side of the nasal septum. With speech, the lateral pharyngeal walls can be observed to bow inward where they appear to meet the area of the nasal septum.

Base View

For the *base view* (also called an *enface view*), the beam enters through the base of the chin and then up through the velopharyngeal port. This allows the examiner to see the entire velopharyngeal sphincter as if looking up through the port (Kuehn & Henne, 2003). With this orientation, the relative contributions of the velum, the lateral pharyngeal walls, and posterior pharyngeal wall to closure can be determined.

For the base view, the patient is placed on the X-ray table in a prone position. The patient is then asked to assume a "sphinx position" by pulling the head up and placing the upper body weight on the arms and elbows (Figure 16–4). The head and the back are then hyperextended so that the X-ray beam can be directed vertically through the base of the chin. The correct positioning of the base view is actually very difficult, because the beam must be directly at right angles to the plane of closure. Otherwise, the port will not be visualized or the dimensions of the port will be severely distorted. The border of the velum is not as easy to appreciate as the pharyngeal walls with this view. Also, the presence of large adenoids can also affect the interpretation of this view (Witt, Marsh, McFarland & Riski, 2000).

Towne's View

For the *Towne's view*, the beam goes down into the port from above. It has been described as an alternative to the base view because it also provides an *en face* orientation, although from above rather than from below (Stringer &

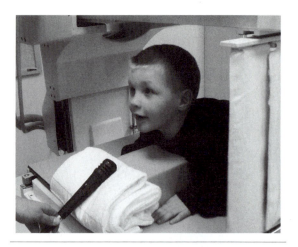

FIGURE 16–4   Patient position for the base view. The patient is placed on the X-ray table in a prone position and then asked to assume a "sphinx position" by pulling the head up and placing the upper body weight on the arms and elbows. The head and the back are then hyperextended so that the X-ray beam can be directed vertically through the base of the chin and then up through the velopharyngeal port. The correct positioning is important because the beam must be directly at right angles to the plane of closure.
Courtesy Ann W. Kummer, Ph.D./Cincinnati Children's Hospital Medical Center & University of Cincinnati College of Medicine

Witzel, 1986, 1989). As such, the Towne's view shows the perimeter of the velopharyngeal valve.

For the Towne's view, the patient is seated upright with the chin tucked and the head hyperflexed (Kuehn & Henne, 2003). The beam goes through the top of the head and intersects the plane of the portal in a perpendicular manner. When the adenoids are large, the Towne's view may provide a better view of the velopharyngeal portal than the base view (La Rossa, Brown, Cohen, & Spackman, 1980; Stringer & Witzel, 1986, 1989).

Oblique View

The *oblique view* might be chosen if a satisfactory base view cannot be obtained due to large adenoids or the inability to hyperextend the neck (Skolnick & Cohn, 1989). The oblique view shows the relationship between movements of structures seen on the lateral view to those seen on the frontal view. It can also be helpful in visualizing asymmetrical movement of the lateral pharyngeal walls, which is actually quite common. In fact, it has been estimated that about 15% of patients with velopharyngeal dysfunction have asymmetrical lateral wall movement (Argamaso, Levandowski, Golding-Kushner, & Shprintzen, 1994; D'Antonio, Muntz, Marsh, Marty-Grames, & Backensto-Marsh, 1988).

The oblique view is performed by having the patient sit facing forward. With the fluoroscopy on, the patient slowly rotates the head and body as a single unit so that it moves 45 degrees to one side, back to the midline, and then 45 degrees to the other side. Because it is important to compare the movements on both sides with each other, the same speech sample should be used.

Use of Contrast Material

A radiopaque contrast substance is needed in order to view the pharyngeal walls adequately on the frontal and base views. The contrast substance most commonly used is a suspension of barium sulfate. This can be purchased as a premixed liquid or as a powder that is mixed with water until it is the consistency of heavy cream (Skolnick & Cohn, 1989). Flavoring can be added to the mixture as well.

A contrast substance is not usually used for the lateral view, however, because the velum and posterior pharyngeal wall are actually better visualized without it. This is due to the fact that there is an air column in the pharynx between the velum and posterior pharyngeal wall. As noted previously, the air is less absorbent of X-ray photons than the soft tissues of the velum and posterior pharyngeal wall. As a result, the air appears black, which provides contrast against the soft tissue density of the velum and posterior pharyngeal wall, which appear white. In addition, the contrast material can actually obscure the point of closure on this view, or mix with mucus and cause the velum to appear longer than it actually is.

When the barium is added for the other views, however, it is sometimes helpful to repeat the lateral view. Barium can make a Passavant's ridge more obvious on the lateral view (Cohn, Rood, McWilliams, Skolnick, & Abdelmalek, 1984). It can also be helpful in determining the patency of an oronasal fistula. If the fistula is patent, the barium can often be seen dripping from the nasal cavity through the fistula to the oral cavity (Clark, D'Antonio, Liu, & Welch, 1992; Skolnick, Glaser, & McWilliams, 1980). In addition, as the patient swallows, barium may be seen going up into the fistula. Finally, barium on the lateral view can sometimes outline a defect in the nasal surface of the velum as a result of a submucous cleft. Because barium can produce artifacts or occasionally obscure structures on the lateral view, it is recommended that lateral videofluoroscopy always be performed without barium first and then again with barium only if specific information is needed.

With all views, barium may be helpful in the identification of small gaps that cannot otherwise be seen due to the resolution of the views. This is because with small gaps, the high pressure of the airflow that is released through the opening can cause bubbling of the barium at the top of the opening. The observation of bubbling, therefore, always indicates a small velopharyngeal gap. However, the absence of bubbling is not similarly diagnostic. When there is a larger velopharyngeal gap, there is less concentrated air pressure going through the opening, and therefore bubbling is less likely to occur.

Before instilling the barium into the nasopharynx, the patient is asked to blow his or her nose to discharge any secretions that could interfere with the exam. One way to instill the barium into the nasal passages is through a soft rubber catheter that is inserted in a nostril and then pushed through the nose to the nasopharynx. A spray of tetracaine in the nose a few minutes prior to inserting the catheter can help to numb the nasal cavity for more comfortable insertion. In addition, a small amount of viscous lidocaine can be applied to the tip of the catheter to help ease it through the nasal meatus. These steps are not required, however, as there is very little discomfort with the catheter insertion. A syringe is then used to place the barium through the catheter (Figure 16–5).

Another method is to simply drip the barium through the nares using a large nose dropper or pipette. The head is hyperextended or the patient is placed in a supine position so that gravity helps to move the barium back to the nasopharynx. The patient is asked to sniff the barium, and the head of the patient is rotated to be sure that the soft palate and pharyngeal walls become adequately coated with the contrast material. This is important because without an adequate and even coating of barium over all the structures, the view may be useless to the examiner. The drip method is usually less frightening to young children, but it can delay the procedure and may not result in adequate coverage of the tissues. Regardless of the method used, approximately 1 to 3 ml of barium is needed in each nostril for adequate coverage.

When barium is introduced in the nasopharynx through the nose, it causes the eyes to water and gives the sensation that is felt when water goes into the nose. A mild burning sensation in the nasopharynx can last for an hour or more following its introduction. Although the barium can cause some discomfort and minor irritation, most children tolerate the procedure fairly well, especially if they are prepared for what to expect. However, if the child cries during this procedure, the secretions can wash the barium down. When that occurs, more barium has to be passed into the nasopharynx for the study.

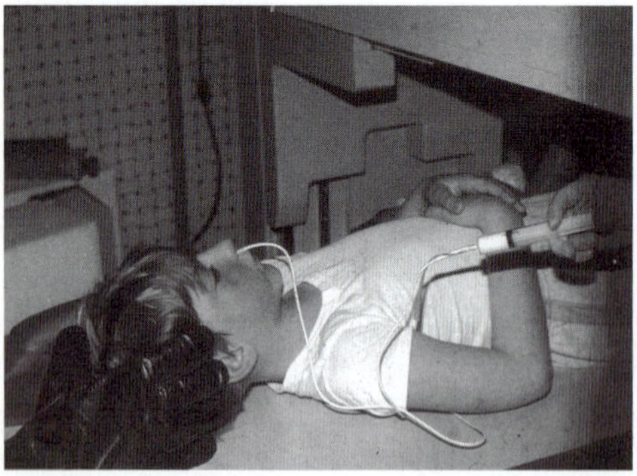

Speech Sample

During the projection for each view, the patient should first be asked to swallow. With the act of swallowing, the velopharyngeal structures come together forcefully and are easy to identify. This helps the X-ray technologist to ensure that the orientation is correct. It can also be useful when the study is interpreted because it orients the evaluators to the location of the structures. The technologist then asks the patient to repeat syllables or standard sentences. A microphone is placed near the patient's head in order to record the speech simultaneously with the visual images (Figure 16–6).

As noted in Chapter 13, the patient should be asked to repeat a combination of sentences loaded with pressure-sensitive phonemes (see Table 11–3), produce a repetition of pressure sensitive syllables, and count from 60 to 70.

Courtesy Ann W. Kummer, Ph.D./Cincinnati Children's Hospital Medical Center & University of Cincinnati College of Medicine

FIGURE 16–5 A method for instilling barium into the nasopharynx is through the use of a large syringe and catheter. The barium is squeezed through the catheter to the nasopharynx.

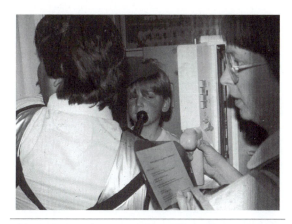

FIGURE 16–6 The X-ray technician asks the patient to repeat syllables and standard sentences. A microphone is placed near the patient's head so that it can record the speech simultaneously with the visual images.
Courtesy Ann W. Kummer, Ph.D./Cincinnati Children's Hospital Medical Center & University of Cincinnati College of Medicine

Because there is an inherent risk with radiation exposure, the speech sample needs to be long enough to obtain needed information, but as short as possible to avoid unnecessary radiation exposure (Isberg, Julin, Kraepelien, & Henrikson, 1989). If the speech sample is carefully chosen, no more than 30 seconds is needed to obtain an adequate speech sample for each view.

INTERPRETATION

Team Interpretation of the Results

A videofluoroscopic speech study can be performed by the X-ray technologist or radiologist. However, the biggest challenge is the analysis and interpretation of the findings and the formulation of appropriate recommendations. For this part of the evaluation, a team approach is definitely preferable. Experience, skill, and careful analysis are required for interpretation of the study.

Although the radiologist or X-ray technologist actually performs the study, both the radiologist and the speech-language pathologist must work together to interpret the study. The radiologist has a thorough understanding of the anatomy, physiology, and imaging of the velopharyngeal structures. The speech-language pathologist also understands the anatomy and physiology but particularly understands the physiology speech and the correlation between velopharyngeal function and the acoustic product of speech. With both perspectives, the interpretation of the study is more complete and accurate.

Interpretation of the Lateral View

On the lateral view, the examiner should observe the length, thickness, and contour of the velum, both at rest and during phonation. During phonation, the velum should elevate to the approximate level of the hard palate. There should be a bend in the velum at a point that is about two-thirds of the distance from the hard palate to the tip of the uvula. This bend, where there is "knee action," is at the point of insertion of the levator veli palatini muscles and occurs as the levator sling contracts to pull the velum up and back. When the velum makes contact with the posterior pharyngeal wall, the extent of contact between the velar eminence (the high point on the top of the "knee") and the vertical part of the velum should be noted (Kuehn & Henne, 2003). The extent of the contact area gives an indication of the firmness of closure. If the contact area is small, it might be assumed that the closure is tenuous.

On the posterior pharyngeal wall, the presence and approximate size of an adenoid pad should be noted. The adenoid pad usually appears as a smooth, convex structure that is either on the same plane as the hard palate or slightly higher. If there is no adenoid mass, the depth and contour of the pharyngeal wall should be assessed. The examiner should note the relative depth of the pharynx during nasal breathing and then observe the anterior motion of the posterior pharyngeal wall, if this occurs, with speech. When a Passavant's ridge is present, it can be viewed during speech as a shelf-like projection on the posterior pharyngeal wall during speech. Tonsillar tissue can be seen somewhat on this view. It appears as an oval mass that is superimposed over the area of the posterior tongue.

Tongue movement during articulation can be assessed from this view. In some cases, patients use the posterior portion of the tongue to assist in elevating the velum during speech as a compensatory strategy. If this is occurring, then the apparent movement of the velum and the resultant closure is actually very deceiving. The movement of the tongue tip, dorsum, the posterior tongue, and even the larynx should be observed to determine whether there are compensatory productions, such as glottal stops, pharyngeal plosives, pharyngeal fricatives, or middorsum palatal stops. Abnormal tongue movement, including backing of articulation or the use of the dorsum for articulation, should be noted.

Evidence of abnormality may include a short velum relative to the posterior pharyngeal wall, a thin velum, or poor knee action of the velum during speech. Figure 16–7 shows a lateral view of a patient with a short velum relative to the posterior pharyngeal wall, resulting in velopharyngeal insufficiency. Figure 16–8 shows a velum with poor movement and little knee action, resulting in velopharyngeal incompetence. An estimate of the size of the velopharyngeal opening as a result of these abnormalities should be noted.

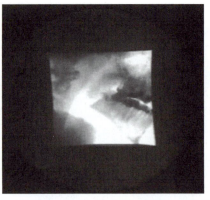

Courtesy Ann W. Kummer, Ph.D./Cincinnati Children's Hospital Medical Center & University of Cincinnati College of Medicine

FIGURE 16–7 Lateral view showing a short velum relative to the posterior pharyngeal wall, which results in velopharyngeal insufficiency.

On the lateral view, the examiner may also see evidence of a patent oronasal fistula if barium is used. Other abnormalities may include a localized indentation on the posterior pharyngeal wall following the removal of the adenoids. The appearance of hypertrophic tonsils or adenoids that intrude into the airway should be noted.

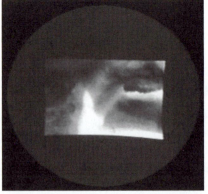

Courtesy Ann W. Kummer, Ph.D./Cincinnati Children's Hospital Medical Center & University of Cincinnati College of Medicine

FIGURE 16–8 Lateral view showing a velum of normal length, but poor movement during speech, which results in velopharyngeal incompetence.

Interpretation of the Frontal View

The purpose of the *frontal view* is to assess the extent of lateral pharyngeal wall motion, the symmetry of movement between the two sides, and the approximate level of maximum movement. In most normal speakers, the point of maximum lateral pharyngeal wall movement is just below the plane of the velar eminence (see Figure 1–14A) (Skolnick & Cohn, 1989). Interpreting this view is a challenge because of the superimposition of the vomer and facial structures. The examiner should also remember that, because this view goes from the front to the back, the lateral wall on the right side of the screen is on the patient's left side and vice versa. The side of deficiency should be reported based on the patient's right or left rather than on the examiner's orientation. Standard markers can be used on the image to reduce reporting errors concerning the side of the body.

The observation of poor lateral wall movement may suggest a problem with velopharyngeal closure. On the other hand, the patient may merely have a coronal pattern of closure, which requires only minimal lateral wall movement. Figure 16–9 shows the frontal view of a patient. The barium-coated lateral pharyngeal walls can be seen on either side of the septum. When there is a small velopharyngeal opening, bubbling of barium is often noted on this view. The examiner should note whether the bubbling is in the midline or skewed to one side.

In some cases, the lateral pharyngeal walls appear asymmetrical in their position at rest and during speech. Asymmetry with lateral wall movement can suggest a velopharyngeal opening on the side with the least amount of movement. Before making this judgment, however, it is important to be sure that the orientation of the view is appropriate and that the head was not turned slightly to give a false

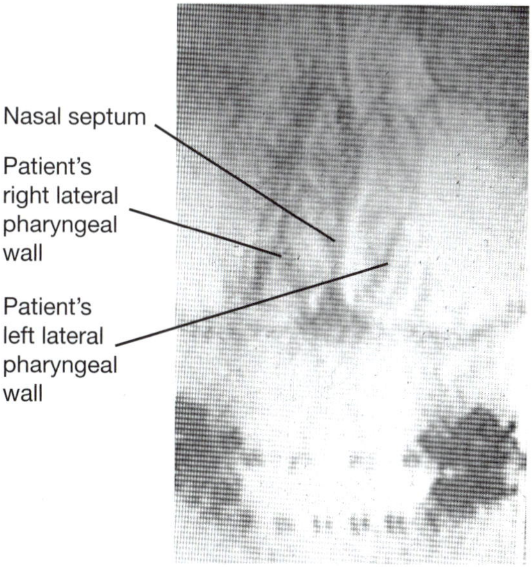

Nasal septum

Patient's right lateral pharyngeal wall

Patient's left lateral pharyngeal wall

FIGURE 16–9 Frontal view showing the nasal septum in midline. The lateral pharyngeal walls are well coated with barium and bow outward during nasal breathing as noted in the frame.

impression. If there is a true asymmetry, this is important to document because it can affect the surgical management.

Interpretation of the Base View

If the head is positioned properly for the base view so that the beam goes directly through the velopharyngeal port, the margins of the port appear as an oval or round structure during nasal breathing. The lateral and posterior pharyngeal walls can be seen easily with this view if there is an adequate coating of barium and the position is correct. The velum, which appears at the top of the oval, is harder to visualize because it does not pick up as much barium.

During speech, the structures can be observed to narrow and then close the lumen as a sphincter. Depending on the basic pattern of closure, a black horizontal line (with a coronal pattern), a vertical line (with a sagittal pattern), or a circle (with a circular pattern)

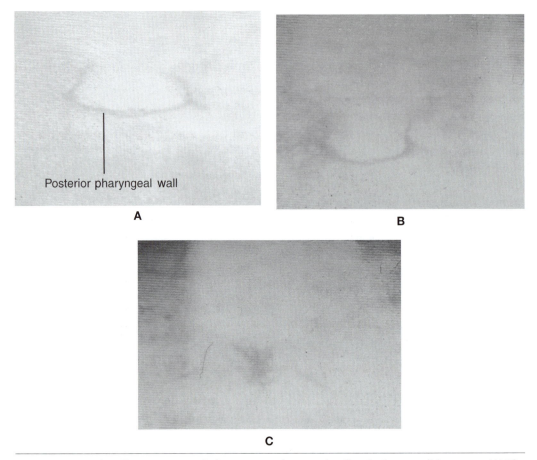

FIGURE 16–10 (A–C) Base view with the posterior pharyngeal wall at the bottom of the screen. (A) The entire port is open for nasal breathing. (B) The port is partly closed. (C) The port is totally closed. This represents a circular pattern of closure.

Courtesy Ann W. Kummer, Ph.D./Cincinnati Children's Hospital Medical Center & University of Cincinnati College of Medicine

remain in the middle of the closure area. Figure 16–10 shows the nasopharyngeal port through the base view. Figure 16–10A shows the port entirely open. The port begins to close in Figure 16–10B and is entirely closed in Figure 16–10C, leaving a small circle. On this view, the examiner should be careful not to confuse movement of the tongue and vocal cords with velopharyngeal movement. In addition, the large foramen magnum can be seen on this view and should not be mistaken for the velopharyngeal port.

When there is velopharyngeal dysfunction, the pharyngeal lumen does not appear to totally close. In fact, an opening during speech is a clear indication of velopharyngeal dysfunction. The examiner should also observe the symmetry of both sides of the port and note asymmetrical movement during speech. As with the frontal view, the left lateral wall is on the right side of the screen and vice versa. With a small velopharyngeal gap, bubbling of barium can often be seen on this view.

Interpretation of the Towne's View

Because the Towne's view is similar to the base view (only looking from above), the same observations and cautions apply. Again, the examiner should note that the patient's left lateral wall is seen on the right side of the screen and vice versa.

Interpretation of the Oblique View

The oblique view can be difficult to interpret due to the superimposition of multiple structures over the area of interest. A coating of barium can make interpretation easier, however, and a swallow prior to the speech sample can help to orient the examiner to the structures of concern. As in the frontal, base, and Towne's view, the patient's right side is seen on the left side of the screen and vice versa.

On the oblique view, the examiner should observe each lateral wall individually. The lateral wall should be viewed at rest and then during speech to determine whether it closes against the velum. A notation should be made if there is an apparent gap between the lateral wall and velum on that side. As with the other views, bubbling of the barium should be noted, because it indicates a small velopharyngeal opening (Sell, Mars, & Worrell, 2006).

Overall Results

Based on the information obtained from all views, the examiner must assimilate the information to make a determination of the extent of closure, the approximate gap size, the gap location, and the basic pattern of closure. This information is especially important because it allows the surgeon to design the surgical correction based on the abnormality.

Interpretation of the various views typically involves subjective analyses only. Direct measurement is difficult to do because the image on the screen is not life-sized and depends on a variety of factors. However, measurements are sometimes needed for research purposes. This can be done by putting a ruler or something of a known dimension in each view. For the view that is of interest, the examiner can then take a stop-frame at rest and once again at the patient's best attempt at closure. Quantifiable measurements can then be made, using as a reference the object with a known dimension (Williams, Henningsson, & Pegoraro-Krook, 1997).

REPORTING THE RESULTS

Some centers report the results of videofluoroscopy with a narrative report, using a few short paragraphs. Other centers use a scale to rate various parameters of structure and function as noted on each view. The first published rating scale was developed by McWilliams-Neely and Bradley (1964). Since that time, others have made additions and modifications to this basic scale.

In 1990, the American Cleft Palate–Craniofacial Association assembled a group of clinicians to develop a standardized method for interpreting and reporting the results from videofluoroscopy and nasopharyngoscopy (Golding-Kushner et al., 1990). They developed a procedure that attempts to quantify the movement of the velopharyngeal structures relative to each structure's resting position and the resting position of the opposing structure. This is done as a ratio rather than as an absolute measurement. For example, the resting position of the velum is at the 0.0 point, and the point of closure against the pharyngeal wall is 1.0. If the velum raises and closes 50%

of the opening, then velar displacement is at a rating of 0.5 along the trajectory toward the posterior pharyngeal wall. This estimation is done for each lateral wall and for the posterior pharyngeal wall as well. Although some may use this system, it is complicated and the inter- and even intra-judge reliability has been an issue. Most importantly, the size of the opening does not usually impact treatment recommendations. Instead, it is the location of the opening and the cause that is most important to determine. Therefore, this rating scale is not widely used.

Regardless of the specific rating scale used or whether a narrative report is done, it is important to be consistent in the observations that are made and in the way that they are reported. This is particularly important if preoperative and postoperative studies are done for comparison.

ADVANTAGES AND LIMITATIONS OF VIDEOFLUOROSCOPY

Videofluoroscopy has the particular advantage of providing a view of the entire length of the posterior pharyngeal wall. It also shows the point at which the velum contacts it during speech. With this view, it is easy to determine whether there is velopharyngeal insufficiency due to a short velum or velopharyngeal incompetence due to poor velar movement. In comparison with nasopharyngoscopy, videofluoroscopy is superior in showing the length of the velum and its upward movement during speech. It also provides a view of the entire length of the posterior pharyngeal wall during closure. As such, it is better than nasopharyngoscopy for looking at the pharynx below the velum during speech (Witt et al., 2000). Videofluoroscopy also allows the examiner to

view the movement of the tongue tip and back of the tongue during speech. The fact that the study is recorded (on video or digital images) allows the study to be viewed by multiple team members after completion of the study.

A primary disadvantage of videofluoroscopy is the radiation exposure, even with the new systems that require lower doses. As with any X-ray procedure, there is always a concern about the amount of radiation exposure associated with the test and its potential to cause somatic or genetic damage. Therefore, the aim of pediatric radiology is to keep the radiation dose to the minimum needed to obtain the required diagnostic information. In 1989, it was estimated that for 1 minute of videofluoroscopy in the lateral view, the radiation exposure is between 0.025 rad and 0.5 rad; and for the frontal and base views, which require a higher radiation level for adequate resolution, the exposure is from 0.125 rad to 1.00 rad (Skolnick & Cohn, 1989). By way of comparison, a single lateral cephalometric X-ray is about 0.25 rad, and a single CT slice is between 1 and 4 rads. Since that time, digital radiographic techniques have significantly reduced the radiation dose, although very little work has been published on the estimated radiation dose used in such examinations (Zammit-Maempel, Chapple, & Leslie, 2007). This may be partly because the radiation dose varies, depending on the patient's size and the thickness of the bones. In general, the radiation dosage for videofluoroscopy is low in comparison with many other types of X-ray procedures (Chan, Chan, & Lam, 2002; Chau & Kung, 2009). However, no amount of radiation is innocuous, and therefore the benefits gained from this procedure must always be weighed against the potential risks, although slight.

Another disadvantage of videofluoroscopy is that the overall resolution of a radiographic procedure is not as good as a direct view. In fact, the ability to visualize structures such as

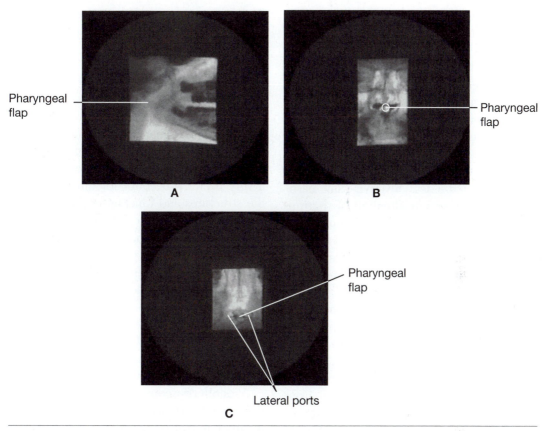

Pharyngeal
flap

A

Pharyngeal
flap

B

Pharyngeal
flap

Lateral ports

C

FIGURE 16–11 (A–C) Videofluoroscopy of a pharyngeal flap. (A) Lateral view that shows the pharyngeal flap as a faint shadow that is low near the base of the tongue. (B) Frontal or AP (anterior–posterior) view that shows the flap in midline and the lateral ports coated with barium. (C) The flap is noted in midline and the open lateral ports can be seen on each side.

Courtesy Ann W. Kummer, Ph.D./Cincinnati Children's Hospital Medical Center & University of Cincinnati College of Medicine

the velum and posterior pharyngeal wall depends on these structures being surrounded by air. However, as the velopharyngeal port narrows for closure, the amount of air between the velum and pharyngeal wall is markedly reduced and finally disappears during contact. Therefore, the ability to distinguish the margins of each structure becomes more difficult, if not impossible. As a result, a small gap is usually not seen. The only clue to its presence may be occasional bubbling of the barium. Gaps as a result of irregular adenoids cannot be seen. In addition, as noted previously, the X-ray beam goes through all of the structures in the plane, so the image represents a sum of all the parts. Therefore, if the velum touches the posterior pharyngeal wall at any point in the coronal plane, it will look as if there is complete closure, even if the velum does not contact the pharyngeal wall at all points. Finally, if the beam is not perfectly perpendicular to the opening, the gap may not be visualized.

Videofluoroscopy is not a good procedure for evaluating the placement and the results of secondary procedures. It is very difficult to see a pharyngeal flap or sphincter pharyngoplasty with this procedure unless there is a very good coating of barium (Figure 16–11A–C). In fact, the presence of either could actually be missed altogether. It is almost impossible to view the ports after these surgeries.

Although some professionals consider videofluoroscopy to be less invasive than nasopharyngoscopy, the introduction of barium into the nasopharynx can be very unpleasant. It can cause watering of the eyes and a burning sensation that can persist for an hour or more. The large equipment can also be frightening to young children.

The final disadvantage is that, although videofluoroscopy shows all of the velopharyngeal structures and their function through the use of multiple views, each individual view is only two-dimensional. Therefore, the examiner must essentially extrapolate information from each view in order to imagine the three-dimensional structure and its function. Videofluoroscopy does not provide a clear view of all the structures as they function in the multidimensional pharynx.

Because of the limitations of videofluoroscopy and the relative advantages of nasopharyngoscopy, this X-ray procedure seems to be used less frequently as a primary means of evaluating velopharyngeal function. Most centers now use nasopharyngoscopy as their primary means of evaluating velopharyngeal function (D'Antonio, Achauer, & Vander Kam, 1993; Kuehn & Henne, 2003; Kummer, Clark,

Redle, Thomsen, & Billmire, 2011; Lertsburapa, Schroeder, & Sullivan, 2010).

SUMMARY

Instrumental assessment is not required for the diagnosis of velopharyngeal dysfunction because this can be determined through a perceptual assessment alone. However, videofluoroscopy is a very useful procedure for directly evaluating the structures and function of the velopharyngeal valve in order to determine the cause of velopharyngeal dysfunction and, in some cases, the location of the opening. In particular, videofluoroscopy is very useful for viewing the movement and knee action of the velum and its level of contact on the posterior pharyngeal wall. Information obtained from videofluoroscopy is used to determine the type of intervention (including the best surgical procedure) that has the greatest chance of success.

Videofluoroscopy is not ideal for evaluating the results of surgery for velopharyngeal insufficiency/incompetence because the new surgical structures and their ports cannot be seen clearly. Videofluoroscopy can be used to determine the presence of obstruction in the vocal tract, particularly if it involves adenoid or tonsillar hypertrophy. Videofluoroscopy is a very useful tool for evaluation of swallowing. In the last few decades, videofluoroscopy is used less as a standard evaluation procedure for individuals who exhibit resonance disorders or characteristics of velopharyngeal dysfunction. This is because most centers now rely more on nasopharyngoscopy.

FOR REVIEW AND DISCUSSION

1. What are the current uses for lateral cephalometric X-rays? Why are lateral cephalometric X-rays no longer used for evaluation of velopharyngeal function?

2. What are the typical views used with videofluoroscopy? For each view, describe the structures that can be evaluated. Why are multiple views necessary?

3. In evaluating an X-ray, what color are the structures and what color is the air? What causes this difference?

4. What radiopaque contrast material is commonly used during a videofluoroscopic

evaluation? Which views require this substance in order to view the structures adequately? How is this substance instilled into the nasopharynx?

5. Describe what the examiner should observe and note when reviewing each of the views.

6. What are the advantages of videofluoroscopy? What are some of the limitations?

REFERENCES

American Speech-Language-Hearing Association (ASHA). (2004). Knowledge and skills needed by speech-language pathologists performing videofluoroscopic swallowing studies. Accessed June 1, 2012, from http://www.asha.org/policy/KS2004-00076.htm.

Argamaso, R. V., Levandowski, G. J., Golding-Kushner, K. J., & Shprintzen, R. J. (1994). Treatment of asymmetric velopharyngeal insufficiency with skewed pharyngeal flap. *Cleft Palate–Craniofacial Journal, 31*(4), 287–294.

Chan, C. B., Chan, L. K., & Lam, H. S. (2002). Scattered radiation level during videofluoroscopy for swallowing study. *Clinical Radiology, 57*(7), 614–616.

Chau, K. H., & Kung, C. M. (2009). Patient dose during videofluoroscopy swallowing studies in a Hong Kong public hospital. *Dysphagia, 24*(4), 387–390.

Clark, D. E., D'Antonio, L. L., Liu, J. R., & Welch, T. B. (1992). Radiographic demonstration of oronasal fistulas in patients with cleft palate with the use of barium sulfate contrast. *Oral Surgery, Oral Medicine, Oral Pathology, Oral Radiology, and Endodontology, 74*(5), 661–670.

Cohn, E. R., Rood, S. R., McWilliams, B. J., Skolnick, M. L., & Abdelmalek, L. R. (1984). Barium sulphate coating of the nasopharynx in lateral view videofluoroscopy. *Cleft Palate Journal, 21*(1), 7–17.

D'Antonio, L. L., Achauer, B. M., & Vander Kam, V. M. (1993). Results of a survey of cleft palate teams concerning the use of nasendoscopy. *Cleft Palate–Craniofacial Journal, 30*(1), 35–39.

D'Antonio, L. L., Muntz, H. R., Marsh, J. L., Marty-Grames, L., & Backensto-Marsh, R. (1988). Practical application of flexible fiberoptic nasopharyngoscopy for evaluating velopharyngeal function. *Plastic and Reconstructive Surgery, 82*(4), 611–618.

Dudas, J. R., Deleyiannis, F. W., Ford, M. D., Jiang, S., & Losee, J. E. (2006). Diagnosis and treatment of velopharyngeal insufficiency: Clinical utility of speech evaluation and videofluoroscopy. *Annals of Plastic Surgery, 56*(5), 511–517; Discussion 517.

Golding-Kushner, K. J., Argamaso, R. V., Cotton, R. T., Grames, L. M., Henningsson, G., Jones, D. L., Karnell, M. P., et al. (1990). Standardization for the reporting of nasopharyngoscopy and multiview videofluoroscopy: A report from an International Working Group. *Cleft Palate Journal, 27* (4), 337–347; Discussion 347–348.

Havstam, C., Lohmander, A., Persson, C., Dotevall, H., Lith, A., & Lilja, J. (2005).

Evaluation of VPI-assessment with video-fluoroscopy and nasoendoscopy. *British Journal of Plastic Surgery, 58*(7), 922–931.

Isberg, A., Julin, P., Kraepelien, T., & Henrikson, C. O. (1989). Absorbed doses and energy imparted from radiographic examination of velopharyngeal function during speech. *Cleft Palate Journal, 26*(2), 105–109.

Kendall, K. A., Leonard, R. J., & McKenzie, S. (2004). Airway protection: Evaluation with videofluoroscopy. *Dysphagia, 19*(2), 65–70.

Kuehn, D. P., & Henne, L. J. (2003). Speech evaluation and treatment of patients with cleft palate. *American Journal of Speech-Language Pathology, 12*, 103–109.

Kummer, A. W., Clark, S. L., Redle, E. E., Thomsen, L. L., Billmire, D. A. (2011). Current practice in assessing and reporting speech outcomes of cleft palate and velopharyngeal surgery: A survey of cleft palate/craniofacial professionals. *Cleft Palate–Craniofacial Journal, 49*(2), 146–152.

Lam, D. J., Starr, J. R., Perkins, J. A., Lewis, C. W., Eblen, L. E., Dunlap, J., & Sie, K. C. (2006). A comparison of nasendoscopy and multiview videofluoroscopy in assessing velopharyngeal insufficiency. *Otolaryngology-Head and Neck Surgery, 134*(3), 394–402.

La Rossa, D., Brown, A., Cohen, M., & Spackman, T. (1980). Videoradiography of the velopharyngeal portal using the Towne's view. *Journal of Maxillofacial Surgery, 8*(3), 203–205.

Lertsburapa, K., Schroeder, J. W., Jr., & Sullivan, C. (2010). Assessment of adenoid size: A comparison of lateral radiographic measurements, radiologist assessment, and nasal endoscopy. *International Journal of Pediatric Otorhinolaryngology, 74*(11), 1281–1285.

Major, M. P., Flores-Mir, C., & Major, P. W. (2006). Assessment of lateral cephalometric diagnosis of adenoid hypertrophy and posterior upper airway obstruction: A systematic review. *America Journal of Orthodontics and Dentofacial Orthopedics, 130*(6), 700–708.

McWilliams-Neely, B. J., & Bradley, D. P. (1964). A rating scale for evaluation of videotape recorded X-ray studies. *Cleft Palate Journal, 1*, 88–94.

Pelo, S., Tassiello, S., Boniello, R., Gasparini, G., & Longobardi, G. (2006). A new method for assessment of craniofacial malformations. *Journal of Craniofacial Surgery, 17*(6), 1035–1039.

Perry, J. L. (2011). Variations in velopharyngeal structures between upright and supine positions using upright magnetic resonance imaging. *Cleft Palate–Craniofacial Journal, 48*(2), 123–133.

Rowe, M. R., & D'Antonio, L. L. (2005). Velopharyngeal dysfunction: Evolving developments in evaluation. *Current Opinion in Otolaryngology & Head & Neck Surgery, 13*(6), 366–370.

Sell, D., Mars, M., & Worrell, E. (2006). Process and outcome study of multidisciplinary prosthetic treatment for velopharyngeal dysfunction. *International Journal of Language Communication Disorders, 41*(5), 495–511.

Shprintzen, R. J. (1995). Instrumental assessment of velopharyngeal valving. In R. J. Shprintzen & J. Bardach (Eds.), *Cleft palate speech management: A multidisciplinary approach* (vol. 4, pp. 221–256). St. Louis, MO: Mosby.

Shprintzen, R. J., Rakof, S. J., Skolnick, M. L., & Lavorato, A. S. (1977). Incongruous movements of the velum and lateral pharyngeal walls. *Cleft Palate Journal, 14*(2), 148–157.

Skolnick, M. L. (1969). Video velopharyngography in patients with nasal speech, with emphasis on lateral pharyngeal motion in velopharyngeal closure. *Radiology, 93*(4), 747–755.

Skolnick, M. L. (1970). Videofluoroscopic examination of the velopharyngeal portal during phonation in lateral and base projections—A new technique for studying the mechanics of closure. *Cleft Palate Journal*, 7, 803–816.

Skolnick, M. L. (1975). Velopharyngeal function in cleft palate. *Clinics in Plastic Surgery*, 2(2), 285–297.

Skolnick, M. L., & Cohn, E. R. (1989). Videofluoroscopic studies of speech in patients with cleft palate. New York: Springer-Verlag.

Skolnick, M. L., Glaser, E. R., & McWilliams, B. J. (1980). The use and limitations of the barium pharyngogram in the detection of velopharyngeal insufficiency. *Radiology*, 135(2), 301–304.

Skolnick, M. L., & McCall, G. N. (1971). Radiological evaluation of velopharyngeal closure. *Journal of the American Medical Association*, 218(1), 96.

Skolnick, M. L., McCall, G. N., & Barnes, M. (1973). The sphincteric mechanism of velopharyngeal closure. *Cleft Palate Journal*, 10, 286–305.

Smith, B. E., & Kuehn, D. P. (2007). Speech evaluation of velopharyngeal dysfunction. *The Journal of Craniofacial Surgery*, 18(2), 251–260.

Stringer, D. A., & Witzel, M. A. (1986). Velopharyngeal insufficiency on videofluoroscopy: Comparison of projections. *American Journal of Roentgenology*, 146(1), 15–19.

Stringer, D. A., & Witzel, M. A. (1989). Comparison of multiview videofluoroscopy and nasopharyngoscopy in the assessment of velopharyngeal insufficiency. *Cleft Palate Journal*, 26(2), 88–92.

Williams, W. N., & Eisenbach, C. R. D. (1981). Assessing VP function: The lateral still technique vs. cinefluorography. *Cleft Palate Journal*, 18(1), 45–50.

Williams, W. N., Henningsson, G., & Pegoraro-Krook, M. I. (1997). Radiographic assessment of velopharyngeal function for speech. In K. R. Bzoch (Ed.), *Communicative disorders related to cleft lip and palate* (vol. 4). Austin, TX: Pro-Ed.

Witt, P. D., Marsh, J. L., McFarland, E. G., & Riski, J. E. (2000). The evolution of velopharyngeal imaging. *Annals of Plastic Surgery*, 45(6), 665–673.

Ysunza, A., Pamplona, M. C., Ortega, J. M., & Prado, H. (2008). Video fluoroscopy for evaluating adenoid hypertrophy in children. *International Journal of Pediatric Otorhinolaryngology*, 72(8), 1159–1165.

Ysunza, A., Pamplona, M. C., Ortega, J. M., & Prado, H. (2011). [Videofluoroscopic evaluation of adenoid hypertrophy and velopharyngeal closure during speech.] *Gaceta Medica de Mexico*, 147(2), 104–110.

Zammit-Maempel, I., Chapple, C. L., & Leslie, P. (2007). Radiation dose in videofluoroscopic swallow studies. *Dysphagia*, 22(1), 13–15.

CHAPTER

17

NASOPHARYNGOSCOPY

INTRODUCTION

Velopharyngeal insufficiency/incompetence (VPI) can be diagnosed based on the characteristics of the speech as determined through a perceptual speech evaluation alone. However, instrumental assessment of the velopharyngeal valve, often done through nasopharyngoscopy, is usually indicated to determine the cause, the approximate size, and particularly the location of the velopharyngeal opening. This information is important to obtain so that the best form of surgical intervention can be determined.

Nasopharyngoscopy (also called *nasendoscopy* or *videonasendoscopy*) is a minimally invasive endoscopic procedure that allows visual observation and analysis of the velopharyngeal mechanism during speech (D'Antonio, Achauer, & Vander Kam, 1993; D'Antonio, Chait, Lotz, & Netsell, 1986; D'Antonio, Muntz, Marsh, Marty-Grames, & Backensto-Marsh, 1988; David, White, Sprod, & Bagnall, 1982; Ramamurthy, Wyatt, Whitby, Martin, & Davenport, 1997; Shetty, Frampton, & Patel, 2009; Smith & Kuehn, 2007; Strauss, 2007). Nasopharyngoscopy can help the examiner assess both the anatomic and physiologic abnormalities that are causing VPI so that the optimal surgical or prosthetic treatment for the patient can be determined. Nasopharyngoscopy is not only a powerful tool in the evaluation of velopharyngeal function, but it is also commonly used in the evaluation of swallowing, upper airway obstruction, and the structure and function of the larynx and vocal cords.

The purpose of the chapter is to explain how nasopharyngoscopy is used in the evaluation of velopharyngeal function. The specific procedures for a nasopharyngoscopy assessment are reviewed, including methods for preparing a child for the exam and then procedures for inserting the endoscope. The interpretation of the observations is discussed as it relates to the diagnosis of VPI and the recommendations for treatment.

ENDOSCOPY

By definition, *endoscopy* is a procedure that allows the visualization of the interior of a canal or hollow organ by means of a special instrument called an *endoscope*. Physicians have used endoscopy for many years to view anatomic structures and physiological function in order to make medical or surgical treatment decisions. Many specially trained speech-language pathologists perform a type of endoscopy, called *nasopharyngoscopy* or *nasendoscopy* to assess the structures and function of the vocal tract. With this procedure, the examiner is able to observe both the anatomical and physiological correlates of speech sound production, resonance, phonation, and swallowing in order to make a determination about the cause of certain disorders. This is important so that appropriate treatment can be recommended or initiated.

Early Endoscopic Procedures

In 1966, Taub (1966) described the use of a panendoscope for the assessment of velopharyngeal function. The *panendoscope* consisted of an optical tube that could be placed in the mouth and then turned upward for visualization of the velopharyngeal sphincter. This early scope had certain distinct disadvantages. Of course, placement of the tube in the mouth interfered with the normal production of speech, and it had an effect on velopharyngeal function as well. However, the optical tube was too big for nasal insertion. Another problem was that the light bulb generated a dangerous amount of heat and there was also an electrical hazard for the individual. Therefore, use of this scope did not gain wide acceptance.

In 1969, Pigott, Bensen, and White (1969) described the use of a rigid endoscope that was slender enough to be inserted through the nose but large enough to allow observation of velopharyngeal portal at rest and during speech. This endoscope provided a wide-angle view of about 70 degrees, which allowed visualization of most of the port (Pigott & Makepeace, 1982). However, despite the large cone of view, this scope could not be maneuvered for additional assessment of the lateral edges of the port or to see farther down into the pharynx or vocal tract. In addition, because the scope was very straight and the diameter of the nasal cavity is not, the rigid scope was very difficult to insert, particularly if the patient had a septal deviation or stenosis of the naris. In addition, the pressure of the scope on the nasal septum and turbinates caused significant pain and therefore was not well tolerated by most patients.

Flexible Fiberoptic Nasopharyngoscopy

In the mid-1970s and the 1980s, the use of a flexible fiberoptic nasopharyngoscope began to appear in the literature. The flexible scope is smaller in circumference than the rigid scope. As a result, it has a more restricted cone of view. However, its smaller size makes it much easier to be passed transnasally and also easier for patients to tolerate. This is particularly advantageous when evaluating young children.

In 1975, a side-viewing flexible endoscope was described by Miyazaki, Matsuya, and Yamaoka (1975). With this design, the scope remained in a horizontal position, and the opening at the side of the scope gave the examiner the same view as with the rigid scope. However, due to the side opening, the scope could not be manipulated easily to provide a view of both the horizontal and vertical aspects of the port.

In the late 1970s and the 1980s, the end-viewing flexible endoscope was described by several authors (Croft, Shprintzen, & Rakoff, 1981; Shprintzen et al., 1979). The tip of this scope is flexible, and with the use of a lever the examiner can turn the tip down like a periscope to view the velopharyngeal port from various angles. It can even be moved farther down the pharynx for a view of the larynx and the vocal folds. This type of endoscope is used today.

Flexible nasopharyngoscopy is now widely used in the evaluation of velopharyngeal function (D'Antonio et al., 1993; Kuehn & Henne, 2003). Most clinicians now feel that the results are superior to those obtained through videofluoroscopy (Lam et al., 2006; Lertsburapa, Schroeder, & Sullivan, 2010) because of the excellent clarity of the nasopharyngoscopy view and the maneuverability of the scope. At this point, most cleft/craniofacial centers in the United States now use nasopharyngoscopy primarily, or even exclusively, over videofluoroscopy for the visual evaluation of velopharyngeal function (Kummer, Clark, Redle, Thomsen, & Billmire, 2011).

Equipment

Nasopharyngoscopy equipment includes a durable and flexible fiberoptic endoscope (Figure 17–1). Endoscopes can be purchased from several manufacturers (KayPENTAX, Machida, Olympus, and Storz).

Scopes vary in the size of the distal tip (Figure 17–2). The smallest scope, often used in pediatrics, has about a 2.2 mm diameter and the largest scope is almost 5 mm diameter. The 3.5 mm scope is commonly used because this size provides a wide scope of vision, yet it is easily tolerated by most individuals, including children. However, for very young children and infants (when the procedure is done to evaluate swallowing), a smaller scope is preferable.

Courtesy KayPENTAX & Ann W. Kummer, Ph.D./Cincinnati Children's Hospital Medical Center & University of Cincinnati College of Medicine

FIGURE 17–1 A flexible fiberoptic nasopharyngoscope. This instrument includes the long tubular endoscope. The body of the instrument, which is held in the examiner's hand, consists of an eyepiece and a control apparatus with a lever or wheel. The control apparatus allows the examiner to move the tip of the scope up and down like a periscope.

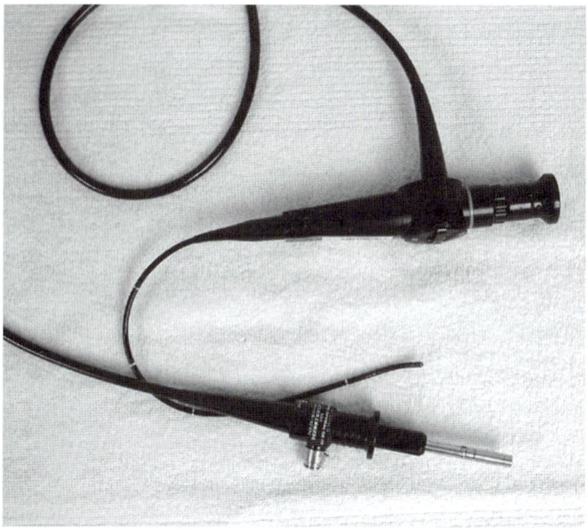

Looking at the insertion end of the fiberscope, one can see the small lens in the middle for obtaining the image and the fiber bundles that encircle the lens for transmitting light to illuminate the anatomic structures of interest. The scope body has slightly tapered tip for easy insertion. The end of the scope is very flexible and can be bent or turned easily without distorting the image.

The body of the scope, which is held in the examiner's hand, consists of an eyepiece and a control apparatus with a lever (Figure 17–3). The control apparatus (lever or wheel) allows the examiner to move the tip of the scope up and down like a periscope. The scope has a cable that is plugged into a high-intensity light source (typically halogen or xenon) for illumination. The flexible fiberoptic

Willging, M.D./Cincinnati Children's Hospital Medical Center & University of Cincinnati College of Medicine

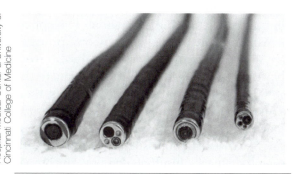

FIGURE 17–2 Nasopharyngoscopes of various sizes. The first scope on the left has a "chip in the tip" camera.

Image Courtesy of Olympus America Inc.

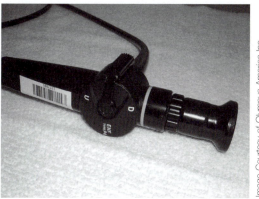

FIGURE 17–3 Eyepiece and control lever for moving the tip of the scope up and down.

nasopharyngoscope and light source are the bare necessities for this examination. With this equipment alone, the examiner can perform a nasopharyngoscopy procedure at bedside or almost anywhere by viewing anatomic structures of interest through the endoscope's eyepiece during the procedure. However, for standard evaluations in a clinic, a complete system that includes a video monitor and a recording system is strongly recommended and may even be required in some cases for appropriate documentation and billing.

With the complete system, a specially designed camera is attached to the eyepiece (Figure 17–4). There are newer "distal chip" endoscopes that come with the CCD camera mounted on the tip of the endoscope. These scopes offer significantly improved resolution compared to the traditional endoscopes so that even fine anatomical features, such as small capillaries, can be seen. However, the traditional fiberoptic scope with a camera mounted to the eyepiece is still far more typical and much less expensive than distal chip scopes.

In addition to the camera, there should be a high-resolution monitor, which provides the examiner with a much better view than the single-person (and single-eye) eyepiece. In addition, the monitor allows others (including the parents and the patient) to see the exam as it is done.

A complete system includes a high-quality digital video recorder and the use of an external microphone. With recording equipment, the videos can be reviewed frame by frame for in-depth analysis and can be reviewed later by the surgeon, who may not be present during the examination. The study can be shown to the patient and family to help them understand the problem and proposed treatment. The recordings allow for pre- and postoperative comparisons, which is important in improving outcomes. Videos and still images can be used in PowerPoint presentations for professional education. Finally, a high-quality color printer can also be useful for a hard copy of still pictures and a report of key examination findings. Figure 17–5 shows a system with a large high-definition monitor, a halogen cold-light source, and video recording equipment (KayPENTAX, Montvale, N.J.).

Clinical Uses for Nasopharyngoscopy

As noted previously, flexible fiberoptic nasopharyngoscopy is now commonly used in clinical settings for the evaluation of velopharyngeal function. Nasopharyngoscopy provides a view of the entire velopharyngeal valve from above. As such, the examiner can evaluate the integrity of the velopharyngeal structures, their movement during speech production, and whether the velopharyngeal valve closes completely when appropriate. If there is VPI (velopharyngeal insufficiency or incompetence), the examiner can determine the size of the opening, the location, and the probable

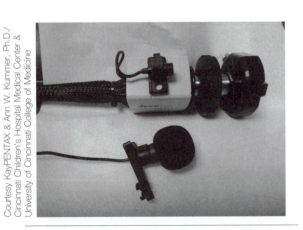

FIGURE 17–4 A very small, lightweight chip camera that can be attached directly to the eyepiece of a nasopharyngoscope.

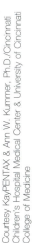

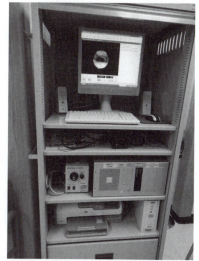

FIGURE 17–5 In addition to the endoscope, camera, and cold light source, a complete system for nasopharyngoscopy should include a computer, monitor, keyboard, speakers, video recording equipment, and a printer.

cause. Even very small gaps are easily visualized with this technique.

In addition to viewing the velopharyngeal port, nasopharyngoscopy allows the examiner to view the nasal surface of the velum. This can reveal defects that are characteristic of a submucous cleft, including dysplastic musculus uvulae muscles or a concavity in the nasal surface of the velum. Because an occult submucous cleft can only be viewed on the nasal surface of the velum, nasopharyngoscopy is the only way to diagnose (other than in surgery). The nasal surface of the hard palate can be evaluated by passing the scope through the inferior meatus. This can show the actual size and extent of an oronasal fistula.

Nasopharyngoscopy allows the examiner to evaluate the pharyngeal walls. A Passavant's ridge may be noted on the posterior pharyngeal wall during speech. In addition, the adenoid pad can be evaluated for size and its

potential to cause upper airway obstruction. The examiner can see protrusions or fissures in the adenoid tissue that may affect the firmness of veloadenoidal closure. If the carotid artery is medially displaced, as is common in velocardiofacial syndrome, this can be noted as pulsations on the posterior pharyngeal wall.

In addition to viewing the velopharyngeal structures, nasopharyngoscopy allows the examiner to view the larynx and vocal cords (Karnell, 1994; Karnell & Langmore, 1998). Because laryngeal abnormalities are often found in individuals with craniofacial anomalies and also because there is a high incidence of vocal nodules in individuals with velopharyngeal insufficiency, an examination of the vocal cords is often done with the nasopharyngoscopy exam.

The information obtained through nasopharyngoscopy is very valuable for treatment planning for VPI. In fact, the observations provide a clear direction for the surgical procedure that is most likely to be successful for each patient (Osberg & Witzel, 1981; Shprintzen et al., 1979). If surgery is not an option, nasopharyngoscopy can help the prosthodontist design and modify an effective speech prosthetic device for the patient (D'Antonio et al., 1988; Hung & Cheng, 1989; Karnell, Rosenstein, & Fine, 1987). See Chapter 20 for more information about prosthetic management.

If surgery is done for VPI (e.g., pharyngeal flap or sphincter pharyngoplasty), nasopharyngoscopy is an excellent tool to evaluate the results (Abdel-Aziz, 2007). If there is residual hypernasality or nasal emission, or if there is evidence of upper airway obstruction after the VPI surgery, nasopharyngoscopy can help the surgeon to determine the appropriate surgical revision procedure.

It should be noted that nasopharyngoscopy is essentially the same procedure that is used for evaluation of swallowing disorders. When done for evaluation of swallowing, it is referred to as the FEES (*fiberoptic endoscopic evaluation of swallowing*) procedure (Aviv et al., 1998; Bastian, 1991, 1993, 1998; Donzelli, Brady, Wesling, & Theisen, 2005; Kidder, Langmore, & Martin, 1994; Langmore, Schatz, & Olsen, 1988; Leder, Acton, Lisitano, & Murray, 2005; Nacci et al., 2008). Also, the scope is passed through the inferior meatus instead of the middle meatus, as is done for evaluation of speech.

Although nasopharyngoscopy is primarily used for diagnostic purposes, it can also be used to provide biofeedback to the patient as part of the evaluation appointment (Brunner, Stellzig-Eisenhauer, Proschel, Verres, & Komposch, 2005; Witzel, Tobe, & Salyer, 1988; Ysunza, Pamplona, Femat, Mayer, & Garcia-Velasco, 1997). It should be noted that biofeedback is only useful when the problem with closure is functional (as in phoneme-specific nasal emission due to misarticulation). It is not effective if the problem is due to abnormal structure. See Chapter 21 for more information about speech therapy.

LEARNING TO PERFORM THE NASOPHARYNGOSCOPY PROCEDURE

Passing the scope for a nasopharyngoscopy procedure can be done by a physician (e.g., an otolaryngologist or plastic surgeon) or by a speech-language pathologist who has been specially trained in this procedure. Adequate training and experience are important so that the procedure can be performed with good results and without causing undue discomfort for the patient.

Training for this procedure is usually not available (or even practical to provide) in a typical university setting. Instead, speech-language pathologists who are interested in performing endoscopy evaluations (whether to evaluate velopharyngeal function, swallowing, or voice) should first review relevant documents on the website of the American Speech-Language, Hearing Association (ASHA 2004a, 2004b, 2004c). Clinical skills can then be obtained by attending specific focused courses, mentoring with an experienced professional, reviewing videotapes of previous exams, and by direct supervised experience.

NASOPHARYNGOSCOPY PREPARATION

The success of the nasopharyngoscopy procedure depends greatly on the child's developmental level and cooperation (Smith & Kuehn, 2007). In order to obtain adequate information about the velopharyngeal valve during nasopharyngoscopy, it is best if the child has connected speech for short sentences. In addition, the child must be able to cooperate enough to repeat words and sentences. With proper preparation, children as young as age 3 are generally able to cooperate sufficiently to obtain a useful nasopharyngoscopy examination.

Information before the Exam Day

In a pediatric setting, preparing the child for what to expect can make the difference between a successful examination and one that is a waste of time, money, and everyone's patience. At Cincinnati Children's, we send the family a coloring book about the procedure a few weeks before the examination (see Appendix 17–1). This helps the child and the parents understand what to expect on the day of the examination, and it allows the parents the opportunity to assist in preparing the child. Giving information in advance also reduces preparation time on the day of the exam. Cooperation tends to improve with age so that obtaining a good examination with adults is usually not a problem. However, even adults can be nervous and apprehensive about the exam. Therefore, giving them information on what to expect before the day of the exam is also helpful.

Perceptual Evaluation

Just before the nasopharyngoscopy evaluation, the speech-language pathologist should complete a perceptual evaluation. This way, information regarding the speech characteristics can be obtained without the discomfort of the scope in place.

The information derived from the perceptual evaluation helps the examiner to determine what needs to be tested in the nasopharyngoscopy evaluation. For example, if the patient demonstrates nasal emission on sibilants only, the examiner should test these sounds in particular and determine whether, through instruction and biofeedback, closure can be obtained by altering the place of production. On the other hand, if hyponasality or cul-de-sac resonance is noted during the perceptual evaluation, the examiner would use nasal sounds and sentences to assess the source of obstruction.

When doing the perceptual assessment before the nasopharyngoscopy, the speech-language pathologist has an opportunity to develop a rapport with the child and help the child to become comfortable in the surroundings (D'Antonio et al., 1986; Lotz, D'Antonio, Chait, & Netsell, 1993). It also provides a chance to practice the speech sample that will be used during the nasopharyngoscopy procedure.

Infection Control

Before even administering the topical anesthetic, the examiner should follow the Standard Precautions for the prevention of the spread of disease (ASHA, n.d.; Centers for Disease Control and Prevention [CDC], 2005, 2013). This is not only for the protection of the individual but also for the protection of the examiner. Following these guidelines, thorough handwashing should be done as the first step. The examiner should then wear gloves for the entire examination. The disinfected endoscope should always be hung or placed on a clean surface when not in use.

Nasal Anesthesia and Decongestion

Although nasopharyngoscopy can be done without topical anesthesia, especially with adults (Frosh, Jayaraj, Porter, & Almeyda, 1998), most clinicians use some form of numbing solution before the procedure. It is also helpful to open up the nasal passages before the examination with a topical decongestant. Before administering a topical anesthetic and/or decongestant, it is best to have the patient blow her nose. Excess secretions can interfere with the topical anesthetic and can also obscure the view of the velopharyngeal valve.

Topical anesthetics are medications that must be ordered by the physician but can be administered by the nurse or the speech-language pathologist. The speech-language pathologist should refer to the ASHA guidelines on the administration of topical anesthetics (ASHA, 2005) before beginning this practice. Several methods for numbing the nasal cavity have been reported in the literature. Shprintzen and Golding-Kushner (1989) described a procedure where cotton packing is soaked in tetracaine and then inserted in the nose and left for approximately 5 minutes. Other centers use a long cotton swab to administer lidocaine gel into the middle meatus. Although these methods may be effective in numbing the nasal cavity, we have found that using a nasal spray is faster, results in better nasal coating, and is less traumatic for children.

At Cincinnati Children's Hospital Medical Center, as well as some other centers, we use a nasal spray bottle to administer a mixture of topical anesthesia and a decongestant (Figure 17–6). The composition of the numbing medicine and decongestant may vary by center. Some authors recommend the use of cophenylcaine (Douglas, 2006; Lennox, Hern, Birchall, & Lund, 1996; Smith & Rockley, 2002), whereas others dispute its benefits (Cain, Murray, & McClymont, 2002; Georgalas, Sandhu, Frosh, & Xenellis, 2005). Some use only a nasal decongestant, such as xylometazoline or oxymetazoline (Jonas et al., 2007; Sadek et al., 2001). Still others recommend the use of water only as a lubricant and argue that a local anesthetic or other lubricant is not necessary (Nankivell & Pothier, 2008; Pothier, Raghava, Monteiro, & Awad, 2006).

At Cincinnati Children's, we use a one-to-one mixture of oxymetazoline (0.025%) and tetracaine (1%), with a dosage of 0.3 mg/kg tetracaine per puff. The pharmacy dispenses this mixture in individual spray bottles that are disposed of after use. Tetracaine is preferred in our setting because it also has a vasoconstrictor action, acts quickly, has infrequent side effects, and does not have a noxious odor. Although tetracaine affects the sensation, it does not affect velopharyngeal movement, so it has no negative effect on the study. Overall, this mixture is very effective in achieving the desired numbing effects while opening up the nasal passages for the scope.

Three puffs of spray are administered to each nostril so that there is adequate coating of the turbinates and the nasal septum. After each nostril is sprayed, the child is asked to close the opposite nostril and then sniff hard to ensure that the solution is well distributed. A wait of only a few minutes is needed before the anesthetic takes effect.

The numbing spray should always be administered with the patient seated upright. If the medication is administered with the child in a reclining position, the spray may enter the hypopharynx and numb the airway, leading to aspiration and coughing episodes. This problem will spontaneously resolve after about 20 minutes, but this should be avoided by keeping the patient upright during administration of the spray (J. Paul Willging, M.D., personal communication, May 12, 2006).

For additional numbing, the sides of the scope can be coated with viscous lidocaine (2%) gel or, as we describe it for children, our "special slime." (It is important to coat just the sides of the scope and not the viewing end.)

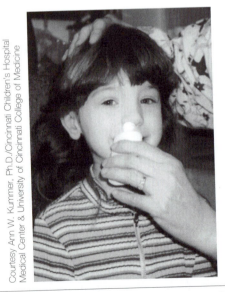

Courtesy Ann W. Kummer, Ph.D./Cincinnati Children's Hospital Medical Center & University of Cincinnati College of Medicine

FIGURE 17–6   The use of a spray bottle to administer both the topical anesthesia and a decongestant prior to the nasopharyngoscopy procedure.

This gel also acts as a lubricant for the scope to slide easily through the nose (Pothier, Awad, Whitehouse, & Porter, 2005). Using this technique, the examiner can ensure that the child has received adequate topical anesthesia to complete the procedure in relative comfort.

Explaining the Procedure

Before inserting the scope, the examiner should carefully explain what will be done and what to expect so that there are no surprises. If the patient is a child, it is important to talk on the child's level and to keep the atmosphere as light as possible. For example, the child can be asked if he ever picks his nose and if so, if it hurts. The size of his "nose-picking finger" can then be compared to the size of the end of the scope, which, of course, is much smaller. You can even tell the child that you will be looking for the biggest "boogers" with your special "booger-picker."

When explaining what to expect, it is important to be honest about what might be felt. For example, the explanation might be as follows:

You will feel the scope in your nose, but because we put the medicine in there, it shouldn't hurt. Instead, you will feel a little pressure and it may feel a little uncomfortable at first. When the scope is almost where it needs to be, there is a tight spot. As the scope goes through it, it might make you want to sneeze. (In fact, many children do sneeze repeatedly at this point, so it's good to stand clear!) It is very important to hold still, though, because if you move your head too much, it might make the scope bang around inside of your nose and that might hurt a little. Once the scope is in place, you need to repeat some silly sentences, and we will watch what

happens on the monitor. When you finish saying all the sentences, we can take the scope out of your nose, and you are done.

Promising a reward at the end of the procedure can also provide some motivation for cooperation.

At times, children delay the procedure out of fear. If the child has further questions on what to expect, these should be answered. However, an extended delay is counterproductive and just increases the fear. The examiner should be mindful of this and be firm about doing the exam to complete it.

With an adult, a nasopharyngoscopy examination can be done in a matter of a few minutes. When working with young children, however, nasopharyngoscopy takes more time and a lot more patience. If the child is prepared in advance and the examiner commits to spend whatever time is necessary, an adequate nasopharyngoscopy study can almost always be obtained for children, even those as young as 3 years of age.

Positioning the Patient

For best results in inserting the scope, the patient should be seated upright in a chair in front of the examiner. Ideally, the patient should be positioned so that she can watch the procedure on the monitor (Figure 17–7). A young child should be seated on the parent's lap. The parent is then instructed to "hug" the child around the arms and hold the child's hands. This prevents the child from grabbing the scope during the procedure. It is also helpful to have another person gently hold the child's head to be sure that it does not move erratically during the exam. At times, it may be necessary for the parent to wrap his or her legs around the child's legs to keep the child from kicking.

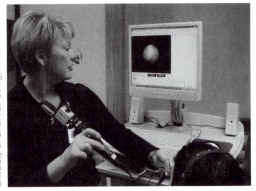

FIGURE 17–7   The nasopharyngoscopy procedure with the patient positioned to see the monitor.

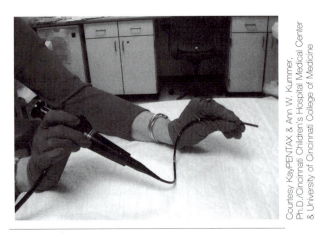

FIGURE 17–8   The best way to hold the scope is to place the viewing end in one hand (usually the dominant hand) with the tip control lever on top for manipulation with either the thumb or the index finger. The thumb and fingers of the other hand should grasp the insertion end of the scope and gently pass it into the nostril.

Nasopharyngoscopy Procedure

With knowledge of the anatomy of the nose and a period of practice, the nasopharyngoscopy procedure is not difficult to perform. It does require patience, however, particularly when evaluating young children. Tips on achieving a successful nasopharyngoscopy examination are described in the following sections.

Passing the Scope

Before inserting the scope, the examiner should check the camera to be sure the image is in focus. This can be done by placing the scope just above something in print and making adjustments in the focus as needed. The camera may also have to be turned slightly to be sure the image is upright. This usually means the cord should be straight down.

The best way to hold the scope is to place the camera end in one hand (usually the dominant hand), with the control lever on top for manipulation with the index finger. The thumb and fingers of the other hand should grasp the insertion end of the scope and gently pass it into the nostril (Figure 17–8). The examiner can rest a hand against the patient's nose or forehead for maximum control during insertion.

The examiner should try to determine the most patent side of the individual's nose for passage of the scope. This can be done by putting the scope at the entrance of each nostril to view the passageway first. Another way is to have the patient close one nostril at a time and then inspire deeply through the other. The nostril with the higher pitch during inspiration is usually the one with the smallest passageway (Shprintzen, 1996). If one side is tried and there is resistance, the examiner should try the other side. When there is a unilateral cleft, usually the unaffected side is the most patent.

For evaluation of velopharyngeal function, the scope is guided up and over the inferior turbinate and through the middle meatus (Figure 17–9). If it goes through the inferior nasal meatus, which is on the floor of the nose,

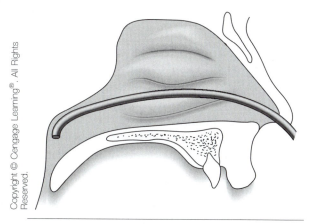

FIGURE 17–9 The scope is usually guided into the middle nasal meatus and then back to the nasopharynx where it periscopes down to view the velum.

it will be on top of the velum when it reaches the port. In this position, the scope usually bounces up and down with velar movement during speech, thus obscuring the examiner's view of velopharyngeal function. (Note: The inferior meatus can be used for FEES, however, because the examiner is viewing residue following the swallow and when the velum is back down.) The superior nasal meatus is too narrow for comfortable passage of the scope. Therefore, the middle nasal meatus is the passage of choice. The middle meatus is large enough for the scope to fit through easily, and because of its position, it allows an unobstructed view of the port from above. The inferior meatus is used to evaluate a hard palate fistula, however.

With practice, passing the scope is usually fast and easy. However, a deviated septum, narrow or stenotic nasal passage, choanal atresia, or even bone spurs can make passage of the scope more challenging. The examiner should avoid contact with the nasal septum, which is sensitive, by carefully observing the passage of the scope through the meatus and adjusting the position of the scope accordingly.

It is always a good idea to tell the patient to let you know whether it hurts or is especially uncomfortable so that appropriate adjustments can be made in the position of the scope. If the field of view appears to be totally white, this is due to the light bouncing off a close object. Therefore, the examiner should withdraw the scope slightly and then reposition it before advancing further. If contact occurs, it will be felt by the examiner as resistance, and it will be felt by the patient as pressure or mild pain. The back of the nose, just in front of the choana, is the narrowest part of the canal and is the area that is usually the most sensitive, even with good anesthetic coverage. As the scope passes through this area, it may cause the eyes to water and may even elicit a few sneezes. Once the scope goes through the choana, the area opens up, and there is less discomfort for the patient.

When the scope is first passed through the choana, it may be oriented in a horizontal position so that the view is across the port and looking toward the posterior pharyngeal wall. To look down on the velopharyngeal port, the end of the scope has to be turned down with the control apparatus (lever or wheel) on the scope. It is very important that the end of the scope be perpendicular to the port rather than looking across it. Otherwise, there can be a significant error in interpretation (Henningsson & Isberg, 1991). The examiner should also be careful not to place the scope too far down so that it is below the area of closure. This would give the false impression of velopharyngeal insufficiency, when the true closure is occurring above the level of view.

Once the scope is turned down, the velum should be viewed at the bottom of the screen and the posterior pharyngeal wall should be at the top. If this is not the case, the camera may have to be turned slightly so that the velum is seen at the bottom of the screen. Because the patient is facing the examiner, the left side of the screen will show the patient's right lateral pharyngeal wall and vice versa.

Even when the scope is in good vertical position, the entire port is usually not seen at one time, particularly if using a smaller diameter scope. To examine the entire area, the hand holding the scope should be rotated slightly from one side to the other. By moving the lever of the scope up and down, and by turning the scope from side to side, the examiner can view all areas of the velopharyngeal port from just one nostril.

Once the velopharyngeal valve has been adequately assessed, the scope can be passed down to the hypopharynx to observe the vocal cords. The individual is asked to prolong an /i/ as long as possible so that vocal fold movement can be observed. If stroboscopy is available, the examiner can view the waveform of the vocal folds. Some children have difficulty with the concept of prolonging the sound. When this occurs, the speech-language pathologist can help by producing the sound simultaneously with the child in a contest to see who can hold it the longest.

During some examinations, the end of the scope becomes foggy or obscured by secretions. When this occurs, it helps to ask the patient to sniff hard and then swallow to try to clear the scope. If that does not work, the examiner should advance the scope slightly into the oropharynx and ask the patient to swallow again. If the scope is still foggy, despite frequent swallows, then it is necessary to remove it, wipe the end with rubbing alcohol, and then try again. For copious secretions in the nasopharynx that interfere with the view of the velopharyngeal port, suctioning through the nose is most effective, if available. Suctioning can be done with the scope in place by putting the suction catheter in the same or opposite naris, but along floor of the nose (inferior meatus).

A successful examination is one in which there has been painless insertion of the scope. There must be good light saturation and good optical quality. There must be appropriate positioning of the scope so that there is good visualization of the velopharyngeal port and nasopharynx. Finally, because the scope of view is limited to a portion of the velopharyngeal area, there must be good manipulation of the scope so that the entire sphincter has been adequately viewed (Shprintzen, 1995). Although published in 1994, the book entitled *Videoendoscopy: From Velopharynx to Larynx* (Karnell, 1994) still provides useful information about this procedure.

Management of Crying

Although there may be some minor discomfort with the nasopharyngoscopy procedure, particularly as the scope goes through the choana, it is definitely not painful. Most children tolerate it very well if they are adequately prepared (Figure 17–10). However, it is natural for a young child to be fearful and therefore cry before and during the examination. Once the scope is in place (which takes only a few seconds), there should be minor discomfort at

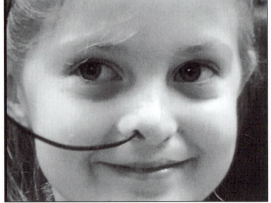

FIGURE 17–10 The scope in place in a patient who obviously has no discomfort.

most. If the child continues to cry, it is important to calm him down for his sake and also for the sake of obtaining an adequate assessment.

Typically, when the child begins crying, all the adults in the room have the tendency to talk to the child at once, and everyone ends up yelling over each other to the child. This has the opposite effect of the one intended. Instead, it is best to tell everyone in the room, including the parents, to be quiet during the examination so that the speech-language pathologist is the only person talking to the child. It is important to talk softly and calmly to the child. If you can get the child to open his eyes to look at you, that usually stops the crying. Distraction techniques can also be useful. It is helpful to have a stuffed animal, puppet, or a bottle of bubbles handy. If the child agrees to blow some bubbles while the scope is in place, the act of blowing will stop the crying. In a firm yet gentle way, the child should be told that he must stop crying and say the words so that the scope can be removed.

Speech Sample

Once the scope is in place, the velopharyngeal port should first be visualized at rest so that all the structures can be observed and the patency of the airway can be noted. The individual is then asked to repeat syllables or sentences so that velopharyngeal function can be directly observed. As noted previously, the speech-language pathologist should determine the type of speech samples needed based on the results of the perceptual evaluation. Unlike videofluoroscopy, there is no inherent danger to the individual with this procedure; therefore, there is no need to restrict the length of time eliciting speech, unless the patient's cooperation is limited. As noted in Chapter 11, the examiner should elicit a combination of sentences loaded with pressure-sensitive pho-

nemes (see Table 11–3), counting, and repetition of syllables for the evaluation of velopharyngeal function.

If hyponasality or upper airway obstruction is a concern, the examiner should assess the patency of the velopharyngeal port during nasal breathing and during the production of nasal sounds. This can be done by having the individual repeat sentences with nasal phonemes, count from 90 to 100, repeat nasal syllables (e.g., /ma, ma, ma/, /mi, mi, mi/, /na, na, na/, /ni, ni, ni/) and then prolong an /m/ as long as possible. The examiner should also have the patient close her mouth and breathe as normally as possible through the nose for at least 30 seconds. Keeping the lips closed, the individual should then be asked to inspire deeply through the nose. During all of these activities, the relative opening of the pharyngeal port should be assessed. If a pharyngeal flap or sphincter pharyngoplasty is in place, the patency of the ports should be carefully examined during nasal breathing and production of nasal sounds. This is done by placing the scope directly above the port.

Occasionally, a child will continue to cry or refuse to talk with the scope in the nose. In these cases, "desperate measures" are needed. For testing velopharyngeal function, sentences like "Stop sticking this scope in my nose!" or "Take this scope out of my nose" may be used. If nasal phonemes are needed, the child can repeat "No, no, no!" or "Not now!"

Potential Complications

Complications with nasopharyngoscopy occur very rarely. However, it is possible for the patient to experience a vasovagal event, causing fainting. Fainting is usually the result of individual anxiety and can be avoided by watching the patient carefully and giving a great deal of reassurance as needed. The fainting response is not limited to the patient. The parent may actually be the one to faint!

If the patient (or parent) appears ashen, the procedure should be terminated immediately. The individual should be placed in a reclining position with the head lower than the legs, or in a sitting position with the head below the knees.

Another rare complication is *epistaxis*, which is a nosebleed. Even when this occurs, the bleeding is usually slight and resolves quickly. A nasal decongestant (oxymetazoline) can help stop the bleeding because it acts as a vasoconstrictor. However, with a little pressure the bleeding stops on its own in most cases (J. Paul Willging, M.D., personal communication, May 12, 2006). Although the risk of medical complication is very slight, nasopharyngoscopy should be performed in a setting where medical support is available.

INTERPRETATION

Once the clinician has been trained in nasopharyngoscopy, it is not difficult to pass the scope through the nose. The biggest challenge is the analysis and interpretation of the findings and the formulation of appropriate recommendations. For this part of the evaluation, a team approach is definitely preferable (D'Antonio et al., 1986; Willging, 2003).

Team Interpretation of the Results

The most appropriate team for nasopharyngoscopy evaluations is the speech-language pathologist and a pediatric otolaryngologist or plastic surgeon. Because speech, resonance, and phonation are highly dependent on the structures of the vocal tract, and many of the problems seen through nasopharyngoscopy are related to the ear, nose, or throat, it is especially helpful to have an otolaryngologist as part of the team. Speech-language pathol-

ogists are trained to evaluate the velopharyngeal structures and function as they relate to the acoustic characteristics of speech, voice, and resonance. The gold standard for determining the need for intervention remains the perceptual quality of the speech. The speech-language pathologist can also determine whether the individual is stimulable, which may suggest correction with speech therapy, or whether the problem is functional, which definitely suggests correction with speech therapy. The speech-language pathologist is essential during the examination to determine the appropriate stimuli to emphasize the velopharyngeal closure defects. Finally, the speech-language pathologist can assist in determining the appropriate recommendations for treatment. The physician can assess the structural aspects of the oral cavity, pharynx, and nasal cavity with respect to the velopharyngeal valve and airway. Physicians are trained to assess the anatomy and physiology with a focus on disease and abnormality. They can determine the appropriate medical or surgical approaches to treatment for any abnormalities that are found. The physician can also identify associated problems, such as middle ear effusion, vocal nodules, and adenotonsillar hypertrophy.

The nasopharyngoscopy assessment is most valuable when it is not just viewed by both professionals, but when it is done live by both professionals working together as a team. It makes no difference who passes the scope, as long as both professionals take a part in the interpretation of the results and formulation of the recommendations. In this way, a separate referral and evaluation are often avoided, and recommendations for treatment can be made on the spot.

Clinical Observations

With the endoscope in place in the nasopharynx, the examiner can view the velopharyngeal structures with the velum at the bottom of the screen and the posterior pharyngeal wall at the top of the screen. The opening to the Eustachian tube can often be seen in the view (Figure 17–11). As noted previously, the view through the scope is from the patient facing the examiner. Therefore, the left side of the screen is the individual's right side and vice versa. This is particularly important to keep in mind when reporting the location of an opening or growth, or reporting asymmetrical movement.

The morphology of the nasal surface of the velum should be carefully scrutinized. If the patient had a cleft palate repair, the examiner should be sure the palate is intact. In some cases, there is an indentation in the posterior border of the velum, which can cause a gap during speech. If the patient has no history of cleft, the velum should be inspected for signs of a submucous cleft palate (Figure 17–12 A–F). This might include a hypoplastic musculus

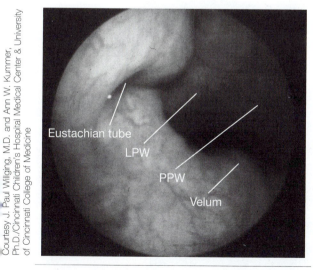

Eustachian tube

LPW

PPW

Velum

FIGURE 17–11 A nasopharyngoscopy view of normal velopharyngeal structures. The nasal surface of the velum is always at the bottom of the screen and the posterior pharyngeal wall is always at the top of the screen. The opening to the Eustachian tube can be seen on the left side of the view.

uvula, which appears as a flattening or concavity in the area where there should be a convex shape. There may also be a depression or a notch in midline at the posterior border, which usually causes a velopharyngeal opening in midline (Gosain, Conley, Marks, & Larson, 1996; Lewin, Croft, & Shprintzen, 1980; Peterson-Falzone, 1985; Shprintzen, 1995; Shprintzen, 1996; Shprintzen & Golding-Kushner, 1989). If there is an oronasal fistula in the hard palate, even this can be seen through the endoscope through the inferior meatus (Figure 17–13).

The adenoid pad should be inspected for its size, surface, and location (Lertsburapa et al., 2010). The adenoid tissue may be large and blocking the nasopharynx, the opening of the choanal (see Figure 8–10), or the opening to one or both Eustachian tubes. It may also have an irregular surface or fissures in the surface that prohibit the velum from achieving a tight veloadenoidal seal (Figure 17–14A–E). This is a particular concern in children who tend to achieve velar contact against the adenoids (Finkelstein, Berger, Nachmani, & Ophir, 1996; Gereau & Shprintzen, 1988; Mason, 1973; Siegel-Sadewitz & Shprintzen, 1986; Williams, Preece, Rhys, & Eccles, 1992). Finally, the examiner should note other unusual findings on the pharyngeal wall, such as the scar band, as seen in Figure 17–15.

If the patient has a Passavant's ridge during speech, this can often be observed only if there is a velopharyngeal opening (Figure 17–16A–C). With complete or nearly complete closure, the Passavant's ridge usually cannot be seen through nasopharyngoscopy because it appears only with velopharyngeal closure and is usually located below the area of closure (Finkelstein et al., 1991; Finkelstein, Lerner, et al., 1993; Witzel & Posnick, 1989).

The morphology of the posterior pharyngeal wall should be examined during quiet

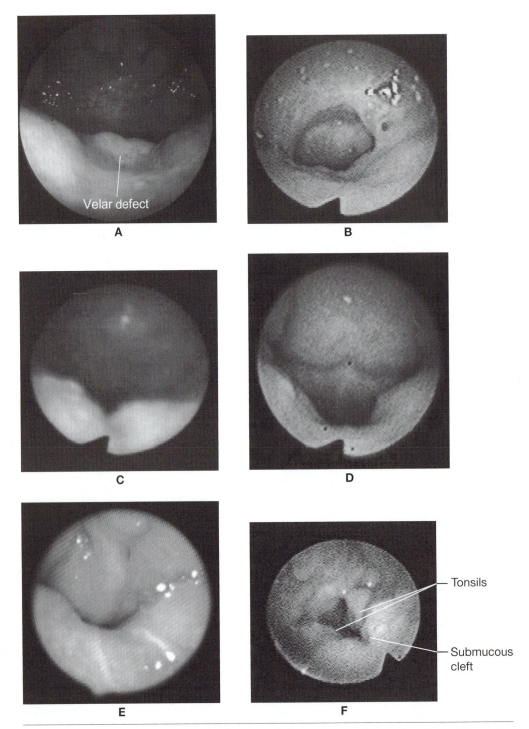

FIGURE 17–12 (A–F)   Examples of submucous clefts, as seen on the nasal surface of the velum through nasopharyngoscopy. Note that in all cases, there is a notch in midline and a depression on the end of the velum where there should be a bulge from the musculus uvulae muscles. In example F, note the large tonsils that are intruding into the oropharynx.

Courtesy J. Paul Willging, M.D. and Ann W. Kummer, Ph.D./Cincinnati Children's Hospital Medical Center & University of Cincinnati College of Medicine

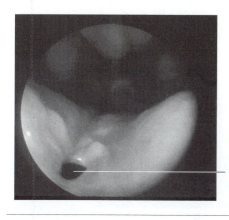

Fistula in the hard palate (nasal surface)

FIGURE 17–13   View of an oronasal fistula as seen through nasopharyngoscopy.

Courtesy J. Paul Willging, M.D. and Ann W. Kummer, Ph.D./Cincinnati Children's Hospital Medical Center & University of Cincinnati College of Medicine

breathing in order to determine whether a pulsating vessel is apparent on the posterior pharyngeal wall. This is particularly important for patients with a diagnosis of velocardiofacial syndrome (or a submucous cleft of unknown origin) because with this syndrome the carotid arteries can be medially displaced, as noted in Figure 17–17. In fact, one or both of the carotid arteries may be seen pulsating on the posterior pharyngeal wall (D'Antonio & Marsh, 1987; Finkelstein, Zohar, et al., 1993; MacKenzie-Stepner, Witzel, Stringer, Lindsay, et al., 1987; Ross, Witzel, Armstrong, & Thomson, 1996; Witt, Miller, Marsh, Muntz, & Grames, 1998).

Hypertrophic tonsils can be so large that they push against and past the posterior faucial pillars and intrude into the pharynx. This can easily be seen through nasopharyngoscopy (Figure 17–12F and Figure 17–18A and B). When this occurs, it can cause both a functional and mechanical interference with lateral pharyngeal wall movement (Finkelstein, Nachmani, & Ophir, 1994; Henningsson & Isberg, 1988; Kummer, Billmire, & Myer, 1993;

MacKenzie-Stepner, Witzel, Stringer, & Laskin, 1987). In rare cases, a tonsil (or both) is so large that it extends up to the area between the velum and posterior pharyngeal wall, thus interfering with velopharyngeal closure (see Figure 7–14B and Figure 7–15C). When hypertrophic tonsils interfere with velopharyngeal function (and also affect the airway), this can be corrected with a tonsillectomy.

The degree of velar, lateral pharyngeal, and posterior pharyngeal wall movement should be observed, and the symmetry of lateral wall movement should be noted. The relative contribution of all of these structures to closure should be assessed. Based on these observations, the basic closure pattern (coronal, circular, or sagittal) can be determined (Croft et al., 1981; Finkelstein, Lerner, et al., 1993; Igawa, Nishizawa, Sugihara, & Inuyama, 1998; Shprintzen, Rakof, Skolnick, & Lavorato, 1977; Siegel-Sadewitz & Shprintzen, 1982; Skolnick, Shprintzen, McCall, & Rakoff, 1975; Witzel & Posnick, 1989).

The adequacy of closure of the velopharyngeal sphincter should be directly assessed during connected speech. If there is a velopharyngeal opening, it is important to determine the size, shape, and location of the opening. These observations can dictate the type of surgical management and the placement of the correction (Shprintzen et al., 1979). Figure 17–19A–M shows various openings with different patterns of closure and therefore different shapes.

A very small opening may not be seen immediately through nasopharyngoscopy. With connected speech, however, there is bubbling of the secretions (Figure 17–19A). Whenever bubbling is noted, the examiner can be sure that it is caused by a velopharyngeal opening, which is usually small in size. This bubbling is due to air pressure being forced through a small velopharyngeal opening. If the opening

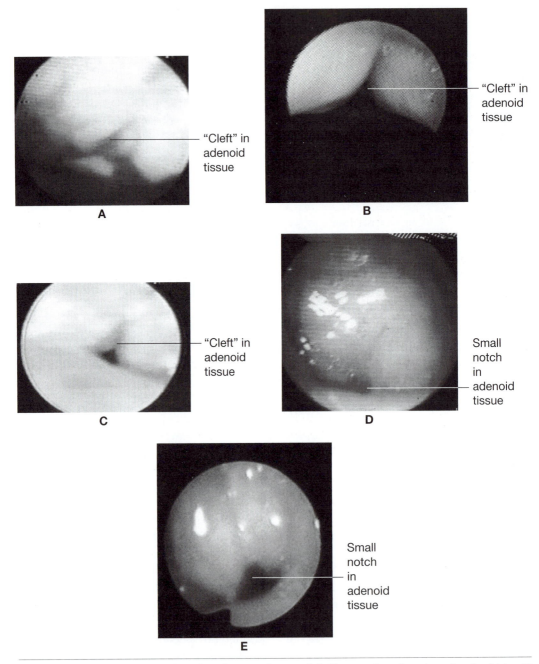

FIGURE 17–14 (A–E) Irregular adenoids. A–C show a "cleft-like" notch in the adenoid pad, which will interfere with a tight velopharyngeal seal. D and E each show a smaller notch in the adenoid, but these notches will also cause velopharyngeal insufficiency during closure.

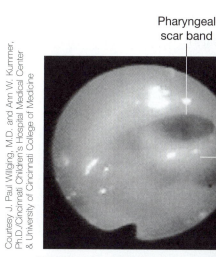

Pharyngeal scar band

Epiglottis

FIGURE 17–15 Scar band on the pharyngeal wall that occurred following an aggressive tonsillectomy.

was larger, there would be less friction and bubbling. The bubbling is perceived as a nasal rustle, also called nasal turbulence (Kummer, Curtis, Wiggs, Lee, & Strife, 1992). The location of the opening (midline, left of midline, in the right corner, etc.) is important to document because it has implications for surgical correction.

It is very common to observe inconsistency in the degree of velopharyngeal movement, and thus the size of velopharyngeal opening, when there is a dysfunctional velopharyngeal valve. With short utterances or with effort, there may be complete closure or just a small opening. With connected speech or with speech segments that are loaded with pressure-sensitive phonemes, however, the opening may be much larger and more consistent. Inconsistent closure may also occur due to fatigue with connected speech or prolonged speaking. In this case, the individual may be able to achieve closure but is not able to maintain it over time. The examiner can assess this by having the patient count or repeat syllables quickly. Closure should be main-

tained throughout the utterance unless there is a nasal phoneme within the utterance. The examiner should observe whether the closure occurs at the beginning of an utterance and then begins to break down toward the end. Inconsistent closure can also be due to abnormal timing and/or coordination of velopharyngeal movement with anterior articulation movement. This is commonly seen with apraxia of speech. In fact, when there is apraxia, the velum may actually elevate inappropriately for nasal sounds and then lower for oral sounds. This can be tested by having the patient repeat multisyllabic words or produce longer, more complex utterances.

When there is inconsistent closure at the sentence level, the examiner should analyze whether the velopharyngeal opening is phoneme specific (occurs only on certain sounds). A phoneme-specific velopharyngeal opening (resulting in phoneme-specific nasal air emission) is caused by faulty articulation (Peterson-Falzone & Graham, 1990). Typically, the patient is substituting a pharyngeal or nasal fricative for the /s/ (and sometimes for other sibilants), causing nasal emission. However, closure is complete and consistent on all other sounds. The examiner should work with the patient to change placement and then note the results on velopharyngeal closure.

For the patient with velopharyngeal dysfunction, the observations noted above will help the examiner to diagnosis the cause of the perceived "nasality" (VPI versus mislearning). This information is used to determine appropriate treatment (i.e., surgery versus speech therapy). If surgery is indicated, it is important to note the size, location, and shape of the opening. This information is helpful when choosing the type of surgical procedure that has the best chance of success for that patient. For a simple checklist of observations through nasopharyngoscopy, see (Table 17–1).

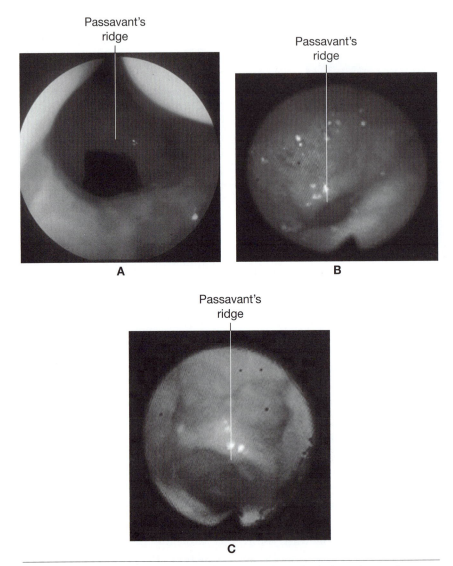

FIGURE 17–16 (A–C) Passavant's ridge as seen from above through nasopharyngoscopy.

Courtesy J. Paul Willging, M.D. and Ann W. Kummer, Ph.D./Cincinnati Children's Hospital Medical Center & University of Cincinnati College of Medicine

Because of the high incidence of vocal nodules or voice disorders in individuals with velopharyngeal dysfunction (D'Antonio et al., 1988; Hirschberg et al., 1995; Lewis, Andreassen, Leeper, Macrae, & Thomas, 1993; Zajac & Linville, 1989), an evaluation of the larynx and vocal cords should also be performed, partic-ularly if dysphonia was noted in the perceptual evaluation. By viewing the vocal folds, the examiner can determine the presence of vocal nodules (Figure 17–20) or a laryngeal web (Figure 17–21), or whether there is thickening or edema of the folds. The movement of the folds can be observed, and the use of

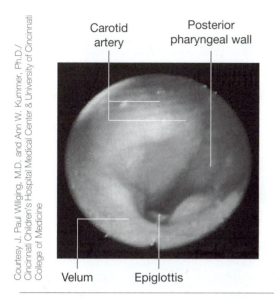

FIGURE 17–17 View of a medially displaced carotid artery, which is commonly seen in patients with velocardiofacial syndrome.

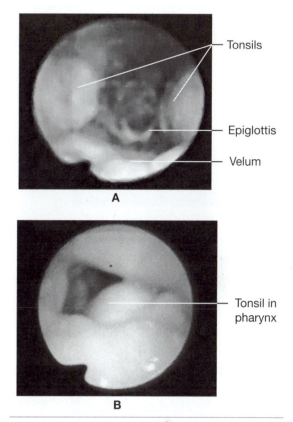

FIGURE 17–18 (A and B) Tonsillar hypertrophy. Note the tonsils in the oropharynx as seen from above through nasopharyngoscopy.

ventricular folds during phonation should be noted if it occurs. Any other anomalies of the vocal folds or their movement should also be noted.

As noted previously, nasopharyngoscopy is a good procedure for evaluation of velopharyngeal function after the patient has undergone a surgical procedure, such as an adenoidectomy, pharyngeal flap (Figure 17–22A–E), sphincter pharyngoplasty (Figure 17–23A and B), or pharyngeal augmentation (see Chapter 18 for details regarding each type of surgery) (Abdel-Aziz, 2007). The examiner should note whether there is complete closure as a result of the surgery or a remaining leak, which may require surgical revision. It should be kept in mind that the closure that is seen through nasopharyngoscopy represents what the patient does with speech and velopharyngeal closure—not what the patient is capable of doing. Because changing structure does not change function, compensatory productions (e.g., pharyngeal

fricatives and glottal stops) will continue after the surgery, and during production, the port will remain open. If this is the case, stimulability testing to change placement should be done to determine the actual potential of the velopharyngeal valve. In addition, the examiner should note the closure of sounds that are correctly articulated. Finally, the postoperative exam should include an assessment of the nasopharyngeal airway. If a port is too narrow for nasal breathing or production of nasal sounds, this should be noted.

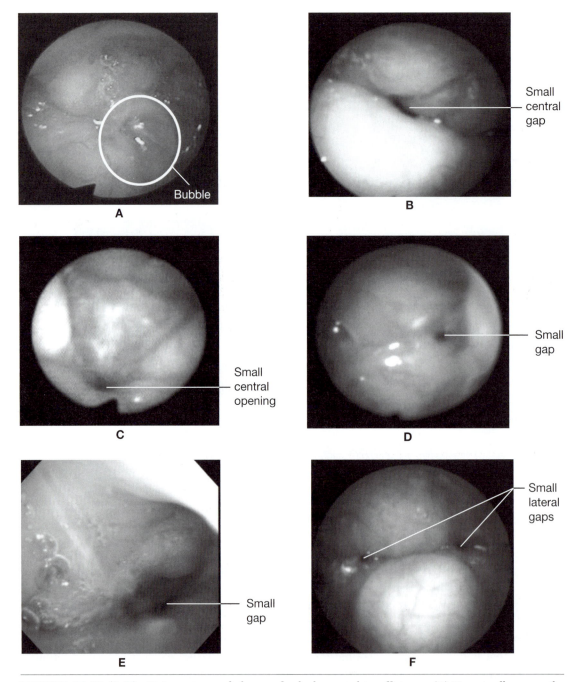

FIGURE 17–19 (A–F) Various sizes and shapes of velopharyngeal insufficiency. (A) Very small gap on the (patient's) left side of midline. (This is on the right side of the figure.) This is noted by the bubbling in that area during speech. (B) Small central gap with a coronal pattern of closure. (C) Small central gap with a circular pattern of closure. (D) Small opening to the (patient's) left of midline. (E) Larger opening to the (patient's) left of midline. (F) Bowtie closure with closure in the midline, but small openings on both sides.

Courtesy J. Paul Willging, M.D. and Ann W. Kummer, Ph.D./Cincinnati Children's Hospital Medical Center & University of Cincinnati College of Medicine

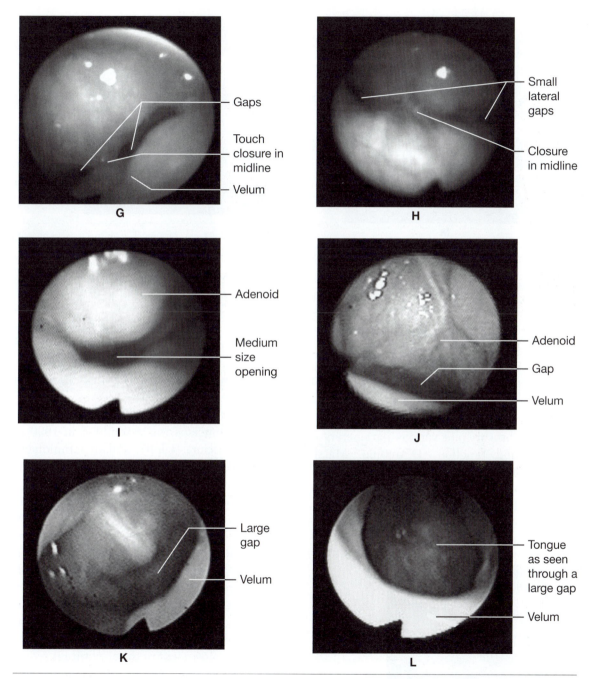

FIGURE 17–19 (G–L) (G) Narrow coronal opening with touch closure in midline. (H) Bowtie closure with medium-size openings on both sides. (I) Medium-size opening with a circular pattern of closure. (J) Medium coronal opening. (K) Large velopharyngeal opening due to short velum. (L) Very large velopharyngeal opening showing the back of the tongue.

Courtesy J. Paul Willging, M.D. and Ann W. Kummer, Ph.D./Cincinnati Children's Hospital Medical Center & University of Cincinnati College of Medicine

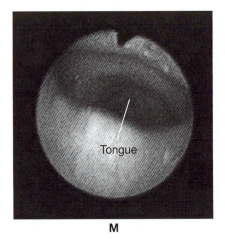

FIGURE 17–19 (M)   Very large velopharyngeal opening showing the back of the tongue.

Courtesy J. Paul Willging, M.D. and Ann W. Kummer, Ph.D./Cincinnati Children's Hospital Medical Center & University of Cincinnati College of Medicine

REPORTING THE RESULTS

As with videofluoroscopic speech studies, some centers report nasopharyngoscopy results with a narrative report. Several authors have suggested using either a numeric scale or a particular form to rate various parameters of structure and function (D'Antonio, Marsh, Province, Muntz, & Phillips, 1989; D'Antonio et al., 1988; Karnell, Ibuki, Morris, & Van Demark, 1983; Sinclair, Davies, & Bracka,

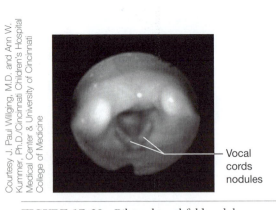

Courtesy J. Paul Willging, M.D. and Ann W. Kummer, Ph.D./Cincinnati Children's Hospital Medical Center & University of Cincinnati College of Medicine

FIGURE 17–20   Bilateral vocal fold nodules.

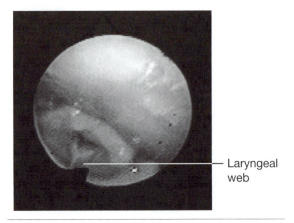

FIGURE 17–21   A laryngeal web in a patient with velocardiofacial syndrome.

Courtesy J. Paul Willging, M.D. and Ann W. Kummer, Ph.D./Cincinnati Children's Hospital Medical Center & University of Cincinnati College of Medicine

1982; Zwitman, Sonderman, & Ward, 1974). What is most important is that there is consistency in the observations that are made in each study and in the way that the studies are reported.

As noted previously, a multidisciplinary group of clinicians was assembled in 1990 by the American Cleft Palate–Craniofacial Association to address the question of standardizing reporting techniques for multiview videofluoroscopy and nasopharyngoscopy (Golding-Kushner et al., 1990). As with videofluoroscopy, the proposed system was to rate the movement of the velum, the posterior pharyngeal wall, and each lateral wall in relation to the structure that it is moving toward. The resting position of the structure is rated as 0.0, and the resting position of the opposing structure is 1.0. Using a ratio, the movement of the structure is scored according to the degree of its movement toward the resting position of the opposing structure. It is unclear how many centers are currently using this system, but its use may be somewhat limited due to its complexity. In

---

TABLE 17–1 Nasopharyngoscopy Rating Form

Velopharyngeal Function

□ **Normal** □ **Abnormal**: □ borderline □ mild □ moderate □ severe □ very severe

Velopharyngeal Opening

Size: □ pinhole □ small □ medium □ large □ very large

Shape: □ circular □ sagittal □ coronal □ bowtie

Location:

□ midline □ R of midline □ R corner □ L of midline □ L corner □ both corners

Consistency: □ consistent □ inconsistent

□ phoneme-specific sounds affected: _____

Effect of stimulation: □ improved closure □ no change

Previous Secondary Surgery: □ None

Type: □ pharyngeal flap □ sphincter pharyngoplasty □ pharyngeal augmentation □ Furlow

Status: □ intact □ too low □ too narrow

Ports during Speech:

Left port: □ open □ stenosed   **Right port:**   □ open □ stenosed

_____   _____

Both ports: □ open □ stenosed   **Central (sphincter) port:** □ open □ stenosed

_____   _____

Additional Findings: (e.g., occult submucous cleft, bubbling of secretions, tonsils in oropharynx, large tonsils, irregular adenoids, medialized carotid arteries, Passavant's ridge, fistula, vocal nodules, laryngeal web, etc.)

_____

_____

Probable Cause

□ VP insufficiency □ VP incompetence □ poor lateral wall movement

□ irregular adenoids: □ phoneme-specific due to misarticulations: _____

Recommendations

□ **Surgical intervention:**

□ pharyngeal flap   □ sphincter pharyngoplasty

□ pharyngeal augmentation   □ palatoplasty

□ adenoidectomy   □ tonsillectomy

□ **Prosthetic intervention:** □ palatal lift □ palatal obturator □ speech bulb

□ **Speech therapy**

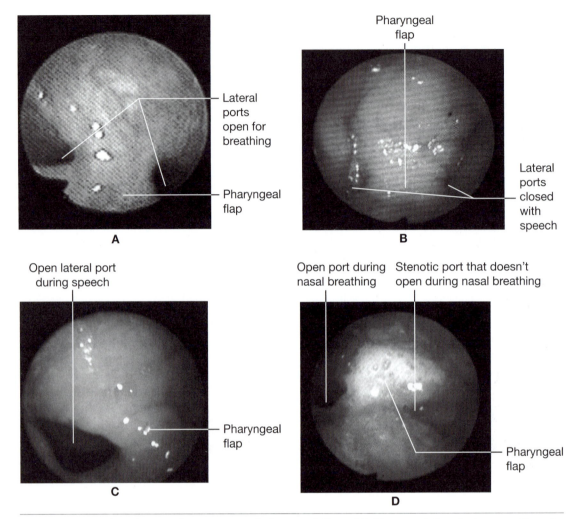

FIGURE 17–22 (A–D) Nasopharyngoscopy of pharyngeal flaps. (A) Pharyngeal flap during rest. Note the lateral ports on each side are patent for normal nasal breathing. (B) Pharyngeal flap during speech with both ports completely closed. (C) Pharyngeal flap with a persistent opening in the (patient's) right port during speech. (D) Pharyngeal flap at rest with the (patient's) right port open for normal nasal breathing, but the (patient's) left port stenosed, causing upper airway obstruction.

Courtesy J. Paul Willging, M.D. and Ann W. Kummer, Ph.D./Cincinnati Children's Hospital Medical Center & University of Cincinnati College of Medicine

addition, the location and cause of the opening is what is important for determining treatment recommendations. Therefore, the ratings may not be of particular value.

The reliability of judgments from nasopharyngoscopy, regardless of the procedure used to report the results, seems to be greatly depen-dent on the experience of the evaluator (D'Antonio et al., 1989). Therefore, working with another experienced examiner initially is important to help the novice evaluator to develop the necessary skills. After that, prac-tice is necessary to hone the skills required for observation and analysis.

Sphincter
pharyngoplasty

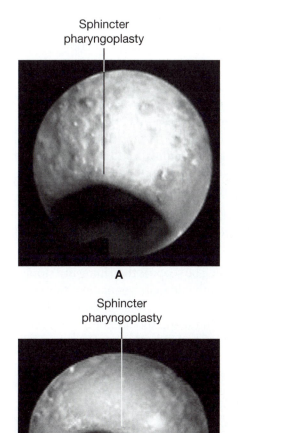

A

Sphincter
pharyngoplasty

Epiglottis

B

FIGURE 17–23 (A and B)   Sphincter pharyngoplasty. (A) This shows a sphincter pharyngoplasty during speech with maximum closure. A large gap remains in midline, despite the presence of the sphincter. (B) This sphincter is too low (note the epiglottis below) and caused sleep apnea, yet is not big enough to close the port during speech.
Courtesy Ann W. Kummer, Ph.D./Cincinnati Children's Hospital Medical Center & University of Cincinnati College of Medicine

Although results are reported to other professionals, they also must be reported to the family. It is very important that the person who counsels the family use clear, easy-to-

understand language. All medical terms should be clearly defined. When discussing the function of the velopharyngeal mechanism, pictures and diagrams must be used. After the initial explanation, it may also be helpful to play the video of the procedure and point out the structures and their function.

CLEANING AND STORING THE ENDOSCOPY

Once the endoscope has been used, care should be taken so that the scope is not placed on a surface that will be touched by others. Instead, the scope should be taken for immediate cleaning and disinfection (McCullagh & Baker, 2000). Guidelines for disinfection of the scope have been developed by the Association for the Advancement of Medical Instrumentation (AAMI, 2010). However, each medical facility should have a specific policy on how endoscopes are reprocessed. Cleaning and high-level disinfection or sterilization is easier and more complete for endoscopes that can be immersed. Therefore, this should be considered when purchasing a new scope.

There are nine steps to reprocessing an endoscope, as noted in the following list (J. Paul Willging, personal communication, May 12, 2006):

1. **Precleaning:** Before disinfection and sterilization, the scope should be carefully cleaned of visible residue with a cloth and enzymatic detergent solution. "Sterile dirt" can still cause infection (Catalone & Koos, 2005).

2. **Transportation to the cleaning facility:** The scope should be placed in a closed, rigid container for the protection of patients, health care workers, and the scope. The cleaning facility must have a separate dirty area to receive the contaminated scope.

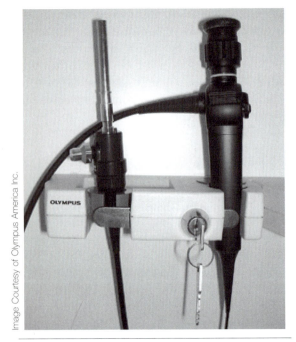

Image Courtesy of Olympus America Inc.

FIGURE 17–24 The scope should ideally be hung when stored for adequate ventilation to prevent moisture buildup and to prevent physical damage.

3. **Leakage testing:** The scope is tested for leakage to ensure the integrity of the external skin. If cleaning materials leak into the core of the scope, the fiberoptic bundles will be severely damaged. If there is a leak, the scope is removed from service until it is repaired.

4. **Manual cleaning:** The scope is immersed in an enzymatic solution and cleaned manually to remove retained debris that can interfere with the capability of germicides to effectively kill microorganisms.

5. **Rinsing:** The endoscope is rinsed to remove residual debris and detergent. The endoscope is then dried to prevent dilution of the chemical germicide during disinfection.

6. **High-level disinfection:** A liquid chemical germicide is used with the required exposure time. These are toxic substances, so personal protection equipment is important (gloves, mask, eye protection, and impervious gown).

7. **Rinsing:** The scope is moved to a designated clean area and thoroughly rinsed in sterile, filtered water. It is important to remove the chemical residue to prevent injury to the skin and mucous membranes of the next patient.

8. **Drying:** The endoscope is dried with a lint-free towel. This inhibits the growth of waterborne organisms.

9. **Storage:** The scope is then hung in a storage cabinet with adequate ventilation to prevent moisture buildup or physical damage (Figure 17–24). The scope should not be stored in the case provided by the manufacturer.

ADVANTAGES AND LIMITATIONS OF NASOPHARYNGOSCOPY

The most commonly used methods for direct visualization of the velopharyngeal mechanism are nasopharyngoscopy and videofluoroscopy (Rowe & D'Antonio, 2005). There are differences in opinion as to the best method of assessment in all cases. The examiner should consider what is more important to visualize in each patient's case, and the relative benefits and risks of each procedure, before determining which type of assessment to use.

One advantage of nasopharyngoscopy over videofluoroscopy is that all structures of the velopharyngeal mechanism can be seen in great detail and almost at the same time. The location, size, shape, and cause of the opening can be determined more easily through nasopharyngoscopy than through videofluoroscopy.

As noted previously, this information is very important for surgical planning. Even very small openings (that cannot be seen with videofluoroscopy) can be seen with nasopharyngoscopy. Finally, the results of surgeries for VPI can be best evaluated through nasopharyngoscopy.

Of course, nasopharyngoscopy is done without radiation; therefore, there is no risk of harmful physical effects to the patient. Because there is no radiation involved, the examiner can take as much time as needed to determine the problem and the appropriate intervention. The procedure can also be repeated as often as needed for pre- and post-treatment assessments. It is well tolerated by most children, even those as young as 3 years old.

Nasopharyngoscopy can be used as a biofeedback tool. The speech-language pathologist can give the individual instructions on placement, and the patient can watch the velopharyngeal results on the monitor as he tries to follow the instructions. This is a particularly powerful procedure for the treatment of certain learned causes of velopharyngeal dysfunction (Brunner et al., 1994; D'Antonio et al., 1988; Kunzel, 1982; Rich, Farber, & Shprintzen, 1988; Shelton et al., 1978; Siegel-Sadewitz & Shprintzen, 1982; Witzel et al., 1988; Witzel, Tobe, & Salyer, 1989; Yamaoka, Matsuya, Miyazaki, Nishio, & Ibuki, 1983; Ysunza et al., 1997). For more information on the use of nasopharyngoscopy for biofeedback, please see Chapter 21.

The risks or limitations associated with nasopharyngoscopy are minimal. The biggest disadvantage of nasopharyngoscopy is that the examiner cannot see the entire length of the pharyngeal wall during speech. In addition, some clinicians argue that videofluoroscopy is less invasive than nasopharyngoscopy. However, introduction of barium in the nasopharynx for videofluoroscopy is also invasive, and the large machinery can be just as frightening to a child as nasopharyngoscopy.

Nasopharyngoscopy requires a moderate degree of cooperation from the individual to successfully complete the study. Getting the scope through to the right place is not difficult. However, getting a child to talk and repeat sentences with the scope in place and without crying can be a challenge. Although nasopharyngoscopy should not be a painful procedure, it can cause some discomfort, especially if the scope hits a nasal spur or the base of the nasal septum. However, with a good coating of topical anesthesia and with previous preparation as to what to expect, the nasopharyngoscopy procedure is usually well tolerated by children as young as 3 years of age. A final disadvantage is that the nasopharyngoscopy equipment is expensive to purchase and maintain.

SUMMARY

Instrumental assessment is not required for the diagnosis of velopharyngeal dysfunction because this can be determined through a perceptual assessment alone. When there is VPI, however, as noted through the perceptual evaluation, nasopharyngoscopy has become a standard secondary evaluation procedure because it is effective in determining the size, shape, location, and cause of the velopharyngeal gap. This information is used to determine the surgical procedure that has the greatest chance of success for the individual patient.

Nasopharyngoscopy is also ideal for evaluating the effectiveness of surgery for VPI because the structures as a result of the surgery can be clearly seen. Nasopharyngoscopy can be used to determine the presence of obstruction in the vocal tract, which can also affect resonance. Finally, it is used to evaluate swallowing and vocal cord anomalies or dysfunction.

FOR REVIEW AND DISCUSSION

1. What equipment is absolutely necessary for a nasopharyngoscopy examination? What additional components are strongly recommended, and why?

2. Why is it important to do a perceptual evaluation of speech before the nasopharyngoscopy exam?

3. Discuss the methods for nasal anesthesia and decongestion.

4. Describe the procedure for passing the scope. What conditions can make passing the scope more challenging? Why is the scope through the middle nasal meatus rather than the inferior nasal meatus or the superior nasal meatus? What should you do if the scope lens becomes cloudy?

5. What determines the appropriate speech samples to use in the exam? Why is it preferable to obtain a sample without the child crying? What are methods to calm the child and stop the crying, if it occurs?

6. What are potential complications during the exam, and how should they be handled?

7. What structures can be viewed through nasopharyngoscopy? What clinical observations can be seen that could affect resonance?

8. What are the advantages of nasopharyngoscopy? What are some of the limitations?

REFERENCES

Abdel-Aziz, M. (2007). Treatment of submucous cleft palate by pharyngeal flap as a primary procedure. *International Journal of Pediatric Otorhinolaryngology*, 71(7), 1093–1097.

American Speech-Language-Hearing Association (ASHA). (n.d.). Infection control in speech-language pathology. Accessed January 19, 2013, from http://www.asha.org/slp/infectioncontrol.htm.

American Speech-Language-Hearing Association (ASHA). (2004a). Knowledge and skills for speech-language pathologists with respect to vocal tract visualization and imaging. Accessed January 19, 2013, from http://www.asha.org/policy/KS2004-00071.htm.

American Speech-Language-Hearing Association (ASHA). (2004b). Vocal tract visualization and imaging: Technical report. Accessed January 19, 2013, from http://www.asha.org/policy/TR2004-00156.htm.

American Speech-Language-Hearing Association (ASHA). (2005). The role of the speech-language pathologist in the performance and interpretation of endoscopic evaluation of swallowing: Technical Report. Accessed January 19, 2013, from http://www.asha.org/policy/TR2005-00155.htm.

Association for the Advancement of Medical Instrumentation (AAMI). (2010). Processing of flexible and semi-rigid scopes. Accessed June 1, 2012, from http://www.aami.org/applications/search/details.cfm.

Aviv, J. E., Kim, T., Thomson, J. E., Sunshine, S., Kaplan, S., & Close, L. G. (1998). Fiberoptic endoscopic evaluation of swallowing with sensory testing (FEESST) in healthy controls [see Comments]. *Dysphagia*, 13(2), 87–92.

Bastian, R. W. (1991). Videoendoscopic evaluation of patients with dysphagia: An adjunct to the modified barium swallow. *Otolaryngology—Head & Neck Surgery*, 104(3), 339–350.

Bastian, R. W. (1993). The videoendoscopic swallowing study: An alternative and partner to the videofluoroscopic swallowing study. *Dysphagia*, 8(4), 359–367.

Bastian, R. W. (1998). Contemporary diagnosis of the dysphagic patient. *Otolaryngology Clinics of North America*, 31(3), 489–506.

Brunner, M., Stellzig, A., Decker, W., Strate, B., Komposch, C., Wirth, C., & Verres, R. (1994). Video-feedback therapy with the flexible nasopharyngoscope. The potentials for modifying velopharyngeal closure and phonation deficiencies in cleft patients. *Fortschritte de Kieferorthopadei*, 55(4), 197–201.

Brunner, M., Stellzig-Eisenhauer, A., Proschel, U., Verres, R., & Komposch, G. (2005). The effect of nasopharyngoscopic biofeedback in patients with cleft palate and velopharyngeal dysfunction. *Cleft Palate–Craniofacial Journal*, 42(6), 649–657.

Cain, A. J., Murray, D. P., & McClymont, L. G. (2002). The use of topical nasal anaesthesia before flexible nasendoscopy: A double-blind, randomized, controlled trial comparing cophenylcaine with placebo. *Clinical Otolaryngology & Allied Sciences*, 27(6), 485–488.

Catalone, B., & Koos, G. (2005). Beyond cleaning: Reprocessing flexible GI endoscopes successfully. *Heathcare Purchasing News*, 29(11), 38–39.

Centers for Disease Control and Prevention (CDC). (2005, May 3). Recommendations for application of standard precautions for the care of all patients in all healthcare settings. Accessed January 19, 2013, from http://www.cdc.gov/sars/guidance/I-infection/app1.html.

Centers for Disease Control and Prevention (CDC). (2013, January 11). Handwashing: Clean hands save lives. Accessed January 19, 2013, from http://www.cdc.gov/handwashing.

Croft, C. B., Shprintzen, R. J., & Rakoff, S. J. (1981). Patterns of velopharyngeal valving in normal and cleft palate subjects: A multiview videofluoroscopic and nasendoscopic study. *Laryngoscope*, 91(2), 265–271.

D'Antonio, L. D., & Marsh, J. L. (1987). Abnormal carotid arteries in the velocardiofacial syndrome [Letter]. *Plastic and Reconstructive Surgery*, 80(3), 471–472.

D'Antonio, L. L., Achauer, B. M., & Vander Kam, V. M. (1993). Results of a survey of cleft palate teams concerning the use of nasendoscopy. *Cleft Palate–Craniofacial Journal*, 30(1), 35–39.

D'Antonio, L. L., Chait, D., Lotz, W., & Netsell, R. (1986). Pediatric videonasoendoscopy for speech and voice evaluation. *Otolaryngology—Head & Neck Surgery*, 94(5), 578–583.

D'Antonio, L. L., Marsh, J. L., Province, M. A., Muntz, H. R., & Phillips, C. J. (1989). Reliability of flexible fiberoptic nasopharyngoscopy for evaluation of velopharyngeal function in a clinical population. *Cleft Palate Journal*, 26(3), 217–225; Discussion 225.

D'Antonio, L. L., Muntz, H. R., Marsh, J. L., Marty-Grames, L., & Backensto-Marsh, R. (1988). Practical application of flexible fiberoptic nasopharyngoscopy for evaluating velopharyngeal function. *Plastic and Reconstructive Surgery*, 82(4), 611–618.

David, D. J., White, J., Sprod, R., & Bagnall, A. (1982). Nasendoscopy: Significant refinements of a direct-viewing technique of the velopharyngeal sphincter. *Plastic and Reconstructive Surgery, 70*(4), 423–428.

Donzelli, J., Brady, S., Wesling, M., & Theisen, M. (2005). Effects of the removal of the tracheotomy tube on swallowing during the fiberoptic endoscopic exam of the swallow (FEES). *Dysphagia, 20*(4), 283–289.

Douglas, R., Hawke, L., & Wormald, P. J. (2006). Topical anaesthesia before nasendoscopy: A randomized controlled trial of co-phenylcaine compared with lidocaine. *Clinical Otolaryngology, 31*(1), 33.

Finkelstein, Y., Berger, G., Nachmani, A., & Ophir, D. (1996). The functional role of the adenoids in speech. *International Journal of Pediatric Otorhinolaryngology, 34*(1/2), 61–74.

Finkelstein, Y., Lerner, M. A., Ophir, D., Nachmani, A., Hauben, D. J., & Zohar, Y. (1993). Nasopharyngeal profile and velopharyngeal valve mechanism. *Plastic and Reconstructive Surgery, 92*(4), 603–614.

Finkelstein, Y., Nachmani, A., & Ophir, D. (1994). The functional role of the tonsils in speech. *Archives of Otolaryngology—Head & Neck Surgery, 120*(8), 846–851.

Finkelstein, Y., Talmi, Y. P., Kravitz, K., Bar-Ziv, J., Nachmani, A., Hauben, D. J., & Zohar, Y. (1991). Study of the normal and insufficient velopharyngeal valve by the "Forced Sucking Test" *Laryngoscope, 101*(11), 1203–1212.

Finkelstein, Y., Zohar, Y., Nachmani, A., Talmi, Y. P., Lerner, M. A., Hauben, D. J., & Frydman, M. (1993). The otolaryngologist and the patient with velocardiofacial syndrome. *Archives of Otolaryngology—Head & Neck Surgery, 119*(5), 563–569.

Frosh, A. C., Jayaraj, S., Porter, G., & Almeyda, J. (1998). Is local anaesthesia actually beneficial in flexible fibreoptic nasendoscopy? *Clinics in Otolaryngology, 23*(3), 259–262.

Georgalas, C., Sandhu, G., Frosh, A., & Xenellis, J. (2005). Cophenylcaine spray vs. placebo in flexible nasendoscopy: A prospective double-blind randomized controlled trial. *International Journal of Clinical Practice, 59*(2), 130–133.

Gereau, S. A., & Shprintzen, R. J. (1988). The role of adenoids in the development of normal speech following palate repair. *Laryngoscope, 98*(3), 299–303.

Golding-Kushner, K. J., Argamaso, R. V., Cotton, R. T., Grames, L. M., Henningsson, G., Jones, et al. (1990). Standardization for the reporting of nasopharyngoscopy and multiview videofluoroscopy: A report from an International Working Group. *Cleft Palate Journal, 27*(4), 337–347; Discussion 347–348.

Gosain, A. K., Conley, S. F., Marks, S., & Larson, D. L. (1996). Submucous cleft palate: Diagnostic methods and outcomes of surgical treatment. *Plastic and Reconstructive Surgery, 97*(7), 1497–1509.

Henningsson, G., & Isberg, A. (1988). Influence of tonsils on velopharyngeal movements in children with craniofacial anomalies and hypernasality. *American Journal of Orthodontics and Dentofacial Orthopedics, 94*(3), 253–261.

Henningsson, G., & Isberg, A. (1991). Comparison between multiview videofluoroscopy and nasendoscopy of velopharyngeal movements. *Cleft Palate–Craniofacial Journal, 28*(4), 413–417; Discussion 417–418.

Hirschberg, J., Dejonckere, P. H., Hirano, M., Mori, K., Schultz-Coulon, H. J., & Vrticka, K. (1995). Voice disorders in children. *International Journal of Pediatric Otorhinolaryngology, 32*(Suppl.), S109–S125.

Hung, C. H., & Cheng, S. Y. (1989). Application of nasopharyngoscopy and videofluoroscopy in the fabrication of a speech aid for soft palate defects. *Journal of the Formosan Medical Association*, 88(8), 812–818.

Igawa, H. H., Nishizawa, N., Sugihara, T., & Inuyama, Y. (1998). A fiberscopic analysis of velopharyngeal movement before and after primary palatoplasty in cleft palate infants. *Plastic and Reconstructive Surgery*, 102(3), 668–674.

Jonas, N. E., Visser, M. F., Oomen, A., Albertyn, R., van Dijk, M., & Prescott, C. A. (2007). Is topical local anaesthesia necessary when performing paediatric flexible nasendoscopy? A double-blind randomized controlled trial. *International Journal of Pediatric Otorhinolaryngology*, 71(11), 1687–1692.

Karnell, M. P. (1994). *Videoendoscopy: From velopharynx to larynx*. San Diego, CA: Singular Publishing Group.

Karnell, M. P., & Langmore, S. (1998). Videoendoscopy in speech and swallowing for the speech-language pathologist. In A. F. Johnson & B. H. Jacobson (Eds.), *Medical speech-language pathology: A practitioner's guide* (pp. 563–584). New York, NY: Thieme.

Karnell, M. P., Ibuki, K., Morris, H. L., & Van Demark, D. R. (1983). Reliability of the nasopharyngeal fiberscope (NPF) for assessing velopharyngeal function: Analysis by judgment. *Cleft Palate Journal*, 20(3), 199–208.

Karnell, M. P., Rosenstein, H., & Fine, L. (1987). Nasal videoendoscopy in prosthetic management of palatopharyngeal dysfunction. *Journal of Prosthetic Dentistry*, 58(4), 479–484.

Kidder, T. M., Langmore, S. E., & Martin, B. J. (1994). Indications and techniques of endoscopy in evaluation of cervical dysphagia: Comparison with radiographic techniques. *Dysphagia*, 9(4), 256–261.

Kuehn, D. P., & Henne, L. J. (2003). Speech evaluation and treatment of patients with cleft palate. *American Journal of Speech-Language Pathology*, 12, 103–109.

Kummer, A. W., Billmire, D. A., & Myer, C. M. (1993). Hypertrophic tonsils: The effect on resonance and velopharyngeal closure. *Plastic and Reconstructive Surgery*, 91(4), 608–611.

Kummer, A. W., Clark, S. L., Redle, E. E., Thomsen, L. L., & Billmire, D. A. (2011). Current practice in assessing and reporting speech outcomes of cleft palate and velopharyngeal surgery: A survey of cleft palate/craniofacial professionals. *Cleft Palate–Craniofacial Journal*, 49(2), 146–152.

Kummer, A. W., Curtis, C., Wiggs, M., Lee, L., & Strife, J. L. (1992). Comparison of velopharyngeal gap size in patients with hypernasality, hypernasality, and nasal emission, or nasal turbulence (rustle) as the primary speech characteristic. *Cleft Palate–Craniofacial Journal*, 29(2), 152–156.

Kunzel, H. J. (1982). First applications of a biofeedback device for the therapy of velopharyngeal incompetence. *Folia Phoniatrica*, 34(2), 92–100.

Lam, D. J., Starr, J. R., Perkins, J. A., Lewis, C. W., Eblen, L. E., Dunlap, J., & Sie, K. C. (2006). A comparison of nasendoscopy and multiview videofluoroscopy in assessing velopharyngeal insufficiency. *Otolaryngology—Head & Neck Surgery*, 134(3), 394–402.

Langmore, S. E., Schatz, K., & Olsen, N. (1988). Fiberoptic endoscopic examination of swallowing safety: A new procedure. *Dysphagia*, 2(4), 216–219.

Leder, S. B., Acton, L. M., Lisitano, H. L., & Murray, J. T. (2005). Fiberoptic endoscopic evaluation of swallowing (FEES) with and without blue-dyed food. *Dysphagia, 20*(2), 157–162.

Lennox, P., Hem, J., Birchall, M., & Lund, V. (1996). Local anaesthesia in flexible nasendoscopy. A comparison between cocaine and co-phenylcaine. *Journal of Laryngology & Otology, 110*(6), 540–542.

Lertsburapa, K., Schroeder, J. W., Jr., & Sullivan, C. (2010). Assessment of adenoid size: A comparison of lateral radiographic measurements, radiologist assessment, and nasal endoscopy. *International Journal of Pediatric Otorhinolaryngology, 74*(11), 1281–1285.

Lewin, M. L., Croft, C. B., & Shprintzen, R. J. (1980). Velopharyngeal insufficiency due to hypoplasia of the musculus uvulae and occult submucous cleft palate. *Plastic and Reconstructive Surgery, 65*(5), 585–591.

Lewis, J. R., Andreassen, M. L., Leeper, H. A., Macrae, D. L., & Thomas, J. (1993). Vocal characteristics of children with cleft lip/palate and associated velopharyngeal incompetence. *Journal of Otolaryngology, 22*(2), 113–117.

Lotz, W. K., D'Antonio, L. L., Chait, D. H., & Netsell, R. W. (1993). Successful nasoendoscopic and aerodynamic examinations of children with speech/voice disorders. *International Journal of Pediatric Otorhinolaryngology, 26*(2), 165–172.

MacKenzie-Stepner, K., Witzel, M. A., Stringer, D. A., & Laskin, R. (1987). Velopharyngeal insufficiency due to hypertrophic tonsils: A report of two cases. *International Journal of Pediatric Otorhinolaryngology, 14*(1), 57–63.

MacKenzie-Stepner, K., Witzel, M. A., Stringer, D. A., Lindsay, W. K., Munro, I. R., & Hughes, H. (1987). Abnormal carotid arteries in the velocardiofacial syndrome: A report of three cases. *Plastic and Reconstructive Surgery, 80*(3), 347–351.

Mason, R. M. (1973). Preventing speech disorders following adenoidectomy by pre-operative examination. *Clinics in Pediatrics, 12*(1), 405–414.

McCullagh, L., & Baker, K. (2000). Endoscope reprocessing: Taking the mystery out of high-level disinfection. *ORL- Head and Neck Nursing, 18*(1), 6–10.

Miyazaki, T., Matsuya, T., & Yamaoka, M. (1975). Fiberscopic methods for assessment of velopharyngeal closure during various activities. *Cleft Palate Journal, 12*, 107–114.

Nacci, A., Ursino, F., La Vela, R., Matteucci, F., Mallardi, V., & Fattori, B. (2008). Fiberoptic endoscopic evaluation of swallowing (FEES): Proposal for informed consent. *ACTA Otorhinolaryngologica Italica, 28*(4), 206–211.

Nankivell, P. C., & Pothier, D. D. (2008). Nasal and instrument preparation before rigid and flexible nasendoscopy: A systematic review. *The Journal of Laryngology & Otology, 122*(10), 1024–1028.

Olympus America. P.O. Box 90582, Corporate Center Dr., Melville, NY, 11747.

Osberg, P. E., & Witzel, M. A. (1981). The physiologic basis for hypernasality during connected speech in cleft palate patients: A nasendoscopic study. *Plastic and Reconstructive Surgery, 67*(1), 1–5.

PENTAX Medical Company. A Division of PENTAX of America. 102 Chestnut Ridge Road, Montvale, NJ, 07645-1856.

Peterson-Falzone, S. J. (1985). Velopharyngeal inadequacy in the absence of overt cleft palate. *Journal of Craniofacial Genetics and Developmental Biology* (Suppl. 1), 97–124.

Peterson-Falzone, S. J., & Graham, M. S. (1990). Phoneme-specific nasal emission in

children with and without physical anomalies of the velopharyngeal mechanism. *Journal of Speech and Hearing Disorders*, 55(1), 132–139.

Pigott, R. W., Bensen, J. F., & White, F. D. (1969). Nasendoscopy in the diagnosis of velopharyngeal incompetence. *Plastic and Reconstructive Surgery*, 43(2), 141–147.

Pigott, R. W., & Makepeace, A. P. (1982). Some characteristics of endoscopic and radiological systems used in elaboration of the diagnosis of velopharyngeal incompetence. *British Journal of Plastic Surgery*, 35(1), 19–32.

Pothier, D. D., Awad, Z., Whitehouse, M., & Porter, G. C. (2005). The use of lubrication in flexible fibreoptic nasendoscopy: A randomized controlled trial. *Clinical Otolaryngology*, 30(4), 353–356.

Pothier, D. D., Raghava, N., Monteiro, P., & Awad, Z. (2006). A randomized controlled trial: Is water better than a standard lubricant in nasendoscopy? *Clinical Otolaryngology*, 31(2), 134–137.

Ramamurthy, L., Wyatt, R. A., Whitby, D., Martin, D., & Davenport, P. (1997). The evaluation of velopharyngeal function using flexible nasendoscopy. *Journal of Laryngology & Otology*, 111(8), 739–745.

Rich, B. M., Farber, K., & Shprintzen, R. J. (1988). Nasopharyngoscopy in the treatment of palatopharyngeal insufficiency. *International Journal of Prosthodontics*, 1(3), 248–251.

Ross, D. A., Witzel, M. A., Armstrong, D. C., & Thomson, H. G. (1996). Is pharyngoplasty a risk in velocardiofacial syndrome? An assessment of medially displaced carotid arteries. *Plastic and Reconstructive Surgery*, 98(7), 1182–1190.

Rowe, M. R., & D'Antonio, L. L. (2005). Velopharyngeal dysfunction: Evolving developments in evaluation. *Current Opinion in Otolaryngology & Head & Neck Surgery*, 13(6), 366–370.

Rutala, W. A. (1996). APIC guideline for selection and use of disinfectants. *American Journal of Infectious Disease Control*, 24, 313–342.

Sadek, S. A., De, R., Scott, A., White, A. P., Wilson, P. S., & Carlin, W. V. (2001). The efficacy of topical anaesthesia in flexible nasendoscopy: A double-blind randomized controlled trial. *Clinical Otolaryngology & Allied Sciences*, 26(1), 25–28.

Shetty, S., Frampton, S., & Patel, N. (2009). Flexible nasendoscopy. [Letter]. *Clinical Otolaryngology*, 34(2), 169–171.

Shprintzen, R. J. (1979). The use of multiview videofluoroscopy and flexible fiberoptic nasopharyngoscopy as a predictor of success with pharyngeal flap surgery. In R. Ellis & F. C. Flack (Eds.), *Diagnosis and treatment of palato-glossal malfunction* (pp. 6–14). London: College of Speech Therapists.

Shprintzen, R. J. (1995). Instrumental assessment of velopharyngeal valving. In R. J. Shprintzen & J. Bardach (Eds.), *Cleft palate speech management: A multidisciplinary approach* (vol. 4, pp. 221–256). St. Louis, MO: Mosby.

Shprintzen, R. J. (1996). Nasopharyngoscopy. In K. R. Bzoch (Ed.), *Communicative disorders related to cleft lip and palate* (vol. 4, pp. 387–409). Austin, TX: Pro-Ed.

Shprintzen, R. J., & Golding-Kushner, K. J. (1989). Evaluation of velopharyngeal insufficiency. *Otolaryngology Clinics of North America*, 22(3), 519–536.

Shprintzen, R. J., Lewin, M. L., Croft, C. B., Daniller, A. L, Argamaso, R. V., Ship, A. G., & Strauch, B. (1979). A comprehensive study of pharyngeal flap surgery: Tailor-made flaps. *Cleft Palate Journal*, 16(1), 46–55.

Shprintzen, R. J., Rakof, S. J., Skolnick, M. L., & Lavorato, A. S. (1977). Incongruous movements of the velum and lateral pharyngeal walls. *Cleft Palate Journal, 14*(2), 148–157.

Siegel-Sadewitz, V. L., & Shprintzen, R. J. (1982). Nasopharyngoscopy of the normal velopharyngeal sphincter: An experiment of biofeedback. *Cleft Palate Journal, 19*(3), 194–200.

Siegel-Sadewitz, V. L., & Shprintzen, R. J. (1986). Changes in velopharyngeal valving with age. *International Journal of Pediatric Otorhinolaryngology, 11*(2), 171–182.

Sinclair, S. W., Davies, D. M., & Bracka, A. (1982). Comparative reliability of nasal pharyngoscopy and videofluorography in the assessment of velopharyngeal incompetence. *British Journal of Plastic Surgery, 35*(2), 113–117.

Skolnick, M. L., Shprintzen, R. J., McCall, G. N., & Rakoff, S. (1975). Patterns of velopharyngeal closure in subjects with repaired cleft palate and normal speech: A multi-view videofluoroscopic analysis. *Cleft Palate Journal, 12*, 369–376.

Smith, B. E., & Kuehn, D. P. (2007). Speech evaluation for velopharyngeal dysfunction. *The Journal of Craniofacial Surgery, 18*(2), 251–261; Quiz 266–257.

Smith, J. C., & Rockley, T. J. (2002). A comparison of cocaine and "co-phenylcaine" local anaesthesia in flexible nasendoscopy. *Clinical Otolaryngology & Allied Sciences, 27*(3), 192–196.

Storz Medical. 1000 Cobb Place Blvd., Bldg. 400, Suite 450, US-Kennesaw, GA, 30144.

Strauss, R. A. (2007). Flexible endoscopic nasopharyngoscopy. *Atlas of the Oral and Maxillofacial Surgery Clinics of North America, 15*(2), 111–128.

Taub, S. (1966). The Taub oral panendoscope: A new technique. *Cleft Palate Journal, 3*, 328–346.

Willging, J. P. (2003). Velopharyngeal insufficiency. *Current Opinion in Otolaryngology & Head & Neck Surgery, 11*(6), 452–455.

Williams, R. G., Preece, M., Rhys, R., & Eccles, R. (1992). The effect of adenoid and tonsil surgery on nasalance. *Clinics in Otolaryngology, 17*(2), 136–140.

Witt, P. D., Miller, D. C., Marsh, J. L., Muntz, H. R., & Grames, L. M. (1998). Limited value of preoperative cervical vascular imaging in patients with velocardiofacial syndrome. *Plastic and Reconstructive Surgery, 101*(5), 1184–1195; Discussion 1196–1199.

Witzel, M. A., & Posnick, J. C. (1989). Patterns and location of velopharyngeal valving problems: Atypical findings on video nasopharyngoscopy. *Cleft Palate Journal, 26*(1), 63–67.

Witzel, M. A., Tobe, J., & Salyer, K. (1988). The use of nasopharyngoscopy biofeedback therapy in the correction of inconsistent velopharyngeal closure. *International Journal of Pediatric Otorhinolaryngology, 15*(2), 137–142.

Witzel, M. A., Tobe, J., & Salyer, K. E. (1989). The use of videonasopharyngoscopy for biofeedback therapy in adults after pharyngeal flap surgery. *Cleft Palate Journal, 26*(2), 129–134; Discussion 135.

Yamaoka, M., Matsuya, T., Miyazaki, T., Nishio, J., & Ibuki, K. (1983). Visual training for velopharyngeal closure in cleft palate patients: A fibrescopic procedure (preliminary report). *Journal of Maxillofacial Surgery, 11*(4), 191–193.

Ysunza, A., Pamplona, M., Femat, T., Mayer, L, & Garcia-Velasco, M. (1997). Video-nasopharyngoscopy as an instrument for visual biofeedback during speech in cleft palate patients. *International Journal of Pediatric Otorhinolaryngology, 41*(3), 291–298.

Zajac, D. J., & Linville, R. N. (1989). Voice perturbations of children with perceived nasality and hoarseness. *Cleft Palate Journal*, 26(3), 226–231; Discussion 231–232.

Zwitman, D. H., Sonderman, J. G, & Ward, P. H. (1974). Variations in velopharyngeal closure assessed by endoscopy. *Journal of Speech and Hearing Disorders*, 39(3), 366–372.

Coloring Book Pages

Coloring book pages to help prepare the child for a nasopharyngoscopy examination:

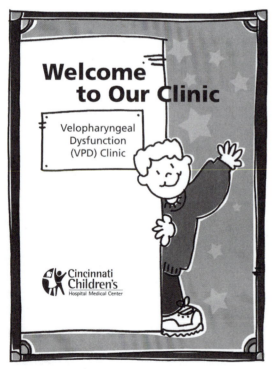

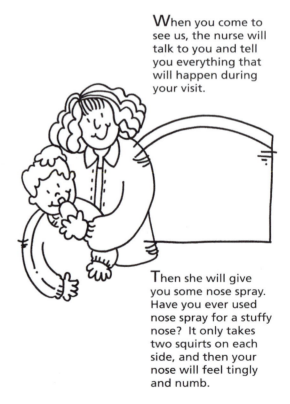

When you come to see us, the nurse will talk to you and tell you everything that will happen during your visit.

Then she will give you some nose spray. Have you ever used nose spray for a stuffy nose? It only takes two squirts on each side, and then your nose will feel tingly and numb.

Next it will be time to see your nose on TV. The doctor will put a long, skinny tube inside your nose. This is called a scope and here is what it looks like.

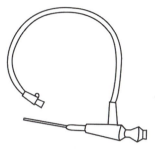

Once the scope is in your nose, the speech pathologist will ask you to repeat some sentences again.

When you are talking, you can watch the inside of your nose on TV. There are parts in there that move... almost like magic.

It is very important to hold still so the tube doesn't bump around inside. If you want, you can sit on someone's lap to help you hold still.

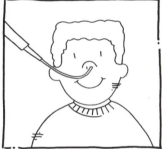

The scope only goes in a little bit.

It doesn't hurt because your nose will be numb from the nose drops.

Sometimes it seems a little scary though... so be brave!

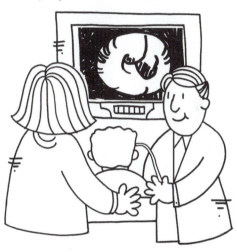

PART 4

TREATMENT PROCEDURES: SPEECH, RESONANCE, AND VELOPHARYNGEAL DYSFUNCTION

CHAPTER

18

SURGICAL MANAGEMENT OF CLEFTS AND VELOPHARYNGEAL INSUFFICIENCY/ INCOMPETENCE (VPI)

DAVID A. BILLMIRE, M.D.

CHAPTER OUTLINE

INTRODUCTION

Cleft lip and palate occur on a spectrum—from the abortive form, such as a form fruste of the lip, a bifid uvula, or an asymptomatic submucous cleft palate—to bilateral complete clefts of the lip and palate. Regardless of the degree of involvement, the surgical principles remain the same. For example, in an incomplete cleft of the lip, although a portion of the lip maybe intact, the underlying muscle, nasal cartilage, and oral sphincter function are usually significantly affected. Therefore, correction requires a complete lip repair. For the same reason, correction of a symptomatic submucous cleft of the palate requires the same type of repair as if it were a complete cleft.

Clefts of lip and palate involve much more than the obvious defect to the lip and roof of the mouth. Their sphere of influence extends to other aesthetic areas, such as the nose and midface, and to other anatomical areas, such as the jaws, teeth, oral sphincter, and velopharyngeal sphincter. In addition, cleft lip and palate often affect the functional areas of breathing, speech, voice, resonance, hearing, feeding, and even the psychological aspects that involve the individual's identity. As much as possible, the surgeon attempts to normalize both the anatomy and physiology, which usually improves the psychological state as well.

Structural defects require physical management, usually in the form of surgery. Although surgical concepts and approaches have become more standardized in the last few years, there is a wide range of interpretation of these "standards" throughout the world, across the country, and even within a single treatment team. Treatment options, timing, surgical techniques, and philosophies are presented in this chapter solely as broad general guidelines. Overall, the successful treatment of the patient with cleft lip and palate hinges not just on the surgery but also on the treatment team's adherence to and completion of a comprehensive program with well-defined goals and objectives.

For those who would like more information about the actual surgical procedures, Virtual Surgery Videos are available free of charge through the Smile Train website under Medical Resources (Smile Train, n.d.).

CLEFT LIP REPAIR

The technique used for cleft lip repair, also known as a *cheilorraphy*, depends on whether the cleft is unilateral or bilateral. In addition, there are variations in the presurgical management and specific techniques chosen based on the surgeon's training, previous experience, and bias. The goals of the cleft lip repair are to bring the skin, muscles (orbicularis oris), and mucous membrane together; to achieve symmetry of the nostrils and Cupid's bow; to achieve a natural border (white roll) between the vermilion and the skin of the upper lip; and to minimize the appearance of the scars. The continuity of the lip after the repair helps to mold the underlying bony structures, particularly the premaxilla. On the other hand, a scarred or tight upper lip can actually have a detrimental effect on maxillary growth.

Presurgical Management

Presurgical management is often done to align the lip and maxillary segments before the formal lip repair. In wide clefts of the lip, whether they are unilateral or bilateral, this presurgical management results in less tension on the lip after it is repaired and can improve the ultimate outcome. Presurgical management is particularly important for bilateral cleft lips, as the protrusion of an unrestrained premaxilla puts tremendous pressure on the repaired lip. Presurgical orthopedics is usually unnecessary, however, for incomplete clefts and those with just a *Simonart's band* (a band of skin without underlying muscle that bridges the cleft just below the nose).

There are a number of options for aligning the lip and maxillary segments before formal surgery. The decision as to which method is used is highly dependent on the experience of the surgeon and the facilities available.

The simplest procedure to pull the segments together is to tape the lip with adhesive tape (see Figure 9-22). This may also be used in conjunction with *dental elastics*, which are small rubber bands to add a dynamic component. With a bilateral cleft lip, a more elaborate headgear (bonnet) with Velcro elastic bands can be used to draw the premaxilla into appropriate position. In some centers, a palatal molding plate is used with the tape or elastics to help guide the segments as they move. This procedure usually is done over a 4- to 6-week period of time and requires caregiver cooperation and careful monitoring.

A second option for aligning the segments is the use of a palatal appliance, which can be either active or passive in nature. A typical active device is the *Latham appliance* (Georgiade & Latham, 1975; Latham, 1980; Latham, Kusy, & Georgiade, 1976; Millard & Latham, 1990; Millard, Latham, Huifen, Spiro, & Morovic, 1999) (see Figure 9-21). This two-piece acrylic dental appliance is pinned to both segments of the palate. On a daily basis, a screw is turned slowly, which draws the two segments together to gradually close the gap. For bilateral clefts, dental chain elastics, which are periodically adjusted by the pediatric dentist, are used to pull the premaxilla into position. If the two maxillary segments are collapsed together with the bilateral cleft, the Latham appliance can be used to pull them apart to make room for the premaxilla. All of this usually takes 3 to 4 weeks to accomplish.

The Latham appliance is often combined with a plate that has an acrylic extension to help mold the nostril. This combination appliance is called a *nasal alveolar molding* device or just *NAM* (Da Silveira et al., 2003). The NAM is also frequently done with a passive device or molding plate that slowly changes the dental arch position by weekly adjustments to the plate. These adjustments are accomplished by adding and removing acrylic in key areas to shape the dental arch. Whether active of passive, the NAM device is labor intensive and requires the skills of a pedodontist or orthodontist. These devices narrow the opening and realign the cleft segments and nasal cartilages before repair so that a better surgical result can be achieved.

The third option for drawing the segments together is a surgical procedure called a *lip adhesion*. This simple straight-line repair of the lip is performed to apply pressure on the segments to help pull them together. A lip adhesion can be used with a molding plate and/ or a NAM. The lip adhesion is usually done at 6 weeks of age, followed by the formal surgical repair of the lip 3 or 4 months later.

Techniques: Unilateral Cleft Lip Repair

By examining an unrepaired unilateral cleft lip deformity, one can see that all the structures are present, including the philtral dimple and both philtral ridges. The cleft passes just to the lateral side of the philtral ridge. On the cleft side, the lip is short and the Cupid's bow is twisted up into the cleft. Early surgical techniques to repair a cleft lip were simple straight-line repairs. This type of repair resulted in a lip that was characteristically short and notched due to contraction with the straight-line scarring.

Currently, there are two major methods for repairing the unilateral cleft lip: the Millard technique (Trier, 1985b; Paranaiba et al., 2009) and the Tennison-Randall technique (Brauer & Cronin, 1983; Lazarus, Hudson, van Zyl, Fleming, & Fernandes, 1998; Leon-Valle, 1980; Tan & Atik, 2007) (Figure 18–1). With both the Millard and the Tennison-Randall techniques, the shortened philtral ridge is lengthened by inserting a "patch" of tissue. In the Millard repair, it is inserted at the top of the lip, just beneath the nose, and in the Tennison-Randall repair it is inserted just above the vermilion boarder of the lip. This brings the ridge down to match the unaffected side.

Millard Technique

The Millard technique, or rotation advancement flap, is used in approximately 80% of cases and is perhaps the most anatomical of the repairs (Stal et al., 2009. It is known as a "cut as you go" technique because adjustments are constantly made during this procedure to bring the lip into balance. The initial incision is placed along the philtral ridge on the cleft side. The incision is carried up along the ridge and beneath the nose in a curvilinear manner. This causes the lip to open up and "rotate" down until the Cupid's bow

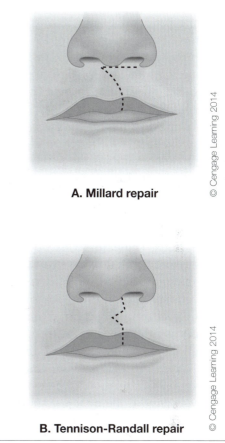

A. Millard repair

© Cengage Learning 2014

B. Tennison-Randall repair

© Cengage Learning 2014

FIGURE 18–1 (A and B) Techniques of unilateral cleft lip repairs. (A) Millard repair. (B) Tennison-Randall repair.

is level (hence the rotation part of the name). As the philtrum rotates into the correct position, it leaves a gap at the top of the lip, beneath the nose. Tissue is therefore advanced into this gap (hence the advancement portion of the name) from the lateral portion of the lip, just beneath the alae. This not only fills the defect but also helps to maintain the length. By increasing or decreasing the amount of rotation, the lip length may be adjusted. Tissue that is lateral to the incision on the philtral ridge is used to lengthen the shortened columella on the cleft side. Figure 18–1A shows the basic technique for the Millard lip repair, and Figure 18–2 is a photograph of this type of repair. Figure 18–3A shows a patient preoperatively, Figure 18–3B shows the patient one day after a Millard repair, and Figure 18–3C shows the patient 6 months postoperatively.

The Millard repair, with its "cut as you go" philosophy, is thought to be the more difficult of the repairs. Additionally, the tissue is inserted at the point of maximum tension where the underlying structures are relatively fixed to the maxilla. In inexperienced hands, this can often lead to a lip that is too short. In very wide clefts, some surgeons do not consider this repair at all, or they resort to a lip adhesion before a formal repair. On the plus side, the normal philtral dimple is preserved; the scar follows and mimics the philtral ridge; and by inserting the tissue at the top of the lip, the result is a better nasal configuration (Becker, Svensson, McWilliam, Sarnas, & Jacobsson, 1998). Revisions when necessary are relatively easy. If the lip is too short, it can simply be re-rotated and lengthened in a second procedure. Because the advantages of this procedure far outweigh its disadvantages, it is the most widely used lip repair done today.

Tennison-Randall Technique

The Tennison-Randall technique, or triangular flap procedure, is used in about 20% of cases and follows from an older technique, the LeMesurier repair or quadrilateral flap technique. The Tennison-Randall procedure is precise and measured, and therefore it is often referred to as a "cookie cutter" technique. Many surgeons like the security of this type of fixed technique. In the Tennison-Randall method, an incision is placed about halfway up through the philtral ridge on the cleft side. This creates a triangular opening (hence the name "triangular flap technique") in the inferior portion of the lip and causes the point of the Cupid's bow to drop into position. A triangular-shaped flap from the lateral portion of the lip is inserted into this triangular-shaped gap in the bottom and most mobile portion of the lip. Significant mobilization in the upper portion of the lip, where tension is the greatest, is thereby avoided.

Despite violating both the philtral ridge and philtral dimple, the results from this procedure

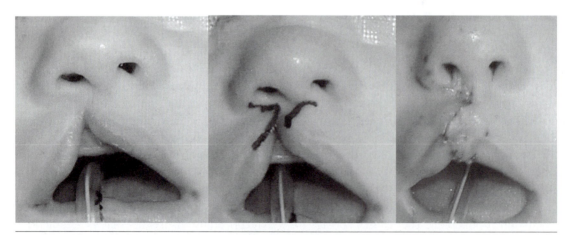

FIGURE 18–2 Photographs of a unilateral Millard lip repair.

Courtesy David A. Billmire, M.D./Cincinnati Children's Hospital Medical Center & University of Cincinnati College of Medicine

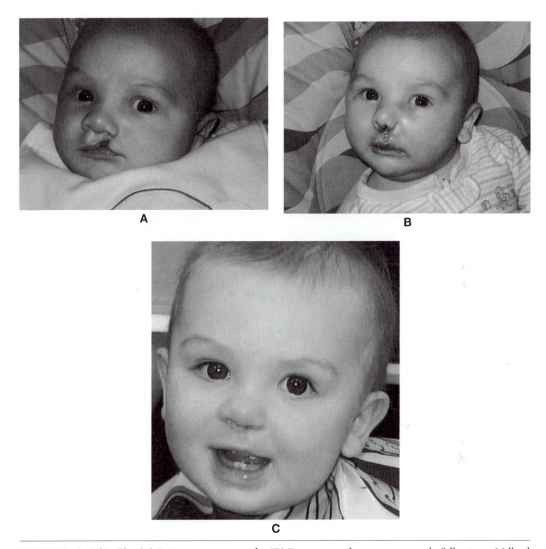

FIGURE 18–3 (A–C)   (A) Patient preoperatively. (B) Patient one day postoperatively following a Millard repair. (C) Patient six months postoperatively.

Courtesy David A. Billmire, M.D./Cincinnati Children's Hospital Medical Center & University of Cincinnati College of Medicine

can be quite good, with good lip configuration and a symmetrical Cupid's bow. The nasal results are usually not as good, however, because the alar base usually remains somewhat splayed. Subsequent nasal reconstruction is compromised because the tissue in the upper part of the lip tends to bunch up as the alar base is brought into its proper position, and therefore there is little possibility of creating a nostril sill. However, because the extra tissue is inserted in the most mobile portion of the lip, this repair is often used for wide clefts.

It is important to remember that the mouth is a sphincter. Just as it is important to reconstruct the velopharyngeal sphincter, it is also important to reconstruct the oral sphincter. Although this may seem intuitively obvious, historically it has been ignored by some surgeons. When there is a cleft lip, the orbicularis oris muscles of the oral sphincter are divided. Instead of creating a complete ring around the mouth, they are discontinuous, and the divided ends are abnormally inserted. In unilateral clefts, the orbicularis oris inserts laterally along the *pyriform aperture* (the opening at the base of the ala) and medially along the anterior nasal spine (at the base of the columella). Regardless of the type of repair chosen, these abnormal insertions have to be taken down and the muscles realigned into the correct orientation. Failure to do so results in distortion of the lip on activation, noticeable depressions, and a poor aesthetic result.

In the past, and to a certain extent even today, there has been debate over whether to address the accompanying nasal deformity of the unilateral cleft lip with the initial lip repair. Historically, it was felt that the nose should not be operated on in infancy because of a concern that its growth potential would be adversely affected. In the last few decades, several surgeons have demonstrated that not only is this concern unfounded, but better long-term results can be achieved by early correction of the nasal deformity at the time of initial lip repair (Salyer, 1986). Therefore, all lip repair techniques now involve some method of repositioning the distorted lower lateral cartilage of the nose and malpositioned alar base. Although these early repairs on the lip and nose do not obviate the need for secondary surgery, they greatly reduce the initial deformity and lessen the extent of subsequent reconstruction.

Techniques: Bilateral Cleft Lip Repair

Repair of a bilateral cleft lip is more frustrating and usually less successful when compared to the unilateral cleft lip repair. The magnitude of the lip and nasal deformities can present formidable challenges to even the most experienced surgeons. Even a cleft limited to the primary palate can result in the unrestrained protrusion of the premaxillary complex. In complete clefts with the premaxilla protruding anteriorly, it is not uncommon for the two lateral segments of the maxilla to collapse behind it. Expansion of the lateral segments is sometimes required in order to allow the premaxilla to drop back into appropriate position.

Broadbent-Manchester Repair and Millard Repair

The two major contemporary methods of bilateral cleft lip repair are the modified Broadbent-Manchester repair and the Millard repair (Figure 18–4A and B). The major difference between the two procedures is the method in which the white roll of the philtrum is created. In the modified Broadbent-Manchester repair, the white roll from the prolabium is preserved. In the Millard repair, the white roll from the lateral elements is used.

In the bilateral cleft, the *prolabium* (the central part of the upper lip, which would have formed the philtrum if there hadn't been a cleft) is prominently located just in front of the premaxilla. Because of the discontinuity of the orbicularis oris in the bilateral cleft lip, the prolabium has no muscle in it. Instead, the orbicularis oris inserts abnormally on either side of the piriform aperture at the alar bases. This lack of muscle tension in the prolabium gives it the appearance of being diminutive in size. In the past, this appearance led to the incorrect assumption that there was a need for extra tissue in the prolabium. As a result, repairs were often done that included adding tissue beneath the prolabium from the lateral lip elements. The resulting scars from this

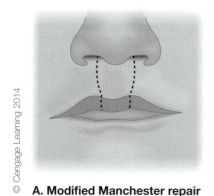

© Cengage Learning 2014

A. Modified Manchester repair

© Cengage Learning 2014

B. Millard bilateral cleft repair

FIGURE 18–4 (A and B) Techniques of bilateral lip repairs. (A) Modified Manchester repair. (B) Millard bilateral cleft repair.

procedure were shaped like a "Y" or a goal post (which is hardly in keeping with the concept of hiding scars in naturally occurring lines). What became evident over time was that the prolabium, when exposed to muscle tension, stretches and becomes tight transversely and very long vertically. The transverse tightness places significant pressure on an already compromised maxilla, often resulting in dramatic retrusion of the upper jaw. In the 1960s, the shortcomings of this type of repair were realized, and it was finally abandoned.

Even though the prolabium appears small in a bilateral cleft, it is routinely made narrower during the repair. Although immediately after the repair the lip looks tight and bunched up, the prolabium begins to stretch out and achieve a more normal size within a few weeks. If care is not taken to initially trim the prolabial segment down, it will be too large once the lip matures.

Although most surgeons now feel that nasal repair in the unilateral lip can be accomplished with the initial lip repair, there is still some controversy in bilateral lips. Traditional methods of lengthening the columella require "banking," or storing the lateral parings. (The *parings* consist of the excess tissue that is trimmed, or "pared" off, from each side of the prolabium during the initial lip repair.) This tissue is banked in either the lip or the floor of the nose for later use. It can usually be seen as small bumps. Use of this prolabial tissue for columella lengthening cannot be done with the initial repair because it would devascularize the remaining prolabial tissue that forms the new philtral dimple. However, Mulliken, Cutting, and others have been successful in developing techniques that use tissue from the elongated nasal rim to form and elongate the columella at the time of the original lip repair, thereby negating the need for a secondary lengthening (Cutting & Grayson, 1993; Cutting et al., 1998; Kohout, Aljaro, Farkas, & Mulliken, 1998; Morovic, & Cutting, 2005; Mulliken & LaBrie, 2012; Stal et al., 2009). This technique may be enhanced by the use of a nasoalveolar molding device.

In the event that the nasal columella is not lengthened during the original lip repair, a secondary procedure is done, usually done between 9 months and 5 years of age. Two methods of columellar lengthening are widely used. In the first method, an incision is made transversely, curving from alar base to alar base just below the banked parings. As the nose is elevated, the floor of the nose with the banked parings is drawn up into the columella, thereby lengthening it. As the nose moves up, the alae move closer together, narrowing the base of the nose. This type of secondary lip repair is referred as a Cronin columellar lengthening procedure.

If no parings were created in the original repair and the full width of the prolabium was used to make the philtral dimple, the resulting dimple will be quite wide once the scars mature. In a sense, the parings were banked in the lip, not the floor of the nose. When this is the case, the lateral parings are created in the second procedure and raised from the lip to lengthen the columella.

Potential Complications

The lip repair can contribute to nasal obstruction if it results in stenosis of the nasal vestibule. This obstruction can cause problems with nasal breathing and sleep, and can even cause abnormal resonance.

Timing of Cleft Lip Repair

Over the years, there has been considerable debate among surgeons about the appropriate timing for cleft lip repair. At one time, repair of the cleft lip was often done shortly after birth and before the child was sent home. It was felt that neonatal repair was appropriate because it allowed the mother to better bond to the infant. In addition, from an anesthetic standpoint, neonates were felt to be most physiologically sound immediately after birth before their own physiological systems became more active. Modern pediatric anesthesia has negated the latter argument, whereas the former remains debatable. Although a few cleft palate centers are reintroducing the concept of repair within the first week of life,

most centers advocate delaying repair and following some variation of the *rule of 10s*. This "rule" is a guideline that says that the infant should be at least 10 weeks of age, weigh at least 10 pounds, and have hemoglobin of 10 grams before the lip repair.

There are several reasons for delaying this initial surgery. First, delaying surgery allows time for investigation of other associated abnormalities or serious problems, which may not be readily apparent at birth. In addition, an acceptable feeding technique must be established and weight gain assured before taking on extensive surgery. Finally, many teams use some form of active or passive nasoalveolar molding devices (NAMs) prior to surgery for best results.

Despite the presence of the cleft lip during the first few months, bonding will occur with the caregivers, which is crucial to the child's development. Given these considerations, in most cleft palate centers at this time, the initial repair of cleft lip is usually accomplished between 10 and 12 weeks of age.

CLEFT PALATE REPAIR

Cleft palate repair (also called *palatoplasty*) is done to close off the oral cavity from the nasal cavity for the benefit of feeding, middle ear function, but most of all for speech. Although the cleft lip repair dates back to antiquity, successful palatal repair dates only from the early nineteenth century. With the advent of anesthesia and specialized instrumentation, success rates of palate repair have improved dramatically.

Presurgical Management

Depending on the center and the surgeon, there may be a preoperative change in the feeding technique. Some surgeons prefer that the child be off the bottle before the surgery, while others will allow bottle-feeding postoperatively. If the surgeon wants the child off the bottle before repairing the cleft, the child can usually be transitioned to a cup. This is done by gradually introducing a cup to the child around 6 months of age. There are commercially available feeding cups, or one can simply use a paper cup. Some surgeons avoid cup feeding but go directly to syringe feeding following the repair. The postoperative precautions can vary in length from just a few days to as long as 3 weeks, depending on the center.

Techniques: Cleft Palate Repair

There are several techniques for cleft palate repair. The commonly used techniques are described as follows.

Von Langenbeck Repair

The von Langenbeck repair, illustrated in Figure 18–5A and B, is one of the oldest and most successful means of palatal closure and is still popular today (Murison & Pigott, 1992; Trier & Dreyer, 1984). In this repair, an incision is made just inside the gum line, starting behind the area of the molars and extending up to the area of the canine tooth. The mucoperiosteum is carefully raised off the bone and, in conjunction with the velum, separated in one large layer. The cleft margin is incised, and the raw edges are brought together and sewn down the middle. The incisions along the gum line are usually left open. With this operation, the levator muscle was typically not addressed (although it can easily be reconstructed), and there was a high incidence of velopharyngeal insufficiency. This set off a search for a procedure that not only closed the opening but also actively lengthened the palate.

Wardill-Kilner V–Y Pushback

A number of approaches for lengthening the palate have been tried (Bae, Kim, Lee, Hwang, & Kim, 2002). Some have caused problems with growth, wound healing, and airway obstruction. One technique that is commonly used is the Wardill-Kilner V–Y pushback procedure, which is illustrated in Figure 18–6. In this procedure, the initial incisions are similar to that of the von Langenbeck—except instead of leaving the mucoperiosteum attached in the front of the mouth, it is cut across as a "V." The resulting open area is "Y" shaped. This frees up the mucoperiosteum of the whole palate and allows it to be pushed back in an attempt to lengthen it. With this procedure, the levator muscle is still not addressed, although it could be, and a high incidence of anterior fistulas has been reported (Moore, Lawrence, Ptak, & Trier, 1988).

Intravelar Veloplasty

Just as a cleft lip disrupts the oral sphincter in the lip and alters the insertion of the sphincter muscles, a cleft palate changes the muscles of the velopharyngeal sphincter. In the patient with cleft palate, the levator veli palatini inserts onto the back of the hard palate instead of fusing together in the midline of the velum to form the levator sling. As noted above, initial palate repairs ignored this muscle and did nothing to correct its orientation.

To normalize the construction of the velopharyngeal sling, *intravelar veloplasty (IVVP)* has been advocated by some surgeons (Brown, Cohen, & Randall, 1983; Dreyer & Trier, 1984). Intravelar veloplasty can be done in conjunction with any type of palate repair. However, whether as an isolated procedure in the treatment of a submucous cleft or in conjunction with any type of palatoplasty, intravelar veloplasty has not been as successful

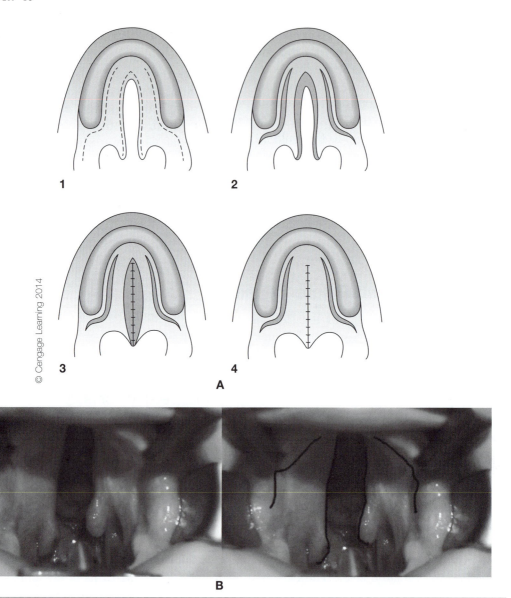

© Cengage Learning 2014

FIGURE 18–5 (A and B)   (A) Technique of the von Langenbeck repair. Note lateral relaxing incisions which are left open. (B) Photograph of the palate marked for von Langenbeck repair. Anterior palate remains attached, forming a bipedicle flap.

as was initially hoped (Brothers, Dalston, Peterson, & Lawrence, 1995; Coston, Hagerty, Jannarone, McDonald, & Hagerty, 1986; Jarvis & Trier, 1988). In fact, some authors have found no difference in velopharyngeal function between palatoplasty with and without intravelar veloplasty (Marsh, Grames, & Holtman, 1989). These results suggest that either there is no beneficial effect of intravelar veloplasty, or the effect is minimal.

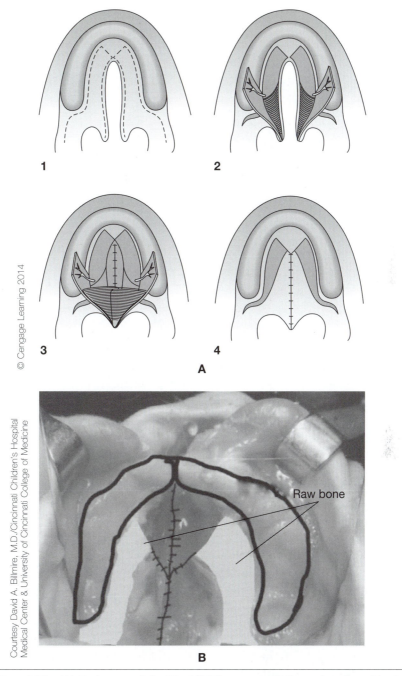

FIGURE 18–6 (A and B)   (A) Technique of the Wardill-Kilner repair. Palate is lengthened by "pushing" back the mucoperiosteum. The raw area is allowed to fill by secondary healing (scarring). (B) Photograph of the Wardill-Kilner repair.

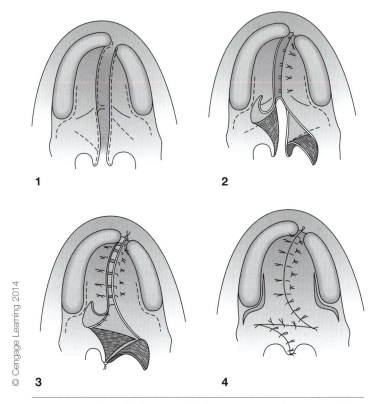

© Cengage Learning 2014

FIGURE 18–7 Technique of the Furlow palatoplasty. Note Z-plasty closure of both nasal side and mirror image on the oral side.

Furlow Z-Palatoplasty

Some investigators have reported better speech outcomes with the Furlow palatoplasty than with other methods (Gunther, Wisser, Cohen, & Brown, 1998). The Furlow palatoplasty involves reconstruction of the levator sling and lengthening the velum by closing it with opposing Z-plasties (Furlow, 1986, 1990, 2009) (Figure 18–7). A *Furlow Z-palatoplasty* is a plastic surgery technique that is used to lengthen tissue. The Furlow Z-plasty is done by borrowing tissue from the width of the velum to add to the length. The resulting scar looks like a "Z." To avoid possible breakdown and fistula, the procedure is done so that the "Z" on the oral surface goes in the opposite direction of the "Z" on the nasal side of the velum. The levator muscles are carried on the "Z's," one on each side, so that when they are moved into position they automatically overlap and form an intravelar veloplasty.

Two-Flap Palatoplasty

The two-flap palatoplasty is a very popular technique introduced by Bardach and Salyer. It involves mobilizing the palatal shelves on the greater palantine arteries and incorporating an intravelar veloplasty. It is very effective and allows the single stage closure of even the widest clefts.

Potential Complications

Achieving a good result in palatal surgery is much more difficult than achieving a good result in lip surgery. Although it may appear that a palate repair is simple in comparison to a lip repair, palate surgery can be quite challenging for several reasons. First, it is technically more demanding than a lip repair. In addition, there is a greater risk of postoperative problems, such as *dehiscence* (a breakdown in the surgical repair), causing a fistula or excessive scarring. If these problems occur, they are difficult to correct. There is a potential for airway compromise or excessive bleeding, which may put the patient's life in jeopardy. Finally, merely closing the palate is not enough. The palate not only serves as a physical barrier between the mouth and nose, but it must also function dynamically for normal speech. In some cases, the palate repair alone is not sufficient for normal velopharyngeal function.

Timing of the Cleft Palate Repair

The timing of the cleft palate repair has been even more controversial than timing of the lip repair. There have been a few cleft teams that advocated for palate repair in the first week of life, but this is extremely controversial. Most centers fall into two major philosophies—early and late. Early is defined as between 6 months and 15 months of age. Late is defined as between 15 months and 24 months of age. Most centers do the repair between 9 and 12 months of age unless the mandible is very small or there are significant airway issues.

In general, it is acknowledged that the earlier the palate repair is done, the lower the incidence of velopharyngeal insufficiency and development of compensatory articulation productions that require speech therapy for correction (Hardin-Jones & Jones, 2005; Murthy,

Sendhilnathan, & Hussain, 2010). However, early repair of the hard palate has raised concerns about the potential effect on maxillary growth and the appearance of the midface. Patients with a history of cleft lip and palate often demonstrate midface retrusion and Class III malocclusion due to a lack of adequate midfacial and maxillary growth. Over the last 50 years, there has been a debate in the literature as to whether this is caused by the inherent nature of the cleft or whether it is the result of the surgical repair of the alveolus and palate.

Believing that midface deficiency is the direct result of the surgical repair of the palate, Schweckendiek (1955) advocated closing just the velum at an early age, usually around 6 months. His patients used an obturator to close the hard palate for speech until the cleft was finally surgically closed around 4 or 5 years of age. His theory was that this procedure promoted velopharyngeal closure while avoiding restriction in maxillary growth (Blocksma, Leuz, & Mellerstig, 1975; Dingman & Grabb, 1971; Perko, 1979; Schweckendiek, 1966, 1968, 1983; Schweckendiek & Doz, 1978; Liao, Yang, Wang, Yun, & Huang, 2010).

In subsequent studies, the results of this two-stage approach have been found to be less than impressive (Pradel et al., 2009; Holland et al., 2007). Several studies have shown that a high percentage of the patients treated with this method failed to develop acceptable speech and required pharyngeal flaps (Bardach, Morris, & Olin, 1984; Cosman & Falk, 1980; Fara & Brousilova, 1988; Fara, Brousilova, Hrivnakova, & Tvrdek, 1992; Jackson, McLennan, & Scheker, 1983). In addition it has been found that with the delayed palatoplasty, the hard palate is more difficult to close (Cosman & Falk, 1980; Jackson et al., 1983), and greater orthodontic effort is needed to achieve an aligned dentoalveolar arch (Fara, Brousilova,

SPEECH NOTES

Interpreting the data regarding the effect of each palatoplasty technique on speech is very difficult. There are many variables to consider, including the timing of surgery, the experience and skill of the surgeon, the experience and skill of the speech-language pathologist in evaluating the speech, and the very definition of success (normal, acceptable, or improved). However, there is general agreement that early repair is better than late repair when considering speech results. In addition, experienced surgeons have a lower incidence of growth disturbance. Most experienced cleft palate centers report an incidence of between 17% and 20% of VPI requiring secondary surgery following the palate repair.

Hrivnakova, & Tvrdek, 1992; Smahel & Horak, 1993). Finally, it has been shown that there is virtually no difference in facial growth between patients who have early palate repair and those who have the two-stage procedure with delayed palate repair (Fara et al., 1992; Smahel & Horak, 1993).

In addition to the concern about midface growth, there is an additional factor that may delay the palate repair. When there is an extremely wide cleft, some inexperienced surgeons may not be comfortable closing the palate in a single stage. Some feel that closing the velum first narrows the remaining cleft of the hard palate for a secondary repair later. As with the classic Schweckendiek technique, the speech results with this delay are less than desirable.

ORONASAL FISTULA REPAIR

A *fistula* is an abnormal opening between two hollow organs in the body. In most cases, a nasolabial fistula is deliberately left in the alveolus (under the lip) at the time of the primary palatoplasty. This *intentional fistula* allows anterior facial growth without restriction from a surgical closure or scarring. This fistula is usually closed in early-to-mid mixed dentition with a bone graft from the rib or iliac crest. This

completes the dental arch and allows eruption and retention of the permanent dentition through the bony support from the graft.

Unintentional oronasal fistulas occur in approximately 5% to 30% of reported series. An unintentional *oronasal fistula* is a persistent opening between the oral and nasal cavity that occurs when the palate fails to heal after a palatoplasty. These fistulas are often blamed on expansion of the dental arch or growth of the patient. However, growth and expansion do not actually cause fistulas. Instead, they can cause existing fistulas to get bigger and become symptomatic. Although fistulas can be asymptomatic, large fistulas can cause significant hypernasality and nasal air emission during speech, as well as regurgitation of food and fluids into the nasal cavity during eating.

Techniques: Oronasal Fistula Repair

Closure of a fistula can be a daunting task. Closure of fistulas is usually attempted with the use of local *autogenous* (the individual's own) tissue first. If there is not adequate local tissue or if the use of local tissue has failed in a previous closure attempt, more complex and difficult procedures may be necessary. Techniques include using flaps of tissue from the turbinates,

Tongue flap

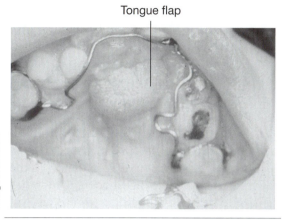

FIGURE 18–8 Fistula repair with a tongue flap. Note the tongue tissue in the anterior portion of the palate.

the buccal surface, and even the tongue (Figure 18–8) (Argamaso, 1990; Assuncao, 1993; Barone & Argamaso, 1993; Busic, Bagatin, & Boric, 1989; Coghlan, O'Regan, & Carter, 1989; Pigott, Rieger, & Moodie, 1984; Posnick & Getz, 1987; Thind, Singh, & Thind, 1992; Penna, Bannasch, Stark, 2007). With the tongue flap procedure, the dorsum of the tongue is sutured into the fistula and left for 2 to 3 weeks to develop its blood supply. At that point, the tongue flap is severed from the rest of the tongue. Although this leaves scarring on the top of the tongue, it does not adversely affect the

movement of the tongue for speech or feeding. The scar on the tongue is usually not well received by patients, however. In addition, the tongue flap can be large and bulky, thus interfering with speech. In these cases, the tongue flap is shaved down in a later procedure.

Potential Complications

Closure of an oronasal fistula can be very difficult, especially if autogenous tissue is used, because it is very thin. Even tongue flaps and buccal flaps can be challenging. As a result, there is about a 37% or more recurrence risk, which gets higher with subsequent repairs (Cohen, Kalinowski, LaRossa, & Randall, 1991). At times, total surgical correction is not possible, and the use of an obturator is recommended instead.

Timing of Oronasal Fistula Repair

The timing of fistula repair varies. It is often done in conjunction with the bone graft to the alveolar arch (around age 6 or 7). If it is large and affecting speech, the closure may be done earlier, or a temporary speech obturator is used until the fistula can be surgically repaired.

SPEECH NOTES

A large oronasal fistula can cause both hypernasality and nasal emission. A fistula that is 15 mm (dime size) or less may cause nasal emission, but not hypernasality. A fistula 5 mm (pea size) or less may not be symptomatic for speech at all, particularly if it is in the middle of the palate.

If the fistula is in the hard palate (as usual), it will not cause nasal emission on velar sounds (/k/, /g/) because the airflow will be horizontal to the opening. It is most likely to cause nasal emission on sibilants sounds, because the tongue movement can send airstream into the fistula. Some patients compensate for a fistula by holding the tongue against the opening to prevent the loss of airflow. This results in a palatal-dorsal production, which can cause a lateral distortion.

SURGERY FOR VELOPHARYNGEAL INSUFFICIENCY/ INCOMPETENCE (VPI)

Velopharyngeal insufficiency following a palatal repair can be due to a number of factors. There may be scarring from the initial palatoplasty, which can shorten the velum, making it impossible to reach the posterior pharyngeal wall during speech. In addition, it can cause muscular dysfunction, resulting in poor movement of the velum. Despite the best palatoplasty procedures, most centers report a 20% to 30% rate of velopharyngeal insufficiency in patients with a history of palate repair.

Velopharyngeal insufficiency can occur due to reasons other than a history of cleft palate. For example, patients with cranial base abnormalities may have a nasopharynx that is deep relative to the position of the velum, causing inadequate velopharyngeal closure. Some patients demonstrate velopharyngeal incompetence, where there is normal velar morphology, but inadequate velopharyngeal closure due to neuromuscular dysfunction.

It is important to note that whether due to an anatomical or neurophysiological cause, *VPI is a surgical disorder*. As such, speech therapy is ineffective for correction of this disorder. On the other hand, correction of the structure through surgery does not correct abnormal speech articulation. Therefore, speech therapy is usually needed postoperatively to correct compensatory errors that developed before correction of VPI.

Successful surgical management of VPI has been a relatively recent accomplishment. Historically, VPI was treated with prosthetic obturation. In the 1970s, however, the use of both videofluoroscopy, and later nasopharyngoscopy, led to a better understanding of the velopharyngeal valve and its function. As a result, better methods of surgical correction have evolved. At this point, surgical correction of VPI is the norm, and prosthetic devices are rarely used, particularly with children.

There are several surgical procedures of the pharynx that are designed to correct VPI. All are considered a type of *pharyngoplasty*. Pharyngoplasty procedures involve introducing something into the velopharyngeal opening to reduce the size of the gap. Therefore, there is always a risk of compromising the upper airway.

The goals of VPI surgery are to "normalize" velopharyngeal closure for speech, while avoiding symptomatic airway compromise. As such, the surgeon tries to ensure that the velopharyngeal port not only closes completely for oral speech but also opens adequately for nasal breathing and the production of nasal sounds (/m/, /n/, /ŋ/).

Presurgical Management

Before considering surgery for VPI, it is important to obtain a speech evaluation that includes an evaluation of velopharyngeal function. This is necessary to confirm the diagnosis of VPI and to rule out velopharyngeal mislearning as the major cause of the speech characteristics. It is also important to ensure that the VPI surgery will make a sufficient difference in the child's speech and communication skills to warrant the surgical risks.

Prior to the surgical procedure to correct VPI, the patient should undergo an evaluation of potential sources of airway obstruction. Particular attention should be paid to the size of the tonsils and the adenoid pad, and the presence of micrognathia (small mandible), as is common in Pierre Robin sequence. Enlarged tonsils, adenoid hypertrophy, or micrognathia may portend airway obstruction in the immediate postoperative period, as well as long-term problems with sleep apnea. Some centers advocate routine tonsillectomy before pharyngoplasty, although this is usually not necessary unless the tonsils are enlarged. If tonsillectomy is indicated, it should precede the pharyngoplasty by at least 6 weeks. Although adenoidectomy is usually not recommended for patients with repaired cleft palate, an adenoidectomy prior to pharyngoplasty may allow the surgeon to position the flap higher in the nasopharynx for better speech results and to avoid port obstruction postoperatively. Because enlargement of the tonsils is often accompanied by enlargement of the adenoids, a conservative adenoidectomy at the time of tonsillectomy is often appropriate. Of course, the characteristics of VPI will worsen until the pharyngoplasty is done.

Patients with velocardiofacial syndrome often have tortuosity of the carotid arteries. As a result, these arteries can course medially so that they are beneath the posterior pharyngeal wall rather than in the normal lateral position (D'Antonio & Marsh, 1987; Finkelstein et al., 1993; MacKenzie-Stepner et al., 1987; Ross, Witzel, Armstrong, & Thomson, 1996). These displaced carotid arteries can often be seen pulsating on the posterior pharyngeal wall through nasopharyngoscopy (Ysunza et al., 2004). Because the abnormal position of these arteries can put them in harm's way with the placement of a pharyngeal flap, a careful examination of the posterior pharyngeal wall is indicated before the surgery. Some surgeons advocate preoperative magnetic resonance angiography (MRA) studies or nasopharyngoscopy to identify the position of the carotid arteries (Krugman & Brant-Zawadski, 1997; Lai, Lo, Wong, Wang, & Yun, 2004; Mitnick, Bello, Golding-Kushner, Argamaso, & Shprintzen, 1996). Others feel that these studies are unnecessary because the

vessels can usually be found by palpating the pharyngeal walls when the patient is in surgery (Mehendale & Sommerlad, 2004; Witt, Miller, Marsh, Muntz, & Grames, 1998).

Following presurgical testing, some patients are found to be poor candidates for surgical intervention of VPI. In fact, VPI surgery may not be appropriate for patients with the following conditions: significant airway obstruction that is not well managed; neurological conditions, particularly those that are progressive; significant cognitive disability; severe hearing loss or deafness; previous oropharyngeal radiation; a bleeding disorder; and in rare cases, a carotid artery that is medialized in the posterior pharynx.

Techniques: VPI Correction

There are several techniques for the correction of VPI. The choice of technique may be determined by the size, location, and cause of the opening, the history of airway obstruction, and also by the surgeon's experience and preference. These techniques are described in the following sections.

Furlow Palatoplasty

The Furlow palatoplasty technique has been found to have a relatively low incidence of VPI. This repair has two advantages—it lengthens the palate with the Z-plasty technique, and it guarantees reconstruction of the levator sling. Because of its success as a primary procedure, the Furlow technique is now being used as a secondary technique to redo the palate when the original repair was another approach (Deren et al., 2005; Lindsey & Davis, 1996; Perkins, Lewis, Gruss, Eblen, & Sie, 2005; Sie & Gruss, 2002; Sie, Tampakopoulou, Sorom, Gruss, & Eblen, 2001; Por, Tan, Change, & Chen, 2010). This is effective in correcting cases of mild VPI or a very narrow velopharyngeal

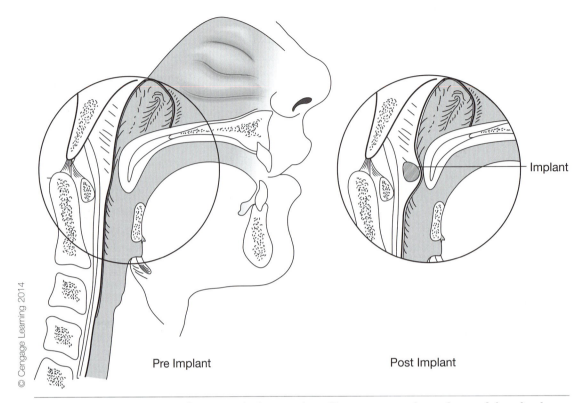

© Cengage Learning 2014

Pre Implant

Post Implant

Implant

FIGURE 18–9 This drawing illustrates velopharyngeal insufficiency prior to the implant, and then the closure that occurs with the augmented posterior pharyngeal wall as a result of an implant.

opening. The Furlow procedure has also become the typical technique used to repair a submucous cleft palate that results in VPI. In some cases, this technique does not give enough length to the velum to correct the VPI, so a type of pharyngoplasty may be needed in addition. In addition, this technique is somewhat prone to fistula development in patients with a history of cleft palate.

Pharyngeal Wall Augmentation

When the velopharyngeal opening is small, no more than 10 mm in diameter, posterior *pharyngeal wall augmentation* has been used by some surgeons (Witt et al., 1997). With this procedure, an implant is surgically placed or injected in the posterior pharyngeal wall in the

area of the velopharyngeal opening. The implant is placed deep in the superior pharyngeal constrictors but superficial to the prevertebral fascia. Figure 18–9 illustrates velopharyngeal insufficiency prior to the implant and then the closure that occurs with the augmented posterior pharyngeal wall. The augmentation can even be done in the posterior border of the velum.

Various materials have been reported for augmentation, including calcium hydroxylapatite, cartilage, fascia, fat, silicone, porous polyethylene, proplast, and even Teflon (Brigger, Ashland, & Hartnick, 2010; Cantarella, Mazzola, Mantovani, Baracca, & Pignataro, 2011; Dejonckere & van Wijngaarden, 2001; Denny, Marks, & Oliff-Carneol, 1993; Furlow,

Williams, Eisenbach, & Bzoch, 1982; Gray, Pinborough-Zimmerman, & Catten, 1999; Remacle, Bertrand, Eloy, & Marbaix, 1990; Terris & Goode, 1993; Trigos, Ysunza, Gonzalez, & Vazquez, 1988; Ulkur et al., 2008; Witt et al., 1997; Wolford, Oelschlaeger, & Deal, 1989; Leuchter, Schweizer, Hohlfeld, & Pasche, 2009). More recently, a gel-like substance called Deflux has been used for pharyngeal augmentation. Deflux has been used for a year as a treatment for vesicoureteral reflux (VUR) (caused by dysfunction of the valve between the ureters and the bladder) and holds promise for pharyngeal augmentation to correct VPI (Shelagh Cofer, M.D., Mayo Clinic, personal communication).

Initially, over-correction is required for all injectable augmentation material because the vehicle solution becomes absorbed. Complications from implantation of foreign materials in the posterior pharyngeal wall include infections, extrusion, reabsorption, and even migration of the material after insertion. Granuloma formation and migration of the material leading to embolus has been associated with Teflon implantation, so it is no longer used. These implants are not always effective because they are often too small or in the wrong location to completely fill the opening and totally correct VPI. On the other hand, over-correction can occur, which may result in hyponasality and upper airway obstruction.

Sphincter Pharyngoplasty

The *sphincter pharyngoplasty* (also called *Orticochea sphincteroplasty*) (Orticochea, 1970, 1983, 1997, 1999) was designed to create a sphincter that encircles the velopharyngeal port (Figure 18–10). Initially, it was felt that this procedure would create a dynamic sphincter as opposed to a passive obturator. However, recent studies have shown that the muscle

fibers in the sphincter are actually passive and that all movements seen postoperatively are caused by the contraction of the superior constrictor muscles and the movement of the velum. The sphincter pharyngoplasty procedure has undergone a series of modifications, and in its most current and widely used form it now exists with the Jackson modification (Jackson, 1985; Jackson, McGlynn, Huskie, & Dip, 1980; Jackson & Silverton, 1977; Losken, Williams, Burstein, Malick, & Riski, 2003; Marsh, 2009; Sie et al., 1998).

In this procedure, bilateral superiorly based myomucosal flaps are raised from the posterior faucial pillars, which include the palatopharyngeus muscles (Marsh, 2009). These flaps are rotated posteriorly and inset into a transverse incision in the nasopharynx, just at the level of velopharyngeal closure. This effectively narrows the pharynx. A small, superiorly based pharyngeal flap can then be raised and attached to the lateral flaps. This leaves a single round opening (port) of about 1 centimeter in diameter in the center of the pharynx. A sphincter pharyngoplasty is usually done bilaterally, but it can also be done unilaterally if the opening is just on one side.

Because the sphincter pharyngoplasty narrows the lateral borders of the velopharyngeal sphincter, it has been advocated for use with coronal gaps that include poor lateral pharyngeal wall motion or for corner gaps due to deep lateral pharyngeal recesses. The sphincter pharyngoplasty can even be done unilaterally if the opening is in just one corner (Lin, Wang, Cheong, & Lo, 2010). This is useful for the treatment of VPI secondary to unilateral palatal paralysis, as occasionally seen in hemifacial microsomia.

Pharyngeal Flap

The *pharyngeal flap* is the most commonly used procedure for correction of VPI (Cable,

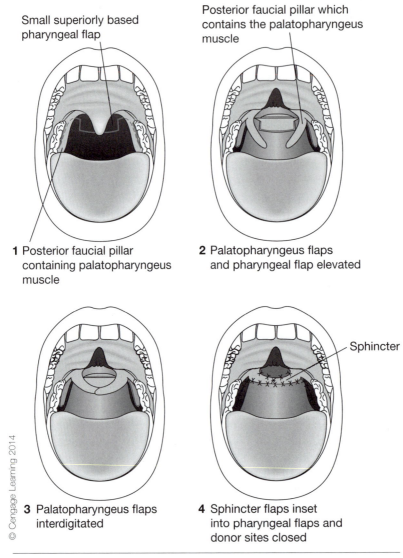

Small superiorly based pharyngeal flap

Posterior faucial pillar which contains the palatopharyngeus muscle

1 Posterior faucial pillar containing palatopharyngeus muscle

2 Palatopharyngeus flaps and pharyngeal flap elevated

3 Palatopharyngeus flaps interdigitated

Sphincter

4 Sphincter flaps inset into pharyngeal flaps and donor sites closed

© Cengage Learning 2014

FIGURE 18–10 A sphincter pharyngoplasty. In this procedure, bilateral myocutaneous flaps are raised from the posterior faucial pillars, which include the palatopharyngeus muscles. These muscles are rotated posteriorly and inset into a transverse incision on the posterior pharyngeal wall, just at the level of velopharyngeal closure. A small superiorly based flap may also be raised and attached to the lateral flaps. This effectively narrows the velopharyngeal port for speech.

Canady, Karnell, Karnell, & Malick, 2004). The pharyngeal flap is designed to be a passive, soft tissue obturator that is placed in the middle of the velopharyngeal port (Tharanon, Stella, & Epker, 1990; Trier, 1985a; Vedung, 1995; Wu & Epker, 1990; Yoshida, Stella, Ghali, & Epker,

1992). As such, it is effective in the management of midline gaps (which are most common following a cleft repair) and large gaps in the anterior–posterior dimension (Saman & Tatum, 2012). With the flap in midline, a port (or opening) is left on each side of the flap to allow for normal nasal breathing, drainage of nasal secretions, and production of nasal sounds. During (oral) speech, the lateral pharyngeal

A

Pharynx prior to a pharyngeal flap

Pharynx with a pharyngeal flap

B

FIGURE 18–11 (A and B) A pharyngeal flap. (A) A lateral view of a pharyngeal flap, as would be seen through lateral videofluoroscopy. The flap is raised from the posterior pharyngeal wall, and then sutured into the velum. (B) A superior view of the pharyngeal flap, as would be seen through nasopharyngoscopy. On the left is a view of the pharynx during nasal breathing before the flap. On the right is a view of the pharynx with a pharyngeal flap during nasal breathing. Note that the pharyngeal flap is in midline and the lateral ports are open on both sides, as would occur during nasal breathing and the production of nasal sounds.

walls move medially to close against the flap, thus completely closing the lateral ports (Forrest, Klaiman, & Mason, 2009).

Figure 18–11A shows a lateral view of a pharyngeal flap, as would be seen by lateral videofluoroscopy. Figure 18–11B shows a diagram of a superior view of the pharynx, as would be seen through nasopharyngoscopy, before and after placement of pharyngeal flap. Note the pharyngeal flap in midline and the open lateral ports on either side. Figure 18–12A–C shows photos of pharyngeal flaps, as viewed through nasopharyngoscopy. In each case, the pharyngeal flap can be seen in midline and the lateral ports can be noted on each side of the flap. In these examples, the ports are open for nasal breathing.

The pharyngeal flap procedure is done by making an incision in the pharyngeal wall that begins at the top of the nasopharynx at the base of the skull, and then goes down to the area near the base of the tongue. The incision then goes across the width of the pharynx between the tonsillar pillars, and up again. This results in a superiorly based flap. The pharyngeal flap includes the mucosal surface and the underlying musculature all the way down to the prevertebral fascia of the spinal column. The blood supply comes in through the attached portion of the flap at the base of the skull. Next, the velum is split up to the hard palate. The flap from the posterior pharyngeal wall is then elevated and sutured into the velum, forming a bridge between the posterior pharyngeal wall and the velum. These superior based pharyngeal flaps are lined with mucosal flaps from the nasal side of the velum. This prevents the natural tendency of a flap to tube and narrow. A port is left on each side of the flap for nasal breathing. To keep the ports patent, stents are sometimes placed in the ports and kept there overnight. They are then removed the next day.

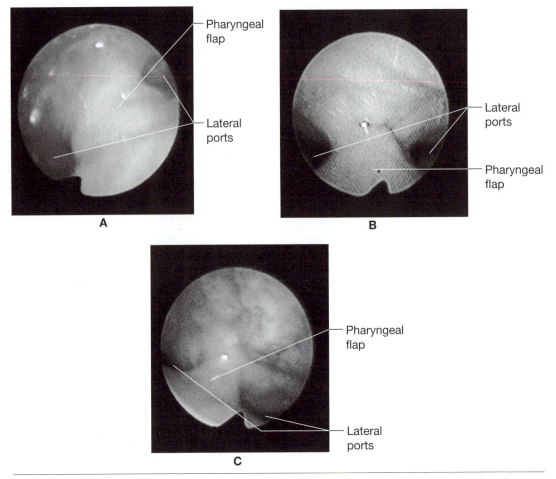

FIGURE 18–12 (A–C) Pharyngeal flaps, as viewed through nasopharyngoscopy during nasal breathing. In each example, note the pharyngeal flap in midline and the open lateral ports on each side.
Courtesy David A. Billmire, M.D./Cincinnati Children's Hospital Medical Center & University of Cincinnati College of Medicine

There are several factors that determine the success of a pharyngeal flap in correcting VPI. One is the vertical position of the flap in the nasopharynx (Skolnick & McCall, 1972). For best results, the flap should be set as high as possible, preferably at the level of the skull base and hard palate, because this is the area of maximum lateral pharyngeal wall movement. In correct position, the flap is high enough that it usually cannot be seen through an intraoral examination.

Another important factor in the success of a flap is its width. A wide flap is preferable to a narrow flap for speech, not only because it increases the possibility of lateral port closure during speech but also because the pharyngeal flap receives its blood supply from its base. Therefore, the wider the base, the greater the blood supply will be.

Flaps should also be made as long as possible because if they are too short, they will be under greater tension. If there is tension or limited blood supply, this can result in more scarring and contraction, which will adversely affect the function of the flap. In general, a pharyngeal flap should be wide, long, and set as high as possible.

The success of a pharyngeal flap depends not only on its size and position but also on the extent of lateral pharyngeal wall movement against it (Argamaso et al., 1980). A topic of some debate is whether the extent of lateral wall movement changes with the introduction of the pharyngeal flap. Some researchers have found no change in lateral wall motion postoperatively (Lewis & Pashayan, 1980), whereas others have reported adaptation of lateral pharyngeal wall adduction to different flap widths (Karling, Henningsson, Larson, & Isberg, 1999).

Because lateral pharyngeal wall motion is the key to the function of the velopharyngeal mechanism following the placement of the flap, patients with a sagittal pattern of closure or good lateral pharyngeal wall movement preoperatively have the best prognosis for total correction of VPI with a pharyngeal flap. Patients with poor lateral wall motion require a wider flap for total correction. The challenge in these cases is to make the flap wide enough for speech, yet not so wide that it causes upper airway obstruction with hyponasality and obstructive sleep apnea. When there is hypotonia, as in velocardiofacial syndrome, or a compromised airway due to retrognathia, the surgeon may need to compromise perfect speech results for a functional airway.

Choice of Procedure

The choice of a surgical procedure to treat VPI involves a number of factors, including the etiology, the pattern of velopharyngeal closure, the size of the opening, and the location of the opening (Armour, Fischbach, Klaiman, & Fisher, 2005; Seagle, Mazaheri, Dixon-Wood, & Williams, 2002; Ysunza et al., 2002; Abdel-Aziz, El-Hoshy, & Ghandour, 2011). Therefore, a preoperative assessment to determine these factors is very important (Witt & D'Antonio, 1993). The selected procedure also depends on the experience and skill of the surgeon, the patient's medical condition, the size of the airway, and previous surgeries. For small openings, treatment may involve augmentation of the posterior pharyngeal wall or a repeat palatoplasty. Larger gaps require some type of flap or sphincter-type procedure.

As any of these procedures may fail, it is important that surgical correction be performed with this possibility in mind. For instance, a posterior wall augmentation can usually be "upgraded" to either a pharyngeal flap or a sphincter pharyngoplasty operation, whereas rolled flaps can only be changed to a sphincter. Although the superiorly based pharyngeal flap is the gold standard and provides the highest chance of success, particularly for children with cleft palate, it carries a higher incidence of airway obstruction and obstructive sleep apnea (Cole, Banerji, Hollier, & Stal, 2008). However, if a flap needs to be taken down due to airway obstruction, it can be easily converted to a simple augmentation, a redo palatoplasty, or a sphincter pharyngoplasty. On the other hand, if a sphincter pharyngoplasty fails to correct VPI, it is not as easy to convert it to a pharyngeal flap.

There is not yet consensus regarding the specific outcomes of one procedure versus the other for correction of VPI (Sloan, 2000). Further research on the outcomes of each procedure for different patient populations is greatly needed. However, centers vary in their criteria for determining success. In some cases, the surgery in considered a success only when the postoperative resonance and velopharyngeal function is normal. In some centers (including ours at Cincinnati Children's Hospital), the surgery is considered a success only when the postoperative speech is normal (aside, that is, from articulation errors). In other cases, success is defined as either "acceptable" speech or improved speech (Lauck, Lee, Kummer, Billmire, & Bandaranayake, 2006; Kummer, Clark, Redle, Thomsen, & Billmire, 2012). Centers also vary in who determines success (the surgeon, the speech-language pathologist, or the family) and the procedures for measuring success (perceptual judgment or instrumental assessment). Until there is standardization of the measurement of success, it will be impossible to compare studies of surgical efficacy.

Potential Complications

Regardless of the type of VPI surgery, there is always a risk of unwanted complications. As noted previously, a pharyngeal augmentation can cause infections due to the fact that a foreign material is placed in the body. There can also be extrusion, reabsorption, and even migration of the material after insertion. A Furlow Z-plasty can cause an oronasal fistula. All of these procedures may result in overcorrection (which causes airway obstruction, sleep apnea, and hyponasality) or undercorrection (which causes persistent VPI).

Immediately after placement of the pharyngeal flap or sphincter, there is significant *edema* or swelling in the pharynx. As a result, most patients exhibit hyponasality and loud snoring during the immediate postoperative period. Temporary sleep apnea is also common, but this usually resolves within 2 to 6 weeks postoperatively, or after the swelling has gone down.

Snoring is the most common consequence of pharyngoplasty, and many patients will snore to some extent for the rest of their lives. Chronic obstructive sleep apnea occurs in a small number of patients, however (Tharanon et al.,

1990; Trier, 1985a; Vedung, 1995; Ysunza, Garcia-Velasquez, Garcia-Garcia, Haro, & Valencia, 1993). Some authors have reported a prevalence of sleep apnea as high as 10% following pharyngeal flap surgery, but a prevalence of 5% or less is probably more common (personal data). The prevalence of sleep apnea may be less following a sphincter pharyngoplasty, but it does occur, particularly if the sphincter is low in the pharynx (Abyholm et al., 2005; de Serres et al., 1999; Saint Raymond et al., 2004; Witt, Marsh, Muntz, Marty-Grames, & Watchmaker, 1996). Regardless of procedure, sleep apnea is the greatest risk for patients who have micrognathia, such as those with Pierre Robin sequence (Abramson, Marrinan, & Mulliken, 1997; Wells, Vu, & Luce, 1999), or for patients with neurological impairment.

Sleep apnea cannot be ignored because it can cause serious health problems if left untreated. Therefore, if sleep apnea is suspected postoperatively, it is usually evaluated with *polysomnography* (a diagnostic test where a number of physiologic variables are recorded during a sleep study). If sleep apnea is confirmed, an evaluation is done to determine the actual cause of the obstruction. For example, the source of the obstruction in a patient with a pharyngeal flap might actually be micrognathia, glossoptosis, or even hypotonia rather than the flap. Nasopharyngoscopy can be helpful in identifying the source of obstruction. For complex cases, however, a sleep MRI is often needed to determine the cause of obstruction.

The treatment of sleep apnea usually involves the use of *continuous positive air pressure* (CPAP). The CPAP device delivers positive air pressure into the airway during sleep through a specially designed mask. This positive air pressure keeps the pharynx patient during sleep. Patients with sleep apnea are restudied about every 6 months, and in most cases the

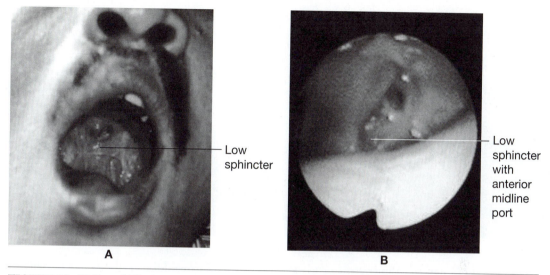

A   **B**

FIGURE 18–13 (A and B)   Unsuccessful sphincter pharyngoplasties. If the sphincter can be seen intraorally, it is almost always too low to eliminate VPI. A low sphincter is also more likely to cause airway obstruction, particularly if it is at the level of the tongue base. In Figure 18–13A, the central port is very narrow, which also causes airway obstruction.

Courtesy David A. Billmire, M.D./Cincinnati Children's Hospital Medical Center & University of Cincinnati College of Medicine

problem resolves within 1 to 2 years. In refractory cases however, the flap is taken down. Fortunately, taking down the flap does not necessarily cause deterioration in speech. The bulk of tissue from the flap, which remains in the posterior pharyngeal wall, continues to provide a pad to assist with velopharyngeal closure. In addition, the speech patterns that the patients learned with the flap in place are often maintained after flap division (Agarwal et al., 2003).

When there is upper airway obstruction and sleep apnea, there is usually an unwanted effect on resonance as well. Obstruction of the nasopharynx can cause hyponasality. Total obturation of the nasopharyngeal port causes denasality. There can even be cul-de-sac resonance, particularly if placement of the flap(s) is too low.

In addition to over-correcting VPI, the pharyngoplasty can also fail to completely correct VPI for a variety of reasons. One of

the most common causes of persistent VPI after surgery is low placement of the pharyngeal flap or sphincter flaps. Figure 18–13 A and B shows two examples of a low-set sphincter pharyngoplasty, and Figure 18–14 A and B shows two examples of a low-set pharyngeal flap. If the flaps can be viewed from an intraoral perspective, they are almost always too low to eliminate VPI. In addition, a low sphincter or pharyngeal flap is more likely to cause airway obstruction, particularly if it is at the level of the tongue base.

Persistent postoperative VPI can also be caused by flaps that are too narrow to adequately obturate the nasopharyngeal port during speech (Figure 18–15). It can even be caused by inadequate lateral pharyngeal wall motion to close the central port of a sphincter or lateral ports of a pharyngeal flap. Patients with velocardiofacial syndrome often have less than ideal postoperative results due to generalized hypotonicity of the velopharyngeal

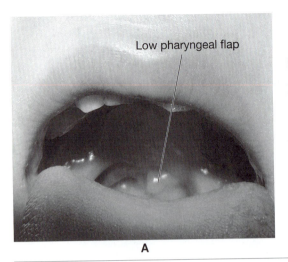
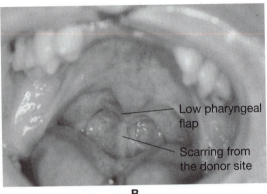

A **B**

FIGURE 18–14 (A and B) Unsuccessful pharyngeal flaps. If the pharyngeal flap can be seen intraorally, it is almost always too low to eliminate VPI. A low pharyngeal flap is also more likely to cause airway obstruction, particularly if it is at the level of the tongue base.

Courtesy David A. Billmire, M.D./Cincinnati Children's Hospital Medical Center & University of Cincinnati College of Medicine

mechanism resulting in poor lateral pharyngeal wall movement (Kasten et al., 1997; Witt, Marsh, Marty-Grames, & Muntz, 1995). Finally, there may be partial or total *dehiscence* (surgical breakdown) of the flap or sphincter days or weeks after the surgery. Figure 18–16 shows an example of a dehisced pharyngeal flap. Remnants of the flap can be seen on the posterior border of the velum.

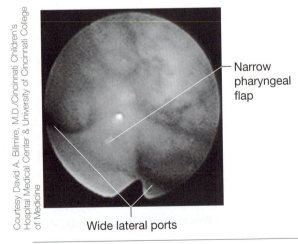

FIGURE 18–15 A narrow pharyngeal flap as noted through nasopharyngoscopy. Note that the lateral ports are wide in comparison to the width of the pharyngeal flap.

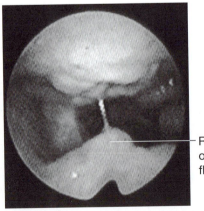

FIGURE 18–16 A dehisced pharyngeal flap. Remnants of the flap can be seen on the posterior border of the velum. The breakdown of the flap has left a large velopharyngeal opening.

Evaluation of postoperative results should begin with a perceptual speech evaluation. If this evaluation reveals hypernasality and/or nasal emission or hyponasality and/or evidence of airway obstruction, a nasopharyngoscopy assessment should also be done. The nasopharyngoscopy gives essential information regarding the location of a persistent gap; the function of the port(s); the function of the velum; the position and integrity of the flap or sphincter; and the airway. Armed with this information, the surgeon can do a revision as needed.

If the flap or sphincter is too low to be maximally effective, the surgeon may attempt to raise the existing flap(s) to a more appropriate position. In other cases, the flap(s) may need to be completely taken down and redone. Surgical revisions may also include opening a port for better breathing if the port is too narrow or has become stenosed due to scarring. More commonly, a port needs to be augmented or closed down further to correct persistent hypernasality or nasal air emission. An auxiliary flap can be raised to augment the primary flap(s) to further close a leaking port.

With pharyngeal flaps, secondary revisions are relatively uncommon. An appropriately placed pharyngeal flap has a greater than 90% chance for normal speech when accompanied by speech therapy (in our series). The overall success rate of the sphincter pharyngoplasty for the elimination of hypernasality and nasal air emission is reported to be only 60% to 85% (James, Twist, Turner, & Milward, 1996; Kasten, Buchman, Stevenson, & Berger, 1997; Riski, Ruff, Georgiade, & Barwick, 1992; Riski, Ruff, Georgiade, Barwick, & Edwards, 1992; Roberts & Brown, 1983; Sie et al., 1998; Witt, D'Antonio, Zimmerman, & Marsh, 1994; Yin et al., 2010). One reason for this may be patient

selection. The sphincter pharyngoplasty narrows the lateral borders of the velopharyngeal port but leaves a midline opening in the anterior–posterior dimension (Ren & Wang, 1993). Therefore, it is likely to be less successful than the pharyngeal flap in correcting VPI due to a history of cleft palate or short velum where the gap is usually in the midline.

Regardless of the pharyngoplasty procedure chosen, the surgery must be followed by a reassessment of the speech so that an appropriate plan of speech therapy can be instituted. Because it takes about 3 months for most of the swelling to resolve and the flap or sphincter to begin to function, this is the best time for the reevaluation. Patients and parents must realize that treating VPI is a two-stage process. The surgery is done first in order to correct the anatomical defect. Following the surgery, speech therapy is required to help the child to eliminate compensatory productions and learn how to use the new mechanism effectively.

Timing of VPI Surgery

Pharyngoplasty procedures can technically be performed at a very young age. In fact, one surgical group used to advocate for simultaneous palatal repair and pharyngeal flap before the first birthday. This is no longer an acceptable practice because it often resulted in significant morbidity, and the procedure was done before it was determined that it was really needed for speech.

Currently, a diagnosis of VPI must be made before considering a pharyngoplasty. This cannot be done definitively until the child begins to produce connected speech and can cooperate with the speech-language pathologist for stimulability testing. In most cases, this is around the age of 3. Some children with a history of cleft palate have normal velopharyngeal function in the preschool years but develop velopharyngeal insufficiency due to a growth spurt or shrinkage of the adenoid pad around puberty. Therefore, longitudinal follow-up of these patients through adolescence is very important.

Evaluation of velopharyngeal function may include nasopharyngoscopy and/or videofluoroscopy, in addition to the speech-language pathologist's examination. The speech-language pathologist's perceptual evaluation is the most critical, however, because surgical decisions are based on the auditory perception of the speech rather than instrumental measures.

Once the patient has been diagnosed with VPI, surgical intervention should be done as soon as possible to avoid the development of strongly habituated compensatory productions, which are harder to correct as the child becomes older. By adulthood, the chance of success, or even improvement, with pharyngoplasty is sig-

nificantly reduced and the risk of complications, such as obstructive sleep apnea, is increased. Therefore, the risks and benefits of pharyngoplasty for adults must be carefully considered.

Although it is generally accepted that early intervention for VPI results in the best speech outcomes, surgical correction must be delayed in some cases. For example, if the child has signs of obstructive sleep apnea, pharyngoplasty should not be done until the airway issues are resolved. In particular, patients with a history of Pierre Robin sequence with micrognathia and upper airway obstruction may not be candidates for pharyngoplasty surgery until the mandible grows or the size of the airway increases. This may require a mandibular advancement procedure, a tongue base reduction, removal of enlarged lymphoid tissue in the nasopharyngeal area, or any combination of these procedures.

SPEECH NOTES

Regardless of the pharyngoplasty procedure chosen (i.e., sphincter pharyngoplasty or pharyngeal flap), best speech results are obtained if the flap(s) is placed high in the nasopharynx (at the level of the skull base). If the flap can be seen during an intraoral evaluation, it is probably too low to be effective for speech and is much more likely to cause sleep apnea because it is at the level of the tongue base.

The challenge of VPI surgery is that it needs to result in a good balance between total obstruction of velopharyngeal port for oral speech, and a sufficiently open velopharyngeal valve for nasal breathing and production of nasal sounds. Over-correction (i.e., small central port after a sphincter pharyngoplasty or small lateral port(s) after pharyngeal flap) can result in airway obstruction and hyponasal speech. Under-correction (i.e., lack of total closure of the port(s) during oral speech) can result in persistent hypernasality and/or nasal emission.

A big problem with under-correction is that, although it may decrease the size of the velopharyngeal port during speech, it could make speech perceptually more distorted. This is because decreasing the port size decreases or eliminates the hypernasality. However, the smaller opening increases the sound of nasal emission/ nasal rustle. When this occurs, a surgical revision can usually be done to further close the remaining gap. (It is best to determine the location of the persistent velopharyngeal gap through nasopharyngoscopy to guide the type and location of the revision surgery.)

SUMMARY

The goals of surgical correction of cleft lip and palate are to normalize the structure for normal feeding, speech, dentition, facial profile, and aesthetics. There are several surgical approaches that can be used to correct each type of cleft. The success of the surgery is dependent upon many factors, including the location, size, and severity of the cleft, type of procedure used, and experience of the surgeon. With the improvement in surgical techniques in recent years, the functional and aesthetic outcomes of surgery have also improved.

VPI continues to be a risk for patients with a history of cleft palate, even after successful palate repair. The treatment of VPI requires close cooperation and teamwork between the surgeon and the speech-language pathologist for the best outcomes. Failure to work cooperatively as a team may result in unnecessary additional surgery, unnecessary speech therapy, or both. It should be remembered that VPI always requires surgery for correction of the structures first and then speech therapy afterward in many cases to correct the function.

FOR REVIEW AND DISCUSSION

1. What is the "rule of 10s," and how does it relate to cleft lip repair?

2. What are the reasons for aligning the maxillary segments before cleft lip surgery? Why is this not done in all cases? What are the different methods?

3. What procedures are done for a unilateral cleft lip repair? What are done for a bilateral cleft lip repair?

4. Discuss the general timing of cleft lip repair. What are the potential advantages and disadvantages of early versus late lip repair?

5. Describe the differences among the von Langenbeck, the Two-Flap, the Wardill-Kilner V–Y pushback, and the Furlow palatoplasty as if you were explaining it to a parent.

6. Discuss the general timing of cleft palate repair. What are the potential advantages and disadvantages of early versus late repair of the palate?

7. List the types of surgeries that can be done for VPI, and describe the basic procedures for each as if you were explaining it to a parent. What factors influence the choice of procedure for the patient?

8. Where should a pharyngeal flap be placed for best speech results and a decreased risk of sleep apnea?

9. Discuss the potential complications of surgery for VPI. Which patients may be at particular risk?

10. What are the problems that can occur with VPI surgery if there is over-correction? What changes in speech production could occur with a sphincter or pharyngeal flap that improves velopharyngeal closure but does not completely close the port during oral speech? If this occurs, what would you recommend?

REFERENCES

Abdel-Aziz, M., El-Hoshy, H., & Ghandour, H. (2011). Treatment of velopharyngeal insufficiency after cleft palate repair depending on the velopharyngeal closure pattern. *The Journal of Craniofacial Surgery, 22*(3), 813–817.

Abramson, D. L., Marrinan, E. M., & Mulliken, J. B. (1997). Robin sequence: Obstructive sleep apnea following pharyngeal flap. *Cleft Palate–Craniofacial Journal, 34*(3), 256–260.

Abyholm, F., D'Antonio, L., Davidson Ward, S. L., Kjoll, L., Saeed, M., Shaw, W., Sloan, G., et al. (2005). Pharyngeal flap and sphincterplasty for velopharyngeal insufficiency have equal outcome at 1 year postoperatively: Results of a randomized trial. *Cleft Palate–Craniofacial Journal, 42*(5), 501–511.

Agarwal, T., Sloan, G. M., Zajac, D., Uhrich, K. S., Meadows, W., & Lewchalermwong, J. A. (2003). Speech benefits of posterior pharyngeal flap are preserved after surgical flap division for obstructive sleep apnea: Experience with division of 12 flaps. *Journal of Craniofacial Surgery, 14*(5), 630–636.

Argamaso, R. V. (1990). The tongue flap: Placement and fixation for closure of postpalatoplasty fistulae. *Cleft Palate Journal, 27*(4), 402–410.

Argamaso, R. V., Shprintzen, R. J., Strauch, B., Lewin, M. L., Daniller, A. L., Ship, A. G., & Croft, C. B. (1980). The role of lateral pharyngeal wall movement in pharyngeal flap surgery. *Plastic and Reconstructive Surgery, 66*(2), 214–219.

Armour, A., Fischbach, S., Klaiman, P., & Fisher, D. M. (2005). Does velopharyngeal closure pattern affect the success of pharyngeal flap pharyngoplasty? *Plastic and Reconstructive Surgery, 115*(1), 45–52; Discussion, 53.

Assuncao, A. G. (1993). The design of tongue flaps for the closure of palatal fistulas. *Plastic and Reconstructive Surgery, 91*(5), 806–810.

Bae, Y. C., Kim, J. H., Lee, J., Hwang, S. M., & Kim, S. S. (2002). Comparative study of the extent of palatal lengthening by different methods. *Annals of Plastic Surgery, 48*(4), 359–362; Discussion 362–364.

Bardach, J., Morris, H. L., & Olin, W. H. (1984). Late results of primary veloplasty: The Marburg Project. *Plastic and Reconstructive Surgery, 73*(2), 207–218.

Barone, C. M., & Argamaso, R. V. (1993). Refinements of the tongue flap for closure of difficult palatal fistulas. *Journal of Craniofacial Surgery, 4*(2), 109–111.

Becker, M., Svensson, H., McWilliam, J., Sarnas, K. V., & Jacobsson, S. (1998). Millard repair of unilateral isolated cleft lip: A 25-year follow-up. *Scandinavian Journal of Plastic and Reconstructive Surgery and Hand Surgery, 32*(4), 387–394.

Blocksma, R., Leuz, C. A., & Mellerstig, K. E. (1975). A conservative program for managing cleft palates without the use of mucoperiosteal flaps. *Plastic and Reconstructive Surgery, 55*(2), 160–169.

Brauer, R. O., & Cronin, T. D. (1983). The Tennison lip repair revisited. *Plastic and Reconstructive Surgery, 71*(5), 633–642.

Brigger, M. T., Ashland, J. E., & Hartnick, C. J. (2010). Injection pharyngoplasty with calcium hydroxylapatite for velopharyngeal insufficiency: Patient selection and technique. *Archives of Otolaryngology—Head & Neck Surgery, 136*(7), 666–670.

Brothers, D. B., Dalston, R. W., Peterson, H. D., & Lawrence, W. T. (1995). Comparison of the Furlow double-opposing Z-palato-plasty with the Wardill-Kilner procedure for isolated clefts of the soft palate. *Plastic and Reconstructive Surgery, 95*(6), 969–977.

Brown, A. S., Cohen, M. A., & Randall, P. (1983). Levator muscle reconstruction: Does it make a difference? *Plastic and Reconstructive Surgery, 72*(1), 1–8.

Busic, N., Bagatin, M., & Boric, V. (1989). Tongue flaps in repair of large palatal defects. *International Journal of Oral Maxillofacial Surgery, 18*(5), 291–293.

Cable, B. B., Canady, J. W., Karnell, M. P., Karnell, L. H., & Malick, D. N. (2004). Pharyngeal flap surgery: Long-term outcomes at the University of Iowa. *Plastic and Reconstructive Surgery, 113*(2), 475–478.

Cantarella, G., Mazzola, R. F., Mantovani, M., Baracca, G., & Pignataro, L. (2011). Treatment of velopharyngeal insufficiency by pharyngeal and velar fat injections. *Otolaryngology—Head & Neck Surgery, 145*(3), 401–403.

Coghlan, K., O'Regan, B., & Carter, J. (1989). Tongue flap repair of oronasal fistulae in cleft palate patients. A review of 20 patients. *Journal of Craniomaxillofacial Surgery, 17*(6), 255–259.

Cohen, S. R., Kalinowski, J., LaRossa, D., & Randall, P. (1991). Cleft palate fistulas: A multivariate statistical analysis of prevalence, etiology, and surgical management. *Plastic and Reconstructive Surgery, 87*(6), 1041–1047.

Cole, P., Banerji, S., Hollier, L., & Stal, S. (2008). Two hundred twenty-two consecutive pharyngeal flaps: An analysis of postoperative complications. *Journal of Oral & Maxillofacial Surgery, 66*(4), 745–748.

Cosman, B., & Falk, A. S. (1980). Delayed hard palate repair and speech deficiencies: A cautionary report. *Cleft Palate Journal, 17*(1), 27–33.

Coston, G. N., Hagerty, R. F., Jannarone, R. J., McDonald, V., & Hagerty, R. C. (1986). Levator muscle reconstruction: Resulting velopharyngeal competence—A preliminary report. *Plastic and Reconstructive Surgery, 77*(6), 911–918.

Cutting, C., & Grayson, B. (1993). The prolabial unwinding flap method for one-stage repair of bilateral cleft lip, nose, and alveolus. *Plastic and Reconstructive Surgery, 91*(1), 37–47.

Cutting, C., Grayson, B., Brecht, L., Santiago, P., Wood, R., & Kwon, S. (1998). Presurgical columellar elongation and primary retrograde nasal reconstruction in one-stage bilateral cleft lip and nose repair. *Plastic and Reconstructive Surgery, 101*(3), 630–639.

D'Antonio, L. D., & Marsh, J. L. (1987). Abnormal carotid arteries in the velocardiofacial syndrome *Plastic and Reconstructive Surgery, 80*(3), 471–472.

Da Silveira, A. C., Oliveira, N., Gonzalez, S., Shahani, M., Reisberg, D., Daw, J. L., Jr., & Cohen, M. (2003). Modified nasal alveolar molding appliance for management of cleft lip defect. *Journal of Craniofacial Surgery, 14*(5), 700–703.

Dejonckere, P. H., & van Wijngaarden, H. A. (2001). Retropharyngeal autologous fat transplantation for congenital short palate: A nasometric assessment of functional results. *Annals of Otology, Rhinology, & Laryngology, 110*(2), 168–172.

Denny, A. D., Marks, S. M., & Oliff-Carneol, S. (1993). Correction of velopharyngeal insufficiency by pharyngeal augmentation using autologous cartilage: A preliminary report. *Cleft Palate–Craniofacial Journal, 30*(1), 46–54.

Deren, O., Ayhan, M., Tuncel, A., Gorgu, M., Altuntas, A., Kutlay, R., & Erdoğan, B.

(2005). The correction of velopharyngeal insufficiency by Furlow palatoplasty in patients older than 3 years undergoing Veau-Wardill-Kilner palatoplasty: A prospective clinical study. *Plastic and Reconstructive Surgery, 116*(1), 85–93; Discussion 94–96.

De Serres, L. M., Deleyiannis, F. W., Eblen, L. E., Gruss, J. S., Richardson, M. A., & Sie, K. C. (1999). Results with sphincter pharyngoplasty and pharyngeal flap. *International Journal of Pediatric Otorhinolaryngology, 48*(1), 17–25.

Dingman, R. O., & Grabb, W. C. (1971). A rational program for surgical management of bilateral cleft lip and cleft palate. *Plastic and Reconstructive Surgery, 47*(3), 239–242.

Dreyer, T. M., & Trier, W. C. (1984). A comparison of palatoplasty techniques. *Cleft Palate Journal, 21*(4), 251–253.

Fara, M., & Brousilova, M. (1988). Long-term experience with 2-stage surgery of cleft palate in total unilateral and bilateral clefts from the aspect of maxillary development. *Rozhledy v. Chirugii, 67*(11), 729–741.

Fara, M., Brousilova, M., Hrivnakova, J., & Tvrdek, M. (1992). Long-term experiences with the two-stage palatoplasty with regard to the development of maxillary arch. *Acta Chirurgiae Plasticae, 34*(3), 138–142.

Finkelstein, Y., Zohar, Y., Nachmani, A., Talmi, Y. P., Lerner, M. A., Hauben, D. J., & Frydman, M. (1993). The otolaryngologist and the patient with velocardiofacial syndrome. *Archives of Otolaryngology—Head & Neck Surgery, 119*(5), 563–569.

Forrest, C. R., Klaiman, P. M., & Mason, A. C. (2009). Posterior pharyngeal flaps. In J. E. Lossee & R. E. Kirschner (Eds.), *Comprehensive Cleft Care* (pp. 649–664). New York: McGraw-Hill.

Furlow, L. T., Jr. (1986). Cleft palate repair by double opposing Z-plasty. *Plastic and Reconstructive Surgery, 78*(6), 724–738.

Furlow, L. T., Jr. (1990). Flaps for cleft lip and palate surgery. *Clinics in Plastic Surgery, 17*(4), 633–644.

Furlow, L. T., Jr. (2009). Correction of velopharyngeal insufficiency by a double-opposing Z-plasty. In J. E. Lossee & R. E. Kirschner (Eds.), *Comprehensive Cleft Care* (pp. 641–647). New York: McGraw-Hill.

Furlow, L. T., Jr., Williams, W. N., Eisenbach, C. R. D., & Bzoch, K. R. (1982). A long term study on treating velopharyngeal insufficiency by Teflon injection. *Cleft Palate Journal, 19*(1), 47–56.

Georgiade, N. G., & Latham, R. A. (1975). Maxillary arch alignment in the bilateral cleft lip and palate infant, using pinned coaxial screw appliance. *Plastic and Reconstructive Surgery, 56*(1), 52–60.

Gray, S. D., Pinborough-Zimmerman, J., & Catten, M. (1999). Posterior wall augmentation for treatment of velopharyngeal insufficiency. *Otolaryngology—Head & Neck Surgery, 121*(1), 107–112.

Gunther, E., Wisser, J. R., Cohen, M. A., & Brown, A. S. (1998). Palatoplasty: Furlow's double reversing Z-plasty versus intravelar veloplasty. *Cleft Palate–Craniofacial Journal, 35*(6), 546–549.

Hardin-Jones, M. A., & Jones, D. L. (2005). Speech production of preschoolers with cleft palate. *Cleft Palate–Craniofacial Journal, 42*(1), 7–13.

Holland, S., Gabbay, J. S., Heller, J. B., O'Hare, C., Hurwitz, D., Ford, M. D., Sauder, A. S., & Bradley, J. P. (2007). Delayed closure of the hard palate leads to speech problems and deleterious maxillary growth. *Plastic and Reconstructive Surgery, 119*(4), 1302–1310.

Jackson, I. T. (1985). Sphincter pharyngoplasty. *Clinics in Plastic Surgery, 12*(4), 711–717.

Jackson, I. T., McGlynn, M. J., Huskie, C. F., & Dip, I. P. (1980). Velopharyngeal incompetence in the absence of cleft palate: Results of treatment in 20 cases. *Plastic and Reconstructive Surgery, 66*(2), 211–213.

Jackson, I. T., McLennan, G., & Scheker, L. R. (1983). Primary veloplasty or primary palatoplasty: Some preliminary findings. *Plastic and Reconstructive Surgery, 72*(2), 153–157.

Jackson, I. T., & Silverton, J. S. (1977). The sphincter pharyngoplasty as a secondary procedure in cleft palates. *Plastic and Reconstructive Surgery, 59*(4), 518–524.

James, N. K., Twist, M., Turner, M. M., & Milward, T. M. (1996). An audit of velopharyngeal incompetence treated by the Orticochea pharyngoplasty. *British Journal of Plastic Surgery, 49*(4), 197–201.

Jarvis, B. L., & Trier, W. C. (1988). The effect of intravelar veloplasty on velopharyngeal competence following pharyngeal flap surgery. *Cleft Palate Journal, 25*(4), 389–394.

Karling, J., Henningsson, G., Larson, O., & Isberg, A. (1999). Adaptation of pharyngeal wall adduction after pharyngeal flap surgery. *Cleft Palate–Craniofacial Journal, 36*(2), 166–172.

Kasten, S. J., Buchman, S. R., Stevenson, C., & Berger, M. (1997). A retrospective analysis of revision sphincter pharyngoplasty. *Annals of Plastic Surgery, 39*(6), 583–589.

Kohout, M. P., Aljaro, L. M., Farkas, L. G., & Mulliken, J. B. (1998). Photogrammetric comparison of two methods for synchronous repair of bilateral cleft lip and nasal deformity. *Plastic and Reconstructive Surgery, 102*(5), 1339–1349.

Krugman, M. E., & Brant-Zawadski, M. (1997). Magnetic resonance angioplasty for prepharyngoplasty assessment in velocardiofacial syndrome. *Cleft Palate–Craniofacial Journal, 34*(3), 266–267.

Kummer, A. W., Clark, S. L., Redle, E. E., Thomsen, L. L., & Billmire, D. A. (2012). Current practice in assessing and reporting speech outcomes of cleft palate and velopharyngeal surgery: A survey of cleft palate/craniofacial professionals. *Cleft Palate–Craniofacial Journal, 49*(2), 146–152.

Lai, J. P., Lo, L. J., Wong, H. F., Wang, S. R., & Yun, C. (2004). Vascular abnormalities in the head and neck area in velocardiofacial syndrome. *Chang Gung Medical Journal, 27*(8), 586–593.

Latham, R. A. (1980). Orthopedic advancement of the cleft maxillary segment: A preliminary report. *Cleft Palate Journal, 17*(3), 227–233.

Latham, R. A., Kusy, R. P., & Georgiade, N. G. (1976). An extraorally activated expansion appliance for cleft palate infants. *Cleft Palate Journal, 13*, 253–261.

Lauck, L., Lee, L., Kummer, A. W., Billmire, D., & Bandaranayake, D. (2006, April). Speech outcomes following surgical management of velopharyngeal dysfunction. Paper presented at the Annual Meeting of the American Cleft Palate–Craniofacial Association, Vancouver, Canada.

Lazarus, D. D., Hudson, D. A., van Zyl, J. E., Fleming, A. N., & Fernandes, D. (1998). Repair of unilateral cleft lip: A comparison of five techniques. *Annals of Plastic Surgery, 41*(6), 587–594.

Leon-Valle, C. (1980). The use of a cutaneous-muscular flap for primary naso-labial repair with a modified Tennison-Randall technique. *British Journal of Plastic Surgery, 33*(2), 266–269.

Leuchter, I., Schweizer, V., Hohlfeld, J., & Pasche, P. (2009). Treatment of velopharyngeal insufficiency by autologous fat injection. *European Archives of Oto-Rhino-Laryngology, 267*(6), 977–983.

Lewis, M. B., & Pashayan, H. M. (1980). The effects of pharyngeal flap surgery on lateral pharyngeal wall motion: A videoradiographic evaluation. *Cleft Palate Journal*, *17*(4), 301–308.

Liao, Y. F., Yang, I. Y., Wang, R., Yun, C., & Huang, C. S. (2010). Two-stage palate repair with delayed hard palate closure is related to favorable maxillary growth in unilateral cleft lip and palate. *Plastic and Reconstructive Surgery*, *125*(5), 1503–1510.

Lin, W. N., Wang, R., Cheong, E. C., & Lo, L. J. (2010). Use of hemisphincter pharyngoplasty in the management of velopharyngeal insufficiency after pharyngeal flap: An outcome study. *Annals of Plastic Surgery*, *65*(2), 201–205.

Lindsey, W. H., & Davis, P. T. (1996). Correction of velopharyngeal insufficiency with Furlow palatoplasty. *Archives of Otolaryngology—Head & Neck Surgery*, *122*(8), 881–884.

Losken, A., Williams, J. K., Burstein, F. D., Malick, D., & Riski, J. E. (2003). An outcome evaluation of sphincter pharyngoplasty for the management of velopharyngeal insufficiency. *Plastic and Reconstructive Surgery*, *112*(1), 1755–1761.

MacKenzie-Stepner, K., Witzel, M. A., Stringer, D. A., Lindsay, W. K., Munro, I. R., & Hughes, H. (1987). Abnormal carotid arteries in the velocardiofacial syndrome: A report of three cases. *Plastic and Reconstructive Surgery*, *80*(3), 347–351.

Marsh, J. L. (2009). Sphincter pharyngoplasty. In J. E. Lossee & R. E. Kirschner (Eds.), *Comprehensive Cleft Care* (pp. 665–671). New York: McGraw-Hill.

Marsh, J. L., Grames, L. M., & Holtman, B. (1989). Intravelar veloplasty: A prospective study. *Cleft Palate Journal*, *26*(1), 46–50.

Mehendale, F. V., & Sommerlad, B. C. (2004). Surgical significance of abnormal internal carotid arteries in velocardiofacial syndrome in 43 consecutive Hynes pharyngoplasties. *Cleft Palate–Craniofacial Journal*, *41*(4), 368–374.

Millard, D. R., Jr., & Latham, R. A. (1990). Improved primary surgical and dental treatment of clefts. *Plastic and Reconstructive Surgery*, *86*(5), 856–871.

Millard, D. R., Latham, R., Huifen, X., Spiro, S., & Morovic, C. (1999). Cleft lip and palate treated by presurgical orthopedics, gingivoperiosteoplasty, and lip adhesion (POPLA) compared with previous lip adhesion method: A preliminary study of serial dental casts. *Plastic and Reconstructive Surgery*, *103*(6), 1630–1644.

Mitnick, R. J., Bello, J. A., Golding-Kushner, K. J., Argamaso, R. V., & Shprintzen, R. J. (1996). The use of magnetic resonance angiography prior to pharyngeal flap surgery in patients with velocardiofacial syndrome. *Plastic and Reconstructive Surgery*, *97*(5), 908–919.

Moore, M. D., Lawrence, W. T., Ptak, J. J., & Trier, W. C. (1988). Complications of primary palatoplasty: A twenty-one-year review. *Cleft Palate Journal*, *25*(2), 156–162.

Morovic, C. G., & Cutting, C. (2005). Combining the Cutting and Mulliken methods for primary repair of the bilateral cleft lip nose. *Plastic and Reconstructive Surgery*, *116*(6), 1613–1619.

Mulliken, J. B. (2009). Repair of bilateral cleft lip and its variants. *Indian Journal of Plastic Surgery*, *42*(Suppl), S79–90.

Mulliken, J. B., & LaBrie, R. A. (2012). Fourth-dimensional changes in nasolabial dimensions following rotation-advancement repair of unilateral cleft lip. *Plastic & Reconstructive Surgery*, *129*(2), 491–498.

Murison, M. S., & Pigott, R. W. (1992). Medial Langenbeck: Experience of a modified von Langenbeck repair of the cleft palate. A preliminary report. *British Journal of Plastic Surgery*, 45(6), 454–459.

Murthy, J., Sendhilnathan, S., & Hussain, S. A. (2010). Speech outcome following late primary palate repair. *Cleft Palate–Craniofacial Journal*, 47(2), 156–161.

Orticochea, M. (1970). Results of the dynamic muscle sphincter operation in cleft palates. *British Journal of Plastic Surgery*, 23(2), 108–114.

Orticochea, M. (1983). A review of 236 cleft palate patients treated with dynamic muscle sphincter. *Plastic and Reconstructive Surgery*, 71(2), 180–188.

Orticochea, M. (1997). Physiopathology of the dynamic muscular sphincter of the pharynx. *Plastic and Reconstructive Surgery*, 100(7), 1918–1923.

Orticochea, M. (1999). The timing and management of dynamic muscular pharyngeal sphincter construction in velopharyngeal incompetence. *British Journal of Plastic Surgery*, 52(2), 85–87.

Paranaiba, L. M., Almeida, H., Barros, L. M., Martelli, D. R., Orsi, J. D., Jr., & Martelli, H., Jr. (2009). Current surgical techniques for cleft lip-palate in Minas Gerais, Brazil. *Brazilian Journal of Otorhinolaryngology*, 75(6), 839–843.

Penna, V., Bannasch, H., & Stark, G. B. (2007). The turbinate flap for oronasal fistula closure. *Annals of Plastic Surgery*, 59(6), 679–681.

Perkins, J. A., Lewis, C. W., Gruss, J. S., Eblen, L. E., & Sie, K. C. (2005). Furlow palatoplasty for management of velopharyngeal insufficiency: A prospective study of 148 consecutive patients. *Plastic and Reconstructive Surgery*, 116(1), 72–80; Discussion 81–84.

Perko, M. A. (1979). Two-stage closure of cleft palate (Progress report). *Journal of Maxillofacial Surgery*, 7(1), 46–80.

Pigott, R. W., Rieger, F. W., & Moodie, A. F. (1984). Tongue flap repair of cleft palate fistulae. *British Journal of Plastic Surgery*, 37(3), 285–293.

Por, Y. C., Tan, Y. C., Chang, F. C., & Chen, P. K. (2010). Revision of pharyngeal flaps causing obstructive airway symptoms: An analysis of treatment with three different techniques over 39 years. *Journal of Plastic, Reconstructive, & Aesthetic Surgery*, 63(6), 930–933.

Posnick, J. C., & Getz, S. B., Jr. (1987). Surgical closure of end-stage palatal fistulas using anteriorly based dorsal tongue flaps. *Journal of Oral Maxillofacial Surgery*, 45(11), 907–912.

Pradel, W., Senf, D., Mai, R., Ludicke, G., Eckelt, U., & Lauer, G. (2009). One-stage palate repair improves speech outcome and early maxillary grown in patients with cleft lip and palate. *Journal of Physiology and Pharmacology*, 60, 37–41.

Remacle, M., Bertrand, B., Eloy, P., & Marbaix, E. (1990). The use of injectable collagen to correct velopharyngeal insufficiency. *Laryngoscope*, 100(3), 269–274.

Ren, Y. F., & Wang, G. H. (1993). A modified palatopharyngeous flap operation and its application in the correction of velopharyngeal incompetence. *Plastic and Reconstructive Surgery*, 91(4), 612–617.

Riski, J. E., Ruff, G. L., Georgiade, G. S., & Barwick, W. J. (1992). Evaluation of failed sphincter pharyngoplasties. *Annals of Plastic Surgery*, 28(6), 545–553.

Riski, J. E., Ruff, G. L., Georgiade, G. S., Barwick, W. J., & Edwards, P. D. (1992). Evaluation of the sphincter pharyngoplasty. *Cleft Palate–Craniofacial Journal*, 29(3), 254–261.

Roberts, T. M., & Brown, B. S. (1983). Evaluation of a modified sphincter pharyngoplasty in the treatment of speech problems due to palatal insufficiency. *Annals of Plastic Surgery, 10*(3), 209–213.

Ross, D. A., Witzel, M. A., Armstrong, D. C., & Thomson, H. G. (1996). Is pharyngoplasty a risk in velocardiofacial syndrome? An assessment of medially displaced carotid arteries. *Plastic and Reconstructive Surgery, 98*(7), 1182–1190.

Ross, R. B. (1987). Treatment variables affecting facial growth in complete unilateral cleft lip and palate. Part I-Part 7. *Cleft Palate Journal, 24*(1), 5–77.

Saint Raymond, C., Bettega, G., Deschaux, C., Lebeau, J., Raphael, B., Levy, P., & PÃpin, J. L. (2004). Sphincter pharyngoplasty as a treatment of velopharyngeal incompetence in young people: A prospective evaluation of effects on sleep structure and sleep respiratory disturbances. *Chest, 125*(3), 864–871.

Salyer, K. E. (1986). Primary correction of the unilateral cleft lip nose: A 15-year experience. *Plastic and Reconstructive Surgery, 77*(4), 558–568.

Saman, M., & Tatum, S. A., III. (2012). Recent advances in surgical pharyngeal modification procedures for the treatment of velopharyngeal insufficiency in patients with cleft palate. *Archives of Facial Plastic Surgery, 14*(2), 85–88.

Schweckendiek, W. (1955). [Zur zweiphasigen Gaumenspalten-operation bei primarem Velumerschluss.] *Fortschritte Kiefer- und Gesichtschtschirurgie, 1*, 73–76.

Schweckendiek, W. (1966). [The technique of early veloplasty and its results.] *Acta Chirurgiae Plasticae, 8*(3), 188–194.

Schweckendiek, W. (1968). [Early veloplasty and its results.] *Acta Oto-Rhino-Laryngologica Belgica, 22*(6), 697–703.

Schweckendiek, W. (1983). [Primary closure of cleft lip and cleft palate.] *Zahnarztl Prax, 34*(8), 317–320.

Schweckendiek, W., & Doz, P. (1978). Primary veloplasty: Long-term results without maxillary deformity. A twenty-five year report. *Cleft Palate Journal, 15*(3), 268–274.

Seagle, M. B., Mazaheri, M. K., Dixon-Wood, V. L., & Williams, W. N. (2002). Evaluation and treatment of velopharyngeal insufficiency: The University of Florida experience. *Annals of Plastic Surgery, 48* (5), 464–470.

Sie, K. C., & Gruss, J. S. (2002). Results with Furlow palatoplasty in the management of velopharyngeal insufficiency. *Plastic and Reconstructive Surgery, 109*(7), 2588–2589; Author reply 2590–2591.

Sie, K. C., Tampakopoulou, D. A., de Serres, L. M., Gruss, J. S., Eblen, L. E., & Yonick, T. (1998). Sphincter pharyngoplasty: Speech outcome and complications. *Laryngoscope, 108*(8, Pt. 1), 1211–1217.

Sie, K. C., Tampakopoulou, D. A., Sorom, J., Gruss, J. S., & Eblen, L. E. (2001). Results with Furlow palatoplasty in management of velopharyngeal insufficiency. *Plastic and Reconstructive Surgery, 108*(1), 17–25; Discussion 26–29.

Skolnick, M. L., & McCall, G. N. (1972). Velopharyngeal competence and incompetence following pharyngeal flap surgery: Videofluoroscopic study in multiple projections. *Cleft Palate Journal, 9*(1), 1–12.

Sloan, G. M. (2000). Posterior pharyngeal flap and sphincter pharyngoplasty: The state of the art. *Cleft Palate–Craniofacial Journal, 37*(2), 112–122.

Smahel, Z., & Horak, I. (1993). The effect of two-stage palatoplasty on facial development in unilateral cleft lip and palate. *Acta Chirurgiae Plasticae, 35*(1/2), 67–72.

Smile Train. (n.d.) Virtual Surgery Videos. Accessed January 19, 2013, from http://www.smiletrain.org/

Stal, S., Brown, R. H., Higuera, S., Hollier, L. H., Jr., Byrd, H. S., Cutting, C. B., & Mulliken, J. B. (2009). Fifty years of the Millard rotation-advancement: Looking back and moving forward. *Plastic & Reconstructive Surgery, 123*(4), 1364–1377.

Tan, O., & Atik, B. (2007). Triangular with ala nasi (TAN) repair of unilateral cleft lips: A personal technique and early outcomes. *The Journal of Craniofacial Surgery, 18*(1), 186–197.

Tan, S. P., Greene, A. K., & Mulliken, J. B. (2012). Current surgical management of bilateral cleft lip in North America. *Plastic & Reconstructive Surgery, 129*(6), 1347–1355.

Terris, D. J., & Goode, R. L. (1993). Costochondral pharyngeal implants for velopharyngeal insufficiency. *Laryngoscope, 103*(5), 565–569.

Tharanon, W., Stella, J. P., & Epker, B. N. (1990). The modified superior-based pharyngeal flap. Part III. A retrospective study. *Oral Surgery, Oral Medicine, Oral Pathology, and Endodontics, 70*(3), 256–267.

Thind, M. S., Singh, A., & Thind, R. S. (1992). Repair of anterior secondary palate fistula using tongue flaps. *Acta Chirurgiae Plasticae, 34*(2), 79–91.

Trier, W. C. (1985a). The pharyngeal flap operation. *Clinics in Plastic Surgery, 12*(4), 697–710.

Trier, W. C. (1985b). Repair of bilateral cleft lip: Millard's technique. *Clinics in Plastic Surgery, 12*(4), 605–625.

Trier, W. C., & Dreyer, T. M. (1984). Primary von Langenbeck palatoplasty with levator reconstruction: Rationale and technique. *Cleft Palate Journal, 21*(4), 254–262.

Trigos, L., Ysunza, A., Gonzalez, A., & Vazquez, M. C. (1988). Surgical treatment of borderline velopharyngeal insufficiency using homologous cartilage implantation

with videonasopharyngoscopic monitoring. *Cleft Palate Journal, 25*(2), 167–170.

Ulkur, E., Karagoz, H., Uygur, F., Celikoz, B., Cincik, H., Mutlu, H., Ciyiltepe, M., et al. (2008). Use of porous polyethylene implant for augmentation of the posterior pharynx in young adult patients with borderline velopharyngeal insufficiency. *Journal of Craniofacial Surgery, 19*(3), 573–579.

Vedung, S. (1995). Pharyngeal flaps after one- and two-stage repair of the cleft palate: A 25-year review of 520 patients. *Cleft Palate–Craniofacial Journal, 32*(3), 206–15; Discussion 215–216.

Wells, M. D., Vu, T. A., & Luce, E. A. (1999). Incidence and sequelae of nocturnal respiratory obstruction following posterior pharyngeal flap operation. *Annals of Plastic Surgery, 43*(3), 252–257.

Witt, P. D., & D'Antonio, L. L. (1993). Velopharyngeal insufficiency and secondary palatal management. A new look at an old problem. *Clinics in Plastic Surgery, 20*(4), 707–721.

Witt, P. D., D'Antonio, L. L., Zimmerman, G. J., & Marsh, J. L. (1994). Sphincter pharyngoplasty: A preoperative and postoperative analysis of perceptual speech characteristics and endoscopic studies of velopharyngeal function. *Plastic and Reconstructive Surgery, 93*(6), 1154–1168.

Witt, P. D., Marsh, J. L., Marty-Grames, L., & Muntz, H. R. (1995). Revision of the failed sphincter pharyngoplasty: An outcome assessment. *Plastic and Reconstructive Surgery, 96*(1), 129–138.

Witt, P. D., Marsh, J. L., Muntz, H. R., Marty-Grames, L., & Watchmaker, G. P. (1996). Acute obstructive sleep apnea as a complication of sphincter pharyngoplasty. *Cleft Palate–Craniofacial Journal, 33*(3), 183–189.

Witt, P. D., Miller, D. C., Marsh, J. L., Muntz, H. R., & Grames, L. M. (1998). Limited value of preoperative cervical vascular imaging in patients with velocardiofacial syndrome. *Plastic and Reconstructive Surgery*, *101*(5), 1184–1195; Discussion 1196–1197.

Witt, P. D., O'Daniel, T. G., Marsh, J. L., Grames, L. M., Muntz, H. R., & Pilgram, T. K. (1997). Surgical management of velopharyngeal dysfunction: Outcome analysis of autogenous posterior pharyngeal wall augmentation. *Plastic and Reconstructive Surgery*, 99(5), 1287–1296; Discussion 1297–1300.

Wolford, L. M., Oelschlaeger, M., & Deal, R. (1989). Proplast as a pharyngeal wall implant to correct velopharyngeal insufficiency. *Cleft Palate Journal*, *26*(2), 119–126; Discussion 126–128.

Wu, J., & Epker, B. N. (1990). The modified superiorly based pharyngeal flap technique. Part II. An anatomic study. *Oral Surgery, Oral Medicine, Oral Pathology*, *70*(3), 251–255.

Yin, H., Zhao, S. F., Zheng, G. N., Li, S., Wang, Y., Zheng, Q., & Shi, B. (2010). Investigation of the optimized surgical procedure for the cleft palate patients over six years old. *West China Journal of Somatology*, *28*(3), 294–297.

Yoshida, H., Stella, J. P., Ghali, G. E., & Epker, B. N. (1992). The modified superiorly based pharyngeal flap. Part IV. Position of the base of the flap. *Oral Surgery, Oral Medicine, Oral Pathology*, *73*(1), 13–18.

Ysunza, A., Garcia-Velasco, M., Garcia-Garcia, M., Haro, R., & Valencia, M. (1993). Obstructive sleep apnea secondary to surgery for velopharyngeal insufficiency. *Cleft Palate–Craniofacial Journal*, *30*(4), 387–390.

Ysunza, A., Pamplona, M. C., Molina, F., Drucker, M., Felemovicius, J., Ramirez, E., & Patiño, C. (2004). Surgery for speech in cleft palate patients. *International Journal of Pediatric Otorhinolaryngology*, *68*(12), 1499–1505.

Ysunza, A., Pamplona, G., Ramirez, E., Molina, F., Mendoza, M., & Silva, A. (2002). Velopharyngeal surgery: A prospective randomized study of pharyngeal flaps and sphincter pharyngoplasties. *Plastic and Reconstructive Surgery*, *110*(6), 1401–1407.

CHAPTER

19

ORTHOGNATHIC SURGERY FOR CRANIOFACIAL CONDITIONS

DEEPAK KRISHNAN, D.D.S

JULIA CORCORAN, M.D.

CHAPTER OUTLINE

INTRODUCTION

Craniofacial conditions, including cleft and craniosynostosis syndromes, affect not only soft tissues but also underlying bony tissues. The craniofacial skeleton can be viewed as scaffolding for the soft tissue envelope of the face. If alveolar, palatal, maxillary, or mandibular segments are missing, unstable, or in poor anatomic relationship to one another, the overlying face appears abnormal, drawing unfavorable attention to the patient. Furthermore, the functions of breathing, swallowing, speaking, and chewing can be impaired.

Orthognathic surgery is a type of surgery that involves the bones of the upper jaw (maxilla) and the lower jaw (mandible). It can address several different problems that occur in patients with clefts or craniosynostosis syndromes. For example, congenital absence of bone in cleft patients can be corrected by bone grafting to improve the alveolar arch and occlusion. Compensation can be made for a lack of midfacial growth in patients with a cleft or craniosynostosis by repositioning the maxilla in a more normal occlusal relationship with the mandible. An inadequate mandible in Pierre Robin sequence or facial asymmetry in hemifacial microsomia can be addressed by mandibular advancement through multiple techniques.

Overall, orthognathic surgery techniques aim to improve the skeletal scaffolding and therefore the soft tissue envelope of the face, as well as underlying function. This chapter briefly explains orthognathic procedures and their potential impact on skeletal and occlusal articulation, speech, resonance, and airway.

ALVEOLAR BONE GRAFTING

One of the greatest improvements in care of the patient with cleft lip and palate has been the routine implementation of alveolar bone grafting (El-Sayed & Khalil, 2010; Eppley & Sadove, 2000; van Aalst, Eppley, Hathaway, & Sadove, 2005). With this procedure, the dental arch of the maxilla is greatly improved, and permanent teeth in the line of the cleft can be maintained.

Purpose

Although *cheiloplasty* (lip repair) restores the continuity of the muscular sphincter of the lip, and palatoplasty restores the continuity of the velopharyngeal sphincter, the alveolus is not addressed routinely by either of these procedures. The alveolar cleft is left untreated for a time to allow for less restricted maxillary growth. This cleft is later repaired with an alveolar bone graft.

An alveolar cleft leaves the lesser and greater palatine segments floating free, which usually leads to lateral crossbite on the side of the cleft (the lesser segment) (Figure 19–1). If left untreated, the anterior gap in the arch can lead to loss of the permanent lateral incisor and canine teeth because of lack of supporting bone for the periodontal ligament that secures the tooth within the alveolus. Furthermore, this gap is usually associated with an oronasal

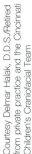

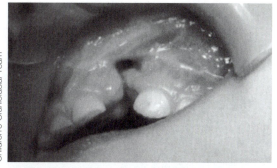

FIGURE 19–1   The bony cleft in the alveolus can be seen as the dark gap between the teeth.

fistula, which can cause liquid and some soft food escape into the nasal cavity (Waite & Waite, 1996). Finally, the crossbite can cause distortion of speech, particularly with the production of sibilants.

The purpose of the alveolar bone graft is to surgically correct the alveolar cleft at the appropriate time in order to provide bony support for eruption and maintenance of the permanent lateral incisor and canine. The bone graft also serves to improve the dental arch.

Techniques

There are two schools of thought regarding alveolar bone grafting. Some surgeons advocate for primary bone grafting, while others prefer a delayed approach. These techniques are discussed as follows.

Primary Bone Grafting

One method of primary alveolar bone grafting is a procedure called a *gingivoperiosteoplasty*. With this procedure, the gingiva and the underlying periosteum of the alveolus on each edge of the cleft are opened. The raw surfaces are then advanced and sewn together. This technique allows the bone progenitor cells found in the gingivoperiosteum to lay down bone as the patient grows. Therefore, bone is

not harvested from elsewhere in the body. Another technique for primary bone grafting is to use a piece of rib graft as a strut across the alveolar cleft and then cover the repair with the gingivoperiosteum. Recent advances in tissue engineering show promise in using recombinant bone morphogenetic protein (r-BMP2) as a substitute for an organic bone graft.

Delayed Bone Grafting

To correct an alveolar cleft, the two alveolar segments are surgically placed in a normal arch alignment and then secured with a bone graft. The bone graft can be harvested from the hip (iliac crest), the marrow cavity of the skull, or other sources. The edges of the cleft are opened, as in a gingivoperiosteoplasty. The floor of the nose is sewn closed, and the bone graft is packed into the space. The gingiva is then repaired over the bone graft. This approach also helps build up the bone deficiency in both the nasal base and para-alar areas.

During the healing phase (the first 6 weeks after the surgery), the patient's palatal segments are held steady by an orthodontic device. Mastication is limited by placing the patient on a diet of soft and pureed foods. Brushing the teeth is replaced by using antimicrobial mouth rinses and a Waterpik® appliance. About 3 months later, when the bone is solidly healed, the orthodontist can then direct the teeth into the appropriate positions along a complete maxillary alveolar arch.

Once healed, the bone graft provides a stable scaffold for the permanent dentition and the upper lip. Figure 19–2A is an intraoperative photo of a patient just before the bone graft. The picture shows the gingival and periosteal tissues reflected off the alveolar cleft. Note how the cleft extends to the floor of the nose. Figure 19–2B is another intraoperative photo of the same patient following the bone graft insertion and filling of the alveolar cleft with

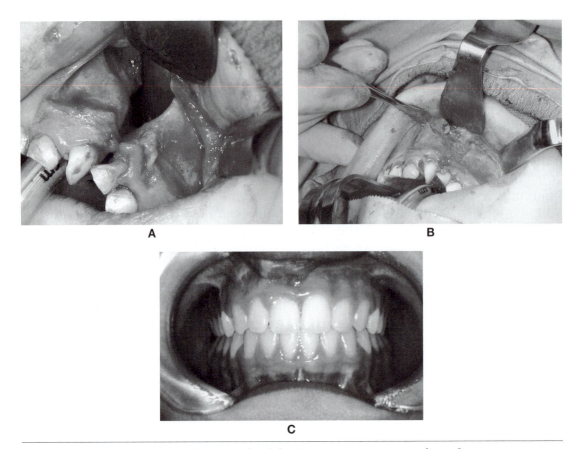

FIGURE 19–2 (A–C) Bone graft for an alveolar cleft. (A) An intraoperative view photo of a patient just prior to the bone graft. Note how the cleft extends to the floor of the nose. (B) An intraoperative photo of the same patient following the bone graft insertion and filling of the alveolar cleft with the graft material. (C) The grafted cleft alveolus following orthodontic therapy that aligned the erupted teeth into perfect form.

Courtesy Deepak Krishnan, D.D.S./University of Cincinnati College of Medicine

the graft material. Figure 19–2C shows a final picture of this grafted cleft alveolus following orthodontic therapy that aligned the erupted teeth into perfect form.

Timing

The timing of alveolar bone grafting is controversial and is often debated vigorously between adherents of each philosophy (Trindade-Suedam et al., 2012). *Primary bone grafting* is done to repair the alveolusis done before the eruption of teeth in the first year—either at the time of palatoplasty or in a separate operation. Surgeons who favor this early, or primary, approach point out that the maxillary arch is aligned appropriately from almost the beginning. The disadvantage of primary bone grafting is that although bone often forms across the alveolar cleft, it may not be of sufficient quantity or quality to support the permanent dentition—necessitating a delayed or secondary bone graft (Dado, 1993; Santiago et al., 1998). This situation can be a concern because the success of bone grafting is directly dependent on good blood flow in the surrounding soft tissues. Scar tissue from the previous primary procedure has a compromised blood supply, thus hindering the bone engraftment.

In contrast to primary bone grafting, *delayed bone grafting* is done when the roots of the permanent lateral incisor or canine (both located at the edges of the cleft) are about two-thirds developed and are ready to descend. Delayed bone grafting is done just in time to provide support for the eruption of these teeth, which usually occurs sometime between 6 and 11 years of age. The actual age of bone grafting is patient specific and depends on the child's dental development (Cohen, Polley, & Figueroa, 1993; Walia, 2011). The pediatric dentist or orthodontist follows the child through serial radiographs to determine when the tooth roots are mature. The lateral incisor erupts earlier than the cuspid. Therefore, the actual timing of the delayed bone graft depends on which tooth is more at risk for that child.

While waiting for maturation, the orthodontist uses an expanding device to put the arch segments into correct alignment. Once aligned, a holding device (a retainer or a lingual arch wire) is used for retention.

Potential Complications

Certain complications can occur with bone grafting. Bleeding and infection are the most common adverse circumstances. However, the bone graft take can be inadequate, causing a breakdown of the repair and persistence of the fistula.

MAXILLARY ADVANCEMENT

Patients with cleft lip and palate, hemifacial microsomia (facioauriculovertebral syndrome), and craniosynostosis syndromes often have maxillary growth problems that lead to concave profiles and malocclusion. These patients are candidates for maxillary advancement, which results in a significant improvement in facial aesthetics and dental occlusion.

Purpose

In patients with clefts or synostosis, the maxillary arch sits behind the mandibular arch, resulting in Angle's Class III malocclusion. A review of the growth patterns of the maxilla and mandible explain why the malocclusion develops.

Children with clefts may initially have a fairly normal occlusal relationship, but they usually develop a Class III relationship with growth. This is due to the fact that maxillary growth in patients with clefts is usually inhibited, presumably because of scar tissue and disturbances to the growth centers from previous surgeries. In addition, mandibular growth normally continues later into life than maxillary growth. Eventually the lack of growth in the maxilla and the normal growth in the mandible place the jaws in Class III malocclusion. The scar tissue may indeed be the causative factor in the transverse as well as anterior–posterior restriction of the maxilla, as is evidenced by its normal growth in unrepaired cleft palates, which are not uncommon in countries with lack of access to care.

Children with craniosynostosis syndromes have restricted maxillary growth because the sutures between the facial bones and the skull bones have closed prematurely and stunted the growth. Children with hemifacial microsomia have a *cant* (slant in occlusion) to the maxilla. The shortened mandible on the affected side leaves inadequate room for the maxilla on that side to grow.

Speech Notes

Maxillary retrusion with Class III malocclusion usually causes oral cavity crowding. As a result, the tongue tip rests in an anterior position relative to the alveolar ridge. This can lead to fronting of lingual-alveolar sounds as an obligatory distortion. It can also lead to the use of compensatory productions, including a palatal-dorsal placement for lingual-alveolar sounds. This placement can lead to a lateral distortion.

When Class III malocclusion is severe, it can even affect bilabial and labiodental sounds, often leading to the use of reverse labiodental production (upper lip against the mandibular teeth) as a substitution for both. See Chapter 9 for more information.

Finally, the relative posterior displacement of the maxilla leads to a small pharyngeal space, which can cause hyponasality and sleep apnea (Demetriades, Chang, Laskarides, & Papageorge, 2010).

A retrodisplaced or small maxilla can cause a shallow orbit due to underdevelopment of the zygoma, as found in syndromic synostosis (Apert and Crouzon syndromes), or complex clefting (Treacher Collins syndrome). Because the orbit is essentially too small, *proptosis* (protrusion) of the globe, with exposure of the cornea, can result in the potential loss of sight.

The purpose of maxillary advancement, therefore, is to bring the maxilla into proper alignment with the mandible, thus correcting the facial profile and Class III malocclusion. This improves the aesthetic and functional problems, including difficulty with speech production.

Techniques

Maxillary advancement can be done through a traditional surgical approach using a Le Fort osteotomy. It can also be done through distraction osteogenesis, which is a relatively new procedure. These techniques are described in the following sections.

Le Fort Osteotomies

Le Fort (1901) originally described the naturally occurring fracture planes in the facial skeleton. These lines of natural weakness in the facial skeleton collapse or break during trauma and are used to describe midfacial fracture patterns. Le Fort's three factures planes are now used by surgeons when they create *osteotomies* (planned surgical cuts) in the maxilla to separate it from the skull and to position it in its appropriate functional and pleasing position. Figure 19–3A illustrates the levels of the three Le Fort osteotomies. Figure 19–3B shows maxillary retrusion and the cuts for a Le Fort I. Figure 19–3C shows the position of the maxilla after the surgery.

The most common osteotomy is the Le Fort I, which includes the maxilla (alveolar arch) only. The maxilla is cut transversely, just above the tooth roots and the base of the nose. This allows the surgeon to move the alveolar arch and palate as a single unit. One can imagine this movement as an edentulous individual being able to move his denture plate forward and out of his mouth. In addition to bringing the midface forward, the maxilla can be rotated to match midlines and tilted to correct a cant. A narrow maxilla can also be widened by further osteotomizing it into segments.

Figure 19–4A and B shows a young girl with severe midface retrusion due to maxillary

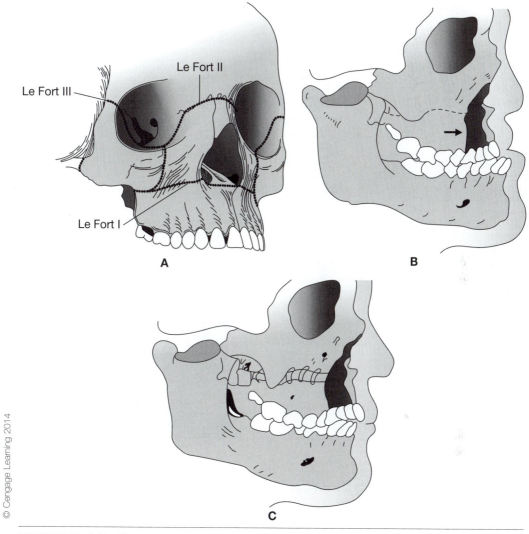

© Cengage Learning 2014

FIGURE 19–3 (A–C) Le Fort osteotomies. (A) This line drawing demonstrates the level of the various Le Fort osteotomies. The Le Fort II osteotomy includes the territory of the Le Fort I osteotomy as well. The Le Fort III osteotomy includes the territory of the Le Fort I and Le Fort II osteotomies as well. (B) Maxillary retrusion and the cuts for a Le Fort I. (C) The position of the maxilla after Le Fort I surgery.

deficiency. Figure 19–4C and D demonstrates the dramatic results of moving this segment of maxilla forward through a Le Fort I advancement. Figure 19–5A–G shows a dramatic improvement in both profile and dental occlusion as a result of a Le Fort I advancement.

If the surgeon needs to reposition the bridge of the nose as well as the teeth (which is commonly needed for patients with Treacher Collins), a Le Fort II osteotomy is done because it includes both the maxilla and the nasal pyramid. If the cheeks have to be

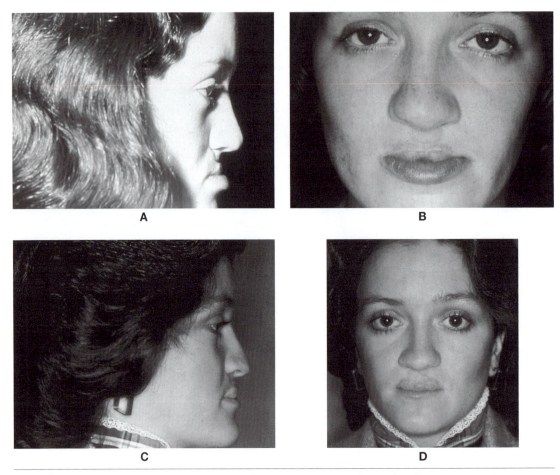

FIGURE 19–4 (A–D) Le Fort I. Figures A and B are preoperative photos that show a young girl with severe midface retrusion due to maxillary deficiency. Figures C and D are postoperative photos that show a remarkable change in profile and facial harmony after the Le Fort I procedure.

Courtesy David A. Billmire, M.D./Cincinnati Children's Hospital Medical Center & University of Cincinnati College of Medicine

brought forward to correct *proptosis* (protrusion of the eye), which is common in patients with Crouzon and Apert syndromes, a Le Fort III osteotomy is done because it includes the maxilla, nasal pyramid, zygomas, and orbital rims. Figure 19–6A and B shows preoperative proptosis, an open bite, and maxillary hypoplasia. Figure 19–6C and D shows the postoperative improvement after Le Fort III advancement was done in this patient. The ultimate goals of maxillary repositioning

include normal occlusion, normal-sized oral and pharyngeal cavities for resonance and breathing, and improved facial proportions.

Orthognathic surgery requires careful planning between the orthodontist and surgeon. The orthodontist and surgeon review the patient's *cephalogram* (also called *cephalometric radiograph*), which is a lateral radiograph of the craniofacial skeleton, in addition to photographs, and study models. They compare the patient's current maxillary placement against

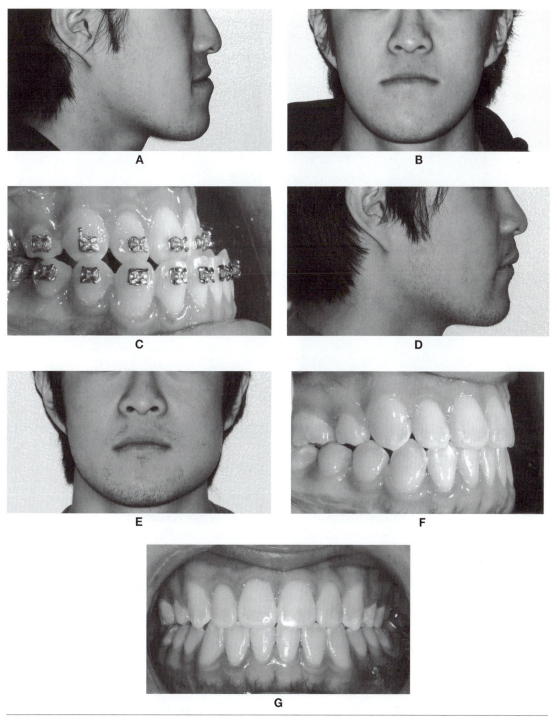

FIGURE 19–5 (A–G)   Le Fort I. Figures A through C show preoperative photos of a young man with maxillary retrusion and dental malocclusion. Figures D through G show dramatic improvement in profile, facial harmony, and dental occlusion as a result of a Le Fort I.

Courtesy Deepak Krishnan, D.D.S./University of Cincinnati College of Medicine

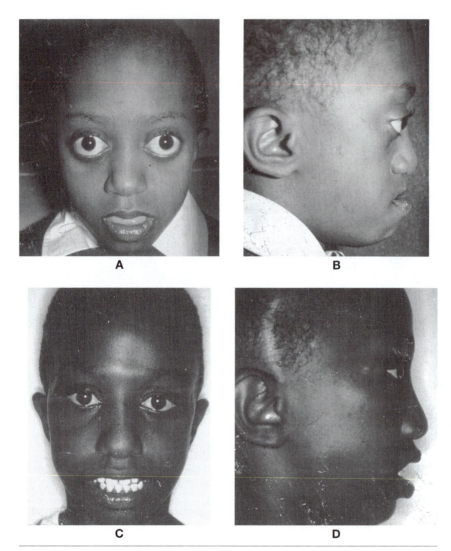

FIGURE 19–6 (A–D) Le Fort III. Figures A and B are preoperative photos of a boy with Crouzon's syndrome. Figures C and D are postoperative pictures after Le Fort III advancement. The changes in the orbits and the occlusion are dramatic.

Courtesy David A. Billmire, M.D./Cincinnati Children's Hospital Medical Center & University of Cincinnati College of Medicine

known normative values to determine how far and at what angle the maxilla must be moved to achieve the desired result. The orthodontist then places the teeth into position. Once the orthodontia is completed, the surgeon performs the procedure on plaster cast models. Guiding surgical stents are made from these models and are used in the operating room to replicate the proposed maxillary position intra-operatively.

During the surgical procedure, the osteotomies are made to release the bone. The surgeon then fixes the maxilla into the advanced position with metal plates and screws. If the advancement is greater than several millimeters, bone grafts are used to support the maxilla and prevent relapse back into its original position. Postoperatively, the jaws are held in occlusion with wire bands. Then, rubber band ligatures are used for 6 to 8 weeks while the maxilla heals in its new position. During this period, the patient is kept on pureed and soft diets. Afterward, final orthodontia is applied to fine-tune the teeth into the most ideal position.

Maxillary Distraction

Distraction osteogenesis is a method of gradually lengthening a bone by taking advantage of the fact that the body heals a fracture by laying down new bone. If the ends of a fracture are gradually separated, the body will create new bone to fill the gap. Distraction osteogenesis has been used relatively recently in orthognathic surgery (Cheung, & Chua, 2006; Cohen, Burstein, & Williams, 1999; Denny, Kalantarian, & Hanson, 2003; Imola & Tatum, 2002; McCarthy, Stelnicki, Mehrara, & Longaker, 2001; Mofid et al., 2001; Swennen, Schliephake, Dempf, Schierle, & Malevez, 2001; Zhou et al., 2007).

All distraction procedures are done by first producing a fracture—either a complete cut (osteotomy) or a partial cut (corticotomy). Distraction for maxillary advancement involves making a planned Le Fort osteotomy and then the placement of either an external or an internal distraction device. An external device anchors onto stable cranial bone and has a large frame that supports the device and its extensions into the maxilla. An internal device is smaller and is concealed within the mouth itself.

After several days of rest (the latent period), the distraction device is activated (the activation period). (The latency period is operator dependent, and the activation period is dependent on the planned new position of the maxilla.) The distraction device is activated to expand and stretch the immature callus over a period of time until the maxillary segment is moved into the desired position. This stretched callus is then allowed to mature and consolidate over time, to become normal bone. This eliminates the need for bone grafts to fill the large gaps (Takigawa, Uematsu, & Takada, 2010). This slow, deliberate advancement allows the body to lay down new bone growth, which solidly bolsters the maxilla in its new position. Figure 19–7A shows an intraoperative view of a patient who has had a maxillary osteotomy so that the maxillary device can be placed in position. Figure 19–7B demonstrates how an external maxillary distraction device attaches to the skull. Figure 19–7C shows an internal maxillary distractor in situ following maxillary osteotomy. Figure 19–8 shows a patient preoperatively, in the distraction device, and then postoperatively.

Advantages of distraction over traditional surgery include a shorter surgical procedure with less blood loss and less postoperative swelling. New bone is generated in the process of distraction, so there is no need to harvest donor bone for bone grafting. Because the advancement is gradual, it can be adjusted somewhat as needed, unlike the single opportunity in the operating room. The gradual nature of the bone repositioning allows soft tissue adaptation to occur over time, which often increases the amount of advancement that can be achieved. Finally, the living bone

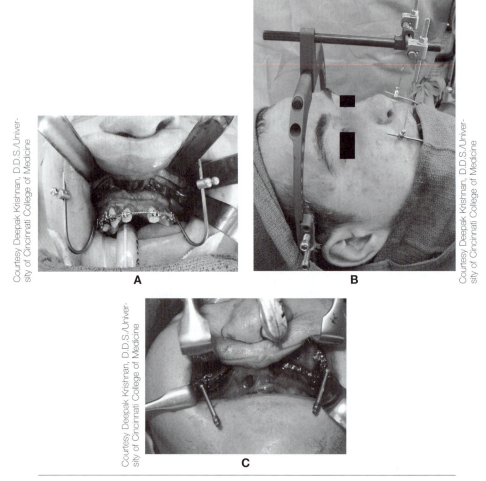

Courtesy Deepak Krishnan, D.D.S./University of Cincinnati College of Medicine

Courtesy Deepak Krishnan, D.D.S./University of Cincinnati College of Medicine

Courtesy Deepak Krishnan, D.D.S./University of Cincinnati College of Medicine

A

B

C

FIGURE 19–7 (A–C)   Maxillary distraction. (A) An intraoperative view of a patient who has had a maxillary osteotomy so that the maxillary device can be placed in position. (B) Shows how an external maxillary distraction device attaches to the skull. (C) An internal maxillary distractor in situ following maxillary osteotomy.

formation in the distraction path helps to prevent relapse.

Disadvantages of distraction include the obvious nature of the hardware and the cumbersome prolonged period of activation that involves the patient wearing the device as well as its daily activation. There may be pain, difficulty sleeping, speech distortion, eating problems, and disruption in the patient's recreational activities (Primrose et al., 2005). There is the potential for hardware to fail and require replacement during the distraction period. A majority of external devices can be removed in the office setting, but internally based hardware may require surgical removal in the operating room.

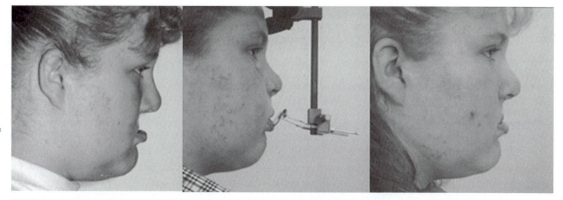

FIGURE 19–8 Distraction osteogenesis as applied to the midface. The left panel demonstrates the preoperative profile. The middle panel shows the patient at the end of distraction in her halo device. The right panel shows the postoperative results.

Timing

Orthognathic surgery of the maxilla cannot be performed until the maxillary sinus is well developed. This is due to the fact that the sinus area of the maxilla is the storehouse for the permanent dentition in young children. Once a child enters mixed dentition (usually between ages 7 and 9), suitable space exists to introduce the surgical saw.

Le Fort III advancement is commonly done during the mixed dentition stage for patients with craniosynostosis syndromes. This surgery helps to improve the airway; close the anterior open bite; increase the oral cavity size; and most importantly, protect the proptotic globes. Because of the shorter operations and lower blood loss as compared to traditional surgery, maxillary distraction as a method of midface advancement is well suited to the younger patient (Cheung & Chua, 2006). Any surgery done at this age will not hold up to future growth however. Therefore, the patient will likely need a Le Fort I advancement, or possibly a repeat Le Fort III advancement, in the teenage years to balance the occlusion, improve facial harmony, and create a convex profile.

Secondary orthognathic surgery for patients with craniosynostosis and primary orthognathic surgery for patients with cleft lip and palate are usually done after the maturity of the facial skeleton and complete eruption of the permanent dentition. Because the mandible is the last bone to mature in the facial skeleton, waiting until mandibular growth is complete assures that the new maxillary placement will be appropriate for the mature facial bones. Consequently, this type of surgery is not done until age 15–16 in girls and age 17–18 in boys. Presurgical orthodontia must be completed before maxillary advancement.

Potential Complications

Potential complications associated with maxillary advancement include major blood loss requiring massive transfusion, infection of the facial soft tissues, relapse of the maxilla, decreased sensation in the upper lip and midface, loss of teeth, loss of gingiva, persistent malocclusion (not correctable with

Speech Notes

Maxillary Advancement

Effect on Speech Sound Production

A primary purpose of maxillary advancement is to normalize the occlusal relationship between the maxillary and mandibular arches. Because malocclusion is a common cause of speech sound distortion, it stands to reason that the correction of the malocclusion could improve the clarity of speech. In fact, many studies have reported improved articulation following maxillary advancement, without intervening speech therapy (Guyette, Polley, Figueroa, & Smith, 2001; Janulewicz et al., 2004; Kummer et al., 1989; Lee, Whitehill, Ciocca, & Samman, 2002; Maegawa, Sells, & David, 1998; McCarthy, Coccaro, & Schwartz, 1979; Trindade, 2003; Vallino, 1990; Ward, McAuliffe, Holmes, Lynham, & Monsour, 2002). It should be noted that this improvement only occurs with *obligatory distortions*, where tongue position (articulation) was normal during production before the surgery, but the structure was abnormal, causing speech sound distortion. When there are *compensatory errors* resulting in abnormal tongue position, the maxillary advancement improves the potential for correction of these errors with speech therapy.

Effect on Airway and Resonance

Advancement of the maxilla, and thus the velum, increases the anterior–posterior dimension of the pharyngeal cavity. This can be beneficial for patients with craniosynostosis syndromes who often have restriction of the pharynx due to the stenotic suture lines between the facial bones and the cranial base. These patients often have hyponasality and upper airway obstruction that can be improved or eliminated with the increased diameter of the pharynx and the reduction of nasal airway resistance (Dalston, 1996; Maegawa et al., 1998; McCarthy et al., 1979; Sharshar & El-Bialy, 2012; Trindade, Yamashita, Suguimoto, Mazzottini, & Trindade, 2003).

Effect on Velopharyngeal Function

For patients with a repaired cleft palate or submucous cleft, maxillary advancement can have a negative effect on velopharyngeal function, even if done gradually through distraction. With the anterior movement of the maxilla and corresponding anterior movement of the velum, there is an increase in the anterior–posterior depth of the velopharyngeal port. If the velum is unable to stretch sufficiently to make up the difference, this will result in the development or worsening of velopharyngeal insufficiency (VPI) (Dalston, 1996; Dalston & Vig, 1984; Haapanen, Kalland, Heliovaara, Hukki, & Ranta, 1997; Heliovaara, Hukki, Ranta, & Haapanen, 2004; Heliovaara, Ranta, Hukki, & Haapanen, 2002; Janulewicz, et al., 2004; Kummer, Strife, Grau, Creaghead, & Lee, 1989; Maegawa et al., 1998; Niemeyer, Gomes Ade; Fukushiro, & Genaro, 2005; Okazaki et al., 1993; Satoh et al., 2004; Watzke, Turvey, Warren, & Dalston, 1990). It would seem that the gradual nature of maxillary advancement through distraction might allow for the velopharyngeal mechanism to adapt to its new situation and minimize post-advancement hypernasality. Studies have shown, however, that there is no significant difference in the risk for velopharyngeal insufficiency between surgical advancement and advancement through distraction (Chanchareonsook, Whitehill, & Samman, 2007; Chua, Whitehill, Samman, & Cheung, 2010; Guyette et al., 2001; Ko, Figueroa, Guyette, Polley, & Law, 1999; Trindade et al., 2003).

(Continues)

(Continued)

Postoperative velopharyngeal insufficiency is most likely to occur in patients with a history of cleft palate or submucous cleft, tenuous velopharyngeal closure initially, and a maxillary advancement that is 10 mm or greater. Some patients have a temporary period of hypernasality and/or nasal emission that corrects itself as the velopharyngeal structures accommodate to their new anatomic relationships. Other patients require either a pharyngeal flap or a sphincter pharyngoplasty to correct the nasality.

Some patients who have already had a pharyngeal flap for correction of VPI pose particular challenges with maxillary advancement. Nasal intubation for the procedure is challenging with the flap in situ. In addition, the tethering of the flap on the velum can make it more difficult to physically mobilize the maxilla forward. Finally, patients with a pharyngeal flap before maxillary advancement seem to have an increased incidence of relapse (retropositioning of the maxilla toward its original location) over time, which is presumably due to the pull of the flap. Therefore, in order to achieve enough maxillary advancement and reduce the risk of relapse, some flaps may require division to release it before the advancement procedure. Fortunately, if the flap has been in place for some time, division of the flap does not always cause deterioration in velopharyngeal function. This is probably due to the residual flap tissue and possibly changes in the inclination of the pharyngeal wall that would have occurred with growth. However, the patient may be at increased risk for a recurrence of VPI after the maxillary advancement surgery.

Before maxillary advancement surgery, it is important to counsel patients, particularly those with a history of cleft palate, regarding the risk of postoperative VPI and the treatment if VPI does occur. In patients with a history of cleft or VPI, a preoperative speech pathology assessment can be helpful in predicting the consequences of maxillary advancement on speech if desired by the patient and family (Phillips, Klaiman, Delorey, & MacDonald, 2005). For patients with no history of cleft who are undergoing elective surgery to improve facial harmony, a simple disclosure of the risk by the surgeon is sufficient.

orthodontia) due to relapse (Kramer et al., 2004), and very rarely blindness. There is also a risk of postoperative velopharyngeal insufficiency (VPI), particularly for those with a history of cleft palate or submucous cleft.

To correct the relapse of the maxilla, maxillary advancement must be performed again, including the presurgical orthodontia. Loss of gingiva can be improved by periodontal correction. Loss of teeth can be masked with bridgework or other prosthetic replacement. Changes in sensation may correct over time, or the patient is no longer bothered by reduced sensation. An additional surgery may be needed to correct postoperative VPI.

MANDIBULAR RECONSTRUCTION

Patients with craniofacial conditions often have micrognathia, requiring mandibular reconstruction. Mandibular reconstruction not only improves the facial aesthetics, but it can also alleviate airway obstruction, and even improve speech production.

Purpose

Micrognathia is associated Pierre Robin sequence, Treacher Collins syndrome (which often includes Pierre Robin sequence), and bilateral hemifacial microsomia (facioauriculo-vertebral syndrome). Patients with unilateral hemifacial microsomia typically present with an asymmetric mandible with hypoplastic or absent portions. On the other hand, patients with cleft lip and palate or craniosynostosis syndromes may appear to have *prognathism* (a condition where the mandible is bigger than the maxilla), even though the mandible is actually normal. This appearance is actually due to the maxillary retrusion and resultant discrepancies in the jaw positions. For individuals with true prognathism, mandibular reconstruction can be done for correction.

Micrognathia and/or a retrognathic mandible, as seen in infants with Pierre Robin sequence, can cause significant airway obstruction. The problems can range from desaturation during feeding and sleep apnea when supine to complete airway obstruction, regardless of position. A priority in the management of these infants is to provide an adequate airway for respiration and for feeding. Simple measures include prone positioning of the baby while sleeping and feeding. More complex methods include placement of a nasalpharyngeal airway (a so-called trumpet) and gavage feedings through an intermittently placed nasogastric tube. Severe cases usually require tracheostomy for airway management and gastrostomy for feeding.

Mandibular advancement is often done to avoid the need for tracheostomy in infants with significant airway obstruction due to micrognathia (Hammoudeh et al., 2012). When applied bilaterally, the distractors pull the mandible, including the base of the tongue, forward. This results in expansion of the pharyngeal space and an improvement in the airway. For those children who have already been treated with tracheostomy, mandibular advancement is often necessary before decannulation can be considered.

Techniques

There are several mandibular reconstruction techniques. The more common methods include mandibular distraction osteogenesis, rib graft reconstruction, free tissue microsurgical reconstruction (free-flap), and mandibular osteotomies, such as the vertical ramus or the sagittal ramus splits.

Mandibular Distraction

Since mandibular distraction osteogenesis was first described in 1992 (McCarthy, Schreiber, Karp, Thorne, & Grayson, 1992), many different approaches have been tried. Devices now have multiple planes, can be internal or external, and have been applied to all of the facial bones. Mandibular distraction can be applied bilaterally to patients with micrognathia or unilaterally for patients with hemifacial microsomia. It can be repeated if needed as the midface grows. Rib grafts used to reconstruct a mandible can also be distracted as if it were native mandible (Corcoran, Hubli, & Salyer, 1997). Mandibular distraction has allowed earlier decannulation of tracheostomized patients, often in the toddler period (Williams, Maull, Grayson, Longaker, & McCarthy, 1999).

To advance the mandible, surgical cuts are made bilaterally in the non-tooth-bearing area of the mandibular body, in the *ramus* or along its angle (Figure 19–9). After several days of rest (the latent period), the distraction device is activated (the activation period). The cut ends of the bone are separated gradually, usually 1 to 2 millimeters daily, until the desired length is achieved. Once the desired advancement is achieved, the device is left in place as a scaffold until the new bone has solidified (the consolidation period). The consolidation period is usually equal to or longer than the period of active distraction. The device is then removed.

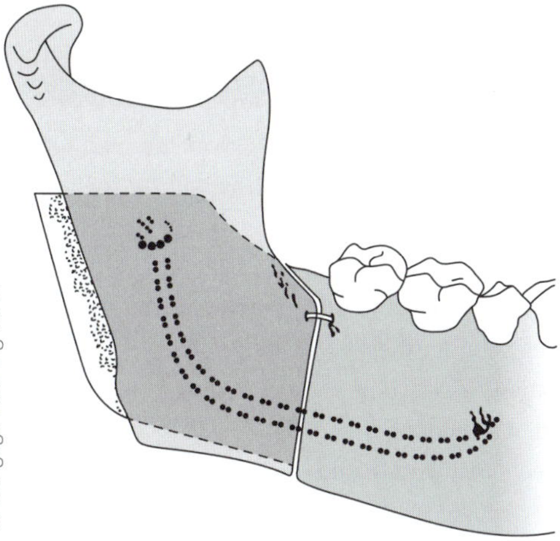

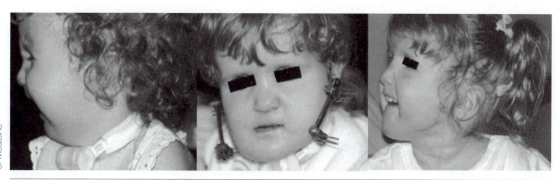

© Cengage Learning 2014

FIGURE 19–9 This line drawing demonstrates the anatomy of a sagittal split osteotomy and the versatility of either advancement, rotation, or set-back that can be obtained.

Variations on this procedure include whether the surgeon approaches the patient externally or intraorally; whether the device is external or internal; whether one or more osteotomies are used; whether the device can move the mandible in one, two, or three dimensions; and finally, whether subsequent fixation devices (often resorbable plates and screws) are used. Figure 19–10 shows a child who was tracheostomy dependent with micrognathia before, during, and after distraction.

In order to determine whether advancement has been sufficient to allow decannulation in a patient with a tracheostomy, the patient is examined just before the end of the active period of distraction. One method of airway evaluation is simply blocking the cannula temporarily with a valve to see whether the child is able to maintain the airway. In addition, lateral cephalograms can be done to demonstrate the increased dimensions of the nasopharyngeal cavity. Perhaps the best way to evaluate the airway, however, is through laryngoscopy and bronchoscopy. This is performed in the operating room by a pediatric otolaryngologist who can attend to the other issues, such as laryngomalacia, and those that result from chronic airway cannulation, including subglottic stenosis and granulation tissue.

Rib Graft Reconstruction

To recreate a hypoplastic or absent mandible, reconstructive surgeons take advantage of the natural structure of the rib, with its bony shaft and cartilaginous tip. The cartilage tip is used to mimic the condyle of the mandible, and the shaft of the rib is used to recreate the ramus and body. The graft is fixed to the mandible with plates and/or screws. The child must have

Courtesy David A. Billmire, M.D./ Cincinnati Children's Hospital Medical Center & University of Cincinnati College of Medicine

FIGURE 19–10 Distraction osteogenesis as applied to the mandible. In this case an external distractor was applied through an intraoral approach. The left panel demonstrates the degree of preoperative micrognathia. The middle panel shows the patient in her distractor. The right panel shows the amount of advancement obtained. Note that the patient has her tracheostomy successfully decannulated.

SPEECH NOTES

The presence of the tracheostomy circumvents subglottic airflow that is necessary for voicing and speech production. Therefore, the earlier decannulation can be done, the better the prognosis will be for speech development.

As noted above and also in Chapter 9, speech sound production is often negatively affected by jaw discrepancies that result in malocclusion. With severe micrognathia or mandibular retrusion, the tongue tip may rest under the palate rather than in its usual position, which is under the alveolar ridge. This can affect the ability to produce lingual-alveolar sounds and sibilants. The patient may compensate by backing these anterior sounds. In addition, bilabial phonemes may be produced with a labiodental placement.

Correcting dental occlusion can correct obligatory speech distortions and improve the potential for correction of compensatory errors.

Deterioration in velopharyngeal function and articulation has been reported immediately following mandibular distraction. This occurs presumably as a result of changes in mandibular height and relationships. However, this deterioration has been found to improve with time (Guyette, Polley, Figueroa, & Cohen, 1996).

---

adequate-sized ribs, which precludes doing this type of reconstruction before 5 or 6 years of age.

A unique problem with rib grafting is the inability to predict postoperative growth patterns. The graft can partially or completely resorb, leaving the patient without any advancement. Alternatively, it can remain the same size so that as the child's other facial bones grow, the asymmetry reproduces itself. Rarely, the rib graft can overgrow and create a secondary asymmetry requiring resection of a portion of the graft. Finally, soft tissue fullness and contour is not provided by this technique, so despite adding facial height and mandibular length, this procedure can leave the patient with an asymmetric appearance.

Free Tissue Transfer (Free-Flap)

The use of a free tissue transfer (free-flap) when reconstructing the mandible is one solution to the lack of soft tissue and the lack of bone growth that occurs with a rib graft. The surgeon can harvest bone only, or both bone and soft tissue with their blood vessels. The free flap is then transferred to the mandible. Donor blood vessels are hooked into the recipient blood vessels of the face, with the aid of the operating microscope. The scapula, with its overlying soft tissue, is often used because it provides a reliable growth center. If only soft tissue is necessary, many donor sites can be used, including the greater omentum from the abdomen.

Sagittal Split Osteotomy

Although many mandibular osteotomies have been designed, the most versatile is the sagittal split osteotomy because it allows advancement, setback, and rotation. The surgeon splits the ramus of the mandible between its inner and outer cortices, separating the condyle and outer cortex of the ramus from the body and the inner cortex. The pieces of the mandible are put into their new positions with the aid of splints, similar to those described for maxillary advancement. Proper interoperative positioning of the mandibular segments is essential to prevent temporomandibular joint problems. The surgeon then secures the segments with rigid fixation hardware. Depending on the stability of the mandibular movement, the patient may require *intermaxillary fixation*, which involves wiring the mandible against the maxilla to keep it closed. The horizontal advancement of the chin, called a *genioplasty*, can be done in conjunction with other mandibular or maxillary osteotomies, or it can be done alone. Although it does not change airway or speech considerations, it does greatly improve facial aesthetics.

Following mandibular advancement, the patient must comply with a physical therapy regiment to prevent stiffness of the temporomandibular joint. In addition, postoperative orthodontia or elastic band therapy may be required for final adjustment of the maxillary and mandibular occlusion.

Timing

Mandibular distraction is commonly done for infants and young children who have micrognathia that causes significant airway obstruction. Mandibular reconstruction is also done for teenagers and adults who have either micrognathia or prognathism for other reasons. Ideally, mandibular reconstruction is done in skeletally mature patients so as to avoid relapse from post-surgical growth.

Potential Complications

Complications with mandibular distraction can include infection of the skin surrounding the device and, on occasion, failure of the device (Corcoran et al., 1997). Unusual complications include facial nerve palsies and fibrous malunion. One complication of this procedure is the permanent damage it inflicts on tooth buds of mandibular molars, which may be immature and microscopic at the time of the distraction. These tooth buds can mature into malformed,

underdeveloped, or malpositioned teeth, which are often challenging to the pediatric dentist as the child ages. Fortunately, problems with relapse have not been reported, despite frequent application of this technique (McCarthy, Stelnicki, & Grayson, 1999).

Mandibular osteotomy is technically challenging and jeopardizes the inferior alveolar nerve during the split. Although almost all patients who undergo this procedure experience numbness in their lower lip, chin, and lower teeth, this is most often temporary, with the sensation returning to normal within a few months. Other potential complications include damage to teeth, malocclusion, and bad splits that necessitate more involved salvage techniques.

SUMMARY

Orthognathic surgery, which involves reconstruction of the maxilla and/or the mandible, can improve several aesthetic and functional problems that occur in patients with clefts or craniosynostosis syndromes. With manipulation of the facial bones, significant improvements can be made in the contours and overall appearance of the face.

Orthognathic surgery often affects speech and resonance. In general, improving the jaw relationships, and thus dental occlusion, has a positive effect on speech, particularly if there were speech distortions or articulation errors due to the abnormal structure. In addition, maxillary advancement can improve airway obstruction and hyponasality in some cases. However, there is a risk of postoperative VPI following maxillary advancement, particularly in patients with a history of cleft palate or submucous cleft. If desired, the speech-language pathologist can help to predict that risk and can also help with the management of VPI if it actually occurs postoperatively.

For Review and Discussion

1. What is orthognathic surgery? What is the goal of this type of surgery? Why do you think it is commonly done for patients with cleft lip and palate?

2. Discuss the reason for alveolar bone grafting, and describe how it is done as if you were explaining it to a parent. Discuss the controversy regarding timing. What are potential complications?

3. Explain the origin of the Le Fort classification system. What is the difference between Le Fort I, Le Fort II, and Le Fort III osteotomies? When is this type of surgery usually done and why?

4. Why do children with a history of cleft lip and palate often benefit from maxillary advancement? What are the potential effects of maxillary advancement on speech and resonance? What are the concerns of maxillary advancement when there is a preexisting pharyngeal flap? Discuss the appropriate timing of this surgery.

5. You have done a speech evaluation on a 17-year-old boy who is scheduled to undergo maxillary advancement. Speech is characterized by obligatory articulation errors due to occlusion and barely audible, inconsistent nasal emission. Describe the potential risks and benefits of this surgery as if you were explaining it to the boy and his family. What kind of follow-up should be done postoperatively?

6. Describe the process of distraction osteogenesis as if you were explaining it to a parent. At what age can this be done? What are the potential advantages of this technique? What are potential complications?

7. In what cases would mandibular advancement be appropriate? What are the potential benefits of this surgery?

8. What are the purposes the following: rib graft reconstruction, free tissue transfer, and mandibular osteotomy?

References

Chanchareonsook, N., Whitehill, T. L., & Samman, N. (2007). Speech outcome and velopharyngeal function in cleft palate: Comparison of Le Fort I maxillary osteotomy and distraction osteogenesis—Early results. *Cleft Palate–Craniofacial Journal*, 44(1), 23–32.

Cheung, L. K., & Chua, H. D. (2006). A meta-analysis of cleft maxillary osteotomy and distraction osteogenesis. *International Journal of Oral & Maxillofacial Surgery*, 35(1), 14–24.

Chua, H. D., Whitehill, T. L., Samman, N., & Cheung, L. K. (2010). Maxillary distraction versus orthognathic surgery in cleft lip and palate patients: Effects on speech and velopharyngeal function. *International Journal of Oral and Maxillofacial Surgery*, 39(7), 633–640.

Cohen, M., Polley, J. W., & Figueroa, A. A. (1993). Secondary (intermediate) alveolar bone grafting. *Clinics in Plastic Surgery*, 20(4), 691–705.

Cohen, S. R., Burstein, F. D., & Williams, J. K. (1999). The role of distraction osteogenesis in the management of craniofacial disorders. *Annals of the Academy of Medicine, Singapore*, 28(5), 728–738.

Corcoran, J., Hubli, E. H., & Salyer, K. E. (1997). Distraction osteogenesis of costochondral neomandibles: A clinical experience. *Plastic and Reconstructive Surgery, 100*(2), 311–315; Discussion 316–317.

Dado, D. V. (1993). Primary (early) alveolar bone grafting. *Clinics in Plastic Surgery, 20*(4), 683–689.

Dalston, R. M. (1996). Velopharyngeal impairment in the orthodontic population. *Seminars in Orthodontics, 2*(3), 220–227.

Dalston, R. M., & Vig, P. S. (1984). Effects of orthognathic surgery on speech: A prospective study. *American Journal of Orthodontics, 86*(4), 291–298.

Demetriades, N., Chang, D. J., Laskarides, C., & Papageorge, M. (2010). Effects of mandibular repositioning, with or without maxillary advancement, on the oro-naso-pharyngeal airway and development of sleep-related breathing disorders. *Journal of Oral and Maxillofacial Surgery, 68*(10), 2431–2436.

Denny, A. D., Kalantarian, B., & Hanson, P. R. (2003). Rotation advancement of the midface by distraction osteogenesis. *Plastic and Reconstructive Surgery, 111*(6), 1789–1799; Discussion 1800–1803.

El-Sayed, K. M., & Khalil, H. (2010). Transpalatal distraction osteogenesis prior to alveolar bone grafting in cleft lip and palate patients. *International Journal of Oral and Maxillofacial Surgery, 39*(8), 761–766.

Eppley, B. L., & Sadove, A. M. (2000). Management of alveolar cleft bone grafting—State of the art. *Cleft Palate–Craniofacial Journal, 37*(3), 229–233.

Guyette, T. W., Polley, J. W., Figueroa, A. A., & Cohen, M. N. (1996). Mandibular distraction osteogenesis: Effects on articulation and velopharyngeal function. *Journal of Craniofacial Surgery, 7*(3), 186–191.

Guyette, T. W., Polley, J. W., Figueroa, A., & Smith, B. E. (2001). Changes in speech following maxillary distraction osteogenesis. *Cleft Palate–Craniofacial Journal, 38*(3), 199–205.

Haapanen, M. L., Kalland, M., Heliovaara, A., Hukki, J., & Ranta, R. (1997). Velopharyngeal function in cleft patients undergoing maxillary advancement. *Folia Phoniatrica et Logopedica, 49*(1), 42–47.

Hammoudeh, J., Bindingnavele, V. K., Davis, B., Davidson Ward, S. L., Sanchez-Lara, P. A., Kleiber, G., Nazarian Mobian, S. S., et al. (2012). Neonatal and infant mandibular distraction as an alternative to tracheostomy in severe obstructive sleep apnea. *Cleft Palate–Craniofacial Journal, 49*(1), 32–38.

Heliovaara, A., Hukki, J., Ranta, R., & Haapanen, M. L. (2004). Cephalometric pharyngeal changes after Le Fort I osteotomy in different types of clefts. *Scandinavian Journal of Plastic and Reconstructive Surgery and Hand Surgery, 38*(1), 5–10.

Heliovaara, A., Ranta, R., Hukki, J., & Haapanen, M. L. (2002). Cephalometric pharyngeal changes after Le Fort I osteotomy in patients with unilateral cleft lip and palate. *Acta Odontologica Scandinavica, 60*(3), 141–145.

Imola, M. J., & Tatum, S. A. (2002). Craniofacial distraction osteogenesis. *Facial Plastic Surgery Clinics of North America, 10*(3), 287–301.

Janulewicz, J., Costello, B. J., Buckley, M. J., Ford, M. D., Close, J., & Gassner, R. (2004). The effects of Le Fort I osteotomies on velopharyngeal and speech functions in cleft patients. *Journal of Oral & Maxillofacial Surgery, 62*(3), 308–314.

Ko, E. W., Figueroa, A. A., Guyette, T. W., Polley, J. W., & Law, W. R. (1999). Velopharyngeal changes after maxillary advancement in cleft patients with distraction osteogenesis using a rigid external distraction device: A 1-year cephalometric follow-up. *Journal of Craniofacial Surgery, 10*(4), 312–320; Discussion 321–312.

Kramer, F., Baethge, C., Swennen, G., Teltzrow, T., Schulze, A., Berten, J., & Brachvogel, P. (2004). Intra- and perioperative complications of the LeFort 1 osteotomy: A prospective evaluation of 1000 patients. *Journal of Craniofacial Surgery, 15*(6), 971–977.

Kummer, A. W., Strife, J. L., Grau, W. H., Creaghead, N. A., & Lee, L. (1989). The effects of Le Fort I osteotomy with maxillary movement on articulation, resonance, and velopharyngeal function. *Cleft Palate Journal, 26*(3), 193–199.

Lee, A. S., Whitehill, T. L., Ciocca, V., & Samman, N. (2002). Acoustic and perceptual analysis of the sibilant sound /s/ before and after orthognathic surgery. *Journal of Oral & Maxillofacial Surgery, 60*(4), 364–372; Discussion 372–363.

Le Fort, R. (1901). Étude experimental sur les fractures de la machoire superieure. Parts I, II, III. *Revue de Chirurgie de Paris, 23,* 201, 360, 479.

Maegawa, J., Sells, R. K., & David, D. J. (1998). Speech changes after maxillary advancement in 40 cleft lip and palate patients. *Journal of Craniofacial Surgery, 9*(2), 177–182; Discussion 183–184.

McCarthy, J. G., Coccaro, P. J., & Schwartz, M. D. (1979). Velopharyngeal function following maxillary advancement. *Plastic and Reconstructive Surgery, 64*(2), 180–189.

McCarthy, J. G., Schreiber, J., Karp, N., Thorne, C. H., & Grayson, B. H. (1992). Lengthening the human mandible by gradual distraction. *Plastic and Reconstructive Surgery, 89*(1), 1–8; Discussion 9–10.

McCarthy, J. G., Stelnicki, E. J., & Grayson, B. H. (1999). Distraction osteogenesis of the mandible: A ten-year experience. *Seminars in Orthodontics, 5*(1), 3–8.

McCarthy, J. G., Stelnicki, E. J., Mehrara, B. J., & Longaker, M. T. (2001). Distraction osteogenesis of the craniofacial skeleton. *Plastic and Reconstructive Surgery, 107*(7), 1812–1827.

Mofid, M. M., Manson, P. N., Robertson, B. C., Tufaro, A. P., Elias, J. J., & Vander Kolk, C. A. (2001). Craniofacial distraction osteogenesis: A review of 3,278 cases. *Plastic and Reconstructive Surgery, 108*(5), 1103–1114; Discussion 1115–1117.

Niemeyer, T. C., Gomes Ade, O., Fukushiro, A. P., & Genaro, K. F. (2005). Speech resonance in orthognathic surgery in subjects with cleft lip and palate. *Journal of Applied Oral Science, 13*(3), 232–236.

Okazaki, K., Satoh, K., Kato, M., Iwanami, M., Ohokubo, F., & Kobayashi, K. (1993). Speech and velopharyngeal function following maxillary advancement in patients with cleft lip and palate. *Annals of Plastic Surgery, 30*(4), 304–311.

Phillips, J. H., Klaiman, P., Delorey, R., & MacDonald, D. B. (2005). Predictors of velopharyngeal insufficiency in cleft palate orthognathic surgery. *Plastic and Reconstructive Surgery, 115*(3), 681–686.

Primrose, A. C., Broadfoot, E., Diner, P. A., Molina, F., Moos, K. F., & Ayoub, A. F. (2005). Patients' responses to distraction osteogenesis: A multicentre study. *International Journal of Oral & Maxillofacial Surgery, 34*(3), 238–242.

Santiago, P. E., Grayson, B. H., Cutting, C. B., Gianoutsos, M. P., Brecht, L. E., & Kwon, S. M. (1998). Reduced need for alveolar bone grafting by presurgical orthopedics and primary gingivoperiosteoplasty. *Cleft Palate–Craniofacial Journal, 35*(1), 77–80.

Satoh, K., Nagata, J., Shomura, K., Wada, T., Tachimura, T., Fukuda, J., & Shiba, R. (2004). Morphological evaluation of changes in velopharyngeal function following maxillary distraction in patients with repaired cleft palate during mixed dentition. *Cleft Palate–Craniofacial Journal, 41*(4), 355–363.

Sharshar, H. H., & El-Bialy, T. H. (2012). Cephalometric evaluation of airways after maxillary anterior advancement by distraction osteogenesis in cleft lip and palate patients: A systematic review. *Cleft Palate–Craniofacial Journal, 49*(3), 255–261.

Swennen, G., Schliephake, H., Dempf, R., Schierle, H., & Malevez, C. (2001). Craniofacial distraction osteogenesis: A review of the literature: Part 1: Clinical studies. *International Journal of Oral & Maxillofacial Surgery, 30*(2), 89–103.

Takigawa, Y., Uematsu, S., & Takada, K. (2010). Maxillary advancement using distraction osteogenesis with intraoral device. *The Angle Orthodontist, 80*(6), 1165–1175.

Trindade-Suedam, I. K., da Silva Filho, O. G., Carvalho, R. M., de Souza Faco, R. A., Calvo, A. M., Ozawa, T. O., Trindade, Jr., A. S., et al. (2012). Timing of alveolar bone grafting determines different outcomes in patients with unilateral cleft palate. *Journal of Craniofacial Surgery, 23*(5), 1283–1286.

Trindade, I. E., Yamashita, R. P., Suguimoto, R. M., Mazzottini, R., & Trindade, A. S., Jr. (2003). Effects of orthognathic surgery on speech and breathing of subjects with cleft lip and palate: Acoustic and aerodynamic assessment. *Cleft Palate–Craniofacial Journal, 40*(1), 54–64.

Vallino, L. D. (1990). Speech, velopharyngeal function, and hearing before and after orthognathic surgery. *Journal of Oral and Maxillofacial Surgery, 48*(12), 1274–1281; Discussion 1281–1282.

van Aalst, J. A., Eppley, B. L., Hathaway, R. R., & Sadove, A. M. (2005). Surgical technique for primary alveolar bone grafting. *Journal of Craniofacial Surgery, 16*(4), 706–711.

Waite, P. D., & Waite, D. E. (1996). Bone grafting for the alveolar cleft defect. *Seminars in Orthodontics, 2*(3), 192–196.

Walia, A. (2011). Secondary alveolar bone grafting in cleft of the lip and palate patients. *Contemporary Clinical Dentistry, 2*(3), 146–154.

Ward, E. C., McAuliffe, M., Holmes, S. K., Lynham, A., & Monsour, F. (2002). Impact of malocclusion and orthognathic reconstruction surgery on resonance and articulatory function: An examination of variability in five cases. *British Journal of Oral & Maxillofacial Surgery, 40*(5), 410–417.

Watzke, L., Turvey, T. A., Warren, D. W., & Dalston, R. (1990). Alterations in velopharyngeal function after maxillary advancement in cleft palate patients. *Journal of Oral and Maxillofacial Surgery, 48*(7), 685–689.

Williams, J. K., Maull, D., Grayson, B. H., Longaker, M. T., & McCarthy, J. G. (1999). Early decannulation with bilateral mandibular distraction for tracheostomy-dependent patients. *Plastic and Reconstructive Surgery, 103*(1), 48–57; Discussion 58–59.

Zhou, L., Wang, X., Yi, B., Ma, L., Ni, D. F., & Jin, Z. Y. (2007). [Upper airway morphologic changes in obstructive sleep apnea hypopnea syndrome patients before and after orthognathic surgery and distraction osteogenesis.] *Zhonghua Kou Qiang Yi Xue Za Zhi, 42*(4), 195–198.

C H A P T E R

20

Prosthetic Management

INTRODUCTION

Individuals with a history of cleft lip, cleft palate, or other craniofacial anomalies often have anatomical problems that affect facial aesthetics, dental arch stability, speech, mastication, and swallowing. These physical and functional problems can also affect the social, emotional, and psychological well-being of the patient in a very negative way.

Historically, patients with cleft lip and palate underwent multiple surgical and habilitative procedures in order to achieve an acceptable aesthetic and functional outcome. Surgical repairs were done later in life than they are today, and the success of the surgical procedures was not as high as it is currently. Despite the best efforts of the surgeon, the patient often had remaining dental and maxillary arch deficiencies and also speech problems due to occlusal anomalies and velopharyngeal insufficiency. Because of these residual problems, prosthetic management was often the most effective form of treatment and therefore was commonly used. In recent years, however, there has been an increase in the understanding of the nature of craniofacial growth and development. In addition, advancements and improvements in surgical techniques have resulted in greatly improved aesthetic and speech outcomes. Therefore, prosthetic devices are no longer needed to achieve optimum results in most patients with a history of cleft lip and palate, particularly those who received early and appropriate surgical intervention (Delgado, Schaaf, & Emrich, 1992; Reisberg, 2000).

Although surgery is usually the option of choice for correction or improvement of many of these structural and functional problems, there still is a need for prosthetic treatment in certain cases. Prosthetic treatment is an excellent option for patients where surgery is not desired or not possible for a variety of reasons.

The overall goal of management, whether it is through surgical or prosthetic treatment, is to obtain the optimum results. Therefore, in choosing a treatment option, it's important to consider not only the preferences of the patient and the expected outcome but also the total amount of time necessary to achieve results, the risks to the patient, and the cost of treatment. A successful treatment option is one that meets the particular needs and expectations of the patient and the family with the least amount of time and the lowest cost.

The purpose of this chapter is to discuss the various types of prosthetic devices available for individuals with a history of cleft lip/palate or other craniofacial conditions. Speech-language pathologists should be well informed about the options for prosthetic management and when it is appropriate for the patient.

PROSTHETIC DEVICES

A *prosthesis*, also called a prosthetic device or appliance, is a fabricated substitute for a body part that is missing or malformed. This substitute may be fixed so that it is essentially permanent, or it can be removable so that the patient can take it out for eating, sleeping, and cleaning. Prosthetic management can be done on a temporary basis before surgical correction or on a permanent basis if surgical correction is not possible or desired by the patient.

Construction of a prosthetic device may be done by an orthodontist or pediatric dentist. However, this work is most often done by a prosthodontist who specializes in the construction of these devices. A *prosthodontist* is a dental professional who deals not only with the restoration of teeth but also with the fabrication of appliances to improve the appearance of missing or malformed oral and facial structures. These devices improve the aesthetics and also assist the patient with certain functions, such as feeding and velopharyngeal closure. The prosthodontist is a very important member of a craniofacial team because he or she can often further improve the speech and appearance of individuals with significant anomalies following the best surgical attempts at correction.

Dental Appliances

Patients who had a cleft of the entire primary palate often have missing teeth, particularly in the line of the cleft. Patient with other craniofacial anomalies are also at risk for missing and malformed teeth, in addition to malocclusion. In these cases, prosthetic management can improve facial aesthetics, mastication, and even speech by the replacement of missing teeth or correction of malocclusion.

There are significant challenges when attempting to replace teeth for individuals with a history of cleft of the primary palate. These challenges may include a shortened upper lip, decreased upper lip mobility due to scarring, protrusion of the premaxilla, spaces created by missing teeth, and supernumerary teeth. Additional problems include jaw discrepancies, an occlusal cant, distortion of the midline of the dentition and face, or scar tissue in the alveolar and palatal areas (Ramstad, 1998). Added to these challenges may be poor dental hygiene, which is common in this population because of neglect as a result of psychological factors.

Replacement of teeth can be done in several ways. A *fixed bridge* is typically used to replace dental segments, and complete *dentures* are used when all of the teeth in an arch must be replaced. If some of the teeth are to be retained but are not functional, overlay dentures are often used. *Overlay dentures* fit over the existing teeth and usually provide more vertical dimension, which improves both function and appearance for individuals who have over closure of the vertical dimension and thus a deep bite. These dental appliances can be combined with any type of speech appliance, if needed. The long-term use of this type of denture can place the underlying teeth at risk for decay and periodontal disease, however.

Although misaligned teeth can make the fabrication of dentures a challenge, tooth extractions are typically avoided unless required for orthodontic purposes. Even a misaligned tooth may serve a purpose in the future, such as providing an anchor for a prosthetic device. Tooth extraction in the cleft area of the dental arch should be especially avoided because it usually results in resorption of the alveolar bone, which widens and deepens the cleft. This tissue and bone loss may exceed that which can be replaced by a fixed partial prosthesis. Therefore, correction would result in a more complex reconstruction than if the tooth is preserved (McKinstry, 1998a).

Facial Prostheses

Individuals with craniofacial anomalies can demonstrate significant facial defects that affect the person's overall appearance to such a degree that their quality of life is greatly impacted. Although surgical intervention often leads to significant improvement, this is not always the case. Acquired facial defects caused by injury or ablative surgery for cancer can be even more challenging, if not impossible, to improve with surgery. Fortunately, prosthetic rehabilitation can make a major difference in the affected person's life, allowing the individual to function normally in society.

Whenever there is a severe facial defect, particularly one that cannot be significantly improved with surgery, a facial prosthesis is a very good option. Even glossectomy patients can benefit from a specially designed prosthesis for the tongue (Mueller et al., 2011).

Figure 20–1 shows the type of person who can benefit from a facial prosthesis. A facial prosthesis can be used to replace missing or disfigured parts of the facial anatomy, resulting in a dramatic improvement in appearance (Grisius, 1991; Lundgren, Moy, Beumer, & Lewis, 1993; Schaaf, 1984). For example, individuals with an aural atresia can benefit from the fabrication of a prosthetic ear. Although the ear will not be functional, it appears very much like a real ear, and thus the anomaly is not noted by others. The same can be done for the eyes or nose and even for the cheek (Singh, Bharadwaj, & Nair, 1997).

A skilled prosthodontist is able to match skin color, tone, and texture so that the prosthesis blends in with the natural tissue. The prosthodontist is also able to shape structures in a way that makes them very realistic in appearance. In addition to using the conventional manual sculpturing techniques, some prosthodontists use optical 3-D imaging and computer-aided design and manufacturing systems to fabricate facial prostheses more precisely (Ahmed, Farshad, & Yazdanie, 2011; Feng et al., 2010; Mueller et al., 2011).

Retention of the prosthesis is often accomplished through the use of *osseointegrated implants* (implants that are drilled in the bone) (Beumer, Roumanas, & Nishimura, 1995; dos Santos et al., 2010; Goiato, dos Santos, Haddad, & Moreno, 2012; Parel, Holt, Branemark, & Tjellstrom, 1986). With the implants in place, the prosthesis can be secured through the use of mechanical clips, magnetic bars, or implants (Chang, Garrett, Roumanas, & Beumer, 2005). Because of what is involved to secure the device, facial prostheses work best for adults who are responsible and motivated. They do not work as well for young children who may be less motivated and are less responsible. In addition, periodic modifications and replacement are necessary for children as they grow.

Feeding Obturators

A *feeding obturator* is a prosthetic appliance that can be used in the first few months of life to assist the infant with cleft palate in feeding (Figure 20–2) (see also Figures 5–8A and B) (Nagda, Deshpande, & Mhatre, 1996; Osuji, 1995; Savion & Huband, 2005; Sultana, Rahman, Nessa, & Alam, 2011). The obturator covers a portion of the infant's unrepaired cleft palate. As such, it keeps the tongue from resting inside the cleft, and it provides a solid surface so that the tongue can achieve compression of the nipple in order to express the milk. It also helps to eliminate the

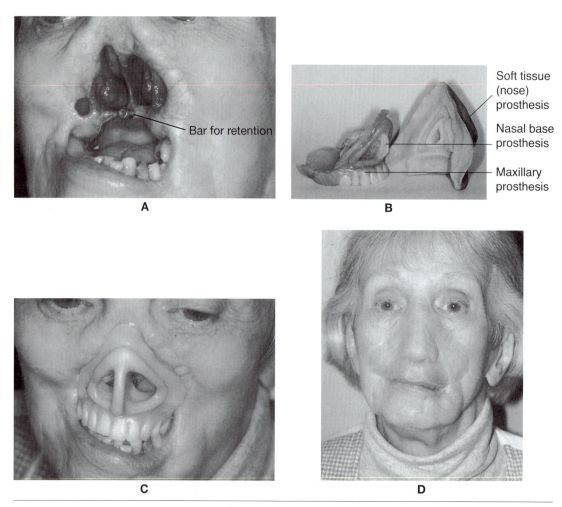

FIGURE 20–1 (A–D) (A) Patient with a history of squamous cell carcinoma. This patient underwent a midface resection that included the anterior maxilla, the upper lip, and the nose. A gold bar spans across the defect and is secured and stabilized by dental implants. When in place, the prosthesis attaches to this bar through the use of two retentive pins. (B) Prosthesis that includes a maxillary obturator and a nasal extension. On the nasal portion, there is a retentive ridge where the silicon prosthesis (nose, cheek, and lip) snaps on for retention. (C) Maxillary and nasal prosthesis in place. The soft tissue nose prosthesis attaches to this base. (D) Both the maxillary and soft tissue prostheses in position. When the patient wears her glasses, this helps to further disguise the facial prosthesis.

Courtesy Gordon Huntress, D.D.S./Cincinnati Children's Hospital Medical Center & University of Cincinnati College of Medicine

regurgitation of liquids into the nose. The appliance occludes the hard palate, but does not obturate the soft palate, however. Therefore, it does not help the infant to achieve suction, which would require complete velopharyngeal closure (McKinstry, 1998b).

The feeding obturator is made of light-cured resins or acrylic and is fabricated using plaster molds (Sultana et al., 2011). It is made so that it fits tightly against the roof of the mouth during feeding. Because the infant does not have teeth to anchor the appliance in place, suction against

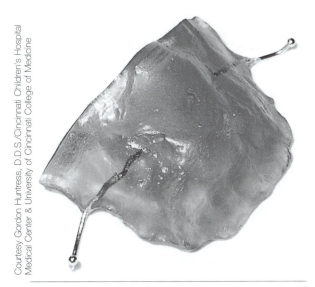

FIGURE 20–2 A feeding obturator.

the palate and a tight fit are particularly important. One or two holes are drilled in the appliance, and dental floss is then tied to the appliance through the holes. These "strings" are attached to the appliance to make it easy for the caregiver to remove it following the feeding.

Although feeding obturators are still used in some centers, most craniofacial centers now feel that they are unnecessary. In fact, there are some obvious disadvantages of using feeding obturators, including the expense and the effort needed to train parents in their use. Fortunately, with only simple modifications most infants with cleft palate can feed adequately and gain weight appropriately (see Chapter 5). Perhaps obturators are more useful for infants with multiple structural anomalies of the airway or certain types of neurological dysfunction (Sidoti & Shprintzen, 1995).

SPEECH APPLIANCES

When surgical correction of velopharyngeal insufficiency/incompetence (VPI) or a symp-

tomatic fistula is not an option, prosthetic management is a good alternative (Gallagher, 1982; Gardner & Parr, 1996). Typically, an interdisciplinary team does an assessment to determine whether the patient is a good candidate for an appliance. The role of the speech-language pathologist is to identify the aspects of speech that may be impacted by the appliance and determine the potential benefit on speech intelligibility. The speech-language pathologist also actively participates in the designing of the appliance to achieve the best speech outcomes. In a position statement of the American Speech-Language-Hearing Association, it was stated that "[P] articipation in the evaluation and treatment of individuals being considered for oral and oropharyngeal prostheses to facilitate speech and swallowing is within the scope of practice of the certified speech-language pathologist" (American Speech-Language-Hearing Association [ASHA], 1993). The knowledge and skills necessary for the speech-language pathologist to assist in the design of a speech prosthesis are outlined in this position statement.

Three types of speech appliances can be used to assist with speech production: a palatal obturator, a palatal lift, and a speech bulb obturator. The palatal obturator is used to close defects of the hard palate or velum; the palatal lift is used for velopharyngeal incompetence; and the speech bulb obturator is used for velopharyngeal insufficiency. Each of these speech appliances is described separately in the following sections.

Palatal Lift

A *palatal lift* prosthesis is a removable device that elevates a passive velum and holds it in place against the posterior pharyngeal wall for speech (Figure 20–3A and B). Because a

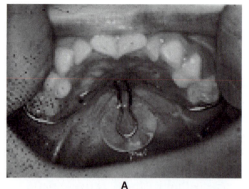

A

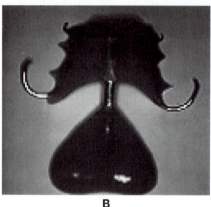

B

FIGURE 20–3 (A and B) A palatal lift. (A) This lift is in the early stages of development. It will gradually be lengthened as the patient learns to tolerate the device. (B) This device is long enough to be positioned so that it elevates the velum at the point of its natural bend.

thickness, and even good lateral pharyngeal wall movement.

The palatal lift device consists of an anterior base that is retained and stabilized by the teeth, and a fingerlike *tailpiece* that extends to the velum. When treatment is first initiated, the tailpiece may reach to the anterior portion of the velum only (Figure 20–3A). As the patient learns to tolerate the device, this extension is gradually lengthened until it reaches the area of the velar dimple at the very least (Figure 20–3B). The extension exerts an upward force against the velum to displace it in a superior and posterior direction. It is important that this tailpiece is positioned correctly so that it can push the velum against the posterior pharyngeal wall in the area of maximum lateral pharyngeal wall movement. With the palatal lift in place, the velum is held against the posterior pharyngeal wall at all times. Because this is the appropriate position for speech, additional velar movement during speech is unnecessary. If the patient has little lateral wall movement, the lift can be widened to further close the lateral borders of the port.

This type of prosthesis works best if the velum is very flaccid so that there is no resistance to the lift. In addition, natural elevation of the velum can cause the prosthesis to become dislodged (Reisberg, 2000). Individuals who have a hyperactive gag reflex or those who are hypersensitive to touch in the area of the soft palate may require desensitization in the area before a palatal lift can be effective. Gentle massage of the soft palate with the index finger can help to increase the person's tolerance for touch in this area. The finger should massage the velum from side to side and then gradually move posteriorly (Daniel, 1982).

palatal lift does not add to length to the velum or fill in a gap, it is not useful for a short velum (velopharyngeal insufficiency). Instead, a palatal lift is indicated in cases of velopharyngeal incompetence, where the velum is of normal length but has inadequate and/or inconsistent velar elevation for closure of the valve. Ideally, there should be adequate velar length and

SPEECH NOTES

A palatal lift can be very effective in the treatment of individuals with velopharyngeal incompetence, which is a neurological impairment that impairs the movement, timing, and coordination of velopharyngeal structures. Velopharyngeal incompetence can be due to a variety of neurophysiological causes (e.g., cerebral palsy, neuromuscular disorders, brain tumors, strokes, traumatic brain injury, etc.), and it accounts for most acquired conditions causing velopharyngeal dysfunction and hypernasality. Velopharyngeal incompetence typically causes moderate to severe hypernasality. In addition to hypernasality, neurophysiological conditions usually cause other speech symptoms that together are characteristic of dysarthria.

Dysarthria is a motor speech disorder that affects all the subsystems of speech, including respiration, phonation, articulation, and velopharyngeal function. There is usually weakness or poor movement of the speech articulators (tongue, lips, jaw and velopharyngeal valve). Typical speech characteristics include slurred, imprecise articulation; slow rate and abnormal prosody; low volume and breathiness; short utterance length; and hypernasality. A palatal lift can be useful for dysarthric patients when hypernasality is the primary contributor to the unintelligibility of speech and when articulation, phonation, and respiration are not severely compromised (Bedwinek & O'Brien, 1985; Esposito, Mitsumoto, & Shanks, 2000; Koidis & Topouzelis, 2003; Shifman, Finkelstein, Nachmani, & Ophir, 2000). A palatal lift can reduce or eliminate hypernasality and can also improve breath support by closing the leak of air through the nose. It can even improve volume by directing sound into the mouth so that it is not absorbed by tissues of the pharynx and even nasal cavity. A palatal lift may even be considered for individuals with severe apraxia that affects velopharyngeal coordination (Hall, Hardy, & LaVelle, 1990).

One disadvantage of a palatal lift is that because the velum is held against the posterior pharyngeal wall at all times, it can potentially interfere with the production of nasal sounds and nasal breathing, particularly if the lift is wide. Nasal breathing can usually be accomplished through openings on either side of the velum, because usually only the middle portion of the velopharyngeal port remains closed. However, hyponasality is often a necessary side effect of forced velopharyngeal closure for adequate oral speech. Fortunately, the palatal lift can be removed during sleep, so obstructive sleep apnea is not a concern.

Palatal Obturator

A *palatal obturator* is a removable prosthetic device that is used to cover an open palatal defect that is symptomatic during speech or is causing nasal regurgitation during feeding (Walter, 2005). The most common use of palatal obturators is to occlude a palatal (oronasal) fistula (Figure 20–4). Although palatal fistulas do not occur as frequently as in the past, they are still a problem for some patients. When a fistula is present, the surgical closure is

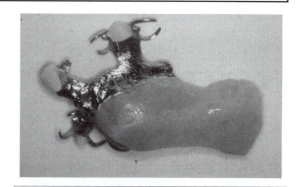

FIGURE 20–4 A palatal obturator. This is designed to fit tightly in the palatal defect. Note the addition of teeth.
Courtesy Gordon Huntress, D.D.S./Cincinnati Children's Hospital Medical Center & University of Cincinnati College of Medicine

often delayed so that it can be done as part of another surgery. With either a delay in surgical correction or a decision not to surgically correct the fistula, obturation can be considered for temporary or permanent correction (Pinborough-Zimmerman, Canady, Yamashiro, & Morales, 1998).

At one time, obturators were used to temporarily occlude hard palate clefts, which were not repaired until facial growth was complete (around age 14 for girls and age 18 for boys). This practice was done by a few treatment centers that subscribed to the theory that early cleft palate closure contributed to a reduction in midfacial growth, causing the high incidence of maxillary deficiency in this population (Schweckendiek, 1966, 1968). To counter this effect, these centers opted to close only the velum at an early age and leave the hard palate open until the teenage years. More recent research has suggested that it is not the early repair that affects maxillary growth, but rather the inherent deficiency in the maxilla. As a result, surgical correction of the hard palate and velum are now done at the same time—usually at around 10 months of age.

A palatal obturator consists of an acrylic body that looks similar to a dental retainer. However, it has additional acrylic on the top of the appliance, which fits tightly into the area of deficiency. This prevents a leak of air pressure or fluid into the nasal cavity. If the obturator has to be large in order to fill in the defect, it can be hollowed out so that its weight does not cause a problem with retention (Blair & Hunter, 1998).

Speech Bulb Obturator

A *speech bulb obturator* (also known as a *speech aid appliance*) is a removable device that is used for the treatment of velopharyngeal insufficiency (Rieger et al., 2009; Tuna, Pekkan, Gumus, & Aktas, 2010). It has even been used for velopharyngeal incompetence (Dutka, Uemeoka, Aferri, Pegoraro-Krook, & Marino, 2011; Shifman et al., 2000; Sun, Li, & Sun, 2002). When the velum is short relative to the depth of the posterior pharyngeal wall, the bulb serves to fill in the velopharyngeal space. Figure 20–5A shows a typical speech bulb obturator. Figure 20–5B shows an obturator in place. Figure 20–5C shows a patient with a very short velum. His speech bulb is in place in Figure 20–5D. The bulb sits high in the nasopharynx to occlude the velopharyngeal port for speech, as can be seen through the X-ray tracing in Figure 20–5E.

As with other types of appliances, a speech bulb obturator can be combined with partial or

SPEECH NOTES

A palatal obturator appliance functions by filling an oronasal opening in order to close off the nasal cavity from the oral cavity. This allows the patient to be able to impound intraoral pressure for the production of speech sounds. When appropriate and implemented at an early age, an obturator can help the child to develop normal articulation placement instead of compensatory productions (Dorf, Reisberg, & Gold, 1985; Raju, Padmanabhan, & Narayan, 2009). This is particularly true if the child receives focused speech stimulation or speech therapy at the same time (Lohmander-Agerskov, Soderpalm, Friede, & Lilja, 1990). If the palatal opening is very large, an obturator can also reduce or eliminate hypernasality.

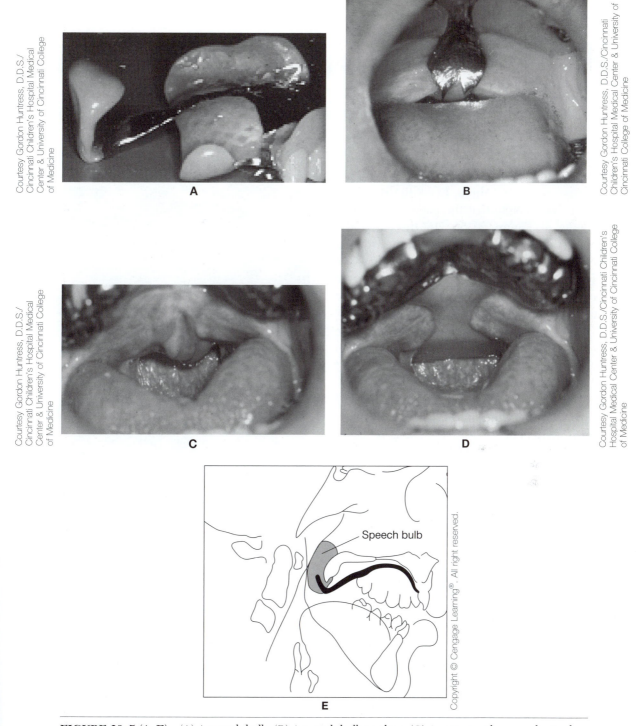

FIGURE 20–5 (A–E)   (A) A speech bulb. (B) A speech bulb in place. (C) A patient with a very short velum and dental implants. (D) A speech bulb obturator in place in the patient seen in Figure 20–5C. Note the dental overlays. (E) The placement of the speech bulb in the pharynx, as can be seen through this X-ray tracing.

SPEECH NOTES

A speech bulb obturator fills a nasopharyngeal gap in order to close off the nasal cavity from the oral cavity for speech. As with a palatal obturator, this allows the patient to be able to impound intraoral pressure for the production of speech sounds. It can also reduce or eliminate hypernasality.

complete dentures (Abreu, Levy, Rodriguez, & Rivera, 2007). Note that the patient has dental implants in Figure 20–5C. In this case, the speech bulb was made with anterior dental overlays, as can be seen in Figure 20–5D. Figure 20–5E is drawing of a lateral view to show the position of the speech bulb in the pharynx.

Although obturators and speech bulbs are used infrequently with children, they are an important method of treatment for adult patients who have who have undergone ablative surgery or radiation for treatment of oropharyngeal cancer or other maxillary tumors (Arigbede, Dosumu, Shaba, & Esan, 2006; Bohle et al., 2005; Chambers, Lemon, & Martin, 2004; Keyf, Sahin, & Aslan, 2003; Rieger, Tang, Wolfaardt, Harris, & Seikaly, 2011; Yenisey, Cengiz, & Sarikaya, 2011). They can also be used for those who have had traumatic injuries to the palate, where surgical correction is not an option. Figure 20–6A shows a patient who underwent a maxillectomy and removal of most of the velum. A palatal speech bulb, combined with a palatal obturator, was used for correction, as can be seen in Figure 20–6B.

The speech bulb obturator usually has an oral base section that clasps to the teeth and then a posterior palatal strap with the bulb on the end. The bulb courses upward to fit behind the velum in the nasopharynx. When it is in place, the speech bulb is not visible from an intraoral perspective.

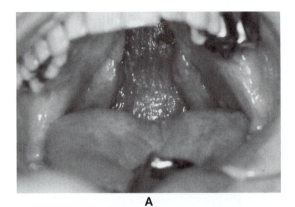

A

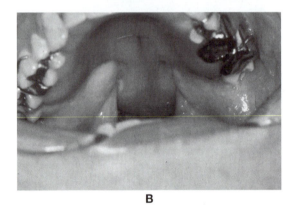

B

FIGURE 20–6 (A and B) (A) This is a patient with a large palatal defect following a maxillectomy and removal of the velum for a malignancy. (B) A combination palatal obturator and speech bulb.

Courtesy Gordon Huntress, D.D.S./Cincinnati Children's Hospital Medical Center & University of Cincinnati College of Medicine

Speech bulb appliances are removed at night, which allows an open airway for normal breathing and reduces the risk of sleep apnea. Although the appliance can help to eliminate nasal regurgitation, many individuals prefer to remove the appliance during meals.

Fabrication of a Speech Appliance

Speech appliances are individually designed to meet the specific needs of the patient. In addition, dental professionals may differ in the techniques and materials that they prefer to use. Although, there is considerable variation among speech devices, there are also many commonalties in the way that they are designed.

Most speech appliances have an anterior *palatal section*, which is the body portion of the appliance. The purpose of this section is to hold the appliance in place against the roof of the mouth. It can also serve as an obturator to close off a defect in the palate. This part of the prosthesis may appear similar to a common orthodontic retainer.

The palatal section is usually made of either acrylic resins or metal. This part of the appliance must be made thick enough to avoid easy breakage, but not so thick as to interfere with speech production. The appliance is formed from a plaster model of the roof of the mouth. It is designed to fit snugly against the contours of the individual's teeth and hard palate so that there is good retention during oral activity. Artificial palatal rugae can be added to assist with tongue tip orientation and articulation (Gitto, Esposito, & Draper, 1999).

The palatal section is held in place by metal wires, which are attached around the teeth for anchorage. The teeth may need to be prepared with buccal lugs on soldered bands, special caps, crowns, or undercuts to adequately retain the wires and the appliance. Retention and stability of an appliance can be a significant challenge for the prosthodontist in patients who do not have adequate maxillary teeth for use as anchors. Fortunately, recent advances in the use of osseointegrated implants have greatly increased the ability to rehabilitate individuals with intraoral anomalies and even those with an edentulous maxillary arch (Grisius, 1991; Hudson & Russell, 1994; Lundqvist & Haraldson, 1992; Lundqvist, Haraldson, & Lindblad, 1992; Parel et al., 1986).

Osseointegrated implants are small cylinders (5 to 6 mm in diameter) that are usually made of titanium. They are fitted into a carefully prepared channel that is drilled into the alveolar bone. At least four implants of a minimum of 10 mm in length are usually recommended in the maxilla of patients with clefts (Ramstad, 1998). Once in place, the bone grows directly around the implant, resulting in *osseointegration* (direct connection between the implant and the bone) and a pseudo root. With these implants embedded in the bone, a speech appliance can be attached and retained. Implants can also be used to support dental restorations. A single implant can support a crown to replace an individual tooth. Multiple implants can be used to support restorations of a row of missing teeth or to secure dentures for an entire dental arch.

In addition to the palatal section, the palatal lift and speech bulb appliances have an extension, or *tailpiece*, that projects posteriorly to close the velopharyngeal port during speech. The palatal section is fabricated first, as it forms the basis of the rest of the prosthesis. In fabricating the tailpiece, the prosthodontist starts with a small bulb and then slowly adds a thin layer of thermoplastic wax compound until the appropriate size and shape are achieved. This is usually done by putting it in the individual's mouth, testing it with speech, and then making modifications as needed. For a speech bulb, the device is inserted and the patient is asked to move his head up and down, then back and forth, in order to mold the bulb appropriately. Wax is gradually added to the bulb until it fits comfortably and works effectively in the pharynx for speech. The challenge is to make the bulb fill the space, while keeping it from causing undue pressure against the soft tissue of the pharynx. The individual must be able to move his head without discomfort or irritation of pharyngeal mucosa. Once the form is finalized, the permanent lift or bulb is made of acrylic. Sometimes speech bulbs must be large, and therefore they become too heavy for the teeth to bear. When this is the case, the bulb can be hollowed out to make it lighter and more stable.

Depending on the needs of the patient, various combinations of appliances can be constructed. For example, the speech appliance may have an oral base section with partial or complete dentures. A palatal obturator can be combined with a palatal lift or speech bulb (Alpine, Stone, & Badr, 1990) (see Figure 20–3B), or it can be used with an expansion appliance (Hobson & Clasper, 1995). A maxillary prostheses and mandibular prostheses can also be combined if this results in increased function. Although these combinations are very beneficial to the patient, the mechanical design of prosthetic appliances should be kept as simple as possible. Wear and tear on the device should be expected, and breakage will occasionally occur. Hence, devices that are simple and easy to repair are best in the long term (Mazahari, 1996). It is also most important that the device be designed so that oral hygiene can be maintained.

Some children and adults learn to accept and tolerate the prosthetic appliance quickly and easily, especially those who are motivated to work for aesthetic or speech improvement. Other patients, particularly young children, are less compliant and even resist wearing a prosthetic device. In these cases, working through the family is the best avenue for achieving compliance and the inherent benefits of the device. Close cooperation between the speech-language pathologist and prosthodontist is also necessary to ensure maximal benefits through prosthetic treatment.

Procedures for Assessment and Modification of a Speech Appliance

A palatal obturator is relatively easy to fit, because it only includes the palatal section and the palatal opening or fistula is not dynamic. In contrast, the palatal lift and speech bulb appliances are used to improve the closure of a dynamic opening in the velopharyngeal port. Therefore, fine adjustments must be made to these appliances so that the velopharyngeal port is closed enough for speech, but not overly closed so that it causes upper airway problems.

The speech-language pathologist can be very helpful to the prosthodontist in providing information on speech and resonance changes that occur as fine adjustments are made to the device. To assess the effectiveness of the speech appliance, the examiner should test the production of pressure-sensitive phonemes (plosives, fricatives, and affricates) in syllable repetition tasks and sentences, as described in Chapter 11. The examiner could use a simple listening tube or straw to detect subtle changes in velopharyngeal closure as the modifications to the device are made. If pressure-sensitive sounds can be produced without nasal air emission and there is no evidence of hypernasality, then the velopharyngeal port is closed adequately for speech. The speech-language pathologist should then assess the ease of nasal breathing with the appliance in place and also test the production of nasal sounds (/m/, /n/, /ŋ/) in repetitive syllables and sentences. Again, a listening tube or straw can help to detect the amount of sound or air that is passing through the nasopharynx. Based on this assessment, the appliance can be modified until an appropriate balance is achieved between closure for oral speech and patency for nasal breathing and the production of nasal phonemes (Rosen & Bzoch, 1997).

In addition to a perceptual assessment, indirect instrumental measures (which provide objective data, but no visualization of the velopharyngeal port) can be used to evaluate the effectiveness of a prosthetic appliance. For example, aerodynamic instrumentation (Reisberg & Smith, 1985; Riski, Hoke, & Dolan, 1989) and nasometry (Pinborough-Zimmerman et al., 1998; Scarsellone, Rochet, & Wolfaardt, 1999) can provide objective information regarding the extent of improvement with the appliance and the relative normalcy of the speech as a result. They also provide information regarding the patency of the airway while the appliance is in place.

Although a perceptual assessment and indirect instrumental assessment techniques are helpful in evaluating the effect of an appliance on speech and airway, these procedures do not give the prosthodontist necessary information if adjustments have to be made. For this information, a direct instrumental approach (where the velopharyngeal valve can be visualized) is needed so that the prosthodontist knows where the appliance should be augmented and where it should be reduced. A lateral cephalometric X-ray and videofluoroscopy have been used for this purpose in the past (Turner & Williams, 1991). However, the best procedure for assessment of an appliance is nasopharyngoscopy.

Using nasopharyngoscopy, the effect of the device can be viewed directly during both nasal breathing and speech. The extent of velopharyngeal closure with the device in place can be easily determined (Rieger, Zalmanowitz, & Wolfaardt, 2006; D'Antonio, Muntz, Marsh, Marty-Grames, & Backensto-Marsh,

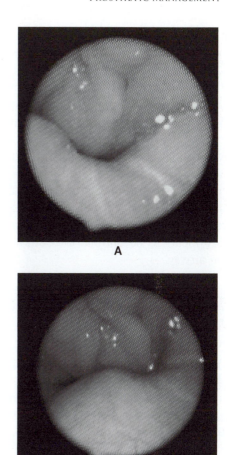

A

B

FIGURE 20–7 (A and B) (A) A velopharyngeal opening, due to velopharyngeal incompetence, as can be seen through nasopharyngoscopy. (B) Greatly improved velopharyngeal competence as a result of placement of a palatal lift.

Courtesy Gordon Huntress, D.D.S./Cincinnati Children's Hospital Medical Center & University of Cincinnati College of Medicine

1988; Karnell, Rosenstein, & Fine, 1987; Rich, Farber, & Shprintzen, 1988; Riski et al., 1989; Turner & Williams, 1991). Figure 20–7A shows the nasopharyngoscopy exam of a patient with velopharyngeal incompetence, resulting in a midline opening. Figure 20–7B shows greatly improved closure as a result of a palatal lift.

An optimal fit often requires trial and error and several adjustments to the appliance. If there is still a leak in velopharyngeal closure, then the appliance can be augmented for that specific area. In addition, the patency of the airway during nasal breathing and production of nasal sounds can be viewed. At times, the airway must be compromised slightly for the best speech benefit. At other times, perfect speech must be compromised for the sake of the airway. With the benefit of a nasopharyngoscopy view, the device can be modified until it appears to be optimal for both speech and the airway.

ADVANTAGES AND DISADVANTAGES OF PROSTHETIC MANAGEMENT

Although surgical correction is usually considered the best option for the treatment of structural defects, there are cases where prosthetic management is more appropriate or necessary. These include patients with a history of cleft for whom surgery must be delayed due to a medical condition or the need to do other procedures first. Prosthetic devices can be used effectively in the management of large soft palate perforations or palatal fistulas. They can also be appropriate for patients with persistent velopharyngeal insufficiency or incompetence after several unsuccessful surgical repairs (Hoffman, 1985). For example, if a pharyngeal flap was done, but the lateral ports do not close sufficiently, a device can be made that has a bulb on each side of the flap to fill in the area of the ports (McKinstry, 1998a). They can even be used on a trial basis in cases where the outcome of surgical correction is unclear. If the prosthodontist is routinely consulted in the initial treatment planning, alternatives to surgical management might be considered for patients with high potential for postsurgical failure (McKinstry & Aramany, 1985).

Speech appliances are sometimes appropriate for patients with structural disorders not related to cleft palate. For example, in rare cases individuals develop velopharyngeal insufficiency following a uvulopalatopharyngoplasty (UPPP), which is done to alleviate snoring and sleep apnea. When this occurs, prosthetic management is often appropriate because there is no risk of causing further sleep problems with this form of correction (Finkelstein, Shifman, Nachmani, & Ophir, 1995). Prosthetic management is particularly useful following cancer treatment, especially if the treatment involved ablative surgery of the maxilla or velum.

Patients with oral carcinomas often require resection of other parts of the mouth as well, including the tongue, the floor of the mouth, or the bone of the mandible. Postoperatively, these patients often encounter problems with chewing and swallowing as well as speech. In these cases, prosthetic treatment may include a tongue prosthesis or other prostheses in addition to the palatal device. Prosthetic management of this type can help to improve articulation, resonance, and swallowing (Pinto & Pegoraro, 2003). Socialization is also enhanced through the improved appearance that these prosthetic devices can provide.

Patients who exhibit normal velopharyngeal anatomy, but demonstrate velopharyngeal incompetence secondary to neuromotor disorders, may not be appropriate surgical candidates. However, as mentioned before, individuals with dysarthria (Bedwinek & O'Brien, 1985; Riski & Gordon, 1979) or apraxia (Hall et al., 1990) may derive significant benefit from a palatal lift. This allows the individual to concentrate on anterior articulation and not be concerned about velopharyngeal articulation.

Prosthetic management is usually most successful with individuals who have adequate dentition for retention of the device and good oral hygiene. Another consideration when trying to fit a palatal lift or speech bulb is the gag reflex. Although the prosthodontist can work to gradually desensitize the patient to the device, a strong gag reflex or oral sensitivity makes successful prosthetic management very difficult, if not impossible, to achieve. Finally, successful prosthetic management is somewhat dependent on good articulation, because corrected velopharyngeal function for speech will not improve intelligibility significantly if the articulation is poor.

Although prosthetic devices have been used successfully by many patients for correction of velopharyngeal dysfunction, they have some distinct disadvantages. Unlike surgery, these devices do not result in a permanent correction. When they are removed, the speech symptoms recur. Prosthetic appliances are expensive and often are not covered by insurance. They can be easily lost or damaged, and they also need to be removed for daily cleaning. Of course, manual dexterity or the assistance of others is important for proper insertion and removal of the device. They may be uncomfortable to wear and can cause ulceration of the surrounding mucosa. Retention of appliances can be a challenge for patients with irregularities in the dentition or missing teeth. In young children, appliances require frequent adjustments as the child grows and as deciduous teeth are lost and permanent teeth erupt, thus increasing the cost. There may be poor compliance, especially with young children.

Because of these limitations, removable prosthetic devices are not well suited for patients who are very young, are developmentally delayed, or have significant physical handicaps. They do not work well for patients who have difficulty managing secretions, who have a strong gag reflex, or who have significant upper airway obstruction. In fact, most patients who are able to undergo surgical correction usually do opt for surgery after a period of prosthetic management (Marsh & Wray, 1980). Despite their limitations, prosthetic devices should always be considered for correction of a palatal defect or velopharyngeal dysfunction when surgery is not an option for medical reasons (McKinstry, 1998a).

PROSTHETIC MANAGEMENT AND SPEECH THERAPY

Speech therapy cannot correct velopharyngeal insufficiency or incompetence or the hypernasality that results. However, once there is sufficient improvement in velopharyngeal function with prosthetic treatment, speech therapy is often required to further improve the speech (Gallagher, 1982). The presence of a speech appliance does not correct misarticulation, but it does improve the ability to impound intraoral air pressure and thus produce oral sounds. Speech therapy is often necessary to help the individual to learn to use this air pressure to produce sounds normally. Therapy is also needed to eliminate any compensatory articulation productions that developed prior to prosthetic management (Pinto, da Silva Dalben, & Pegoraro-Krook, 2007).

Prosthetic devices have also been used as a form of therapy to attempt to improve velopharyngeal function. This type of therapy, called *reduction therapy*, is done in hopes of stimulating increased movement of the velopharyngeal structures in order to avoid surgery or reduce the extent of the surgery that is needed. When a palatal lift is used in reduction therapy, the length of the lift is gradually reduced, or the wearing time of the lift is gradually decreased, in hopes of stimulating velar movement. However, it has been shown that the passive elevation of the velum actually reduces levator veli palatini muscle activity (Nohara, Kotani, Sasao, Ojima, Tachimura, & Sakai, 2010; Tachimura, Nohara, Fujita, Hara, & Wada, 2001). Therefore, this use of a lift may ultimately be more harmful than beneficial if the goal is to increase velar movement.

More commonly, reduction therapy is done with a speech bulb in the nasopharynx. The size of the bulb is gradually reduced in hopes of gradually increasing velar and lateral wall movement. The ultimate goal is to improve velopharyngeal function so that surgical management is either not needed, or the extent of management, such as the size of the pharyngeal flap, is reduced. Some authors have reported some success in improving lateral wall motion with this procedure (Golding-Kushner, Cisneros, & LeBlanc, 1995). However, these results are not always maintained, and most individuals still require surgical intervention for correction (Witt et al., 1995; Wolfaardt, Wilson, Rochet, & McPhee, 1993). Considering this fact, and the time and expense of the prosthesis and speech therapy, surgical correction may still be the most

appropriate and effective option for correction of velopharyngeal dysfunction when possible.

SUMMARY

Prosthetic management is not required in the habilitation of individuals who have repaired clefts as frequently as in years past. With the advances in surgical procedures and improvement in the timing of surgery, the outcomes of surgical intervention are usually superior to those that can be obtained with prosthetic management. However, in certain cases there is a definite need for prosthetic management, particularly when surgical intervention is not an option. Prosthetic management can be very effective in improving the individual's appearance and speech. Speech appliances can be effective in improving or eliminating hypernasality and nasal emission from either a fistula or an open velopharyngeal valve. When fabricating a palatal lift or a speech bulb, it is important to balance the needs for speech with the needs for a nasal airway. The ultimate goal of prosthetic management is to help the patient to achieve the best possible outcome with the device.

FOR REVIEW AND DISCUSSION

1. What types of patients could benefit from a facial or oral prosthetic device? Why do you think prosthetic devices are actually used less than they were 20 years ago? Which professionals are trained to construct these devices?

2. What is the purpose of a dental appliance? What are the different types? How do you think dental appliances could affect speech?

3. What is the purpose of a facial prosthesis? How is it retained?

4. Describe the construction and retention of a feeding obturator. Why is now used infrequently for most children born with cleft lip and/or cleft palate?

5. Describe the three types of speech appliances that are used for improvement of resonance. What is the appropriate indication for each? Why is a palatal lift

inappropriate for a child with velopharyngeal insufficiency?

6. What are the components of most speech appliances? What materials are used? How are they retained?

7. Describe ways that the speech-language pathologist should work with the prosthodontist (or dental professional) in order to achieve the best outcome with a speech appliance.

8. What are the clinical indications and contraindications for the use of prosthetic devices for speech?

9. How have prosthetic devices been used as part of the speech therapy process? Discuss the controversy regarding this practice.

REFERENCES

Abreu, A., Levy, D., Rodriguez, E., & Rivera, I. (2007). Oral rehabilitation of a patient with complete unilateral cleft lip and palate using an implant-retained speech-aid prosthesis: Clinical report. *Cleft Palate–Craniofacial Journal*, *44*(6), 673–677.

Ahmed, B., Farshad, A. F., & Yazdanie, N. (2011). Rehabilitation of a large maxillofacial defect using acrylic resin prosthesis. *Journal of College of Physicians and Surgeons Pakistan*, *21*(4), 254–256.

Alpine, K. D., Stone, C. R., & Badr, S. E. (1990). Combined obturator and palatal-lift prosthesis: A case report. *Quintessence International*, *21*(11), 893–896.

American Speech-Language-Hearing Association (ASHA). (1993). Position statement and guidelines for oral and oropharyngeal prostheses, *ASHA*, *35*(Suppl. 10), 14–16.

Arigbede, A. O., Dosumu, O. O., Shaba, O. P., & Esan, T. A. (2006). Evaluation of speech in patients with partial surgically acquired defects: Pre and post prosthetic obturation. *Journal of Contemporary Dental Practice*, *7*(1), 89–96.

Bedwinek, A. P., & O'Brien, R. L. (1985). A patient selection profile for the use of speech prostheses in adult dysarthria. *Journal of Communication Disorders*, *18*(3), 169–182.

Beumer, J., III, Roumanas, E., & Nishimura, R. (1995). Advances in osseointegrated implants for dental and facial rehabilitation following major head and neck surgery. *Seminars in Surgical Oncology*, *11*(3), 200–207.

Blair, F. M., & Hunter, N. R. (1998). The hollow box maxillary obturator. *British Dental Journal*, *184*(10), 484–487.

Bohle, G., III, Rieger, J., Huryn, J., Verbel, D., Hwang, F., & Zlotolow, I. (2005). Efficacy of speech aid prostheses for acquired defects of the soft palate and velopharyngeal inadequacy—Clinical assessments and cephalometric analysis: A Memorial Sloan-Kettering Study. *Head & Neck*, *27*(3), 195–207.

Chambers, M. S., Lemon, J. C., & Martin, J. W. (2004). Obturation of the partial soft palate defect. *Journal of Prosthetic Dentistry*, *91*(1), 75–79.

Chang, T. L., Garrett, N., Roumanas, E., & Beumer, J., III., (2005). Treatment satisfaction with facial prostheses. *Journal of Prosthetic Dentistry*, *94*(3), 275–280.

Daniel, B. (1982). A soft-palate desensitization procedure for patients requiring palatal lift prostheses. *Journal of Prosthetic Dentistry*, *48*(5), 565–566.

D'Antonio, L. L., Muntz, H. R., Marsh, J. L., Marty-Grames, L., & Backensto-Marsh, R. (1988). Practical application of flexible fiberoptic nasopharyngoscopy for evaluating velopharyngeal function. *Plastic and Reconstructive Surgery, 82*(4), 611–618.

Delgado, A. A., Schaaf, N. G., & Emrich, L. (1992). Trends in prosthodontic treatment of cleft palate patients at one institution: A twenty-one year review. *Cleft Palate–Craniofacial Journal, 29*(5), 425–428.

Dorf, D. S., Reisberg, D. J., & Gold, H. O. (1985). Early prosthetic management of cleft palate. Articulation development prosthesis: A preliminary report. *Journal of Prosthetic Dentistry, 53*(2), 222–226.

dos Santos, D. M., Goiato, M. C., Pesqueira, A. A., Bannwart, L. C., Rezende, M. C., Magro-Filho, O., & Moreno, A. (2010). Prosthesis auricular with osseointegrated implants and quality of life. *Journal of Craniofacial Surgery, 21*(1), 94–96.

Dutka, J. C., Uemeoka, E., Aferri, H. C., Pegoraro-Krook, M. I., & Marino, V. C. (2011). Total obturation of the velopharynx for treatment of velopharyngeal hypodynamism: Case report. *Cleft Palate–Craniofacial Journal, 49*(4), 488–493.

Esposito, S. J., Mitsumoto, H., & Shanks, M. (2000). Use of palatal lift and palatal augmentation prostheses to improve dysarthria in patients with amyotrophic lateral sclerosis: A case series. *Journal of Prosthetic Dentistry, 83*(1), 90–98.

Feng, Z. H., Dong, Y., Bai, S. Z., Wu, G. F., Bi, Y. P., Wang, B., & Zhao, Y. M. (2010). Virtual transplantation in designing a facial prosthesis for extensive maxillofacial defects that cross the facial midline using computer-assisted technology. *International Journal of Prosthodontics, 23*(6), 513–520.

Finkelstein, Y., Shifman, A., Nachmani, A., & Ophir, D. (1995). Prosthetic management of velopharyngeal insufficiency induced by uvulopalatopharyngoplasty. *Otolaryngology—Head & Neck Surgery, 113*(5), 611–616.

Gallagher, B. (1982). Prosthesis in velopharyngeal insufficiency: Effect on nasal resonance. *Journal of Communication Disorders, 15*(6), 469–173.

Gardner, L. K., & Parr, G. R. (1996). Prosthetic rehabilitation of the cleft palate patient. *Seminars in Orthodontics, 2*(3), 215–219.

Gitto, C. A., Esposito, S. J., & Draper, J. M. (1999). A simple method of adding palatal rugae to a complete denture. *Journal of Prosthetic Dentistry, 81*(2), 237–239.

Goiato, M. C., dos Santos, D. M., Haddad, M. F., & Moreno, A. (2012). Rehabilitation with ear prosthesis linked to osseointegrated implants. *Gerodontology, 29*(2), 150–154.

Golding-Kushner, K. J., Cisneros, G., & LeBlanc, E. (1995). Speech bulbs. In R. J. Shprintzen & J. Bardach (Eds.), *Cleft palate speech management* (pp. 352–363). St. Louis, MO: Mosby.

Grisius, R. J. (1991). Maxillofacial prosthetics. *Current Opinions in Dentistry, 1*(2), 155–159.

Hall, P. K., Hardy, J. C., & LaVelle, W. E. (1990). A child with signs of developmental apraxia of speech with whom a palatal lift prosthesis was used to manage palatal dysfunction. *Journal of Speech and Hearing Disorders, 55*(3), 454–460.

Hobson, R. S., & Clasper, R. (1995). A combined obturator and expansion appliance for use in patients with patent oral-nasal fistula. *British Journal of Orthodontics, 22*(4), 357–359.

Hoffman, S. (1985). Correction of lateral port stenosis following a pharyngeal flap operation. *Cleft Palate Journal, 22*(1), 51–55.

Hudson, J. W., & Russell, R., Jr. (1994). Contributions within dental science to cleft lip/palate management: A literature review. *Compendium, 15*(1), 116, 118–120, 122; Quiz 126.

Karnell, M. P., Rosenstein, H., & Fine, L. (1987). Nasal videoendoscopy in prosthetic management of palatopharyngeal dysfunction. *Journal of Prosthetic Dentistry, 58*(4), 479–484.

Keyf, F., Sahin, N., & Aslan, Y. (2003). Alternative impression technique for a speech-aid prosthesis. *Cleft Palate–Craniofacial Journal, 40*(6), 566–568.

Koidis, P. T., & Topouzelis, N. (2003). Palatal lift prosthesis for palatopharyngeal closure in Wilson's disease. *Orthodontics & Craniofacial Research, 6*(2), 101–103.

Lohmander-Agerskov, A., Soderpalm, E., Friede, H., & Lilja, J. (1990). Cleft lip and palate patients prior to delayed closure of the hard palate: Evaluation of maxillary morphology and the effect of early stimulation on pre-school speech. *Scandinavian Journal of Plastic and Reconstructive Surgery and Hand Surgery, 24*(2), 141–148.

Lundgren, S., Moy, P. K., Beumer, J., III. & Lewis, S. (1993). Surgical considerations for endosseous implants in the craniofacial region: A 3-year report. *International Journal of Oral and Maxillofacial Surgery, 22*, 272–277.

Lundqvist, S., & Haraldson, T. (1992). Oral function in patients wearing fixed prosthesis on osseointegrated implants in the maxilla: A 3-year follow-up study. *Scandinavian Journal of Dental Research, 100*(5), 279–283.

Lundqvist, S., Haraldson, T., & Lindblad, P. (1992). Speech in connection with maxillary fixed prostheses on osseointegrated implants: A three-year follow-up study. *Clinics in Oral Implants Research, 3*(4), 176–180.

Marsh, J. L., & Wray, R. C. (1980). Speech prosthesis versus pharyngeal flap: A randomized evaluation of the management of velopharyngeal incompetency. *Plastic and Reconstructive Surgery, 65*(5), 592–594.

Mazahari, M. (1996). Prosthetic speech appliances for patients with cleft palate. In S. Berkowitz (Ed.), *Cleft lip and palate with introduction to other craniofacial abnormalities: Perspectives in management* (vol. 2, pp. 177–194). San Diego, CA: Singular Publishing Group.

McKinstry, R. E. (1998a). Cleft palate prosthetics. In R. E. McKinstry (Ed.), *Cleft palate dentistry* (pp. 206–235). Arlington, VA: ABI Professional Publications.

McKinstry, R. E. (1998b). Presurgical management of cleft lip and palate patients. In R. E. McKinstry (Ed.), *Cleft palate dentistry* (pp. 33–66). Arlington, VA: ABI Professional Publications.

McKinstry, R. E., & Aramany, M. A. (1985). Prosthodontic considerations in the management of surgically compromised cleft palate patients. *Journal of Prosthetic Dentistry, 53*(6), 827–831.

Mueller, A. A., Paysan, P., Schumacher, R., Zeilhofer, H. F., Berg-Boerner, B. I., Maurer, J., Vetter, T., et al. (2011). Missing facial parts computed by a morphable model and transferred directly to a polyamide laser-sintered prosthesis: An innovation study. *British Journal of Oral & Maxillofacial Surgery, 49*(8), e67–71.

Nagda, S., Deshpande, D. S., & Mhatre, S. W. (1996). Infant palatal obturator. *Journal of the Indian Society of Pedodontics & Preventive Dentistry, 14*(1), 24–25.

Nohara, K., Kotani, Y., Sasao, Y., Ojima, M., Tachimura, T., & Sakai, T. (2010). Effect of a speech aid prosthesis on reducing muscle fatigue. *Journal of Dental Research*, 89(5), 478–481.

Osuji, O. O. (1995). Preparation of feeding obturators for infants with cleft lip and palate. *Journal of Clinical Pediatric Dentistry*, 19(3), 211–214.

Parel, S. M., Holt, G. R., Branemark, P. I., & Tjellstrom, A. (1986). Osseointegration and facial prosthetics. *International Journal of Oral and Maxillofacial Implants*, 1(1), 27–29.

Pinborough-Zimmerman, J., Canady, G., Yamashiro, D. K., & Morales, L., Jr. (1998). Articulation and nasality changes resulting from sustained palatal fistula obturation. *Cleft Palate–Craniofacial Journal*, 35(1), 81–87.

Pinto, J. H., da Silva Dalben, G., & Pegoraro-Krook, M. I. (2007). Speech intelligibility of patients with cleft lip and palate after placement of speech prosthesis. *Cleft Palate–Craniofacial Journal*, 44(6), 635–641.

Pinto, J. H., & Pegoraro-Krook, M. I. (2003). Evaluation of palatal prosthesis for the treatment of velopharyngeal dysfunction. *Journal of Applied Oral Science*, 11(3), 192–197.

Raju, H., Padmanabhan, T. V., & Narayan, A. (2009). Effect of a palatal lift prosthesis in individuals with velopharyngeal incompetence. *International Journal of Prosthodontics*, 22(6), 579–585.

Ramstad, T. (1998). Fixed prosthodontics. In R. E. McKinstry (Ed.), *Cleft palate dentistry* (pp. 236–262). Arlington, VA: ABI Professional Publications.

Reisberg, D. J. (2000). Dental and prosthodontic care for patients with cleft or craniofacial conditions. *Cleft Palate–Craniofacial Journal*, 37(6), 534–537.

Reisberg, D. J., & Smith, B. E. (1985). Aerodynamic assessment of prosthetic speech aids. *Journal of Prosthetic Dentistry*, 54(5), 686–690.

Rich, B. M., Farber, K., & Shprintzen, R. J. (1988). Nasopharyngoscopy in the treatment of palatopharyngeal insufficiency. *International Journal of Prosthodontics*, 1(3), 248–251.

Rieger, J., Bohle, G. III., Huryn, J., Tang, J. L., Harris, J., & Seikaly, H. (2009). Surgical reconstruction versus prosthetic obturation of extensive soft palate defects: A comparison of speech outcomes. *International Journal of Prosthodontics*, 22(6), 566–572.

Rieger, J. M., Tang, J. A., Wolfaardt, J., Harris, J., & Seikaly, H. (2011). Comparison of speech and aesthetic outcomes in patients with maxillary reconstruction versus maxillary obturators after maxillectomy. *Otolaryngology—Head & Neck Surgery*, 40(1), 40–47.

Rieger, J. M., Zalmanowitz, J. G., & Wolfaardt, J. F. (2006). Nasopharyngoscopy in palatopharyngeal prosthetic rehabilitation: A preliminary report. *International Journal of Prosthodontics*, 19(4), 383–388.

Riski, J. E., Hoke, J. A., & Dolan, E. A. (1989). The role of pressure flow and endoscopic assessment in successful palatal obturator revision. *Cleft Palate Journal*, 26(1), 56–62.

Rosen, M. S., & Bzoch, K. R. (1997). Prosthodontic management of the individual with cleft lip and palate for speech habilitation needs. In K. R. Bzoch (Ed.), *Communicative disorders related to cleft lip and palate* (vol. 4, pp. 153–168). Austin, TX: Pro-Ed.

Savion, L., & Huband, M. L. (2005). A feeding obturator for a preterm baby with Pierre Robin sequence. *Journal of Prosthetic Dentistry*, 93(2), 197–200.

Scarsellone, J. M., Rochet, A. P., & Wolfaardt, J. F. (1999). The influence of dentures on nasalance values in speech. *Cleft Palate–Craniofacial Journal*, 36(1), 51–56.

Schaaf, N. G. (1984). Maxillofacial prosthetics and the head and neck cancer patient. *Cancer, 54*(11, Suppl.), 2682–2690.

Schweckendiek, W. (1966). [The technique of early veloplasty and its results.] *Acta Chiruriae Plasticae, 8*(3), 188–194.

Schweckendiek, W. (1968). [Early veloplasty and its results.] *Acta Oto-Rhino-Laryngologica Belgica, 22*(6), 697–703.

Shifman, A., Finkelstein, Y., Nachmani, A., & Ophir, D. (2000). Speech-aid prostheses for neurogenic velopharyngeal incompetence. *Journal of Prosthetic Dentistry, 83*(1), 99–106.

Sidoti, E. J., & Shprintzen, R. J. (1995). Pediatric care and feeding of the newborn with a cleft. In R. J. Shprintzen & J. Bardach (Eds.), *Cleft palate speech management* (pp. 63–74). St. Louis, MO: Mosby.

Singh, V. P., Bharadwaj, G., & Nair, K. C. (1997). Direct observation of tongue positions in speech—A patient study. *International Journal of Prosthodontics, 10*(3), 231–234.

Sultana, A., Rahman, M. M., Nessa, J., & Alam, M. S. (2011). A feeding aid prosthesis for a preterm baby with cleft lip and palate. *Mymensingh Medical Journal, 20*(1), 22–27.

Sun, J., Li, N., & Sun, G. (2002). Application of obturator to treat velopharyngeal incompetence. *Chinese Medical Journal (English), 115*(6), 842–845.

Tachimura, T., Nohara, K., Fujita, Y., Hara, H., & Wada, T. (2001). Change in levator veli palatini muscle activity of normal speakers in association with elevation of the velum using an experimental palatal lift prosthesis. *Cleft Palate–Craniofacial Journal, 38*(5), 449–554.

Tuna, S. H., Pekkan, G., Gumus, H. O., & Aktas, A. (2010). Prosthetic rehabilitation of velopharyngeal insufficiency: Pharyngeal obturator prostheses with different retention mechanisms. *European Journal of Dentistry, 4*(1), 81–87.

Turner, G. E., & Williams, W. N. (1991). Fluoroscopy and nasoendoscopy in designing palatal lift prostheses. *Journal of Prosthetic Dentistry, 66*(1), 63–71.

Walter, J. D. (2005). Obturators for cleft palate and other speech appliances. *Dental Update, 32*(4), 217–218.

Witt, P. D., Rozelle, A. A., Marsh, J. L., Marty-Grames, L., Muntz, H. R., Gay, W. D., & Pilgram, T. K. (1995). Do palatal lift prostheses stimulate velopharyngeal neuromuscular activity? *Cleft Palate–Craniofacial Journal, 32*(6), 469–475.

Wolfaardt, J. F., Wilson, F. B., Rochet, A., & McPhee, L. (1993). An appliance-based approach to the management of palatopharyngeal incompetency: A clinical pilot project. *Journal of Prosthetic Dentistry, 69*(2), 186–195.

Yenisey, M., Cengiz, S., & Sarikaya, I. (2011). Prosthetic treatment of congenital hard and soft palate defects: A clinical report. *Cleft Palate–Craniofacial Journal, 49*(5), 618–621.

C H A P T E R

21

Speech Therapy

INTRODUCTION

Individuals with a history of cleft lip/palate or craniofacial anomalies are at risk for certain speech and resonance disorders secondary to velopharyngeal insufficiency or incompetence (VPI), oral anomalies, and dental malocclusion. Even with early surgical repair, the majority of preschoolers with cleft palate will demonstrate difficulties with speech sound development (Hardin-Jones & Jones, 2005). In addition to cleft palate, velopharyngeal dysfunction can occur due to a variety of other reasons.

As has been discussed in other chapters, when the velopharyngeal valve is defective, speech may be characterized by hypernasality and nasal air emission. In addition, inadequate intraoral pressure as a result of nasal emission can result in weak consonant production, short utterance length, and the development of compensatory articulation productions. It is important to determine the underlying cause of these speech characteristics through perceptual and instrumental methods, because the cause has a direct impact on the selection of the appropriate treatment method.

It is very important to understand that speech therapy does not correct hypernasality or nasal emission due to velopharyngeal insufficiency (abnormal structure) or even velopharyngeal incompetence (abnormal neurophysiology). Speech therapy only corrects abnormal function (speech sound placement) that may result from these disorders. It is also important to note that oral-motor exercises (blowing, sucking, or any other nonspeech activities) are totally ineffective in correcting resonance or velopharyngeal function and therefore should not be used for this purpose. Instead, standard speech therapy techniques to change articulation placement are indicated.

The purpose of this chapter to convey all needed information regarding speech therapy for individuals with cleft palate, dental/occlusal anomalies, or various types of velopharyngeal dysfunction. As a result of this information, the speech-language pathologist should be able to treat these individuals (usually children) with both competence and confidence.

SPEECH THERAPY VERSUS PHYSICAL MANAGEMENT

When there are structural anomalies in the cavities of the vocal tract (oral, nasal, and pharyngeal cavities), there is a risk for errors and distortions in speech sound production, in addition to a risk for abnormal resonance (see Chapter 7 for more information). In some cases, speech therapy is appropriate for correction. In other cases, physical management (surgery or a prosthetic device) is indicated. It is very important to determine the appropriate form of management for the child based on the structural anomalies and the characteristics of the speech.

For Obligatory Distortions

Obligatory distortions are those that occur when function (i.e., articulation) is normal, but the structure is abnormal. The abnormal structure is, therefore, the sole cause of the distortion of speech and/or resonance. It is very important to note that hypernasality and nasal emission are usually obligatory distortions due to VPI. Hyponasality and cul-de-sac resonance are also typically obligatory distortions due to a blockage somewhere in the vocal tract. Obligatory distortions can also occur due to dental anomalies. For example, sibilant productions can be distorted if the teeth are in a position to interfere with the air stream, even though tongue placement is normal.

Because obligatory distortions are due to abnormal structure, they can only be eliminated by correcting the structure. Speech therapy is not indicated for obligatory distortions because the articulation placement (function) is normal (Kummer, 2011; Trost-Cardamone, 1997). In fact, for ethical reasons, the speech-language pathologist must refuse to offer speech therapy for an individual who has a structural anomaly that is causing the speech distortion. The only exception to this rule is if the structure cannot (or will not) be corrected. In that case, speech therapy may be appropriate in order to help the person develop compensatory strategies to improve the intelligibility of speech.

Some individuals can demonstrate a small or inconsistent velopharyngeal opening. As such, it may be tempting to try speech therapy for these individuals. However, if the cause is a structural defect, they may be able to achieve closure with extra effort (as in the therapy session), but they usually are not able to maintain this closure due to the extra effort that it requires throughout the day. Therefore, surgical management is usually more appropriate, even though the opening is small. The decision to consider surgical management for a small opening should be made based on how much the defect affects the quality and

intelligibility of speech. Only the family and child can determine whether its effect on speech warrants the surgical procedure.

For Compensatory Errors

Compensatory errors are those that occur when articulation placement (function) is altered in response to the abnormal structure. For example, when there is VPI and therefore a lack of adequate oral pressure for certain speech sounds, oral placement may be changed to the pharynx where there is adequate airflow. Thus, common compensatory productions for VPI include pharyngeal fricatives, pharyngeal plosives, and glottal stops. Compensatory speech errors can also be developed with other structural anomalies, such as dental malocclusion. For example, if an anterior crossbite causes crowding of tongue tip movement for lingual-alveolar sounds, the person may move the tongue backward, resulting in a palatal-dorsal articulation production. Compensatory speech productions are functional errors. Therefore, they always require speech therapy to change the articulation to a normal placement.

Some surgeons (and even some speech-language pathologists) advocate speech therapy to change articulation placement of compensatory errors before surgical correction of the VPI. (Ironically, these professionals would never suggest speech therapy to correct compensatory productions before repairing a cleft palate.) Although changing placement before correction of the structure is possible in some cases, it is very difficult, time-consuming, and therefore expensive. Even if successful, the change in placement usually results in a loss of intelligibility. (After all, compensatory errors are used to increase intelligibility.) Because of these issues, correcting the structure before speech therapy should be done whenever possible. This provides the child with the equipment to learn to produce sounds normally. Once structure is normalized, correction of the compensatory productions is much faster, easier, and less frustrating for both the child and the therapist.

With an Oronasal Fistula

The effect of an oronasal fistula on speech is determined by its size and location. If the oronasal fistula is symptomatic for speech, the child may compensate by either backing to the valve behind the fistula before the air escapes through it, or holding the tongue against the fistula to prevent nasal escape. These errors cannot be easily corrected with speech therapy as long as the fistula remains.

Ideally, surgical correction of a symptomatic oronasal fistula is needed before speech therapy should be initiated. However, the oronasal fistula closure is often done in conjunction with the bone graft at around age 6 or 7 so that it doesn't require a separate procedure. If the child is much younger and speech is affected, it is often worth using a palatal obturator to occlude the fistula for normal speech development and/or for speech therapy. The obturator is only used until the fistula is surgically closed.

Before VPI Surgery

If the child has VPI, it is usually better to wait until after the VPI surgery before beginning speech therapy to correct compensatory productions. Given the fact that compensatory productions develop because there is inadequate oral pressure for normal productions, correcting these productions in the presence of VPI is very difficult.

Typically, VPI surgery is done between the ages of 3 and 5. Of course, the earlier it is done, the better it is for speech. However, the surgery may be delayed for certain patients, such as those with Pierre Robin sequence and airway obstruction, and those with other structural anomalies or neurological disorders. If the surgery is on hold and there is concern that the child is developing compensatory productions, speech therapy can still be done with certain modifications.

The child needs to have enough air pressure in the oral cavity to work on pressure-sensitive consonant sounds. If there is not enough air pressure to work on placement, the speech-language pathologist can plug the child's nose during therapy, either manually or preferably with a nose clip. In addition, the child should wear the nose clip at home as much as possible, not just during practice. This allows the child to get the feel of oral pressure with speech, which can help with carryover.

After VPI Surgery

As noted previously, hypernasality and nasal emission are usually obligatory distortions that cannot be corrected with speech therapy. One notable exception is when there is continued nasality despite surgical correction of VPI.

Changing structure through VPI surgery does not change function, such as articulation placement. Therefore, if the child used productions to compensate for VPI before the surgery, these productions will continue to be used following the surgery. It should be remembered that to compensate for VPI, speech sounds are usually produced in the pharynx, where there is airflow. With this placement, the velopharyngeal valve must stay open for the release of air and sound. Therefore, there will still be the perception of hypernasality and/or nasal emission. In this case, speech therapy to correct compensatory productions by normalizing placement will eliminate the nasality, assuming the velopharyngeal valve is fully functional as a result of the surgery.

Continued hypernasality postoperatively may also occur if there was a large velopharyngeal opening preoperatively, with little lateral pharyngeal wall movement. Once a pharyngeal flap is placed in the midline, it may take a while for the lateral walls to move around the flap, because they had nothing to move against before the surgery. Sometimes, the lateral walls begin to function spontaneously after the surgery. In other cases, speech therapy (particularly with auditory feedback) is needed.

Finally, there may be residual hypernasality or nasal emission because the surgery was not totally successful. If this persists, despite normal articulation placement and auditory feedback, the child should be sent back for further evaluation and consideration of a surgical revision.

For Velopharyngeal Mislearning

Velopharyngeal mislearning is a cause of developmental misarticulations that cause nasal emission and sometimes hypernasality, despite normal velopharyngeal structure and physiology. For example, the substitution of ŋ/l and ŋ/r can increase the perception of nasality in connected speech. Changing the place and manner of production of these sounds leads to a change in overall resonance. In addition, the production of a pharyngeal fricative as a substitution for certain sibilants can lead to phoneme-specific nasal air emission. Again, speech therapy to normalize placement eliminates the nasal emission. Therefore, if the nasality is truly due to faulty placement rather than abnormal structure, speech therapy will be effective. (For more information about velopharyngeal mislearning and phoneme-specific nasal emission, see Chapter 7.)

Finally, speech therapy is appropriate when there is hypernasality or nasal emission due to oral-motor dysfunction, particularly apraxia. With inconsistent articulation of the anterior structures, there is also inconsistent articulation of the velopharyngeal valve. This results in variable resonance. Articulation therapy is therefore effective in improving the coordination of speech sound production.

When in Doubt

There are times when the cause of hypernasality or nasal emission is uncertain. In these cases, it is always best to do a trial period of speech therapy (Golding-Kushner, 2001; Hardin, 1991; Tomes, Kuehn, & Peterson-Falzone, 1996; Ysunza, Pamplona, & Toledo, 1992; Ysunza-Rivera, Pamplona-Ferreira, & Toledo-Cortina, 1991). It usually takes only a few weeks to determine whether the therapy will be effective. If either hypernasality or nasal air emission are noted with normal articulation, surgical intervention will likely be needed.

SPEECH THERAPY TECHNIQUES

Speech therapy is effective when the nasality is due to misarticulations. As noted above, the speech-language pathologist rarely, if ever, provides speech therapy for hypernasality and nasal emission in the absence of misarticulation, because when that occurs, these characteristics are usually due to VPI and not due to velopharyngeal mislearning. The only exceptions are residual hypernasality and/or nasal emission after VPI surgery and, in some cases, hypernasality secondary to dysarthria. In addition, therapy can be done while waiting for VPI surgery, although it is more effective after the surgery.

General Principles

Treating misarticulations that are the functional sequelae of velopharyngeal valving disorders and/or malocclusion is done through standard articulation therapy. The goal of therapy is correct placement (and sometimes manner) of production (Kummer, 2011).

The speech therapy techniques used with this population are not very different from the techniques that are used in therapy for other speech sound disorders. The following basic steps for correction are suggested:

- **Determine the first phonemes to target.** Determine which phonemes to target first.

  - **Select sounds in which the child is most stimulable.** If the child is stimulable for correct production, the sound will be easiest to correct. Therefore, working on this sound will give the child early success.

  - **Select sounds that will have the biggest impact on intelligibility.** In some cases, a developmental sequence may not be the best approach. For example, you may want to start with the /s/ sound when working with a 3-year-old, in order to promote the development of the other sibilants, rather than starting with an /f/ sound, which would have less of an impact on intelligibility.

  - **Select anterior sounds before posterior sounds.** Anterior sounds are more visible than other sounds and therefore easier for the child to correct.

  - **Select continuant cognate before a movement sounds.** With a continuant sound, the child can hold the placement. Therefore, /n/ is easier than /d/, and /ʃ/ is easier than /tʃ/.

- **Select the voiceless sound in isolation before the voiced cognate (which requires a vowel).** Voiceless sounds (e.g., /p/, /f/, or /s/) have one less feature than the voiced sound.

- **Be sure the child can discriminate between the correct and incorrect sounds.** Develop (or ensure) auditory and visual (whenever possible) discrimination between the correct and incorrect production. This may require initial work on auditory, visual, and sometimes tactile-kinesthetic discrimination between correct and incorrect productions.

- **Establish placement of production first.** Establish correct placement and then manner of production (including voicing).

- **Work on continuants and voiceless phonemes first in isolation.** These sounds can be produced in isolation, without the vowel. Therefore, work on these sounds in isolation, and have the child prolong the placement.

- **Work on voiced plosives in syllables.** For voiced plosives (e.g., /b/, /d/, /g/), work on the sound in a simple syllable with an easy vowel e.g., /bɑ/).

- **Begin with the sound in the initial position.** In general, begin with the sound in the initial position, unless the child is more stimulable for the final position. For the /r/, however, always begin with the final position (the final /ɚ/ is a continuant) and then move to the initial position, which requires movement.

- **Use /h/ to transition the consonant to the vowel.** If there is difficulty transitioning from the consonant to the vowel, separate the consonant and vowel by adding an /h/ before the vowel (e.g., /p/

.../hɑ/). Gradually, close the time gap between the two in order to achieve the syllable (e.g., /pɑ/).

- **Once placement is obtained, work on sound in the initial position.** Begin with syllables with various vowels; then work on single syllabic words; and finally, work on multisyllabic words.

- **Determine whether the medial or final position is easiest next.** Once the speech sound is produced correctly in the initial position, determine whether the child is more stimulable for production of that sound in the medial or final position. Choose the position that is easiest for the child, and make that the next step.

- **For medial position, break the word up initially into syllables.** For example, if the target is /k/ and the word is "baker," have the child produce each syllable individually, but in sequence. For example, she should say "ba...ker." Gradually, bring the two syllables closer together. The use of visuals (e.g., a red block for the first syllable and a blue block for the second syllable) can be helpful.

- **The phonemic context of a medial sound can change its production.** It is important to work on the sound, and not the letter, of medial phonemes. For example, in American English, the /t/ in words that end with /n/ (e.g., "kitten," "button," "mitten," etc.) is usually not aspirated but instead is co-articulated with a glottal stop.

- **When working on the final position, break up the word.** Introduce the final word position of the sound by first breaking up the syllable or word. For example, if the target sound is /k/ and the work is "bake," the child should say "baaaa...k."

- **When working on the final word position, combine it with a word that starts with a vowel.** If the word following the final consonant starts with a vowel, it makes the final consonant similar to an initial sound. For example, you could have the child say "Bake it." Have the child pause while holding the /k/ before going on to the next sound.

- **Work on sounds in categories.** If there are several errors in a class of speech sounds, work on sounds in phonological categories based on place or manner of production. This usually results in faster progress because several sounds can be corrected at once (Pamplona, Ysunza, & Espinosa, 1999).

- **When moving to the next sound in a category, change one feature at a time.** When the sound is in a related group of phonemes (e.g., plosives or bilabials), be sure to take small steps when moving to the next sound by changing only one feature at a time (e.g., placement, manner, or voicing).

- **For consonant blends, divide the clusters into individual components.** If the first sound is a continuant, that sound should be prolonged before moving on to the next sound. For example, for the word "snake," the child should say "ssss...nake." For the word "flag," the child should say. "fffff...lag" If the first sound is a plosive, the plosive should be made into a syllable. For example, for the word "play," the child should say "pa...lay."

- **When /s/ is combined with a typically voiceless consonant, the voiceless consonant becomes voiced.** When the /s/ is combined with a /p/, /t/, or /k/, these plosives are produced as their voiced cognates. Examples of this include the following:

- spell = s...bell

- stop = s...dop

- skate = s...gate

Again, it is important to work on the speech sound, not the written letter.

- **Work on the sound in carrier phrases.** When working on carrier phrases, it is helpful to start with the sound at the beginning of the carrier phrase. For example, when working on /l/, the carrier phrase may be "Let me ..." To make it harder, the target sound may be within the carrier phrase, such as "I like ..." or "I love ..." or "I like ..., but I don't like ..." The sound can even complete the carrier phrase, such as "I have a (ladder)."

- **Work on the sound in novel sentences.** Have the child produce a word with the sound in novel sentences. Correct only the targeted sound or sounds.

- **Obtain as many correct productions of the sound in a session as possible.** Correcting abnormal speech sound production requires motor learning, which occurs through feedback, and motor memory, which occurs through many repetitions (e.g., practice). Therefore, once the child is able to produce the sound accurately, speech therapy should incorporate drill work in order to achieve as many correct productions as possible in the session.

- **Work on carryover using unstructured speech.** While trying to produce the target sound correctly, have the child tell a story, relay an incident, describe a picture, give instructions, and so on. Also, have the child read out loud while trying to produce each word with the target sound correctly. Correct only errors on the targeted sound or sounds.

- **Involve the parents and caregivers (including babysitters) in the process.** Success of therapy, and particularly of carryover, depends on the frequency of practice at home. The parents should be given instructions for incorporating practice in their daily lives. Several short practice sessions each day can significantly improve progress, even if each practice session lasts only a few minutes.

Biofeedback

Biofeedback is a technique for making unconscious or autonomic physiological processes perceptible to the senses in order to manipulate them by conscious mental control. Biofeedback techniques are based on the principle that a desired response can be learned when it is determined that a specific thought process can produce that physiological response.

Different types of biofeedback techniques have been used in medicine for years and have been found to be effective for certain uses, such as reducing tension, decreasing heart rate, and even decreasing pain. In recent years, biofeedback techniques have been applied in speech pathology, particularly in the area of voice (Cavalli & Hartley, 2010; Maryn, De Bodt, & Van Cauwenberge, 2006; Rossiter, Howard, & DeCosta, 1996; Van Lierde, Claeys, De Bodt, & Van Cauwenberge, 2004), fluency (Saltuklaroglu, Dayalu, Kalinowski, Stuart, & Rastatter, 2004), and dysarthria (Marchant, McAuliffe, & Huckabee, 2008; Murdoch, Pitt, Theodoros, & Ward, 1999).

There are several ways to provide biofeedback of velopharyngeal function. The feedback can be auditory, visual, or tactile-kinesthetic. The biofeedback can be low-tech or high-tech using sophisticated instrumentation. The clinician must keep in mind that biofeedback will only be successful if the individual is anatomically and physiologically capable of achieving normal velopharyngeal closure. In addition, the individual needs to be old enough to actively participate and cognitively understand the feedback, and then determine what needs to be done to achieve a desired result.

Low-Tech Therapy Tools

There are several low-tech tools that can help to provide sensory stimulation and feedback (Kummer, 2011). These tools can be useful when working to correct misarticulations through therapy. Although all forms of sensory feedback can be helpful, auditory feedback is usually most effective because this is how speech is normally learned.

Straw

A simple bending straw can serve as the most useful therapy tool in a speech-language pathologist's "toolbox." Fortunately, it is cheap (less than a penny each), widely available (even in the cafeteria), and disposable (so you don't have to clean it!). The benefit of a straw is the same as that of a stethoscope in that it amplifies sound. In speech therapy, it can amplify the sound of the airstream (nasal or oral) and the phonated sound (resonance). To provide the child with feedback regarding hypernasality or nasal emission, have the child put one end of the straw at the entrance of a nostril and the other end in his ear (Figure 21–1). (The straw will need to be bent one more time.) When nasality occurs, it is very loud. The child should then be asked to the make adjustment in articulation to eliminate the nasality. To provide the child with feedback regarding oral

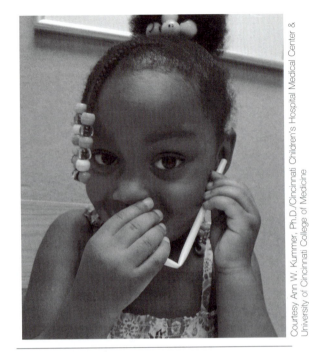

Courtesy Ann W. Kummer, Ph.D./Cincinnati Children's Hospital Medical Center & University of Cincinnati College of Medicine

FIGURE 21–1 Use of a straw. To provide the child with feedback regarding hypernasality or nasal emission, have the child put one end of the straw at the entrance of a nostril and the other end in his ear. When hypernasality or nasal air emission occurs during speech, it can be heard loudly through the tube.

airstream, put the end of the straw in the front of the incisors (Figure 21–2). The child will be able to hear the airflow during the production of oral sounds, particularly sibilants. (The sound of the airstream will be heard without putting the other end of the straw in the ear.) Have the child try to push the airstream through the straw.

Listening Tube

A "listening tube" can be used in exactly the same way as a straw. It can provide loud auditory feedback of nasality when one end is placed in the child's nostril and the other end is placed near the child's ear (Figure 21–3A and B). It can also provide feedback regarding

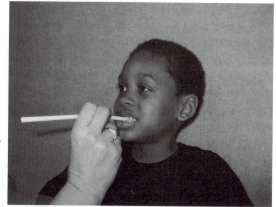

FIGURE 21–2 To promote anterior airflow during production of /s/ and other sibilants, put a straw in front of the child's incisors and have him or her try to produce the sound until he or she can hear the airflow through the straw. (This also works for correction of a lateral lisp.)

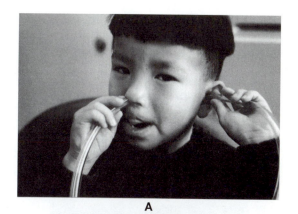

A

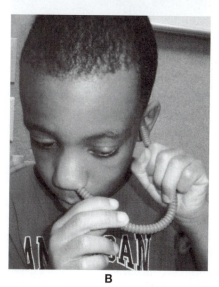

B

oral airflow when one end is placed in front of the child's lips or teeth and the other end is placed near the child's ear (Figure 21–4). A listening tube can consist of virtually any kind of flexible tubing. Suction tubing works particularly well (Figure 21–3). In addition, tube whistles work well and can double as a prize for the child at the end of the session (Figure 21–3B and Figure 21–4). The advantage of a tube is that it is longer. Therefore, when the child is listening for nasal emission, it is a little easier to use than a straw. The disadvantage is that it is less available, and it must be either disinfected for further use or used by only one child.

Oral & Nasal Listener™ (ONL)

Although a straw or a simple listening tube provides the child with feedback regarding resonance and nasal emission, the placement of the tubing in a nostril makes it harder for the clinician to hear the sound at the same time. This affects the clinician's ability to provide appropriate feedback and instruction. To solve this

FIGURE 21–3 (A and B) Use of a "listening tube." The child places one end of the tube at the entrance to a nostril and the other end by the ear. When hypernasality or nasal air emission occurs, they can be heard loudly through the tube. This provides excellent auditory feedback. The child is instructed to eliminate the sound in his or her ear when producing the oral sounds.

problem, the Oral & Nasal Listener™ (ONL) (Super Duper®) was developed at Cincinnati Children's Hospital Medical Center. It is basically a dual stethoscope, which allows both the child and the speech-language

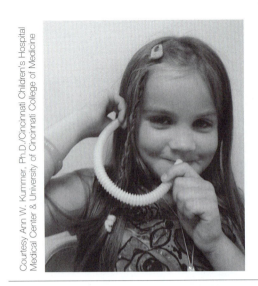

Courtesy Ann W. Kummer, Ph.D./Cincinnati Children's Hospital Medical Center & University of Cincinnati College of Medicine

FIGURE 21–4 Use of a tube to provide feedback of oral pressure. The child is asked to produce the sound so that it is loud in his or her ear.

pathologist to hear the nasality and also oral airflow at the same time and at the same volume (Figure 21–5A).

To provide the child with feedback regarding hypernasality and/or nasal emission, the end of the tube is placed in the child's nostril. The child is then asked to use that feedback to eliminate the nasality. The speech-language pathologist can then give appropriate feedback to the child and monitor progress with the therapy (Figure 21–5B).

To provide the child with feedback regarding oral airflow, the funnel is added to the end of the tube and is placed in front of the mouth. The ONL amplifies the oral speech sounds and allows the child to easily hear the difference between weak consonants or hypernasal vowels and those that are oral. With the ONL, the child can better compare her own productions with the models provided by the clinician (Figure 21–5C). (This also works very well for children who have hearing problems or are easily distracted in therapy.)

Although practice at home is critically important for progress and ultimate carryover, parents are often unsure about what they are hearing and how to give feedback. With the ONL, the parents can easily hear abnormal nasal emission and hypernasality, so they can provide more effective feedback and also know when the child is making progress. This makes the practice at home much more effective.

Air Paddle

A little paddle can be cut from a piece of paper and serve as a visual feedback device for oral air pressure. The air paddle is placed in front of the child's mouth during the production of pressure-sensitive phonemes (Figure 21–6). The child is asked to produce the sound with enough air pressure to force the air paddle to move. This works best for plosives but is less effective for fricatives.

See-Scape

The See-Scape is a pneumatic device that is sold by several distributors (Pro-Ed; Mayer Johnson; Slosson Educational Publications; AliMed, etc.). A "nasal olive" is placed in the child's nostril. The nasal olive is attached to a flexible tube that is connected to a rigid plastic vertical tube. The child is asked to produce pressure-sensitive consonants (plosives, fricatives, and affricates) without allowing the Styrofoam float to rise in the tube (Figure 21–7). (Note that the float will rise during the production of nasal phonemes and with nasal breathing at the end of the utterance.)

There are several significant problems with this device. First, it is very expensive! The retail cost of over $100 is not insignificant. Second, children love to see the Styrofoam float rise in the tube. They have less incentive to keep it from moving in the tube. Perhaps the

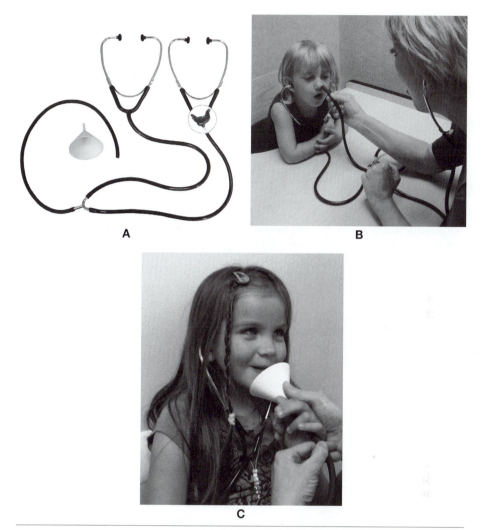

FIGURE 21–5 (A–C) (A) The Oral & Nasal Listener (ONL) (Super Duper Publications at www.superduperinc.com). (B) The Oral & Nasal Listener was designed to allow the child and the speech-language pathologist (or the parent) to hear the nasal emission or hypernasality in an amplified manner and at the same time. With this device, the adult is able to give the child appropriate feedback. Otherwise, it is hard for the adult to hear the nasal emission because the tube is in the child's nose. (C) With the funnel, the oral sound is amplified for the child. Again, the adult can hear what the child hears. This device is useful for not only work on resonance and nasal emission, but it can also be used for working on articulation, particularly for children who need amplified feedback. (*The Oral & Nasal Listener was developed by Jonathon Cross, Jessica Link, and Ann Kummer at Cincinnati Children's Hospital Medical Center and is patented under the name Nasoscope, 12/2/03, patent number: 6656128.*)

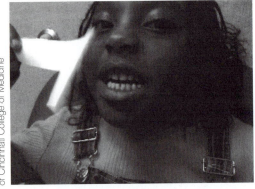

Courtesy Ann W. Kummer, Ph.D./Cincinnati Children's Hospital Medical Center & University of Cincinnati College of Medicine

FIGURE 21–6 Use of an air paddle to encourage an increase in oral pressure during production of plosives. The child is instructed to try to make the paper move with each plosive production.

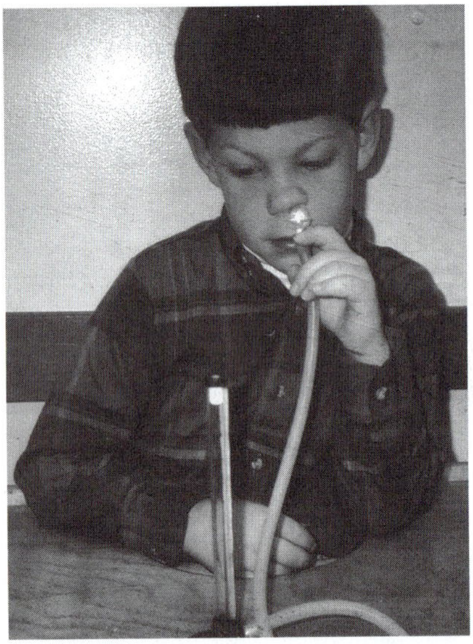

Courtesy Ann W. Kummer, Ph.D./Cincinnati Children's Hospital Medical Center & University of Cincinnati College of Medicine

FIGURE 21–7 Use of the See-Scape. The child is instructed to put the nasal olive in one nostril. The child is then asked to try to produce pressure consonants repetitively without allowing the foam stopper to rise in the tube.

biggest concern, however, relates to infection control. Although this device should be thoroughly cleaned and disinfected between uses, this is not easily done, particularly with the Styrofoam float.

High-Tech Therapy Tools

Speech therapy, even with children, requires minimal resources and virtually no equipment. However, when equipment is available, particularly equipment that is found in a hospital setting, there are some benefits to its use in treatment.

Digital Recording Equipment

Audio recordings can be used to help the child discriminate between normal and nasal speech. Different samples of normal speech and speech with nasality can be used. In addition, recordings of the child's good and "not so good" productions can also be used to help the child self-evaluate his own productions.

Nasometer

The Nasometer (KayPENTAX, Montvale, N.J.) provides the child with visual feedback that can help in eliminating compensatory errors and errors that cause phoneme-specific nasal air emission. It can also be used to modify resonance in certain cases of velopharyngeal incompetence due to neuromotor dysfunction (Bae, Kuehn, & Ha, 2007; Heppt, Westrich, Strate, & Mohring, 1991). The clinician can set a threshold line to serve as the child's visual target. The target can be adjusted downward as the child becomes more proficient in reaching the goal.

The Nasometer software includes lists of sentences that are useful in therapy. These sentences are grouped according to phoneme and degree of difficulty in achieving velopharyngeal closure. Statistics regarding performance can help the clinician to track the child's progress over time with serial records (see Chapter 14 for more information).

Pressure-Flow Instrumentation

The pressure-flow instrumentation can be used to provide visual feedback, which can be helpful in eliminating compensatory errors, such as glottal stops and pharyngeal fricatives. It can also be used to facilitate a change in articulation errors that cause phoneme-specific nasal air emission (see Figure 15–20). Aerodynamic instrumentation can also be useful for providing feedback regarding breath support. Finally, pressure-flow instrumentation can provide objective documentation of therapy progress (see Chapter 15 for more information).

Nasopharyngoscopy

Nasopharyngoscopy provides visual feedback regarding the actions of the velopharyngeal mechanism during speech (Brunner, Stellzig-Eisenhauer, Proschel, Verres, & Komposch, 2005; Bzoch, 2004; Rich, Farber, & Shprintzen, 1988; Siegel-Sadewitz & Shprintzen, 1982; Witzel, Tobe, & Salyer, 1988, 1989; Ysunza, Pamplona, Femat, Mayer, & Garcia-Velasco, 1997). This can help the child to develop a degree of active control of the velopharyngeal movements for opening and closing the valve (Brunner et. al., 2005; Bzoch, 2004). Nasopharyngoscopy is the only practical method for direct visualization of the velopharyngeal mechanism for biofeedback because it is well tolerated by most children and does not involve radiation (O'Sullivan, Finger, & Zwerdling, 2004; Santos, Cipolotti, D'Avila, & Gurgel, 2005).

As a biofeedback tool, nasopharyngoscopy is appropriate for children who have the physical ability to achieve velopharyngeal closure but demonstrate phoneme-specific nasal emission or hypernasality due to faulty articulation (Witzel et al., 1988). Nasopharyngoscopy may also be useful in helping children to increase lateral pharyngeal wall movement following a pharyngeal flap procedure (Paal, Reulbach,

Strobel-Schwarthoff, Nkenke, & Schuster, 2005; Siegel-Sadewitz & Shprintzen, 1982; Witzel et al., 1989; Ysunza et al., 1997). However, research suggests that nasopharyngoscopy may only be effective as an adjunct to traditional speech therapy (Neumann & Romonath, 2011).

The biofeedback procedure begins by helping the child to identify the velopharyngeal structures on the video monitor. The child is then instructed to swallow, blow, or produce a sound repetitively that results in complete closure. The action of the velopharyngeal mechanism is pointed out to the child. Therapy then focuses on achieving velopharyngeal closure for the phonemes where closure is normally incomplete. This is done not only by using the visual feedback but also by changing the place of production for these sounds, with techniques noted above.

Once the placement is changed and the child is able to achieve closure on the target phoneme, it is sometimes helpful to have the child go back and forth between the "good production" and the "bad production" to be able to feel, see, and hear the difference. This helps to develop voluntary control. Once the placement is achieved and the sound can be reproduced with correct placement easily, then the child is ready for traditional speech therapy (see Chapter 17 for more information).

Specific Therapy Techniques

Whenever possible, clinical decision making should incorporate the principles of evidence-based practice (EBP) (American Speech-Language-Hearing Association [ASHA], 2005). EBP is the integration of practitioner expertise with current research to provide quality clinical care. The therapy techniques that are offered here are based primarily on this author's extensive experience and expertise.

Research is always needed on the efficacy of specific techniques in comparison with others.

The following section describes some specific therapy techniques that are helpful for correction of articulation productions that are produced in the pharynx—either as compensatory productions or merely mislearning.

GLOTTAL STOP

A glottal stop is produced by vocal fold adduction and a sudden release, resulting in a voiced grunt-like sound. A glottal stop is often substituted for oral plosives when there is inadequate oral pressure due to VPI.

The following suggestions are offered for eliminating the glottal stop:

Awareness

Tell the child that you are going to eliminate the "jerk" in her neck during the sound production.

Feedback

- **Visual feedback:** Have the child watch her neck in a mirror during production of the glottal stop. The child will notice an obvious movement in the neck area in front of the larynx. Then have the child produce a prolonged vowel or a nasal-vowel syllable in order to notice the difference. Have the child watch your neck as you produce the plosive without the glottal stop.

- **Tactile feedback:** Have the child place her hand on her neck, over the larynx, during the production of a syllable where she would normally produce a glottal stop (Figure 21–8). Tell her to feel the "jerk" during production. Then have her feel her neck during a prolonged vowel or a nasal-vowel syllable (e.g., /mɑ/) in order to feel the difference. Have the child feel your neck as you produce the plosive without the glottal stop.

- **Auditory feedback:** Have the child listen to your productions of plosives without the glottal stop, and then plosives with co-articulation of the glottal stop. Perhaps have the child point to a happy face or sad face to indicate the correct versus incorrect production.

Production

1. Have the child produce a voiceless plosive (e.g., /p/) without the vowel. (A glottal stop is voiced. Therefore, it does not occur until transition from a voiceless phoneme to the voiced vowel.)

2. Have the child produce the voiceless plosive and then the vowel preceded by an /h/ (e.g., /p...hhhhɑ/ for /pɑ/, and /p...hhhho/ for /po/). The /h/ is voiceless, and this keeps the vocal cords open and prevents the production of a glottal stop. Gradually decrease the transition time from the consonant to the /h/ and then the vowel. As the transition is decreased, the /h/ essentially disappears so that the syllable is produced normally without a glottal stop.

3. Once syllables beginning with voiceless plosives are produced easily, move to voiced plosives. Have the child "whisper" the voice plosive while feeling the neck, watching in a mirror, and hearing the sound.

4. Have the child "whisper" the voice plosive and then the vowel preceded by an /h/. Gradually add "smooth" voicing and transition to the vowel with an inserted /h/. Continue to have the child watch, look, and feel for feedback.

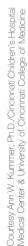
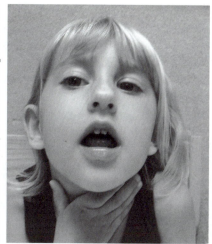

Courtesy Ann W. Kummer, Ph.D./Cincinnati Children's Hospital Medical Center & University of Cincinnati College of Medicine

FIGURE 21–8   To eliminate glottal stops, have the child feel his or her neck for the "jerk" during production. Then have the child feel the difference with the production of /p/.

PHARYNGEAL PLOSIVE

A pharyngeal plosive is produced when the posterior base of the tongue articulates against the posterior pharyngeal wall. A pharyngeal plosive can be a compensatory production for VPI. It is typically substituted for velar phonemes (/k/ or /g/).

The following suggestions are offered for eliminating the pharyngeal plosive and replacing it with the appropriate velar placement.

Awareness

Tell the child that his current sound is produced in his throat. The goal is to make the sound in the back of the mouth instead.

Feedback

- **Visual feedback:** Have the child watch his mouth in a mirror during production of the pharyngeal plosive. Then have the child watch your mouth as you produce a velar sound (/k/ or /g/).

- **Tactile feedback:** Have the child place his hand at the top of his neck, just under his chin during the production of a syllable where he would normally produce a pharyngeal plosive (same as in Figure 21–8). Tell him to feel the "jerk" during production. Then have him feel your neck during production of a velar sound in order to feel the difference.

- **Auditory feedback:** Have the child listen to your productions of velars. If you can imitate a pharyngeal plosive, have the child indicate the correct versus incorrect production.

Production

1. Establish placement by starting with an /ŋ/. If the child can't produce an /ŋ/, put a tongue blade on the mid-part of the tongue. Push down and back slightly. Then put your thumb under the base of the chin, which is under the base of the tongue, and press up firmly. Have the child produce the sound with the help of this manipulation. Also, have the child try to produce the velar with the nose closed. (A nose clip can be helpful.) This prevents the production of the pharyngeal plosive, which requires nasal airflow.

(Continues)

(Continued)

2. Once placement for the /ŋ/ has been obtained, have the child produce an /ŋ/ and then drop the tongue. This should be done repetitively to work on an up-and-down movement of the back of the tongue, rather than a back-and-forth movement, which occurs with the pharyngeal plosive.

3. Have the child close his nose, take a breath, place the tongue in an /ŋ/ position, and then drop the tongue quickly for a /k/ sound. Alternatively, the child can produce an /ŋ/ and drop the tongue for a /g/.

4. Once the child is able to do this a few times, have the child do it without the nose closed.

PHARYNGEAL OR NASAL FRICATIVE/AFFRICATE

A pharyngeal or nasal fricative (or affricate) is usually substituted for a sibilant sound, particularly /s/ and /z/. They can be compensatory productions that require speech therapy after surgical correction of VPI, or they can be mislearned productions that cause phoneme-specific nasal air emission. Regardless of the original cause, the methods for correction are the same.

Before discussing specific therapy techniques, it is important to recognize that the /t/ is developed prior to sibilant phonemes, and it serves as a "building block" sound. The /s/ and /ʃ/ sounds are related to the /t/. They are both produced with the tongue tip under, or just behind, the alveolar ridge. In fact, if you produced a /t/ with the teeth closed and prolong it, it turns into an /s/ with the appropriate tongue placement. The /t/ sound is a component of the /ʧ/ sound (/t/ + /ʃ/ = /ʧ/) and its voiced cognate, /d/ is a component of the /j/ sound (/d /+ /ʒ/ = /dʒ/). Therefore, in most cases, the child needs to be able to produce the /t/ and /d/ sounds before being able to produce sibilants sounds correctly.

The following suggestions are offered for eliminating the pharyngeal plosive and replacing it with the appropriate velar placement.

Awareness

Tell the child that her current sound is produced in her throat. The goal is to make the sound in the front of the mouth with the tongue instead.

Feedback

- **Visual feedback:** Have the child watch her tongue tip movement in a mirror during production of the /t/ sound. Then have the child watch your mouth as you produce a /t/ sound.

- **Tactile feedback:** Have the child produce the sound as she normally does (pharyngeal or nasal), and then have her pinch her nostrils closed. The child will feel the nasal blockage. Then ask the child to place her hand in front of your mouth as you produce the /t/ sound and then an /s/ sound. Tell the child to note the feel of the airstream as a result of this sound production. Then have the child put her hand in front of her own mouth while she tries to produce a /t/ and /s/ and feel the airstream. (The child should wash her hands or use a waterless disinfectant on her hands immediately after this procedure.)

(Continues)

(Continued)

- **Auditory feedback:** Put the end of a straw or tube in the child's nose and the other end in the child's ear. Have the child produce the sound as she normally does (pharyngeal or nasal). The child will hear significant nasal air emission through the tube. Have the child produce another oral sound that is normally produced correctly. Make sure the child notes that there is no nasal air emission during production of an orally produced sound. It is sometimes helpful to put the end of the straw or tube in your nose and the other end in the child's ear. Produce the /s/ sound normally and have the child note that there is no audible nasal air emission through the tube.

Production

For /s/:

1. Have the child try to produce the /s/ sound with the nostrils occluded and then open in order to get the feel for oral rather than pharyngeal airflow (Figure 21–9).

2. Have the child produce a /t/ sound, noting the tongue tip movement.

3. Then have the child produce the /t/ with the teeth closed, which results in /ts/.

4. Have the child increase the duration of the production until it becomes /tssss/.

5. Have the child prolong the sound. Have the child note the position of the tongue and the feel of the airstream flowing over the tongue tip during production.

6. Finally, eliminate the tongue tip movement for the /t/ component.

And/Or:

1. Put one end of a straw or tube in the child's nostril and the other end in the child's ear (Figure 21–1).

2. Have the child produce the /t/ with her teeth closed.

3. Tell the child to be sure she doesn't hear anything coming through the tube.

And/Or:

1. Put a straw in just in front of the incisors (Figure 21–2).

2. Have the child produce a /t/ sound while consciously trying to push air into the straw. If the air goes through the straw, this will be heard.

3. Have the child do the same thing with her teeth closed. This results in an /s/ sound.

For /ʃ/, /ʧ/ and /ʤ/:

1. Start with /ʧ/, because this sound contains a /t/ and is voiceless. Follow the same procedures as noted above for /s/, but have the child round the lips during production. Tell the child that this is a sneeze sound with the teeth closed.

2. Once the /ʧ/ sound is mastered, work on the /ʤ/ in the same way, but start with a /d/ sound.

3. Once /ʧ/ is mastered, have the child prolong the sound and note the position of the tongue and feel the airstream flowing over the tongue tip during production.

4. Finally, eliminate the tongue tip movement for the /t/ component.

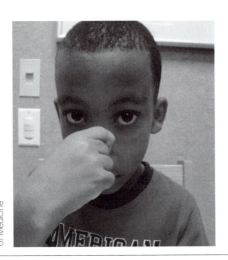

Courtesy Ann W. Kummer, Ph.D./Cincinnati Children's Hospital Medical Center & University of Cincinnati College of Medicine

FIGURE 21–9 Nose pinch or cul-de-sac technique. The child is asked to pinch his or her nostrils during the production of pressure sounds to eliminate the nasal air emission. The child is told to feel the increase in oral airflow and pressure. The child is then instructed to produce the sounds in the same way with the nostrils unoccluded.

PALATAL-DORSAL PRODUCTION (MIDDORSUM PALATAL STOP)

A palatal-dorsal production (also called a middorsum palatal stop) is substituted for lingual-alveolars (/t/, /d/, /n/, or /l/), and also for sibilants (/s/, /z/, /ʃ/, /ʧ/, and /ʤ/). This placement can result in a lateral distortion on all of these sounds. Middorsum palatal stops are often compensatory errors for tongue tip crowding caused by an anterior crossbite or Class III malocclusion.

For lingual-alveolars:

Awareness

Tell the child that his current sound is produced with the middle of the tongue. The goal will be to make the sound with the tongue tip instead.

Feedback

- **Visual feedback:** Have the child watch his tongue tip movement in a mirror during production of the /t/ sound. Then have the child watch your mouth as you produce a /t/ sound. Note that the child's tongue tip will be down during production instead of up.

- **Tactile feedback:** Have the child produce the sound as he normally does. Then have the child use a tongue blade to touch the part of the tongue that articulates against the palate. Have the child then touch the tongue tip, which will be used for the new articulation

- **Auditory feedback:** Put the end of a straw just in front of your central incisors (Figure 21–2). Produce a /t/ sound, making sure that the airstream goes through the straw. Have the child note the sound of air through the straw. Then produce the /t/ sound with a lateral lisp. (Hold the tongue up so the air is emitted laterally.) Note that the air does not go through the straw. You can move the straw to the side of the dental arch until you find where the airstream is actually being emitted (Figure 21–10).

(Continues)

(Continued)
Production

1. Have the child bite on a tongue blade (Figure 21–11).

2. Tell the child to put the tongue tip on the tongue blade and then back down.

3. Then, have the child produce an /n/ sound, using the tongue tip, and hold the sound. Have him note the placement.

4. Have the child work on achieving that placement and then dropping the tongue. This can be done silently and then with voicing.

5. Have the child take a deep breath, achieve the /n/ placement, hold it, and then drop the tongue to produce a plosive (/t/ or /d/).

6. Place a straw in front of the child's incisors. Tell the child to use the tongue tip to push the air through the straw during production of /t/.

For Sibilants:

(Note: The child must be able to produce a /t/ sound correctly before attempting to correct the sibilants.)

Awareness

Tell the child that his current sound is produced with the middle of the tongue touching the roof of the mouth. This causes air to go out the sides of the mouth. The goal is to make the sound so the air goes over the tip of the tongue instead.

Feedback

- **Visual feedback:** Have the child watch his tongue tip movement in a mirror during production of the /t/ sound. Tell the child that for the /s/ sound, the air goes just between the tongue tip area used for a /t/.

- **Tactile feedback:** Have the child produce the sound as he normally does. Then have the child use a tongue blade to touch the part of the tongue that articulates against the palate. Have the child then touch the tongue tip, which will be used for the new articulation.

- **Auditory feedback:** Put the end of a straw just in front of your central incisors. Produce an /s/ sound, making sure that the airstream goes through the straw. Have the child note the sound of air through the straw. Then produce the /s/ sound with a lateral lisp. (Hold the tongue up so the air is emitted laterally.) Note that the air does not go through the straw. You can move the straw to the side of the dental arch until you find where the airstream is actually being emitted.

Production

1. Place the straw at the front of the child's closed incisors during production of the /s/ and note the lack of airstream through the straw (Figure 21–2).

2. Move the straw to the side of the child's dental arch during production of the /s/, and find the place where the airstream can be heard through the straw (Figure 21–10).

3. Have the child put the straw at the front of his closed incisors and produce a /t/ while keeping the teeth closed. Tell the child to push the air into the straw.

4. Have the child close the teeth, produce the /t/, and prolong it until it is a /tssssss/. This can be done while trying to push the air through the straw.

(Continues)

(Continued)

5. Have the child feel the airflow over the tongue and hear the air through the straw.

6. Then have the child achieve the position for /s/ and /ʃ/ without starting with the /t/.

7. The /ʧ/ sound may be easier to achieve than an /s/ in some cases. This is because the /ʧ/ contains a /t/ sound. The child should be told to close the teeth, round the lips, produce a /t/, and prolong it. Have the child feel the airstream over the tongue. Then have the child find the same position to produce an /ʃ/ without starting with a /t/.

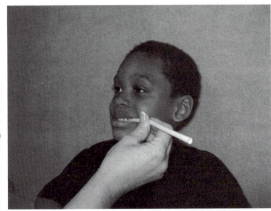

Courtesy Ann W. Kummer, Ph.D./Cincinnati Children's Hospital Medical Center & University of Cincinnati College of Medicine

FIGURE 21–10 To eliminate a lateral distortion, put a straw on the side of the dental arch until you hear air going through the straw during a sustained /s/. Then place the straw in the front of the child's dental arch and note that there is no air going through the straw. Have the child produce a /t/ sound and push the air into the straw. Then have the child do the same with the teeth closed until it produces an /s/.

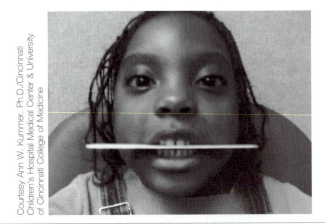

Courtesy Ann W. Kummer, Ph.D./Cincinnati Children's Hospital Medical Center & University of Cincinnati College of Medicine

FIGURE 21–11 To eliminate palatal-dorsal articulation of lingual-alveolar sounds, have the child bite on a tongue blade. Then have the child try to produce the sounds with the tongue tip articulating on the tongue blade.

NASALIZED (OR OTHERWISE DISTORTED) /ɚ/ AND /R/

The final /ɚ/ sound is produced by articulating the sides of the posterior tongue against the gum under the molars. The middle portion of the tongue forms a boat-like shape through which sound resonates. If the child raises the entire back of the tongue, the sound becomes an /ŋ/ sound, which results in nasal resonance. Of course, another common error is when the back of the tongue does not raise on each side. Regardless of the error, the following techniques help to achieve appropriate placement.

It should be noted that the final /ɚ/ is a continuant, where the initial /r/ requires achieving the /ɚ/ placement first, and then moving the tongue forward. Therefore, it is important to establish normal production of /ɚ/ before working on initial /r/.

Awareness

Tell the child that the /ɚ/ sound is produced with the sides of tongue touching the roof of the mouth. Using your hand, show the child how the shape of the tongue forms a boat. In addition, the back of the tongue must touch the gums near the back teeth (Figure 21–12).

Feedback

- **Visual feedback:** Produce the /ɚ/ sound. Using a flashlight, have the child note that the back of your tongue is up on both sides.

- **Tactile feedback:** Using a tongue blade, lightly scratch the sides of the child's tongue toward the back. This causes the tongue to tingle for a few seconds. Have the child produce the sound as usual. Ask the child to determine whether the tingly part of his tongue is down or up or whether the middle part of the tongue is up.

- **Auditory feedback:** Auditory training and discrimination is particularly important when working on /ɚ/ so that the child can ultimately achieve the right acoustic quality. Have the child listen to your correct production of /ɚ/ and then your incorrect production of /ɚ/. Have the child listen carefully and indicate correct versus incorrect productions.

Production of /ɚ/

1. With a tongue blade, stimulate both sides of the tongue toward the back (Figure 21–13A). Then stimulate the gum ridge just under or behind the maxillary molars. This causes tingling of both. Tell the child to put the two together.

2. If necessary, manually assist the child with placement. Put your thumb under the base of the chin, which is under the base of the tongue, and press up firmly. If you feel resistance, have the child make it loose until you can push up easily. To achieve lip placement at the same time, use your middle finger to push under the chin, while squeezing the cheeks with your thumb and forefinger to obtain lip rounding (Figure 21–13B).

Production of /r/

1. Once the final /ɚ/ is established, demonstrate with your hand how the tongue tip moves forward for the initial /r/.

2. Tell the child that the /r/ is produced with the tongue and not the lips. Demonstrate the difference in the lips when producing /r/ and /w/.

(Continues)

(Continued)

3. Have the child place his hands on his cheeks and watch his lips in a mirror. Have the child produce a /w/ sound. He should feel the movement of the cheeks, due to the movement of the lips, and also see the movement of the lips in a mirror. Tell the child that with /r/, there should be no movement of the tongue only and not the face or lips.

4. While watching in a mirror and with his hands on his cheeks, have the child begin by producing the final /ɚ/. Then have the child move the tongue forward for initial /r/, while making sure that there is no movement felt in the cheeks or seen with his lips.

And/Or

1. If the child continues to raise the entire back of the tongue for /ɚ/, resulting in an /ŋ/, close the child's nose during production of the sound. That makes the /ŋ/ sound impossible to produce.

2. Have the child think of forming the back of the tongue around a tube so that sound can go through the middle.

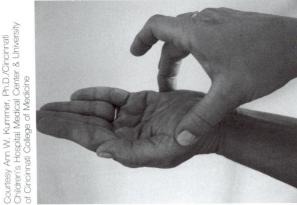

Courtesy Ann W. Kummer, Ph.D./Cincinnati Children's Hospital Medical Center & University of Cincinnati College of Medicine

FIGURE 21–12   Working on the /ɚr/ phoneme. Show the child with your hands how the tongue makes a boat shape and how the back of the tongue must articulate on the gums near the upper molars.

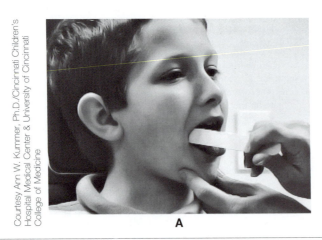

Courtesy Ann W. Kummer, Ph.D./Cincinnati Children's Hospital Medical Center & University of Cincinnati College of Medicine

A

FIGURE 21–13 A   Stimulate the back of the tongue on both sides and then the upper gums on both side just behind the molars.

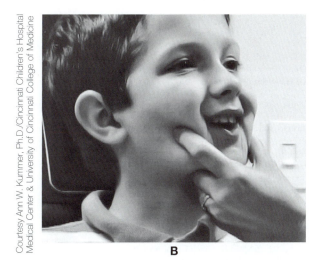

Courtesy Ann W. Kummer, Ph.D./Cincinnati Children's Hospital Medical Center & University of Cincinnati College of Medicine

B

FIGURE 21–13 B To encourage appropriate placement for final /ər/, use your middle finger to push up firmly under the child's chin, near the neck. This pushes against the base of the tongue. With the index finger and thumb, squeeze the cheeks to promote lip rounding.

NASALIZED PHONEMES

Nasalized vowels and consonants can be obligatory distortions due to VPI. If that is the case, therapy is inappropriate. However, they can persist after correction of VPI, or they can be phoneme-specific errors due to mislearning in the absence of a structural anomaly. Phoneme-specific hypernasality is most common on high vowels, particularly /i/, and can occur due to substitution of ŋ/l or for ŋ/ɚ.

Awareness

Tell the child that not enough sound can get into his mouth because the back of her tongue blocks it. The goal is to get the back of the tongue down in order to open the back of the mouth. This allows more sound to come out the mouth.

Feedback

- **Visual feedback:** Using a flashlight, have the child look in your mouth as you say /æ/ with your tongue out as far as possible. Have the child note how the back of your tongue is down so that all the sound can come out. (Mentioning the velum is not necessary or effective because the child has little, if any, active control over its movement.)

- **Tactile feedback:** Have the child place her fingers on the side of the nose while producing the sound as he normally does. The child will be able to feel vibration from the hypernasality. Have the child produce an oral sound that he does not nasalize. Have the child note that there is no vibration (Figure 21–14).

- **Auditory feedback:** Produce the targeted sound for the child. Then close your nose while you produce the sound. Point out that there is no difference in the sound when the nose is closed. Have the child produce the sound as she normally does and then do it again with the nose closed. Point out that there is a change in the sound because it is coming out of the nose.

(Continues)

(Continued)
Production

1. Begin with correct placement of the sound, using the nasal cognate of the oral target (e.g., /m/ for bilabial, /n/ for lingual-alveolars, and /ŋ/ for velars). Have the child feel the placement while prolonging the sound.

2. Have the child achieve that placement and then silently open the lips or drop the tongue as appropriate.

3. Have the child pinch her nostrils and whisper while achieving the placement and then opening the lips or dropping the tongue (same as in Figure 21–9). A nose clip can be used during therapy and practice (Figure 21–15). Have the child note the increase in oral airflow and pressure.

4. Have the child try to produce the sounds in the same way with the nostrils unoccluded.

And/Or:

1. Ask the child to produce a big yawn, which causes the back of the tongue to go down and the velum to go up.

2. Have the child take note of the "stretch" in the back of the mouth.

3. Have the child co-articulate the affected sound (e.g., /l/ or /i/) with a yawn. (The /i/ is hard to do with a yawn, but the child should be thinking about the feel of getting it down with a yawn.

4. Gradually have the child make the co-articulate yawn a little smaller.

5. Have the child produce the new sound with the nose open and then closed. If there is a difference, have the child try to make the sound the same with the nose open and with it closed.

And/Or:

For nasalized vowels, particularly with dysarthria:

1. While the child is producing a vowel sound, preferably /ɑ/, use a tongue blade to lift the velum up. This should be done by gradually stimulating first the hard palate and then the velum with the tongue blade so that the gag reflux is not activated. If the child has a very active gag reflex, this technique is not appropriate. (Note: If there is a significant difference in resonance with elevation using the tongue blade, the child may be a good candidate for a palatal lift.) Have the child listen to the difference in production through a tube or straw.

2. Next, have the child try to produce oral-nasal contrasts with the vowel while receiving feedback through a tube or straw.

The above techniques are only effective if the child has the physical ability (adequate structure and neurophysiological abilities) to produce the speech sounds. In addition, speech therapy should continue only if the child is making progress. If hypernasality and/or nasal emission persist, despite normal articulation placement, velopharyngeal function should be evaluated (or reevaluated). This should be done by VPI specialists (not a general practice otolaryngologist or plastic surgeon), particularly those associated with a cleft or craniofacial team. Speech therapy should be discontinued if there has not been demonstrable progress over the past several months.

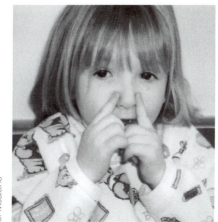

FIGURE 21–14 Tactile feedback for nasal air emission or hypernasality. By having the child lightly touch the side of his or her nose, the child will be able to feel the vibration that occurs with hypernasality or nasal air emission.

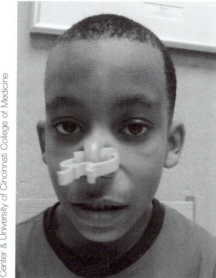

FIGURE 21–15 Nose clip. A nose clip can be used during therapy and practice at home if the child has VPI and surgery is being delayed. This helps increase in oral airflow and pressure so that the child can work on articulation placement.

Oral-Motor Exercises ... They Do *Not* Work!

In the past, clinicians used a variety of oral-motor "exercises" in hopes of strengthening the muscles of the velopharyngeal valve to improve function for speech (Berry & Eisenson, 1956; Kanter, 1947; Massengill, Quinn, Pickrell, & Levinson, 1968; Muttiah, Georges, & Brackenbury, 2011; Van Riper, 1963). Several investigators even tried to stimulate velopharyngeal movement through the use of electrical "exercisors" (Cole, 1971, 1979; Lubit & Larsen, 1969, 1971; Massengill, Quinn, & Pickrell, 1971; Peterson, 1974; Tash, Shelton, Knox, & Michel, 1971; Weber, Jobe, & Chase, 1970; Yules & Chase, 1969). However, these exercises were not effective (Kuehn & Henne, 2003; Powers & Starr, 1974; Ruscello, 1982, 2008).

Later research showed significant differences in the velopharyngeal closure patterns of speech and nonspeech activities, suggesting that nonspeech "exercises" could not possibly be effective in improving velopharyngeal function for speech (Flowers & Morris, 1973; Golding-Kushner, 2001; Moll, 1965; Peterson, 1973; Peterson-Falzone, Trost-Cardamone, Karnell, & Hardin-Jones, 2006; Shprintzen, Lencione, McCall, & Skolnick, 1974). In addition, children with a history of cleft have a structural abnormality—not weakness of the musculature that would respond to exercise. Even if exercises could improve velopharyngeal function, the child would have to continue the exercises for the rest of his life in order to maintain that improvement!

Given current knowledge and the need to adhere to an evidence-based practice, procedures that should not be used in the treatment of speech disorders related to VPI include blowing, sucking, whistling, gagging, swallowing, cheek puffing, icing, stroking, palatal massage, electrical stimulation, playing wind instru-

ments, or any type of oral-motor exercises (Golding-Kushner, 2001; Kummer, 2011; Lof, 2008, 2011; McCauley, Strand, Lof, Schooling, & Frymark, 2009; Ruscello, 2008a, 2008b; Watson & Lof, 2008). Unfortunately, even though there is a total lack of evidence in the literature to support the efficacy of nonspeech exercises in improving velopharyngeal function (or even speech), and although it does not even make sense to use exercises for structural abnormalities, some clinicians continue to incorporate these exercises in their treatment (Lof & Watson, 2008; Watson & Lof, 2009).

SPECIAL PROCEDURES

There are a few special treatment procedures that warrant mention here. These procedures are controversial and require additional research.

Continuous Positive Airway Pressure (CPAP)

A *continuous positive airway pressure (CPAP)* device is an instrument that consists of a flow generator, a valve mechanism, a hose, and a nasal mask. Airflow and air pressure are delivered to the nasal cavity, and thus the pharynx, through the hose and nasal mask. CPAP has been found to be useful in the treatment of individuals with obstructive sleep apnea (OSA) because the positive pressure prevents the collapse of the pharyngeal airway during sleep.

Kuehn (1991, 1997) described the use of CPAP as a means for treating hypernasality. He suggested that CPAP could provide resistance training for the velopharyngeal muscles by having them work actively against the positive air pressure. Based on the principles of exercise physiology, CPAP therapy is designed to overload the muscles by subjecting them to a greater level of resistance than usual during velar elevation for speech. Once the muscles adapt to a certain level of pressure, the pressure is increased. Through this progressive resistance training, it is theorized that the muscles gain strength and become more resistance to fatigue. An important difference between this procedure and other muscle training procedures is that this is done during speech and for speech activities only.

Kuehn, Moon, and Folkins (1993) compared electromyographic activity of the levator veli palatini during the use of CPAP and with atmospheric air pressure only. There was a significant increase in the activity of the levator muscle with an increase in the intranasal pressure, suggesting that this muscle actively reacts to the resistance and possibly increases in strength. One study found a reduction in the degree of hypernasality in some children (Kuehn et al., 2002).

Some caveats of this form of treatment include the fact that child selection is very important. Perhaps this form of treatment is best suited for cases with mild velopharyngeal incompetence where there is poor velar movement, as in the traumatic brain injury population (Cahill et al., 2004). It is unlikely to be successful if there is more than mild velopharyngeal incompetence or if there is a structural defect. In cases where improvement from CPAP therapy is noted, another unknown is whether it is sustained when the exercises are no longer done. Further research is needed to determine the short-term and long-term efficacy of this technique.

Prosthesis Reduction Therapy

Some authors have described the use of a temporary speech prosthesis as a means of improving velopharyngeal function (Golding-

Kushner, Cisneros, & LeBlanc, 1995; Israel, Cook, & Blakeley, 1993; McGrath & Anderson, 1990; Sell, Mars, & Worrell, 2006; Wolfaardt, Wilson, Rochet, & McPhee, 1993). The procedure is to use a palatal lift or speech bulb for a period of time and then gradually reduce its size in hopes of promoting an increase in velopharyngeal movement. However, research has not shown that the lift promotes an increase in muscle function. In fact, it actually negates the need for velopharyngeal function, so it could be argued that the velar muscles could actually be negatively affected. Neither device has been found to eliminate the need for further surgery (Tachimura, Nohara, Fujita, Hara, & Wada, 2001; Yorkston et al., 2001). Therefore, this type of management is still controversial, especially because prosthetic devices are expensive and compliance with children is difficult (see Chapter 20 for more information).

MOTOR LEARNING AND MOTOR MEMORY

The acquisition of a new motor program requires a combination of both motor learning and motor memory. As a new motor program is learned, new connections and pathways are formed in the brain (Maas et al., 2008; Schmidt & Lee, 2005), thus enhancing the ability to execute the new motor skills easily and automatically. Speech requires motor movements that are fast, complex, automatic, and effortless. Speech is developed, therefore, through both motor learning and motor memory.

Motor Learning

Motor learning is the acquisition of new motor skills in order to be able to execute complex motor movements and motor sequences.

Motor learning is dependent on feedback through a "trial and error" approach. It is the feedback that helps with the development and ultimate refinement of the motor program.

Motor learning is necessary for an individual to be able to perform complicated motor movements and sequences without conscious thought. Examples of skills that require motor learning include playing a musical instrument (e.g., the piano); learning a dance (e.g., salsa); learning to play a sport (e.g., kicking the ball in soccer); and, of course, learning to produce speech sounds in sequence for connected speech.

If a child has not learned to produce certain speech sounds correctly on his own, speech therapy is necessary to alter the incorrect motor pattern. In speech therapy, the child is first taught how to produce the sound correctly through instruction and a period of trial and error with constant feedback. This is the motor learning phase of speech therapy.

Motor Memory

Motor memory is what develops the automaticity of the newly learned motor movement Motor memory is dependent on repetition (e.g., practice). It also makes the new learning relatively permanent, although this learning can degrade with a lack of use.

Speech learning (or relearning in the case of speech disorders) is greatly dependent on practice. Of course, there is always some practice that takes place in a therapy session after motor learning has taken place. However, if the child is able to produce the speech sound easily in the therapy session, the majority of the practice should take place at home in the natural environment. Given the cost of speech therapy (to the parents, insurance providers, and taxpayers), each therapy session should be geared primarily toward learning new skills.

Using the analogy of piano lessons, it can be said that new learning should take place in the lesson (therapy session). Practice should take place every day at home. In fact, if you don't practice the piano at home, you make very little progress in learning to play the piano. The same can be said about the relationship between speech practice at home and speech progress.

In designing a practice schedule, the practice frequency and intensity should take into consideration the following for best results:

- **Practice Frequency:** Frequent, distributed practice sessions can facilitate both short-term performance and long-term memory. In fact, it is better to have frequent, albeit short, practice sessions than infrequent, yet longer, sessions.

- **Practice Intensity:** The length of a practice session is less important than the number of responses elicited during the session. In fact, it is the number of correct responses elicited (in therapy or at home) that is directly related to the rate of progress, not the time spent. As such, drill work is most effective in developing motor learning and motor memory. A practice session can be as short as a minute or less, particularly if it is done frequently throughout the day.

Although it is important to design the practice schedule for maximum benefit in the shortest amount of time, the child's needs, attention, and tolerance level should also be considered. Another consideration is the time that the family has to work with the child at home. Parents are more likely to be successful in practicing with the child if they are instructed on how to incorporate short sessions into their regular daily activities. For example, a few minutes of practice can be done during a meal or while giving the child a bath, playing with the child, or doing daily chores around the house. Practice can be done while riding in the car, where the child has nothing else to do. For older children, practice can be incorporated into homework by having the child read aloud.

In summary, frequent short practice sessions throughout the day and week are better than a few long sessions. Drill is effective in achieving as many responses from the child as possible. One practice "session" at home can be as little as a minute or less. Practice should be incorporated into daily activities at home. This makes it more do-able for parents and also helps with the carryover process.

Carryover

Successful carryover of new speech productions into everyday conversational speech is the measure of the true success of therapy. However, carryover is often the most frustrating aspect of therapy because it can be the most difficult to achieve in a therapy session. Carryover success depends on several factors. First, the new speech production must be very easy for the child to produce in connected speech. Second, the child must be able to self-monitor and self-correct. Finally, there must be help from the teachers at school and the family at home to monitor the child's speech and to correct the misarticulations periodically, when necessary.

The best way to obtain teacher and family member involvement in the carryover stage is to engage them as partners in the treatment process from the very beginning. They should be strongly encouraged to observe therapy sessions whenever possible. In addition, it is important to give parents specific strategies for practicing speech sound production at home. In this way, they will be more aware of the child's speech goals and more helpful in

monitoring and correcting the child's speech during the carryover stage.

TIMETABLE FOR INTERVENTION AND GOALS

Involvement of the speech-language pathologist in the care of the child with a cleft or other craniofacial condition begins soon after birth and may extend into adulthood. The intensity of involvement is greatest in the preschool years, particularly between ages 3 and 5. However, adolescents and even adults will sometimes need speech therapy.

Infants and Toddlers

During the first few weeks of life, feeding is necessarily the first priority. Once effective feeding has been established, the next priority is language development. The parents should be counseled that during the first 3 years, they should concentrate on the "quantity" of speech (how much the child can understand, how many different words the child uses, and how many words are used in utterances) and not worry as much about the "quality" of speech (articulation, resonance, and intelligibility).

The speech-language pathologist for the cleft palate/craniofacial team is responsible for counseling families on methods of both speech sound stimulation and language stimulation during this critical period of time. Because the parents are the primary instructors of speech and language for the child, they should be advised on how to be most effective in that job (Amorosa & Endres, 2004; Hahn, 1989; O'Gara & Logemann, 1990; Pamplona & Ysunza, 2000; Phillips, 1990; Skeat, Eadie, Ukoumunne, & Reilly, 2010; Stevens, Watson, & Dodd, 2001). Therefore, the families should always be given both verbal instructions and a printed home program on speech and language stimulation, especially because children with clefts are at greater risk (Antonarakis & Kiliaridis, 2009; Hardin, 1991). If language does not develop normally, or if there are feeding problems, therapy should be initiated immediately.

Although articulation and resonance are not the primary focus of the first 3 years, there are some things that parents should do to stimulate early phonemic development. Parents should be shown how to encourage vocalizations by imitating the child's cooing and babbling. If there is a cleft palate, they should be instructed on how to encourage the production of plosives once the cleft is repaired. The speech-language pathologist should actively teach the parents ways to work with the child on normal sound production in order to try to prevent the development of compensatory articulation productions (Golding-Kushner, 2001). If there is hypernasality or nasal air emission during production, the parent can be shown how to gently pinch the child's nostrils during sound imitation to allow for more normal production.

Preschool Children

By the age of 3, most children are communicating with complete sentences, although errors in syntax and morphology are common. The child should be using nasal and plosive sounds, some fricatives, and even affricate phonemes. Therefore, this is an appropriate time to evaluate speech, resonance, and velopharyngeal function and, if indicated, begin treatment. If it is determined that secondary surgical intervention is needed, this is best done between the ages of 3 and 5. Although speech therapy can be initiated to work on placement errors before surgery for VPI, the therapy will be easier and less frustrating for the child if the surgery is done first. In addition, progress will be much faster, and as a result the therapy will be more cost-effective.

Parents and even older siblings should be active in the treatment process for the best results. Therefore, they should be encouraged to observe therapy. If possible, one spouse should videotape the session for the other spouse to view at home. As noted above, progress is much faster if the parents are involved and there is frequent practice in between the therapy sessions (Pamplona & Ysunza, 2000; Pamplona, Ysunza, & Jimenez-Murat, 2001; Pamplona, Ysunza, & Uriostegui, 1996).

The goal of physical management and speech therapy in the preschool years is to attain age-appropriate speech, or close to it, by the time the child enters kindergarten. This is important for several reasons. Most importantly, preschool children are more receptive to acquiring new speech patterns and correcting abnormal speech patterns than older children. This is due to the plasticity of the brain in the first few years, which makes the brain more receptive to learning these skills (Dowling, 2004). Also, during the first 5 years, speech patterns are not strongly habituated and are therefore easier to change. With early private speech therapy, parents are available so that they can be active partners in the therapeutic process. Finally, early correction avoids the social and emotional problems that come from teasing in the school-age years.

There are several practical reasons for early intervention in a specialty center. One reason is that funding for private speech therapy through medical insurance is more available for preschool children than for school-age children. In addition, individual therapy with frequent access to the parents can be offered in a hospital or specialty center. Finally, there are usually specialists in craniofacial anomalies and VPI to provide the therapy.

School-Age Children

School-age children who continue to have speech problems typically receive therapy through their school. At this point, VPI should have been corrected, if it was present. If there is still hypernasality or nasal emission, the child should be referred to the craniofacial team for evaluation (or reevaluation) and consideration of physical management.

When therapy is required for this age group, it is usually for the correction of compensatory errors related to either VPI or dental malocclusion. Either way, correction is difficult, if not impossible, as long as the structural anomaly is still present. It must be said again that speech therapy is not appropriate for obligatory errors.

One dilemma in this age group is that if there is either a Class II or a Class III malocclusion, which is common in children with cleft palate or craniofacial anomalies, correction requires orthognathic surgery. However, this surgery usually is not done until after facial growth is complete, which is around age 14 for girls and around age 18 for boys. In the meantime, the speech distortion persists. Again, speech therapy for compensatory errors is very difficult and usually ineffective until after the structural anomaly has been corrected, and obligatory errors cannot be corrected with speech therapy. Therefore, the child with speech distortions may be in a "holding pattern" until the surgical correction. It is important to help parents, teachers, and health care professionals understand why speech therapy is not appropriate when this occurs. Certainly, the speech-language pathologist should not be pressured into providing speech therapy if there is not a reasonable expectation that improvement can be made, as this would be an ethical violation.

Some cleft palate or craniofacial centers offer summer camps or residential programs for school-age children who continue to demonstrate speech problems that are correctable with therapy (D'Mello & Kumar, 2007; Pamplona et al., 2005; Nash, Stengelhofen, Toombs, Brown, & Kellow, 2001). The purpose of this type of program is to provide intensive speech therapy while giving the children opportunities to interact with others who have similar problems and experiences. The biggest disadvantages of this mode of intervention are cost and logistics.

Adolescents and Adults

Speech therapy is sometimes required after the patient undergoes orthognathic surgery. In addition, an adolescent or adult with a history of cleft or craniofacial condition occasionally decides to seek improvement in his or her speech. If the primary problem is uncorrected VPI, surgical or prosthetic intervention should be done first. If the person's articulation is essentially normal, then there should be significant improvement in speech with physical management alone.

If there are many compensatory productions (with or without VPI), however, then the outcome of treatment is less certain. The person should be informed that the prognosis for changing speech production patterns at older ages is somewhat guarded because the critical period of speech learning has passed and also because of the strong habit and strength of the current speech productions (Wang, Jiang, Wu, Chen, & Li, 2003). The person should be counseled that speech therapy will not be effective unless there is consistent, daily practice at home. Overall, the severity of the speech and the individual's motivation must be considered before recommending surgical intervention and speech therapy at this point.

THE ULTIMATE GOAL

In past generations, the goal of treatment for individuals with a history of cleft palate was acceptable or intelligible speech, because normal speech was usually not obtainable. Over the past few decades, however, there has been an increase in knowledge of the nature of the velopharyngeal mechanism. In addition, there have been advances in evaluation techniques and instrumentation and also in surgical techniques. Therefore, most children born with cleft palate at this time ultimately attain normal speech. If there are additional craniofacial anomalies, uncorrectable structural problems, or neurological problems, then the prognosis for perfect speech is more guarded. Regardless, all efforts should be made to achieve normal speech (without nasal emission) and resonance (without hypernasality or hyponasality) through appropriate treatment whenever possible. The goal of merely "improved" or "acceptable" speech is not acceptable.

SUMMARY

Speech therapy is appropriate for the correction of articulation errors that are caused by VPI (compensatory errors), particularly after correction of the structure. Therapy is also appropriate for misarticulations due to mislearning, which cause phoneme-specific hypernasality or nasal emission. Therapy is not appropriate for obligatory distortions, including consistent hypernasality or nasal emission, which is usually caused by VPI. These distortions self-correct with normalization of the structure. When in doubt regarding the cause of the speech characteristics and appropriate recommendations, a trial period of speech therapy can be done to determine the individual's response to therapy.

The therapy procedures for compensatory speech errors are no different than those used for other placement errors. Oral-motor exercises, including those that involve blowing and sucking, are totally inappropriate for a variety of reasons (Golding-Kushner, 2001).

Therapy should continue as long as the child is making progress. If the child is not responding to therapy, referral to a craniofacial team for further evaluation (or reevaluation) of velopharyngeal function should be considered. Surgical intervention or revision may be necessary.

FOR REVIEW AND DISCUSSION

1. Discuss the appropriate focus and intervention strategies for the following developmental stage: infants and toddlers, preschool children, school-age children, adolescents and adults. Explain why early intervention and early stimulation are critically important.

2. In what cases is speech therapy appropriate for children with a history of cleft palate? When is speech therapy inappropriate for correction of abnormal speech in this population?

3. Why is speech therapy almost always ineffective in correcting hypernasality or nasal emission? Why do you think that clinicians still keep children in speech therapy for these problems? If a physician refers a child to you for correction of

consistent hypernasality, what would you do and why?

4. Under what circumstances is speech therapy appropriate for nasal emission or hypernasality? What would you do if no progress was made after 2 months of therapy?

5. Discuss methods of auditory, visual, and tactile feedback that can be used as part of therapy. Which methods would be the most effective and why?

6. What is the nose cul-de-sac technique? How can it be used in therapy?

7. The child has a history VPI that was corrected by a pharyngeal flap. Speech is characterized by ŋ/l and nasal emission on s/z only. All other speech sounds are produced normally without hypernasality or nasal emission. Why is there still nasality on the /l/ sound and nasal emission on s/z? What speech therapy techniques might be used for these misarticulations?

8. How can a straw be used to correct inconsistent nasal emission? How can it be used to correct a lateral lisp?

9. Describe therapy approaches for correction of the following: a glottal stop, a pharyngeal fricative, lateral distortion, phoneme-specific nasal air emission, and ŋ/l substitution.

10. Describe various high-tech and low-tech methods of providing biofeedback as part of the therapy process. What are the advantages and disadvantages of each?

11. What is CPAP therapy? What is the theory behind it? Why would it be inappropriate for a child with a submucous cleft or short velum?

12. Why are oral-motor exercises, including blowing and sucking exercises, ineffective in the treatment of velopharyngeal dysfunction? Why do you think some clinicians still use them?

13. How would you explain to parents why their involvement is critically important to the success of therapy?

14. What would you do if a 6-year-old boy was referred to you for a lateral lisp and you found the problem is due to the placement of the teeth relative to the tongue?

REFERENCES

American Speech-Language-Hearing Association (ASHA). (2005). *Evidence-based practice in communication disorders.* Accessed April, 20, 2006, from http://www.asha.org/policy/PS2005-00221/.

Amorosa, H., & Endres, R. (2004). [Group training for parents of young children with specific developmental speech and language disorder (SDLD).] *Psychiatrische Praxis, 31*(Suppl. 1), S129–131.

Antonarakis, G. S., & Kiliaridis, S. (2009). Internet-derived information on cleft lip and palate for families with affected chil-dren. *Cleft Palate–Craniofacial Journal, 46*(1), 75–80.

Bae, Y., Kuehn, D. P., & Ha, S. (2007). Validity of the Nasometer measuring the temporal characteristics of nasalization. *Cleft Palate–Craniofacial Journal, 44*(5), 506–517.

Berry, M. F., & Eisenson, J. (1956). *Speech disorders: Principles and practices of therapy.* New York: Appleton-Century-Crofts.

Brunner, M., Stellzig-Eisenhauer, A., Proschel, U., Verres, R., & Komposch, G. (2005). The effect of nasopharyngoscopic biofeedback in patients with cleft palate and velopharyngeal dysfunction. *Cleft Palate–Craniofacial Journal, 42*(6), 649–657.

Bzoch, K. R. (Ed.) (2004). *Communicative disorders related to cleft lip and palate.* Austin, TX: Pro-Ed.

Cahill, L. M., Turner, A. B., Stabler, P. A., Addis, P. E., Theodoros, D. C., & Murdoch, B. E. (2004). An evaluation of continuous positive airway pressure (CPAP) therapy in the treatment of hypernasality following traumatic brain injury: A report of 3 cases. *Journal of Head Trauma Rehabilitation, 19*(3), 241–253.

Cavalli, L., & Hartley, B. E. (2010). The clinical application of electrolaryngography in a tertiary children's hospital. *Logopedics, Phoniatrics, Vocology, 35*(2), 60–67.

Cole, R. M. (1971). Direct muscle training for the improvement of velopharyngeal function. In K. Bzoch (Ed.), *Communicative disorders related to cleft lip and palate* (pp. 250–256). Boston: Little, Brown and Company.

Cole, R. M. (1979). Direct muscle training for the improvement of velopharyngeal activity. In K. Bzoch (Ed.), *Communicative disorders related to cleft lip and palate* (2nd ed., pp. 328–340). Boston: Little, Brown and Company.

D'Mello, J., & Kumar, S. (2007). Audiological findings in cleft palate patients attending speech camp. *Indian Journal of Medical Research, 125*(6), 777–782.

Dowling, J. E. (2004). *The great brain debate: Nature or nurture?* Washington, DC: Joseph Henry Press.

Flowers, C. R., & Morris, H. L. (1973). Oral-pharyngeal movements during swallowing and speech. *Cleft Palate Journal, 10,* 181–191.

Golding-Kushner, K. J. (2001). *Therapy techniques for cleft palate & related disorders.* Englewood Cliffs, NJ: Thomson Delmar Learning.

Golding-Kushner, K. J., Cisneros, G., & LeBlanc, E. (1995). Speech bulbs. In R. J. Shprintzen & J. Bardach (Eds.), *Cleft palate speech management* (pp. 352–375). St. Louis, MO: Mosby.

Hahn, E. (1989). Directed home language stimulation program for infants with cleft lip and palate. In K. R. Bzoch (Ed.), *Communicative disorders related to cleft lip and palate* (3rd ed., pp. 313–319). Boston: Little, Brown and Company.

Hardin, M. A. (1991). Cleft palate. Intervention. *Clinics in Communication Disorders, 1*(3), 12–18.

Hardin-Jones, M. A., & Jones, D. L. (2005). Speech production of preschoolers with cleft palate. *Cleft Palate–Craniofacial Journal, 42*(1), 7–13.

Heppt, W., Westrich, M., Strate, B., & Mohring, L. (1991). Nasalance: A new concept for objective analysis of nasality. *Laryngorhinootologie, 70*(4), 208–213.

Israel, J. M., Cook, T. A., & Blakeley, R. W. (1993). The use of a temporary oral prosthesis to treat speech in velopharyngeal incompetence. *Facial and Plastic Surgery, 9*(3), 206–212.

Kanter, CE. (1947). The rationale for blowing exercises for patients with repaired cleft palates. *Journal of Speech Disorders, 12,* 281.

Kuehn, D. P. (1991). New therapy for treating hypernasal speech using continuous positive airway pressure (CPAP). *Plastic and Reconstructive Surgery, 88*(6), 959–966; Discussion 967–969.

Kuehn, D. P. (1997). The development of a new technique for treating hypernasality: CPAP. *American Journal of Speech-Language Pathology, 6*(4), 5–8.

Kuehn, D. P., & Henne, L. J. (2003). Speech evaluation and treatment for patients with cleft palate. *American Journal of Speech-Language Pathology, 12*, 103–109.

Kuehn, D. P., Imrey, P. B., Tomes, L., Jones, D. L., O'Gara, M. M., Seaver, E. J., Smith, B. E., et al. (2002). Efficacy of continuous positive airway pressure for treatment of hypernasality. *Cleft Palate–Craniofacial Journal, 39*(3), 267–276.

Kuehn, D. P., Moon, J. B., & Folkins, J. W. (1993). Levator veli palatini muscle activity in relation to intranasal air pressure variation. *Cleft Palate–Craniofacial Journal, 30*(4), 361–368.

Kummer, A. W. (2011). Speech therapy for errors secondary to cleft palate and velopharyngeal dysfunction. *Seminars in Speech and Language, 32*(2), pp.191–199.

Lof, G. L. (2008). Controversies surrounding nonspeech oral motor exercises for childhood speech disorders. *Seminars in Speech and Language, 29*(4), 253–255.

Lof, G. L. (2011). Science-based practice and the speech-language pathologist. *International Journal of Speech-Language Pathology, 13*(3), 189–196.

Lof, G. L., & Watson, M. M. (2008). A nationwide survey of nonspeech oral motor exercise use: Implications for evidence-based practice. *Language Speech Hearing Services Schools, 39*(3), 392–407.

Lubit, E. C., & Larsen, R. E. (1969). The Lubit palatal exerciser: A preliminary report. *Cleft Palate Journal, 6*, 120–133.

Lubit, E. C., & Larsen, R. E. (1971). A speech aid for velopharyngeal incompetency. *Journal of Speech and Hearing Disorders, 36*(1), 61–70.

Maas, E., Robin, D. A., Austermann Hula, S. N., Freedman, S. E., Wulf, G., & Ballard, K. J. (2008). Principles of motor learning in treatment of motor speech disorders. *American Journal of Speech-Language Pathology, 17*, 277–298.

Marchant, J., McAuliffe, M. J., & Huckabee, M. L. (2008). Treatment of articulatory impairment in a child with spastic dysarthria associated with cerebral palsy. *Developmental Neurorehabilitation, 11*(1), 81–90.

Maryn, Y., De Bodt, M., & Van Cauwenberge, P. (2006). Effects of biofeedback in phonatory disorders and phonatory performance: A systematic literature review. *Applied Psychophysiology and Biofeedback, 31*(1), 65–83.

Massengill, R. Jr., Quinn, G. W., & Pickrell, K. L. (1971). The use of a palatal stimulator to decrease velopharyngeal gap. *Annals of Otology, Rhinology, and Laryngology, 80*, 135–137.

Massengill, R. Jr., Quinn, G. W., Pickrell, K. L., & Levinson, C. (1968). Therapeutic exercise and velopharyngeal gap. *Cleft Palate Journal, 5*, 44–47.

McCauley, R. J., Strand, E., Lof, G., Schooling, T., & Frymark, T. (2009). Evidence-based systematic review: Effects of nonspeech oral motor exercises on speech. *American Journal of Speech Language Pathology 18*(4), 343–360.

McGrath, C. O., & Anderson, M. W. (1990). Prosthetic treatment of velopharyngeal incompetence. In J. Bardach & H. L. Morris (Eds.), *Multidisciplinary management of cleft lip and palate* (pp. 809–815). Philadelphia: W. B. Saunders.

Moll, K. L. (1965). A cinefluorographic study of velopharyngeal function in normals during various activities. *Cleft Palate Journal, 2*, 112.

Murdoch, B. E., Pitt, G., Theodoros, D. G., & Ward, E. C. (1999). Real-time continuous visual biofeedback in the treatment of speech breathing disorders following child-hood traumatic brain injury: Report of one case. *Pediatric Rehabilitation, 3*(1), 5–20.

Muttiah, N., Georges, K., & Brackenbury, T. (2011). Clinical and research perspectives on nonspeech oral motor treatments and evidence-based practice. *American Journal of Speech Language Pathology, 20*(1), 47–59.

Nash, P., Stengelhofen, J., Toombs, L., Brown, J., & Kellow, B. (2001). An alternative management of older children with persisting communication problems. *International Journal of Language & Communication Disorders, 36*(Suppl.), 179–184.

Neumann, S., & Romonath, R. (2011). Effectiveness of nasopharyngoscopic biofeedback in clients with cleft palate speech-a systematic review. *Logopedics Phoniatrics Vocology, 37*(3), 95–106.

O'Gara, M. M., & Logemann, J. A. (1990). Early speech development in cleft palate babies. In J. Bardach & H. L. Morris (Eds.), *Multidisciplinary management of cleft lip and palate* (pp. 717–726). Philadelphia: W. B. Saunders.

O'Sullivan, B. P., Finger, L., & Zwerdling, R. G. (2004). Use of nasopharyngoscopy in the evaluation of children with noisy breathing. *Chest, 125*(4), 1265–1269.

Paal, S., Reulbach, U., Strobel-Schwarthoff, K., Nkenke, E., & Schuster, M. (2005). Evaluation of speech disorders in children with cleft lip and palate. *Journal of Orofacial Orthopedics, 66*(4), 270–278.

Pamplona, M. C., & Ysunza, A. (2000). Active participation of mothers during speech therapy improved language development of children with cleft palate. *Scandinavian Journal of Plastic and Reconstructive Surgery and Hand Surgery, 34*(3), 231–236.

Pamplona, M. C., Ysunza, A., & Espinosa, J. (1999). A comparative trial of two modalities of speech intervention for compensatory articulation in cleft palate children, phonologic approach versus articulatory approach. *International Journal of Pediatric Otorhinolaryngology, 49*(1), 21–26.

Pamplona, M. C., Ysunza, A., & Jimenez-Murat, Y. (2001). Mothers of children with cleft palate undergoing speech intervention change communicative interaction. *International Journal of Pediatric Otorhinolaryngology, 59*(3), 173–179.

Pamplona, M. C., Ysunza, A., Patiño, C., Ramirez, E., Drucker, M., & Mazon, J. J. (2005). Speech summer camp for treating articulation disorders in cleft palate patients. *International Journal of Pediatric Otorhinolaryngology, 69*(3), 351–359.

Pamplona, M. C., Ysunza, A., & Uriostegui, C. (1996). Linguistic interaction: The active role of parents in speech therapy for cleft palate patients. *International Journal of Pediatric Otorhinolaryngology, 37*(1), 17–27.

Peterson, S. J. (1973). Velopharyngeal closure: Some important differences. *Journal of Speech and Hearing Disorders, 38*, 89.

Peterson, S. J. (1974). Electrical stimulation of the soft palate. *Cleft Palate Journal, 11*, 72–86.

Peterson-Falzone, S. J., Trost-Cardamone, J. E., Karnell, M. P., & Hardin-Jones, M. A. (2006). *The clinician's guide to treating cleft palate speech.* St. Louis, MO: Mosby Elsevier.

Phillips, B. J. (1990). Early speech management. In J. Bardach & H. L. Morris (Eds.), *Multidisciplinary management of cleft lip and palate* (pp. 732–736). Philadelphia: W. B. Saunders.

Powers, G. L., & Starr, C. D. (1974). The effect of muscle exercises on velopharyngeal gap and nasality. *Cleft Palate Journal, 11*, 28.

Rich, B. M., Farber, K., & Shprintzen, R. J. (1988). Nasopharyngoscopy in the treatment of palatopharyngeal insufficiency. *International Journal of Prosthodontics, 1*(3), 248–251.

Rossiter, D., Howard, D. M., & DeCosta, M. (1996). Voice development under training with and without the influence of real-time visually presented biofeedback. *Journal of the Acoustical Society of America, 99*(5), 3253–3256.

Ruscello, D. M. (1982). A selected review of palatal training procedures. *Cleft Palate Journal, 19*(3), 181–193.

Ruscello, D. M. (2008a). An examination of non-speech oral motor exercises for children with velopharyngeal inadequacy. *Seminars in Speech and Language, 29*(4), 293–303.

Ruscello, D. M. (2008b). Nonspeech oral motor treatment issues related to children with developmental speech sound disorders. *Language Speech and Hearing Services in Schools, 39*(3), 380–391.

Saltuklaroglu, T., Dayalu, V. N., Kalinowski, J., Stuart, A., & Rastatter, M. P. (2004). Say it with me: Stuttering inhibited. *Journal of Clinical and Experimental Neuropsychology, 26*(2), 161–168.

Santos, R. S., Cipolotti, R., D'Avila, J. S., & Gurgel, R. Q. (2005). [Schoolchildren submitted to video nasopharyngoscopy examination at school: Findings and tolerance.] *Jornal de Pediatria (Rio J), 81*(6), 443–446.

Sell, D., Mars, M., & Worrell, E. (2006). Process and outcome study of multidisciplinary prosthetic treatment for velopharyngeal dysfunction. *International Journal of Language Communication Disorders, 41*(5), 495–511.

Shprintzen, R. J., Lencione, R. M., McCall, G. N., & Skolnick, M. L. (1974). A three-dimensional cinefluoroscopic analysis of velopharyngeal closure during speech and nonspeech activities in normals. *Cleft Palate Journal, 11*, 412–428.

Siegel-Sadewitz, V. L., & Shprintzen, R. J. (1982). Nasopharyngoscopy of the normal velopharyngeal sphincter: An experiment of biofeedback. *Cleft Palate Journal, 19*(3), 194–200.

Skeat, J., Eadie, P., Ukoumunne, O., & Reilly, S. (2010). Predictors of parents seeking help or advice about children's communication development in the early years. *Child Care Health Dev, 36*(6), 878–887.

Stevens, L., Watson, K., & Dodd, K. (2001). Supporting parents of children with communication difficulties: A model. *International Journal of Language Communication Disorders, 36*(Suppl.), 70–74.

Tachimura, T., Nohara, K., Fujita, Y., Hara, H., & Wada, T. (2001). Change in levator veli palatini muscle activity of normal speakers in association with elevation of the velum using an experimental palatal lift prosthesis. *Cleft Palate–Craniofacial Journal, 38*(5), 449–454.

Tash, E. L., Shelton, R. L., Knox, A. W., & Michel, J. F. (1971). Training voluntary pharyngeal wall movements in children with normal and inadequate velopharyngeal closure. *Cleft Palate Journal, 8*, 277–290.

Tomes, L., Kuehn, D., & Peterson-Falzone, S. (1996, April). Behavioral therapy for speakers with velopharyngeal impairment. *NCVS Status and Progress Report, 9*, 159–180.

Trost-Cardamone, J. E. (1997). Diagnosis of specific cleft palate speech error patterns for planning therapy of physical management needs. In K. R. Bzoch (Ed.),

Communicative disorders related to cleft lip and palate (*vol. 4*, pp. 313–330). Austin, TX: Pro-Ed.

Van Lierde, K. M., Claeys, S., De Bodt, M., & Van Cauwenberge, P. (2004). Outcome of laryngeal and velopharyngeal biofeedback treatment in children and young adults: A pilot study. *Journal of Voice, 18*(1), 97–106.

Van Riper, C. (1963). *Speech correction: Principles and methods* (4th ed.). New York: Prentice-Hall.

Wang, G. M., Jiang, L. P., Wu, Y. L., Chen, Y., & Li, Q. Y. (2003). [A preliminary study on speech therapy for adult cleft palate patients.] *Shanghai Kou Qiang Yi Xue, 12*(2), 81–84.

Watson, M. M., & Lof, G. L. (2008). Epilogue: What we know about nonspeech oral motor exercises. *Seminars in Speech and Language, 29*(4), 339–344.

Watson, M. M., & Lof, G. L. (2009). A survey of university professors teaching speech sound disorders: Nonspeech oral motor exercises and other topics. *Language Speech Hearing Services Schools, 40*(3), 256–270.

Weber, J., Jobe, R. P., & Chase, R. A. (1970). Evaluation of muscle stimulation in the rehabilitation of patients with hypernasal speech. *Plastic and Reconstructive Surgery, 46*, 173–174.

Witzel, M. A., Tobe, J., & Salyer, K. (1988). The use of nasopharyngoscopy biofeedback therapy in the correction of inconsistent velopharyngeal closure. *International Journal of Pediatric Otorhinolaryngology, 15*(2), 137–142.

Witzel, M. A., Tobe, J., & Salyer, K. E. (1989). The use of videonasopharyngoscopy for biofeedback therapy in adults after pharyngeal flap surgery. *Cleft Palate Journal, 26*(2), 129–134; Discussion 135.

Wolfaardt, J. F., Wilson, F. B., Rochet, A., & McPhee, L. (1993). An appliance-based approach to the management of palatopharyngeal incompetency: A clinical pilot project. *Journal of Prosthetic Dentistry, 69*(2), 186–195.

Yorkston, K. M., Spencer, K. A., Duffy, J. R., Beukelman, D. R., Golper, L. A., Miller, R. M., Strand, E., et al. (2001). Evidence-based practical guidelines for dysarthria: Management of velopharyngeal function. *Journal of Medical Speech-Language Pathology, 9*(4), 257–273.

Ysunza, A., Pamplona, C., & Toledo, E. (1992). Change in velopharyngeal valving after speech therapy in cleft palate patients. A videonasopharyngoscopic and multiview videofluoroscopic study. *International Journal of Pediatric Otorhinolaryngology, 24*(1), 45–54.

Ysunza, A., Pamplona, M., Femat, T., Mayer, L., & Garcia-Velasco, M. (1997). Videonasopharyngoscopy as an instrument for visual biofeedback during speech in cleft palate patients. *International Journal of Pediatric Otorhinolaryngology, 41*(3), 291–298.

Ysunza-Rivera, A., Pamplona-Ferreira, M. C., & Toledo-Cortina, E. (1991). [Changes in valvular movements of the velopharyngeal sphincter after speech therapy in children with cleft palate. A videonasopharyngoscopic and videofluoroscopic study of multiple incidence]. *Boletin Medico del Hospital Infantile de Mexico, 48*(7), 490–501.

Yules, R. B., & Chase, R. A. (1969). A training method for reduction of hypernasality in speech. *Plastic and Reconstructive Surgery, 43*(2), 180–185.

INTERDISCIPLINARY CARE

CHAPTER

22

THE TEAM APPROACH

INTRODUCTION

I ndividuals with craniofacial anomalies, including cleft lip and palate, often demonstrate multiple complex issues. These issues may include early feeding and nutritional problems; developmental delay or learning disabilities; hearing loss; obstructive sleep apnea; neurological problems; dentofacial and orthodontic abnormalities; aesthetic issues; psychosocial problems; and of course, speech, language, resonance, and voice disorders. It is not possible for one professional to deal with all of these areas of concern. In fact, these patients usually have the need for medical, surgical, dental, and allied health (including speech pathology) services. Not only do these patients require treatment from a variety of professionals—the treatment occurs over a very long period of time. The entire habilitative process can last from infancy into adulthood. Because of the complexity of needs, the number of professionals needed, and the amount of time for treatment to be completed, team care is the best method to provide the care and to achieve the best treatment outcomes. In addition, even the most knowledgeable of families prefer a coordinated team approach to multiple individual appointments and procedures (Jeffery & Boorman, 2001).

The main purpose of this chapter is to impress upon the reader the importance of the team approach in the management of patients with cleft lip/palate or other craniofacial anomalies. This chapter includes information about various types of teams, a list of typical team members, and a description of team structure and function. The advantages of the team approach are discussed, along with common problems with this type of clinical management. Finally, information is given on how to find a specialty team in order to refer a child for further assessment and intervention when appropriate.

NEED FOR TEAM MANAGEMENT

There are many qualified professionals throughout the United States and the world who can care for patients with craniofacial anomalies. However, as part of the habilitation process, it is common that the treatment of one professional has an impact on the treatment of other professionals. In addition, the sequence of treatment from each discipline must be considered for a variety of reasons. Therefore, services to this population of patients must be provided in a coordinated and integrated manner over a period of years for maximum benefit to the patient.

To accomplish coordinated and integrated care, the team approach to management is required for these patients. With the team approach, the patient is more likely to receive quality services, continuity of care, and long-term follow-up in order to achieve the best ultimate outcome (Austin et al., 2010; Capone & Sykes, 2007; Vargervik, Oberoi, & Hoffman, 2009; Vlastos et al., 2009; Wellens & Vander Poorten, 2006; Will, Aduss, Kuehn, & Parsons, 1989). In addition, the team approach allows the care to focus on the whole child, and not just the cleft or one particular abnormality. Not only does the interdisciplinary team care provide the best overall outcomes for the patient, but this approach is also the most efficacious and cost-effective way to manage the treatment (Vargervik et al., 2009). Therefore, the coordinated, multidisciplinary approach for the management of these patients is now widely accepted as a basic standard of care (David, Anderson, Schnitt, Nugent, & Sells, 2006; Schnitt, Agir, & David, 2004; Thomas, 2000; ACPA, 2009).

The importance of team management for patients with cleft lip and palate was first recognized by H. K. Cooper, who founded the Lancaster Cleft Palate Clinic in the early 1930s (Krogman, 1979). Many cleft palate or craniofacial teams were formed across the country in subsequent years. In 1987, the Surgeon General of the United States recognized the need for a team approach to the management of patients with special health care needs, and articulated this need in a report (Surgeon General's Report, 1987). This report emphasized that these children require comprehensive, coordinated care provided by health care systems that are accessible and responsive to the patients and their families.

In response to this report, the Maternal and Child Health Bureau provided funding to the American Cleft Palate–Craniofacial Association (ACPA) to develop recommended practices in the care of patients with craniofacial anomalies. To accomplish this, a large group of various professionals from around the country was convened for a consensus conference in 1991. This meeting resulted in the publishing of a comprehensive document by the ACPA called *Parameters for Evaluation and Treatment of Patients with Cleft Lip/Palate or other Craniofacial Anomalies*, which has since been revised (ACPA, 2009). One of the fundamental principles contained in this document is that the management of patients with craniofacial anomalies is best provided by an interdisciplinary team of specialists, especially when these specialists see a significant number of patients each year and therefore develop expertise through experience (p. 7).

There is general consensus among professionals regarding the importance of a team approach to the care of patients with cleft lip/palate or craniofacial anomalies. This approach has the advantages of access to multiple disciplines, centralization of services, long-term treatment planning from birth to adulthood, better continuity of care, comprehensive documentation from all professionals involved in the patient's care, interdisciplinary evaluations, follow-up studies, and interdisciplinary research and quality assurance (Akinmoladun & Obimakinde, 2009). The team approach makes the care of patients easier for the provider and more effective for the patient. The goal of the cleft or craniofacial team, therefore, is to ensure that care is provided in a coordinated and consistent manner with the proper sequence of evaluations and treatments. This should be done with consideration for the patient's overall developmental, medical and psychological needs (ACPA, 2010).

CHARACTERISTICS OF TEAMS

There are many cleft palate/craniofacial teams in various cities across the country. They are similar in their belief that patients with clefts and/or other craniofacial conditions require integrated care from many different professionals. They often differ in many aspects however, including the type and size of the team, team membership and structure, team leadership, processes, and even in quality.

Types of Teams

A team of professionals can be multidisciplinary or interdisciplinary, depending on the working relationship of the members and the structure of the team. A *multidisciplinary team* is a group of professionals from various disciplines who work independently in evaluating and treating patients with complex medical needs. The members of this type of team have well-defined roles and cooperate with each other, but there is little communication and interaction among the team members (Bardach et al., 1984; Butler, Samman, & Gollogly, 2011; Strauss, 1999; Thomas, 2000). The biggest problem with a multidisciplinary team is that the patient receives a series of evaluations and recommendations, but there is no integration of the information or recommendations.

On the other hand, an *interdisciplinary team* is a group of professionals from various disciplines who work together to coordinate the care of the patient. With this model, there is collaboration, interaction, communication, and cooperation among the different specialists who are involved in the patient's care. There may or may not be a joint evaluation, but there definitely is a joint plan of care. This is developed when all members of the team come together to discuss the findings, impressions, and recommendations. The final plan of care is negotiated and based on the integration of all the recommendations (Moller, 2001; Strauss, 1999). With this approach, one person can outline the sequence of procedures and approximate timelines for the patient and the family, and one document represents the entire team. There is also evidence to suggest that patients who do not receive team care are less likely to receive all the services that they need (Austin et al., 2010). Therefore, the interdisciplinary team model is felt to be the most effective one for management of patients with craniofacial anomalies.

A cleft palate or craniofacial team that works together for a period of time may even evolve into a *transdisciplinary team*. This type of team has members that truly understand each other's disciplines and how they relate to the total care of the patient. Although transdisciplinary team members cannot perform duties across disciplines, they have enough understanding of the various disciplines in order to see the "big picture." This can certainly impact the quality of care provided to the patient and the family.

Cleft palate or craniofacial teams often serve as the primary *treating team* for their patients. In larger centers, however, the team may also serve as a *consulting team*. In the role of a consulting team, the team members provide a second opinion as a group regarding the total care of the patient. This is forwarded to the treating professionals for consideration and follow-up. The treating professionals may be in the local community or far away. Regardless, there must be excellent communication between the consulting team and the treating practitioners.

Team Membership and Structure

In order to meet the complex needs of the patients and their families, cleft palate or craniofacial teams typically include medical, surgical, dental, and allied health professionals (Kasten et al., 2008). Table 22–1 lists the various professionals who are often members of a cleft or craniofacial team, and it gives a description of each professional's role in the management of these patients.

In the Parameters document, ACPA has established basic standards for what constitutes a cleft or craniofacial team (ACPA, 2009). One standard requirement for meeting the ACPA standards is that each team must have a coordinator, who is usually a nurse or other health care

TABLE 22–1 Professional Roles within a Cleft Palate or Craniofacial Anomaly Team

Audiologist: The audiologist is the person who is responsible for testing the child's hearing and middle ear function. Because individuals with craniofacial anomalies are at high risk for structural ear anomalies, middle ear disease, and hearing loss, the audiologist works with the otolaryngologist in monitoring the hearing and middle ear function of these individuals.

Dentist (Pediatric): The role of the pediatric dentist (sometimes called a *pedodontist*) is to be responsible for the general care of the child's teeth and the prevention and treatment of tooth decay. The pediatric dentist ensures that the child develops habits of good oral hygiene, despite the cleft or malocclusion, for the promotion of healthy teeth and gums. Even the primary teeth are important to protect and preserve because they act as placeholders for the permanent teeth. The pediatric dentist may be involved in the management of misaligned cleft segments prior to the lip closure. When the child is in the primary or mixed dentition stages, the pediatric dentist is often the one to improve early malocclusion, which often includes moving the maxillary segments through palatal expansion.

Geneticist: A geneticist (also called a *dysmorphologist*) is responsible for assessing patients with a history of cleft, velopharyngeal dysfunction, or craniofacial anomalies for a pattern that indicates a known syndrome or cause. If a syndrome is identified, the geneticist counsels the family regarding the diagnosis, the recurrence risk for additional offspring of both the family and the patient, and the prognosis.

Nurse: The nurse's role on the team is to assess the child's overall physical development. The nurse can determine whether the child is growing normally and is in good general health. The nurse is often the professional who assists the family in developing compensatory feeding techniques. Finally, the nurse is usually the professional who counsels the family regarding surgical procedures and answers their specific questions.

Oral Surgeon: The oral surgeon is the specialist who usually does the bone grafts to the alveolar cleft areas when there is deficient bone in the line of the cleft. This professional also performs the orthognathic surgeries, including maxillary expansions and mandibular setbacks, to normalize the occlusion between the maxillary and mandibular arches.

Orthodontist: The orthodontist is responsible for aligning misplaced teeth, in addition to correcting dental and skeletal malocclusion. The orthodontist works to normalize jaw relationships in order to achieve normal dental function and to improve facial and dental aesthetics.

Otolaryngologist: The otolaryngologist, also known as the ear, nose, and throat specialist (ENT), is responsible for monitoring middle ear function and hearing, and treating middle ear disease, which is common in children with a history of cleft or craniofacial anomalies. The otolaryngologist also manages the upper airway obstruction, which is particularly important for infants with Pierre Robin sequence. The otolaryngologist assesses the structural aspects of the oral cavity, oropharynx, nasal cavity, and upper airway, and treats conditions such as adenotonsillar hypertrophy, pharyngeal masses, and vocal fold abnormalities. The otolaryngologist may be the surgeon involved in the nasal and oral repairs and reconstruction. Finally, some otolaryngologists do surgeries for velopharyngeal insufficiency/incompetence.

Pediatrician: The pediatrician is responsible for assessing the patient's overall medical health, growth, and development. The pediatrician determines whether there are other related or unrelated medical conditions that must be addressed, particularly those that can impact plans for surgical intervention.

Plastic Surgeon: The plastic surgeon is responsible for the surgical repair of the lip and palate, and surgical reconstruction of facial and cranial anomalies. Surgery for correction of velopharyngeal insufficiency/incompetence is usually done by the plastic surgeon. The plastic surgeon may perform bone grafts and orthognathic surgery on the jaws. The aim of plastic surgery is to repair the structural defects so that there is an improvement in the patient's overall facial aesthetics, function, and speech.

Prosthodontist: The prosthodontist is involved with the restoration of natural teeth or the replacement of missing teeth. The prosthodontist develops devices to replace or improve the appearance of oral and facial structures that cannot be adequately improved with surgery or dental care. The prosthodontist can manufacture and fit devices to assist with velopharyngeal closure, if surgery is not an option.

Psychologist: The psychologist assesses the patient's psychosocial needs, and assists the patient and family in dealing with the medical, social, and emotional challenges that occur due to the patient's anomalies and other medical conditions. The psychologist often assists the physician in determining the emotional preparedness of the patient for each surgical procedure.

Pulmonologist: Because many children with clefts and craniofacial anomalies have airway issues and sleep problems, the pulmonologist evaluates and monitors the patient's airway and sleep. If obstructive sleep apnea is suspected, the pulmonologist will order a sleep study.

(Continues)

TABLE 22–1   (Continued)

Social Worker: The social worker helps families deal with the many challenges and problems that they often experience when trying to manage the child's special needs. The social worker may be the one to coordinate appointments and may also assist the families in dealing with insurance and other funding sources. The social worker may help the family to manage their stress and emotional reactions to the many problems and issues associated with the child's treatment.

Speech-Language Pathologist (SLP): The speech-language pathologist counsels the parents or guardians regarding what to expect regarding communication development and how to work with the child at home. The speech-language pathologist evaluates feeding and swallowing, general development, speech, language, resonance, and velopharyngeal function. The speech-language pathologist provides therapy for communication problems and disorders of feeding or swallowing.

Team Coordinator: The team coordinator typically represents the team in any interactions with parents, other health care professionals, and the community. This person is responsible for scheduling patients for each team meeting. The coordinator compiles the recommendations from each professional and puts this together in a comprehensive team report. The coordinator helps to counsel the family regarding the team recommendations and ensures that there is follow-up on recommended treatment.

professional. This person facilitates the scheduling of all team meetings as well as the documentation of team findings and recommendations for each patient. The coordinator ensures that the recommendations are implemented and may also be the person who represents the team in communicating with the patient or family. Other requirements include regular team meetings and participation in continuing education programs about clefts or craniofacial anomalies.

In addition to the professionals on the team, the parents or family are also key players in determining the treatment plan for the patient. It is important that the professionals on the team gain the support and cooperation from the families. In fact, all decisions for treatment must be based on the patient's and family's wishes, in addition to the clinical indications (Johansson & Ringsberg, 2004; Sharp, 1995; Vanz & Ribeiro, 2011). If the family members are not active participants in the decision-making process, compliance with the team's recommendations can be affected (Pannbacker & Scheuerle, 1993; Paynter, Jordan, & Finch, 1990; Paynter, Wilson, & Jordan, 1993). On the other hand, appropriate family involvement can significantly improve compliance with

the recommendations, which can ultimately improve the outcomes of treatment.

As part of the basic standards, ACPA determined which professionals should be members of the team in order to qualify as either a cleft palate team (CPT) or a craniofacial team (CFT) and be listed as such in the team directory. The ACPA minimum standards for team membership are as follows (ACPA, 2009):

- **Cleft Palate Team (CPT):** ACPA has determined that a Cleft Palate Team (CPT) must have a surgeon, an orthodontist, a speech-language pathologist, and at least one additional specialist. Other members might include an audiologist, geneticist (dysmorphologist), nurse, oral surgeon (maxillofacial surgeon), otolaryngologist (ear, nose, and throat specialist), orthodontist, pediatrician, prosthodontist, psychologist, or social worker. ACPA also requires this type of team to evaluate at least 50 patients per year and have at least one surgeon who operates on at least 10 primary clefts per year.

- **Craniofacial Team (CFT):** A Craniofacial Team, as defined by ACPA, must consist of a craniofacial surgeon, an orthodontist, a mental health professional, and speech-language pathologist. Other members may include a neurologist, a neurosurgeon and/or an ophthalmologist, in addition to those professionals included in a cleft team.

ACPA has some additional categories as follows:

- **Evaluation and Treatment Review Team (ERT):** This team provides evaluation services, but not clinical care.

- **Low Population Density Team (LPD):** This team provides clinical care in rural regions where there are few services available.

- **Interim Team (I-CPT or I-CFT):** This team provides clinical care and is in transition.

- **Geographical Listed Teams (GLT):** This category is used for teams that do not fall under the previous categories.

ACPA has made no specific recommendations for a team structure for children who have abnormal resonance (with or without a history of cleft palate) as the primary presenting concern. Patients with velopharyngeal dysfunction, regardless of etiology, are often managed effectively by a cleft palate or craniofacial team. However, a subset of these professionals can form a specialty team as follows:

- **VPI Team:** A team for evaluation of velopharyngeal function should include a speech-language pathologist, an otolaryngologist or a plastic surgeon, and ideally a geneticist. The geneticist is important, because many children with VPI of unknown origin have a previously unidentified syndrome, which is most commonly velocardiofacial syndrome.

Team Leadership

The qualifications, personality, and skill of the team leader are highly important in determining the function and success of the team. There is little room for authoritarianism in clinical team leadership. Instead, the leader must be able to ensure that all team members are respected equally and that their opinions are heard and considered for the best patient outcome. Having a dominant team member can result in decisions that are made based upon that person's opinion rather than on team consensus. It is the responsibility of the team leader to be sure that this does not happen and that all members' opinions are heard and considered before decisions regarding the patient's care are made (Strauss & Broder, 1985). The most effective teams function by consensus, even though each professional may view the needs of the patient differently (Noar, 1992; Strauss, 1999).

Team Responsibilities

To provide a truly integrated system of patient care, the ACPA has made a number of recommendations regarding the responsibilities of the team in its Parameters document (ACPA, 2009). For example, it is recommended that each team should have an office with an administrative assistant or coordinator and a designated phone number. The office should maintain all team documents and patient records. Patients should be evaluated at regular intervals, depending on the needs of the patient and the family. Although the patients may be examined individually by the professionals on the team, regularly scheduled team meetings must be held for discussion and negotiation of the plan of care. Communication of recommendations to the patient and family must be made verbally and in written form. There must be ongoing communication with the direct care providers in the patient's home community. The team should provide patients with information regarding resources for other services and financial assistance as needed. Finally, the teams should provide educational programs for families, other care providers, and the general public.

In a diverse society, team members must be sensitive to the ethnographic and cultural characteristics of the families that they serve. These factors may determine the way in which families understand and view the medical issues, and the way they follow the recommendations of the team (Louw, Shimbambu, & Roemer, 2006). To provide the most effective services, team intervention must be family focused and culturally sensitive.

Team Process

The cleft or craniofacial team typically becomes involved in the management of the child's needs soon after birth. This begins with parent counseling and the management of feeding issues and airway problems in the neonatal period. Team care should then continue until the physical growth of the individual has been completed, which is usually between the ages of 18 and 21. Care can continue through adulthood if there are remaining medical, surgical, dental, psychological, or communication problems that can be improved or resolved by the team members.

The method of scheduling and evaluating patients as a team varies in different settings. In most cases, each professional evaluates the patient through a separate consultation or screening, but this often occurs on the same day in a clinic setting. When the evaluations are done in a clinic, there is the opportunity for several professionals to work together in evaluating the patient (Figure 22–1). The team members then meet to discuss impressions and recommendations and to negotiate a

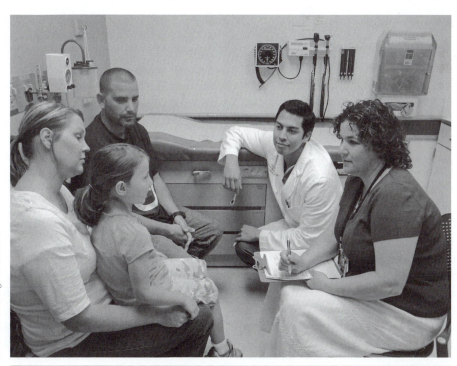

Courtesy Ann W. Kummer, Ph.D./Cincinnati Children's Hospital Medical Center & University of Cincinnati College of Medicine

FIGURE 22–1   The team approach to assessment.

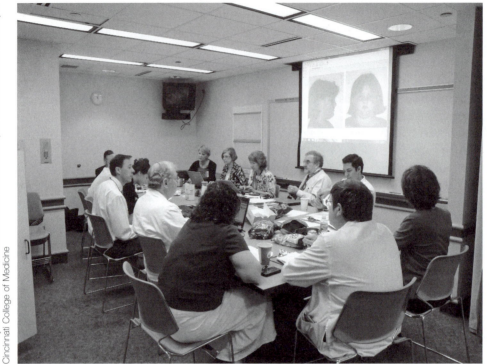

FIGURE 22–2 Team members of the Craniofacial Center at Cincinnati Children's Hospital Medical Center. Face-to-face discussions in team conferences are important for coordinated patient care.

plan of treatment (Figure 22–2). The treatment priorities and appropriate sequence of treatment is then determined. The coordinator, or another designated team member, is responsible for communicating the recommendations with the family and making sure that appropriate appointments are scheduled.

Although the team coordinator may be the primary contact person for the family, each person on the team is responsible for counseling the family about the plan of treatment relative to that person's discipline. It has been shown that when the family members are involved and informed regarding the health care decisions for their children, this can reduce stress and improve treatment outcomes

(Paynter, Edmonson, & Jordan, 1991; Walesky-Rainbow & Morris, 1978). The ultimate treatment plan is determined by the recommendations of the team members; the concerns, needs, and goals of the patient and family; and the limitations and restrictions of the third-party payment sources.

Team Quality

The quality of the services provided by a team is difficult to measure or quantify. In many cases, quality is determined solely by the perception of the "customers." Although this is an important indicator of quality, there are other more measurable ways to assure quality of services.

The guidelines listed in the Parameters document (ACPA, 2009) can help a team achieve and maintain the basic requirements for an appropriate team, as determined by professional consensus from around the country.

As a way to verify the quality of the care provided by teams, ACPA and its related organization, the Cleft Palate Foundation (CPF), have developed an approval process. The purpose of this process is to provide:

- "Standards that identify essential characteristics of quality for Team composition and functioning in order to facilitate the improvement of team care" and

- "Accurate information to patients and families/caregivers regarding services provided by those Teams that meet specified standards"

The Commission on Approval of Teams (CAT) is charged with reviewing applications of teams against these standards (ACPA, n.d.).

Another way to ensure quality is for the team to develop and participate in a performance improvement program. In a 1999 survey of cleft and craniofacial teams in the North America, 50% reported that they have a quality assurance program in place to measure treatment outcomes (Strauss, 1999). Hopefully, that number has increased in more recent years. A quality (now usually called performance improvement) program provides a mechanism for teams to monitor, self-evaluate, and improve various aspects of their patient care. Clinical pathways and algorithms of care have also been developed by some teams. The quality of the team is greatly determined by the quality of each individual member. It is important that all members of the team be licensed and certified in their individual areas of specialty. The education and experience required for specialization are determined by the various professional associations, specialty boards, and licensure boards. Each team must ensure that all members possess not only the appropriate and current credentials for practice but also the requisite experience and skill in the evaluation and treatment of patients in the specialty area of craniofacial anomalies. If the professionals are not well trained in this specialty area, their good intentions may not be enough to result in good decisions. In fact, these "experts" can actually do more harm than good due to their lack of specialty experience in the area of craniofacial anomalies (Sidman, 1995).

Another factor that affects the quality of a team is the number of patients seen per year and the number of team meetings per year. This has an impact on the experience base of the team and on the time commitment given by the team members to craniofacial anomalies. In addition, teams with a large patient base usually have more members than those with few patients and also have more disciplines represented on the team. Therefore, it is more likely that the patient's various treatment needs will be adequately and appropriately served. Of course, when the patient requires services by professionals not represented on the team, members must have the knowledge and resources to refer the patient to appropriate professionals outside of the immediate team.

The stability of the team and how long team members serve on the team can also be a factor to consider. Because the patient's treatment typically begins at birth and may continue until adulthood, the consistency and longevity of team members become important for the consistency and continuity of care.

It is especially important that all members of the team stay current with recent developments in their respective disciplines, particularly in the area of cleft and craniofacial care. Active membership in the American Cleft Palate–Craniofacial Association and attendance at annual meetings of this association and other similar associations (local, national, and international) is the best way to be informed and stay current. In addition, it is important to be familiar with the literature regarding the current techniques used for the evaluation and treatment of craniofacial anomalies. An interest in continuous learning helps the team members to provide the best possible care for the patients.

Finally, the extent to which the team involves the parents or caregivers in the decision-making process affects the overall team quality. It has been found that when parents have a high opinion of the team and the services provided, compliance with recommendations is greatest. In contrast, when parents have a low opinion of the team, compliance can be negatively affected (Paynter et al., 1990).

ADVANTAGES OF AND POTENTIAL PROBLEMS WITH THE TEAM APPROACH

With complex conditions, such as clefts and craniofacial anomalies, it seems obvious that there are many advantages of the team approach to management of care. Certainly, the advantages are significant. However, because teams consist of human beings, there are problems that occasionally occur. These problems must be recognized and addressed for the team to be optimally effective in treating the patients that its members serve.

Advantages of the Team Approach

The team approach to management offers many advantages to the patient and the patient's family (ACPA, 2009; Chen, Chen, Wang, & Noordhoff, 1988; Colburn & Cherry, 1985;

Kline, 1997; Lang, Neil-Dwyer, Evans, & Honeybul, 1998; Pinsky & Goldberg, 1977; Sharp, 1995; Stal, Chebret, & McElroy, 1998; Strauss, 1998; Strauss, 1999; Strohecker, 1993; Capone & Sykes, 2007). First of all, the team offers an evaluation of the whole child that is completed through the individual evaluations of many professionals. The team evaluation is comprehensive, yet done with fewer visits and usually at a lower cost than individual evaluations. The plan of care is devised by professionals who work together and understand each other's disciplines. There is shared decision making among the team members, and decisions are based on more information than one professional would have compiled independently (Sharp, 1995). There is usually better follow-up and monitoring of care because this is a primary responsibility of the team coordinator. The team coordinator also serves as the main contact person on the team, who can assist the family and address their questions or concerns. Teams usually consist of experts in the field who can provide state-of-the-art care. Teams promote better services through parent groups, special camps, and the provision of pamphlets and other educational materials.

There are also many advantages of the team approach for the professionals. The team approach increases interprofessional communication and helps to develop good working relationships among the team members. It increases the knowledge of each professional. One of the most significant advantages of the team approach is that it makes it possible to keep good serial records (Brogan, 1988). The team can also be an effective vehicle for collaboration in research and publications. Some states have developed networks of teams for the purpose of collaboration in research endeavors and continuing education (Abdoney, Habal, Scheuerle, & Rans, 1988; Will & Aduss, 1987; Will & Parsons, 1991).

Finally, it can save time for the provider by expediting the collaboration process.

Potential Problems with the Team Approach

Although the advantages of the team approach far outweigh the disadvantages, there are some common inherent problems associated with interdisciplinary teams. One factor that can affect the function of the team is the perceived or ascribed status of various team members relative to other members. This can be based on characteristics such as age, gender, discipline, experience, or accomplishments (Cohn, 1991). If team members are not considered equals in status on the team, then the individuals with the ascribed higher status will tend to exert more influence on the decisions of the group than those members of lower status (Cohn, 1991). This can have a negative impact on the quality of the group decision making. For the team to be effective, there must be an atmosphere of equality and mutual respect among all of the team members.

Problems can also occur if the individual roles are not clearly defined within the team. If the roles are not clear, there may be interdisciplinary competition or "turf issues." For example, there is often an overlap of skills among the plastic surgeon, the oral surgeon, and the otolaryngologist. As a team, it is helpful to define who does what, when it's done, and under what circumstances. This avoids conflicts over such things as who does the bone graft, who does the orthognathic surgery, or who does the secondary surgery for velopharyngeal dysfunction.

A different but equally disruptive problem occurs when there are members on the team who are hypersensitive to feedback. This can be a problem, for example, when a surgical procedure was not as successful as was hoped and needs to be revised. Team members must be able to speak honestly without concern of "stepping on toes" or "hurting someone's feelings." They must also be able to express differences of opinion without hesitation.

Disagreements in the philosophy of care or in treatment protocols can have a major impact on the team's performance. Communication among members regarding procedures and protocols must take place so that there is consensus regarding the standards of care and continuum of care within the team. If necessary, an algorithm of care can be developed to help team members reach consensus on the management of various diagnoses and patient concerns.

All of the potential problems of the interdisciplinary team can and should be overcome for the team to be successful. This requires ongoing communication, honesty, and mutual respect. Ultimately, the focus of the team should be on the care and well-being of the patients, and not on the individual agendas and egos of the team members.

How to Be an Effective Team Member

Effective interdisciplinary team members are usually those who are very competent and knowledgeable in their particular discipline. When working on an interdisciplinary team that requires specialty knowledge, such as a craniofacial team, each member must have specialty expertise in that area. At the same time, an effective team member must show a strong interest in the knowledge of other disciplines, as well as a desire to learn from other disciplines.

All team members should show respect for others and their opinions, especially when there is disagreement. Each team member must feel free to express his or her honest

CASE REPORT

The Value of the Team Approach

The value of a team approach to clinical management is illustrated by the following case history: Barbara was born with a bilateral complete cleft lip and cleft palate. The lip and palate repairs were done at the appropriate time. She had speech therapy in grade school but was discharged from therapy with the notation that she was "doing as well as can be expected, given her velopharyngeal mechanism." Unfortunately, she was not followed by a craniofacial team at the time, and no referral was made for further assessment and treatment.

Barbara was finally seen at the age of 16 by the craniofacial team at Cincinnati Children's Hospital Medical Center. Following the team evaluation, many treatment recommendations were made.

- The orthodontist reported that the patient had a Class III malocclusion with anterior open bite and linguoverted maxillary incisors. His recommendation was to align the maxillary arch with orthodontics.

- The speech-language pathologist reported that the speech was characterized by hypernasality and significant nasal emission. A large velopharyngeal opening was noted on nasopharyngoscopy. Barbara also had obligatory distortions and compensatory articulation errors as a result of both the malocclusion and the VPI. Given those findings, the speech-language pathologist recommended a pharyngeal flap for correction of velopharyngeal insufficiency (VPI). This was to be followed by postoperative speech therapy to correct the compensatory articulation errors.

- The oral surgeon reported that, with the discrepancy between the position of the maxillary and mandibular arches, a Le Fort I maxillary advancement was indicated to move the maxilla in appropriate position.

- The plastic surgeon reported that there was redundant vermilion in the line of the cleft and that the Cupid's bow needed revision with an Abbe flap.

- The psychologist reported that one of the things that really bothered Barbara about herself was her flattened nose.

Given all of these concerns and recommendations, the plan of care had to be designed with the best overall results in mind. To achieve that goal, the appropriate sequencing of procedures had to be determined.

In this case, the first step was for the orthodontist to bring the teeth into alignment in preparation for the orthognathic (jaw) surgery. Bringing the teeth into proper alignment made the occlusion and profile actually worse, but doing so would yield the best ultimate results. The next step was for the oral surgeon to perform a Le Fort I maxillary advancement. This normalized the occlusion and gave more support for the upper lip and base of the nose. Once the jaws were in alignment, the plastic surgeon did a pharyngeal flap to correct the velopharyngeal insufficiency, and then he performed the lip and nose revision. About 6 weeks after the surgery, Barbara began speech therapy to correct the remaining compensatory articulation errors. She was discharged from therapy with normal speech after less than 2 months of therapy.

With this planned sequence, Barbara had the best overall outcome for both aesthetics and speech. On the other hand, if the pharyngeal flap had been done before maxillary advancement, the position and effectiveness of the flap could have been compromised with the maxillary advancement. The maxillary advancement could also have had a detrimental effect on the lip and nose if those revisions had been done first. Hence it can be seen that the sequence and coordination of treatment is very important for patients who require care from multiple specialists.

opinion, without the fear of offending someone. It is important to place quality patient care and appropriate patient management first and not be willing to compromise because of concern about personal feelings or agendas. When mistakes are made, as they will be, it is important that each team member feel comfortable enough to be able to admit mistakes, without worry about undue criticism. In addition, the team members must be comfortable enough with each other to be able to admit what they don't know in order to further learning and professional competence.

It is important that team members be dependable and reliable, because all professionals are very busy. It is not well received when one person holds up the process or lets the other members down.

Finally, the use of humor can be very effective in developing camaraderie and also helps to enhance respect and working relationships among team members. Team members who use humor in their interactions with each other usually work more effectively together, and this has a positive effect on the quality of services that are ultimately provided to the patients.

RESOURCES FOR SERVICES

Finding a cleft palate/craniofacial team is a challenge for many families. Once a team is found, the next concern is funding for the services. Fortunately, resources can be found on the websites for the American Cleft Palate–Craniofacial Association (ACPA, 2010, 2013) and the Cleft Palate Foundation (CPF, 2013).

How to Find a Cleft Palate or Craniofacial Team

There are cleft palate/craniofacial teams in most major cities and even many midsize cities around the country. There are also cleft/craniofacial teams in larger cities of developed countries and even in some developing countries. Most teams are associated within a teaching hospital or pediatric hospital.

In general, the team has to see the patient for evaluation and consultation only once or twice a year during the active treatment process, so it is not essential that the team be located near the patient's home. Routine treatment, such as general dental care, orthodontics, speech therapy, and pediatric care can usually be provided by professionals in the patient's own community, as long as there is regular communication and consultation with the team members.

The Cleft Palate Foundation (CPF) website has information for parents on team care and also maintains a list of cleft palate and craniofacial teams by geographical area (Cleft Palate Foundation, 2012). Information regarding ACPA, CPF, and other organizations that provide information for families is listed in Appendix A of this book.

Funding Sources

Funding for the evaluation and treatment of cleft lip, cleft palate, and other craniofacial anomalies can come from a variety of sources. Private insurance companies will usually cover most of the expenses associated with the medical care of the patient if the patient was born when the policy was in effect. Financial assistance can also be obtained through federal and state programs such as Champus, Medicaid, the Children's Special Health Services for the state, the Bureau of Vocational Rehabilitation, and through selected Shriners' Hospitals across the country. Some private and nonprofit organizations provide funds or special services to meet the needs of children with clefts or craniofacial anomalies. Resources for financial aid can often be obtained through a social worker or team coordinator.

Identifying sources of funding and making sure that there is adequate funding are important components in treatment planning. Recommending many expensive procedures that are not covered by insurance and are out of the family's financial reach is truly a disservice to the patient and the family and can add to their stress.

CHALLENGES TO THE SPECIALTY TEAM CONCEPT

With changes in health care financing, there are some additional challenges to the team approach for the management of complex patients. Although the managed care system was designed to help control the cost of health care, many critics would argue that this is hard to do when most of the managed care organizations exist as for-profit corporations. In fact, in many cases, the investors and the administrators of these organizations are reaping substantial profits. This may occur at the expense of the patients, who are not always receiving the services that they need. Critics of managed care would also argue that this system discourages the use of specialists in the care of complex disorders (Strauss, 1999). In fact, there are financial disincentives for primary care providers to seek specialty care for their patients. The managed care organizations seek to control costs by limiting the number and type of professionals that the patient can see and the number and type of procedures that the patient can have. This certainly has an impact on the specialty team approach.

An additional concern is that some third-party payers limit access to physicians who are outside the network. If there are no specialists within the network to cover the particular medical needs, this may seriously affect the quality of care provided to the patient. This is an even greater problem when a whole team of professionals is required for quality care.

Some patients or parents are unable to move or change jobs due to a concern about changing insurance coverage. Managed care organizations often refuse to cover preexisting conditions when the policy is new. As a result, the care of patients with cleft palate or craniofacial anomalies may not be covered. In addition, there is an incentive for managed care organizations to seek to enroll groups of patients who are a low financial risk because they have few health problems. This may result in excluding the individuals who really need insurance coverage for medical services.

As the health care system in the United States continues to evolve, it is difficult to predict the future and what it holds for specialty team care or even general medical care. With the help of the efforts of professionals and various advocacy groups, it is hoped that the system will be refined so that the specific needs of the patient become a priority.

SUMMARY

Over the last 50 years, the team approach to the management of individuals with craniofacial anomalies has evolved from a good idea to the accepted standard of care, not only in this country but also internationally. Although there are some inherent difficulties that can occur when a group of professionals must work closely together, the advantages of this approach far outweigh the disadvantages. Without the team approach to management, the treatment of patients would become fragmented, and the outcomes would be negatively affected. Hopefully, as our health care system continues to evolve, the team approach to the care of patients with clefts, craniofacial anomalies, and all other complex medical conditions will be supported and even enhanced.

FOR REVIEW AND DISCUSSION

1. Why is team management preferable to individual management of children with craniofacial anomalies?

2. List the typical members of a cleft palate/ craniofacial team and their specific roles.

3. How soon should a child be seen by a cleft team and for how long?

4. What guidelines are available for standards of team care, and where can they be found?

5. Your patient is 4 years old and has a collapsed maxillary arch, anterior cross-bite, and midface retrusion. He has very poor oral hygiene and large tonsils. Speech is characterized by consistent nasal emis-sion and compensatory productions. The child is very afraid of doctors and cries every time he comes to the hospital. Discuss the interdisciplinary management of this child. Which professionals should be involved in treatment, and how can one type of treatment affect the other treatments?

6. What are the particular advantages and potential problems that health care providers might experience when providing care through an interdisciplinary team?

7. What could you do to be an effective team member?

REFERENCES

Abdoney, M., Habal, M. B., Scheuerle, J., & Rans, N. P. (1988). Cleft palate teams and the craniofacial centers in Florida: A state network. *Florida Dental Journal*, 59(2), 25–27, 53.

Akinmoladun, V. I., & Obimakinde, O. S. (2009). Team approach concept in management of oro-facial clefts: A survey of Nigerian practitioners. *Head & Face Medicine*, 5, 11.

American Cleft Palate–Craniofacial Association (ACPA). (2009). Parameters for evaluation and treatment of patients with cleft lip/palate or other craniofacial anomalies. Accessed January 20, 2013, from http://www.acpa-cpf.org/uploads/site/Parameters_Rev_2009.pdf.

American Cleft Palate–Craniofacial Association (ACPA). (2010). Standards for cleft palate and craniofacial teams, Revised March 31, 2010. Accessed January 20, 2013, from http://www.acpa-cpf.org/team_care/standards/.

American Cleft Palate–Craniofacial Association (ACPA). (n.d.). Commission on approval of teams. Accessed January 20, 2013, from http://www.acpa-cpf.org/team_care/commission_on_approval_of_teams.

Austin, A. A., Druschel, C. M., Tyler, M. C., Romitti, P. A., West, I. I., Damiano, P. C., Robbins, J. M., et al. (2010). Interdisciplinary craniofacial teams compared with individual providers: Is orofacial cleft care more comprehensive and do parents perceive better outcomes? *Cleft Palate–Craniofacial Journal, 47*(1), 1–8.

Bardach, J., Morris, H., Olin, W., McDermott-Murray, J., Mooney, M., & Bardach, E. (1984). Late results of multidisciplinary management of unilateral cleft lip and palate. *Annals of Plastic Surgery, 12*(3), 235–242.

Brogan, W. F. (1988). Team approach to the treatment of cleft lip and palate. *Annals of the Academy of Medicine, Singapore, 17*(3), 335–338.

Butler, D. P., Samman, N., & Gollogly, G. (2011). A multidisciplinary cleft palate team in the developing world: Performance and challenges. *Journal of Plastic, Reconstructive & Aesthetic Surgery, 64*(11), 1540–1541.

Capone, R. B., & Sykes, J. M. (2007). The cleft and craniofacial team: The whole is greater than the sum of its parts. *Facial Plastic Surgery, 23*(2), 83–86.

Chen, Y. R., Chen, S. H., Wang, C. Y., & Noordhoff, M. S. (1988). Combined cleft and craniofacial team: Multidisciplinary approach to cleft management. *Annals of the Academy of Medicine, Singapore, 17*(3), 339–342.

Cleft Palate Foundation (CPF). (2013). Cleft Palate Foundation homepage. Accessed January 20, 2013, from http://www.cleftline.org/parents/about_team_care.

Cohn, E. R. (1991). Commentary on team acceptance of recommendations by Dixon-Wood et al. *Cleft Palate–Craniofacial Journal, 28*(3), 290–292.

Colburn, N., & Cherry, R. S. (1985). Community-based team approach to the management of children with cleft palate. *Child Healthcare, 13*(3), 122–128.

David, D. J., Anderson, P. J., Schnitt, D. E., Nugent, M. A., & Sells, R. (2006). From birth to maturity: A group of patients who have completed their protocol management. Part II. Isolated cleft palate. *Plastic and Reconstructive Surgery, 117*(2), 515–526.

Jeffery, S. L., & Boorman, J. G. (2001). Patient satisfaction with cleft lip and palate services in a regional centre. *British Journal of Plastic Surgery, 54*(3), 189–191.

Johansson, B., & Ringsberg, K. C. (2004). Parents' experiences of having a child with cleft lip and palate. *Journal of Advanced Nursing, 47*(2), 165–173.

Kasten, E. F., Schmidt, S. P., Zickler, C. F., Berner, E., Damina, L. A. K., Christian, G. M., Workman, H., et al. (2008). Team care of the patient with cleft lip and palate. *Current Problems in Pediatric Adolescent Health Care, 38*(5), 139–158.

Kline, R. M., Jr. (1997). Management of craniofacial anomalies. *Journal of the South Carolina Medical Association, 93*(9), 336–341.

Krogman, W. M. (1979). The cleft palate team in action. In H. K. Cooper, R. L. Harding, W. M. Krogman, M. Mazaheri, & R. T. Millard (Eds.), *Cleft palate and cleft lip: A team approach to clinical management and rehabilitation of the patient* (pp. 144–161). Philadelphia: W. B. Saunders.

Lang, D. A., Neil-Dwyer, G., Evans, B. T., & Honeybul, S. (1998). Craniofacial access in children. *Acta Neurochirurgica, 140*(1), 33–40.

Louw, B., Shibambu, M., & Roemer, K. (2006). Facilitating cleft palate team participation of culturally diverse families in South Africa. *Cleft Palate–Craniofacial Journal, 43*(1), 47–54.

Moller, K. T. (2001). Interdisciplinary care for persons with cleft lip and palate in the year 2001. *Northwestern Dental Research, 80*(1), 29–36, 51.

Noar, J. H. (1992). A questionnaire survey of attitudes and concerns of three professional groups involved in the cleft palate team. *Cleft Palate–Craniofacial Journal*, 29(1), 92–95.

Pannbacker, M., & Scheuerle, J. (1993). Parents' attitudes toward family involvement in cleft palate treatment. *Cleft Palate–Craniofacial Journal*, 30(1), 87–89.

Paynter, E. T., Edmonson, T. W., & Jordan, W. J. (1991). Accuracy of information reported by parents and children evaluated by a cleft palate team. *Cleft Palate–Craniofacial Journal*, 28(4), 329–337.

Paynter, E. T., Jordan, W. J., & Finch, D. L. (1990). Patient compliance with cleft palate team regimens. *Journal of Speech and Hearing Disorders*, 55(4), 740–750.

Paynter, E. T., Wilson, B. M., & Jordan, W. J. (1993). Improved patient compliance with cleft palate team regimes. *Cleft Palate–Craniofacial Journal*, 30(3), 292–301.

Pinsky, T. M., & Goldberg, H. J. (1977). Potential for clinical cooperation between dentistry and speech pathology. *International Dental Journal*, 27(4), 363–369.

Schnitt, D. E., Agir, H., & David, D. J. (2004). From birth to maturity: A group of patients who have completed their protocol management. Part I. Unilateral cleft lip and palate. *Plastic and Reconstructive Surgery*, 113(3), 805–817.

Sharp, H. M. (1995). Ethical decision-making in interdisciplinary team care. *Cleft Palate–Craniofacial Journal*, 32(6), 495–499.

Sidman, J. D. (1995). The team approach to cleft and craniofacial disorders—The down side. *Cleft Palate–Craniofacial Journal*, 32(5), 362.

Stal, S., Chebret, L., & McElroy, C. (1998). The team approach in the management of congenital and acquired deformities. *Clinics in Plastic Surgery*, 25(4), 485–491, vii.

Strauss, R. P. (1998). Cleft palate and craniofacial teams in the United States and Canada: A national survey of team organization and standards of care. The American Cleft Palate–Craniofacial Association (ACPA) Team Standards Committee. *Cleft Palate–Craniofacial Journal*, 35(6), 473–480.

Strauss, R. P. (1999). The organization and delivery of craniofacial health services: The state of the art. *Cleft Palate–Craniofacial Journal*, 36(3), 189–195.

Strauss, R. P., & Broder, H. (1985). Interdisciplinary team care of cleft lip and palate: Social and psychological aspects. *Clinics in Plastic Surgery*, 12(4), 543–551.

Strohecker, B. (1993). A team approach in the treatment of craniofacial deformities. *Plastic Surgery Nursing*, 13(1), 9–16.

Surgeon General's Report. (1987, June). *Children with special needs*. Washington, DC: Office of Maternal and Child Health, U.S. Department of Health and Human Services, Public Health Service.

Thomas, P. C. (2000). Multidisciplinary care of the child born with cleft lip and palate. *ORL—Head & Neck Nursing*, 18(4), 6–16.

Vanz, A. P., & Ribeiro, N. R. (2011). [Listening to the mothers of individuals with oral fissures]. *Revista da Escola de Enfermagem da USP*, 45(3), 596–602.

Vargervik, K., Oberoi, S., & Hoffman, W. Y. (2009). Team care for the patient with cleft: UCSF protocols and outcomes. *Journal of Craniofacial Surgery*, 20 (Suppl. 2), 1668–1671.

Vlastos, I. M., Koudoumnakis, E., Houlakis, M., Nasika, M., Griva, M., & Stylogianni, E. (2009). Cleft lip and palate treatment of 530 children over a decade in a single centre. *International Journal of Pediatric Otorhinolaryngology*, 73(7), 993–997.

Walesky-Rainbow, P. A., & Morris, H. L. (1978). An assessment of informative-counseling procedures for cleft palate children. *Cleft Palate Journal*, 15(1), 20–29.

Wellens, W., & Vander Poorten, V. (2006). Keys to a successful cleft lip and palate team. *Belgian ENT, Head and Neck Surgery*, 2(Suppl. 4), 3–10.

Will, L. A., & Aduss, M. K. (1987). Illinois Association of Craniofacial Teams: A new state organization. *Cleft Palate Journal*, 24(4), 339–341.

Will, L., Aduss, M. K., Kuehn, D. P., & Parsons, R. W. (1989). The team approach to treating cleft lip/palate and other craniofacial anomalies in Illinois. *Illinois Dental Journal*, 58(2), 112–115.

Will, L. A., & Parsons, R. W. (1991). Characteristics of new patients at Illinois cleft palate teams. *Cleft Palate–Craniofacial Journal*, 28(4), 378–383; Discussion 383–384.

C H A P T E R

23

CLEFT CARE IN DEVELOPING COUNTRIES

INTRODUCTION

Cleft lip and palate (CLP) is one of the most common of all birth defects. It is estimated that every 3 minutes a child is born into the world with a cleft (Operation Smile, n.d.). There are well over a quarter of a million babies born each year with cleft lip and palate. In fact, many babies will be born with a cleft during the time that it takes to read this chapter.

In developed nations, such as the United States, children born with cleft lip and/or palate typically receive surgical treatment at an early age. In fact, the visible defect (the cleft lip) is usually repaired at around 3 months of age. The palate is usually repaired around 10 months of age. In developing countries, however, individuals born with clefts often do not receive corrective surgery for a variety of reasons. As a result, they are forced to live their entire lives with the visible stigma of cleft lip and the functional problems that go along with cleft palate.

The purpose of this chapter is to provide information on current issues with cleft palate care in developing countries and on how some international organizations are attempting to meet the needs of the world's population of individuals with cleft lip and palate. In addition, this chapter provides information for clinicians who are interested in helping this cause.

CLEFTS IN DEVELOPING COUNTRIES

The prevalence of clefts varies with geography, ethnicity, and socioeconomic status (Mossey et al., 2011). Although clefts occur in all countries and in all races, they occur most frequently in people of indigenous American Indian descent and second most frequently in those of Asian descent. Therefore, countries with these populations have the largest number of affected individuals. In addition, clefting is multifactorial and affected by certain exogenous factors, such as malnutrition and exposure to environmental toxins. Of course, both are common in developing countries that have a great deal of poverty. Because of the above factors, clefts are particularly prevalent in poor countries of Central America, South America, Asia, and in India.

Despite the fact that clefts are common in many developing countries, there is not always a good understanding of the cause of clefts and the fact that this is a treatable condition. Unfortunately, thousands of newborn babies with clefts have been abandoned or killed because the parents believed that the child was a curse (Figure 23–1). In fact, children with clefts in Uganda are given the name "Ajok," which literally means "cursed by God" (Smile Train, n.d.). In China, with its "one child" social policy, children with clefts, particularly those who are girls, are commonly abandoned or put up for adoption soon after the birth.

There are also millions of children and adults around the world who are currently living with an unrepaired cleft because of a variety of reasons. There is often limited access to specialized health care, particularly in remote areas. There may be a lack of hospitals that provide cleft care, a lack of enough trained

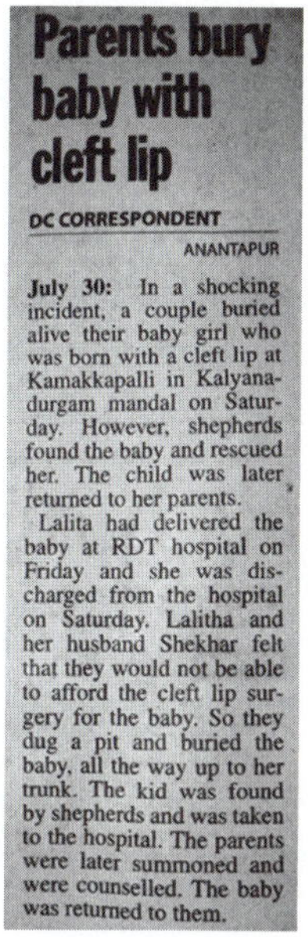

Courtesy of Srinivas Gosla Reddy, M.B.B.S., B.D.S., M.D.S., Ph.D./ Hyderabad, India

Parents bury baby with cleft lip

DC CORRESPONDENT

ANANTAPUR

July 30: In a shocking incident, a couple buried alive their baby girl who was born with a cleft lip at Kamakkapalli in Kalyana-durgam mandal on Satur-day. However, shepherds found the baby and rescued her. The child was later returned to her parents.

Lalita had delivered the baby at RDT hospital on Friday and she was dis-charged from the hospital on Saturday. Lalitha and her husband Shekhar felt that they would not be able to afford the cleft lip sur-gery for the baby. So they dug a pit and buried the baby, all the way up to her trunk. The kid was found by shepherds and was taken to the hospital. The parents were later summoned and were counselled. The baby was returned to them.

FIGURE 23–1 Article in the Deccan Chronicle, the largest circulated English daily in South India, Sunday, July 30, 2011.

surgeons, or even inadequate funding for equipment and technology.

In many cases, the parents have had no formal education and may not know that clefts can be surgically repaired (Aziz, Rhee, & Redai, 2009; Gupta, Bansal, Dev, & Tyagi, 2010). It is not uncommon for a cleft palate to be left unrepaired because the parents do not understand how it affects speech and commu-nication. Even when parents want surgical correction for their child, many families in developing countries do not have the financial resources to pay for the surgery, or even transportation to go to a hospital where there is free care. Because of these problems and the fact that a cleft is not a fatal condition, many individuals in developing nations go through life with unrepaired clefts (Bermudez, 2004).

Individuals with unrepaired clefts experi-ence all of the aesthetic and functional

problems that go with this condition. Many are ostracized from society due to various superstitions, the social stigma of a cleft lip, and the speech and feeding problems with a cleft palate. In many countries, affected children are not allowed to attend school. Even if allowed, families often don't send them to school because of the social stigma. As a result, affected individuals in developing countries are often uneducated and unemployable. In addition, because cleft lip and palate affects facial appearance and speech, affected individuals suffer difficulties with social inter-action and communication with others. Over-all, people with unrepaired clefts lead lives filled with isolation, shame, and heartache (Smile Train, n.d.).

INTERNATIONAL CLEFT CARE

To address the needs of children who are born with clefts or craniofacial conditions from around the world, several not-for-profit organ-izations have been formed in the United States and in other countries. Some are very large organizations (e.g., Operation Smile, ReSurge International [formerly Interplast], Rotaplast International, and Smile Train), whereas others are relatively small and go to only a few places a year (e.g., Operation of Hope/ Operacion Esperanza). International care is also provided by groups of surgeons and nurses who go to the same place each year for a few weeks to donate their time. With the help of these international organizations, volunteers, and donors, millions of children born with cleft lip and/or palate in developing countries have received free cleft care.

Most organizations and international teams have two main goals in providing international care. One goal is to provide direct service for affected individuals. However, 100 surgeries will

Reflections on the Article: Parents Bury Baby with Cleft Lip

By

Srinivas Gosla Reddy M.B., B.S., M.D.S, FDSRCS (Edin.), Ph.D.

Director, GSR Institute of Craniomaxillofacial and Facial Plastic Surgery,
Hyderabad 500059
Andhra Pradesh, India
www.craniofacialinstitute.org

As I read this article, I grimaced, shook my head and left the breakfast table. "Parents bury baby with cleft lip." I realize that I labor under illusions, because as a practicing cleft and craniofacial surgeon, I am powerless at that level to stop this monstrosity.

We all claim that to perform cleft surgery, we need to hone skills under the strictest discipline. But, why are we so powerless at the grass root level? It almost feels as though the snakes on the caduceus are slithering away from us as fast as possible—in shame.

In my experience, parents and children with craniofacial deformities arrive not only with an anxiety regarding surgery, but also a host of misconceptions regarding their future. I have learnt that it is essential to be determined, enthusiastic; to employ common sense, reliability, and sensitivity to everyday practice. But then, there are days when I look at the petty humilities and the predicaments that my patients bring to me. I also realize the sheer destitution and despair that are the hallmarks of the cleft stigma in India, and swear that if I was any less than 100% committed, I would have changed professions a long time ago.

"Parents bury baby with cleft lip"

This headline is blazing crimson in my mind. Where are we going wrong? We wake up, we drive to work, we tootle about in our little surgical realm, and we drive home. But who goes to the grass root level to convince people that a cleft can be corrected?

What is the need of the day is for like-minded, honest, hardworking people to stand behind each other and back up the ones who dare to make a difference.

STARTING TODAY

only help 100 patients (and their families). Therefore, these organizations recognize that to make a lasting impact, it is important to build local capacity by training and supporting in-country professionals to provide the same services. By teaching local surgeons cleft lip and palate repair techniques, and empowering those who are already trained, surgeons can treat patients in their own country and train others to do the same (Hubli & Noordhoff, 2012). With this type of support, the need for ongoing international help will gradually be diminished and ultimately eliminated (Abenavoli, 2005; Ruiz-Razura, Cronin, & Navarro, 2000).

One of the largest international organizations is Operation Smile. Operation Smile assembles national and international teams of volunteer doctors and other professionals, and then sends these teams and surgical equipment to various countries around the world. Between 1982 (when it was founded) and 2011, Operation Smile has provided over 200,000 free cleft surgeries in over 80 countries (Operation Smile, n.d.). Operation Smile also donates medical equipment and provides year-round medical treatment through 13 Comprehensive Care Centers around the world. Finally, Operation Smile trains doctors and local medical professionals in its partner countries so they are empowered to treat their own local communities.

Smile Train is another large international organization. Although it occasionally sends teams to a country in need, Smile Train's primary focus is on training and equipping local doctors and surgical centers to provide comprehensive cleft care. Between 1999 (when it was founded) and 2011, Smile Train has supported over 700,000 free cleft surgeries in over 80 countries (Smile Train, n.d.). As part of its training focus, Smile Train funded the Virtual Surgery Videos (vols. 1 and 2), which is the first surgical educational tool to use virtual technology and advanced 3-D animation software. (These DVDs are available for free on their website.) To raise awareness about the plight of children with clefts, Smile Train funded the documentary entitled "Smile Pinki," featuring a girl from rural India whose life was dramatically changed when she received free surgery to correct her cleft lip. This documentary won an Academy Award in 2008. It is also available for free on the Smile Train website: http://www.smiletrain.org/order/order-smile-pinki.html.

THE ROLE OF THE SPEECH-LANGUAGE PATHOLOGIST

There is a great need for speech-language pathology services in developing countries. One reason is that many countries have few or no speech-language pathologists. In addition, families often do not have transportation or the financial means to access services, even when they are available in their country. Despite this great need, there are significant challenges to providing meaningful services internationally through a cleft palate mission trip.

On a Surgical Mission Trip

It would seem that the speech-language pathologist would be a key member of a cleft palate mission team, especially because the primary reason to repair a cleft palate is for speech. In fact, the role of the speech-language pathologist on most surgical missions is rather limited. One reason is that a speech evaluation is not needed to determine that an unrepaired cleft lip or palate needs to be repaired. In addition, secondary surgery for velopharyngeal insufficiency or incompetence is rarely done on these trips because the focus is usually on the large number of children with unrepaired clefts. In addition, secondary surgery for VPI includes risks of airway obstruction and sleep apnea that require postoperative follow-up. This is usually not available after a surgical mission. Finally, although speech therapy is usually needed following a palate repair, it cannot be done during the time of the surgical mission trip.

The speech-language pathologist helps the mission team by screening patients to determine those who have the best chance of success with a palate repair if there is not enough time in the surgery schedule to treat every patient. The speech-language pathologist also works with the dentist/prosthodontist on fitting speech devices and counsels families on speech stimulation before the surgery or while the child is in surgery. Perhaps the most important role of the speech-language pathologist, however, is to train other professionals in speech therapy techniques to provide some intervention after the surgery.

Providing Speech Therapy

The cleft palate mission concept works well for patients who require a lip repair, because the surgery is done primarily for aesthetic reasons and requires little follow-up. For patients undergoing cleft palate repair, however, postoperative speech therapy is usually needed for best outcomes. This is particularly true if the child has developed compensatory articulation productions, because these will not change with palate repair only.

Unfortunately, very few children in developing countries have the opportunity to receive speech therapy following a palate repair (Kuehn & Henne, 2003) because in many countries speech-language pathologists are not available or affordable for most families.

To try to resolve the lack of access to speech therapy services, some innovative models of service delivery are in the early stages of development. One model is based on intensive speech camps to train parents and caregivers on speech sound production and stimulation. For example, RSF-EARTHSPEAK (2012) provides weeklong training sessions for parents or caregivers. Speech sounds that are specific to the native language are presented in a developmental sequence. The child learns to imitate the production of early sounds in babbling sequences and then to produce later sounds in more complex phonemic combinations. Unfortunately, there is no way to determine those who can't produce the sounds due to velopharyngeal insufficiency. Also, there is no published research to date to validate the outcomes of this approach.

Another approach that is being trialed is the use of local community workers to help serve the need. The community workers are trained to provide the basics of speech stimulation and speech therapy (Prathanee, Dechongkit, & Manochiopinig, 2006). Perhaps the approach that has the most potential entails providing speech therapy sessions remotely through telemedicine (Furr et al., 2011; Glazer et al., 2011; Whitehead et al., 2012). This may be an effective way to provide care to underserved populations around the world in the very near future. In addition, there is a growing, although limited, presence of speech-language pathologists in the developing world, particularly at community centers (Noordhoff, 2009). The number of trained speech-language pathologists may increase if opportunities are provided for online education and training.

Providing Education and Training

The need for education is not limited to the surgical team members. Many countries do not have speech-language pathologists. However, they may have psychologists or other health care professionals who are interested in learning what they can to help children with speech disorders. Even when there are local speech-language pathologists (or similar professionals), these individuals may not be well trained in cleft management. Therefore, the most important role for speech-language pathologist in international care is to provide education and training for other professionals regarding the evaluation and treatment of patients with cleft palate and/or velopharyngeal dysfunction. (Education of other professionals may or may not be possible during the time of a surgical mission.) Individual and group training, seminars, lectures, handouts, and books are greatly appreciated by the local professionals.

To provide training, the speech-language pathologist must be very knowledgeable about the management of this population (Hartley & Wirz, 2002). Even with several years of clinical experience, most speech-language pathologists are at a loss when it comes to working with children with clefts, unless they have had specific experience in this area. Therefore, those who are interested in working internationally in this area should seek additional specialty training and experience in pediatrics, cleft palate, velopharyngeal dysfunction, and resonance disorders (D'Antonio & Landis, 1994; Ducote, 1998, 2005; Ducote & Juul, 1998; Noordhoff, 2009). The *Parameters for Evaluation and Treatment of Patients with Cleft Lip/Palate or other Craniofacial Anomalies*, published by the American Cleft Palate–Craniofacial Association (ACPA, 2009b), should be reviewed for a basic understanding of the sequence and standards of care for individuals affected by a cleft. In addition, the speech-language pathologist should listen to and study the videos of patients with hypernasality and/or nasal emission that are associated with this book and speech samples that are on the American Cleft Palate–Craniofacial Association website (ACPA, n.d.[b]).

Although didactic learning is important, clinical knowledge and experience with the cleft population is also important when teaching others. Clinical experience is particularly important when a person is called upon to make decisions regarding candidates for secondary management of velopharyngeal insufficiency, if that is done on cleft missions.

CLEFT LIP/PALATE SURGICAL MISSIONS

As noted previously, many organizations send teams of medical professionals to countries with less-developed health care. Over a period of weeks, these teams provide services to individuals with cleft lip and palate who cannot otherwise obtain or afford the surgery.

In 1997, an International Task Force on Volunteer Cleft Missions outlined recommendations for volunteer cleft missions based on (1) mission objectives, (2) organization, (3) personal health and liability, (4) funding, (5) use of trainees in volunteer cleft missions, and (6) public relations. They agreed that the main goals for these missions are "to provide top-quality surgical service, train local doctors and staff, develop and nurture fledgling cleft programs, and finally, make new friends" (Yeow et al., 2002). More recently, the American Cleft Palate–Craniofacial Association (ACPA, n.d.[a]) published standards on its website for international care. These standards are "aimed towards assuring that international exchanges or mission-based cleft lip, cleft palate and craniofacial care are delivered in a safe and high quality manner."

Typical Team Members

A small team may consist of a few surgeons, nurses, and anesthesiologists. It may include some professionals from the local hospital in the surgeries. Other organizations (e.g., Operation Smile) send a large group of people to the country so that there is no need for local professionals. Professional team members usually include the following:

- Anesthesiologists and/or nurse anesthetists
- Child life specialist

- Dentist and/or orthodontist and/or prosthodontist
- Intensivist and/or pediatrician
- Medical students and/or residents
- Nurses—surgical, post anesthesia care, postoperative
- Plastic surgeons and/or otolaryngologists
- Speech-language pathologist

In addition to the clinical professionals, many additional people may be included to provide coordination and support, including the following:

- Biomedical technician
- Education coordinator
- Interpreters
- Medical records workers
- Team coordinator
- Volunteers

In many cases, team members do not know each other before the mission and hence have not developed the trust and respect that come from working on a well-established team over time. However, all are committed to one purpose, and that is helping as many patients as possible. This is done by working very long days under less than ideal conditions. This shared dedication and experience actually helps the team to bond and work well together in a very short period of time (Fagan & Jacobs, 2009).

Typical Schedules

Surgical missions are at least a week in length, but most are ten days or longer. During the first few days, patients are evaluated to determine which ones are candidates for surgery, dental treatment, or prosthetic devices. During this time, the nurses set up the operating and recovery rooms.

Once the screening of patients is complete and the operating rooms are ready, the rest of the days are devoted to direct treatment, including surgeries and dental or prosthodontic treatment. A few of the nurses and physicians usually stay a few extra days after others have left, to provide postoperative care for the last surgical patients.

Due to the sheer volume of patients who are usually present for surgery, the majority of the surgeries tend to be primary lip and palate repairs. Therefore, if the palate is not sufficient after the primary surgery and the patient exhibits velopharyngeal insufficiency (VPI), many patients are not offered surgery again because of a lack of adequate resources. One mission group that was performing surgeries in the Philippines was concerned about the high rate of VPI with their palate repairs and the difficulty of doing secondary surgery. Therefore, they began doing a simultaneous sphincter pharyngoplasties with the palate repair. They reported better speech outcomes as a result of this practice (Saboye, Chancholle, Tournier, & Maurette, 2004).

Speech Screening Procedures

On most mission trips, there are hundreds of patients, including older children and even some adults, who need to be evaluated for possible surgery (Figure 23–2A–H). These patients often travel long distances to be seen and are willing to wait for hours, and even days, in hopes of receiving treatment. They wait in long lines for their child to be evaluated and for a determination as to whether their child will be included in the surgery schedule (Figure 23–3A and B).

Because of the volume of patients that need to be seen, the screening has to be very fast

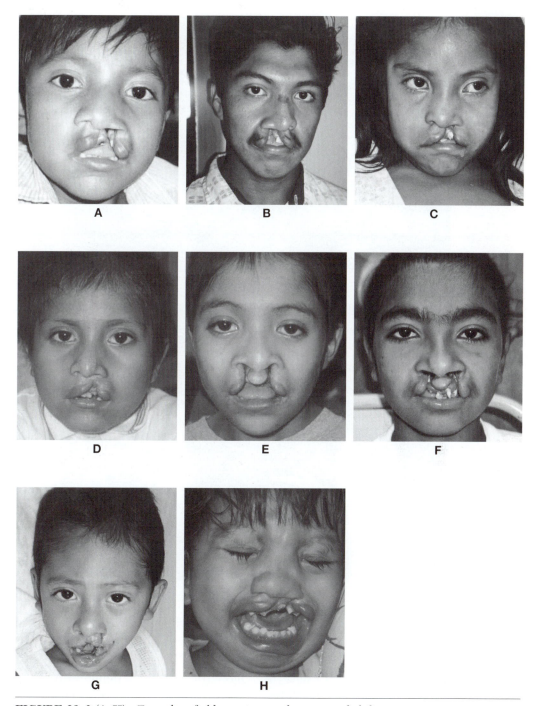

FIGURE 23–2 (A–H)   Examples of older patients with unrepaired clefts.

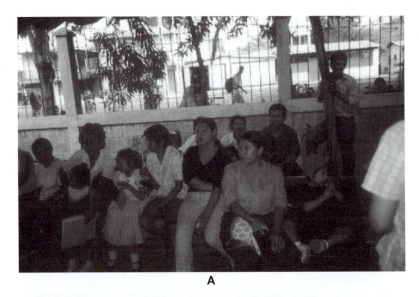

A

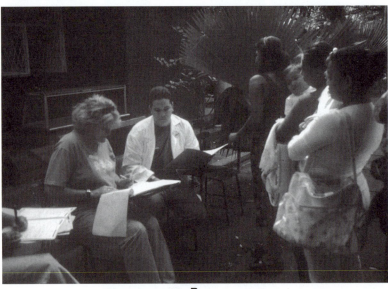

B

FIGURE 23–3 (A and B)   Patients waiting for screening.
Courtesy Ann W. Kummer, Ph.D./Cincinnati Children's Hospital Medical Center & University of Cincinnati College of Medicine

and efficient. It's not uncommon to have to screen 100 or more patients in one day. Assuming a 10-hour day, this leaves 6 minutes per patient if there are no breaks for lunch or the restroom. Realistically, there may be no more than 3 to 5 minutes to do a speech assessment on each patient. This is particularly challenging if the speech-language pathologist is not fluent in the language and has to work through an interpreter.

To make the process as quick and efficient as possible, the following are some suggestions:

- Before the patient comes to you, have a translator fill in identifying information and the answers to a few questions on a screening form.

- Have a volunteer manage the line and keep patients coming quickly, with their screening forms in hand.

- Do an intraoral examination first. With an open cleft palate, you don't need to assess speech because you already know the individual needs a palate repair. Particularly note the presence of a cleft, fistula, or previous velopharyngeal surgery.

- Ask the patient to count to 20 in his or her language. Have the patient repeat syllables with high-pressure phonemes repetitively (e.g., /pɑ, pa, pɑ/, /pi, pi, pi/, /sɑ, sa, sɑ/, /si, si, si/, etc.).

- Evaluate for the presence of obligatory and compensatory articulation productions, hypernasality, and nasal emission.

- Complete the screening form, and add comments as needed.

- Include recommendations for the following: surgery and type, prosthetic device and type, speech therapy, and parent counseling regarding speech-language stimulation techniques.

- For babies with open palates who are not yet candidates for a palate repair, give a written handout consisting of feeding instructions and suggestions for modifying the nipples. Have an interpreter review the instructions. Make sure the interpreter tells the parent to use boiled or bottled water for cleaning and for dry formula.

Speech Procedures during Surgery Days

Because therapy is not a quick fix, and kids who are undergoing surgery cannot participate in therapy, speech therapy is not a focus during a surgical mission. Instead, the speech-language pathologist should work with a dentist, orthodontist, or prosthodontist to (1) determine those patients who are candidates for prosthetic devices; (2) make sure that the devices fit appropriately to maximize speech; and (3) help the patient learn to use the device.

Counseling families is another task to be done during surgery week (Figure 23–4). The families may have various beliefs regarding the cause of the cleft, including God's will, past sins, becoming pregnant during a full moon, or having hiccups during pregnancy (Weatherley-White, Eiserman, Beddoe, & Vanderberg, 2005). Therefore, counseling regarding the cause and the importance of good nutrition during pregnancy can be of benefit to the families. The speech-language pathologist should also counsel parents regarding methods of speech and language stimulation for children under the age of 3, and methods of speech correction for children over the age of 3 who are undergoing palate repair. Handouts written in parents' language are particularly helpful. Even if the parents are illiterate, they can usually find someone in their town to read for them.

A suggested procedure for doing group counseling is as follows:

- Set up a space near the surgical waiting area.

- Obtain the surgery schedule for the day.

- Talk with parents in groups of five to seven while their children are in surgery.

- Try to use the same interpreter. After doing the interpretation many times, some

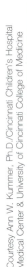

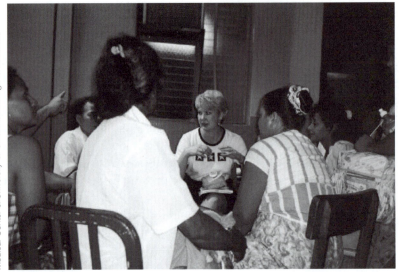

Courtesy Ann W. Kummer, Ph.D./Cincinnati Children's Hospital Medical Center & University of Cincinnati College of Medicine

FIGURE 23–4 Counseling families in groups.

interpreters can then do the counseling on their own.

- Using the surgery schedule, check off the patient's name after the parents have been counseled.

- The day after surgery, meet patients who have had a palate repair or flap/sphincter and their parents as a group. Repeat counseling, but direct it toward the older children. Demonstrate normal airflow and simple therapy correction techniques, using a straw for auditory feedback.

Surgery days are an appropriate time to do lectures and in-service training for local professionals. It can even be valuable to visit local schools for consultations or even have an open speech clinic for children in the area with any type of speech disorders.

If there is any downtime between working on speech appliances, counseling families, and teaching, it is expected that the speech-language pathologist and all other team members will assist with other aspects of the team's work as needed (Ducote, 2005) (Figure 23–5).

Expected Costs

As a volunteer on surgical missions, the team member is usually expected to cover some of the costs of travel. This may be done by paying a set amount up front or by paying directly for a portion of airfare, hotel, and food. Typically, several meals are provided by the mission organization or host country, particularly breakfast and lunch during screening and surgery days.

In addition to direct costs of travel, lodging, and food, there is also the cost of time away from work for the volunteer team members. Most employers require their employees to take vacation days for their time away for mission trips.

Concerns and Criticisms of Surgical Missions

Although most organizations subscribe to the goals of quality care and education, some achieve these goals better than others. There have been criticisms about the way some of the organizations operate (Silver, 2000). These criticisms include those listed here:

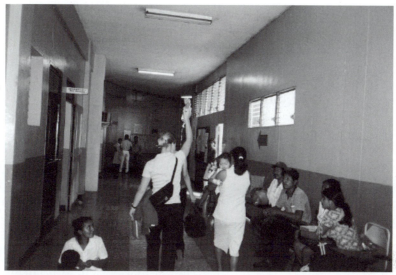
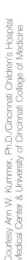

Courtesy Ann W. Kummer, Ph.D./Cincinnati Children's Hospital Medical Center & University of Cincinnati College of Medicine

FIGURE 23–5   Helping out with other duties when necessary. In this case, the child needed someone to hold the IV bag while he walked to surgery because poles and gurneys were unavailable in the hospital.

- More focus on direct care and less focus on training local professionals

- Not using qualified local surgeons, which would be far less costly than sending surgeons from outside the country

- Using volunteer professionals who are not considered experts in cleft care (e.g., using cosmetic surgeons who do not do cleft palate repairs in their practice in the United States)

- Using missions as a training ground for residents who need more surgical experience

- Doing too many surgeries in order to keep the numbers high

- Performing cosmetic surgery during the mission

- Performing surgery on children who would not be considered healthy enough to qualify for surgery in the United States

- Not having records available for returning patients

- Not providing adequate follow-up after the team leaves

- Not providing enough training of in-country professionals

- Having a high rate of fistulas or velopharyngeal insufficiency after palate repair

- Spending too much money on administration and overhead and not enough money on direct patient care

One major issue is that about 20% to 30% of patients who undergo palate repair in the United States have velopharyngeal insufficiency following the surgery. For several reasons, this rate may actually be much higher on mission trips. Unfortunately, there is rarely a mechanism for postoperative speech evaluations or opportunities for secondary surgery for velopharyngeal insufficiency for these patients (Aziz et al., 2009).

Another concern is that there are no studies of outcomes from these missions, so the actual success rates and complication rates are unknown. Because of this, there is an urgent need for more randomized clinical trials to evaluate both the outcomes of treatment and the complications so that clinical guidelines and protocols can be developed based on strong evidence (Lee, 1999).

Because some organizations are better than others, the prospective team member or donor should learn as much as possible about the organization and also consider the following factors:

- Reputation of the organization

- Financial support of the organization

- Quality of procedures, policies, and structure

- Qualifications of the team members

- Method and priority systems for choosing cases

- Number of procedures typically done per surgeon

- Types of procedures done on a mission (e.g., cosmetic vs. reconstructive)

- Method of record keeping

- Method for follow-up

- Experience of those who have been on other mission trips

- Focus on teaching and training of in-country professionals for sustainability

WORKING WITH AN INTERPRETER

If the speech-language pathologist is not fluent in the country's language, a good interpreter is essential when providing care on a surgical mission trip or providing direct education for local professionals.

On a surgical mission, the speech-language pathologist should meet with the interpreter(s) as soon as possible after arriving at the mission site. Spending time with the interpreter before seeing patients will help the process to go more smoothly and save a great deal of time during screening. Ideally, the interpreters should be given some written "scripts" of what will be asked or said during the evaluation and later during the family counseling (Ducote, 1998, 2005; Ducote & Juul, 1998). It is important to make sure that the interpreter understands the information and the procedure that you want to follow. During the session with the family, the interpreter should convey the information in the first person, as if talking directly to the person. For specific tips in working with an interpreter, see Table 23–1.

In addition to reviewing what the interpreters will say, it is also good to learn some words and phrases from the interpreters. Knowing how to introduce yourself can

---

TABLE 23–1   Tips for Working with an Interpreter

- Address remarks and questions directly to the listener, not to the interpreter.

- Use simple terms and short sentences.

- Avoid technical language, idioms, expressions, and slang.

- Pause frequently so that the interpreter can keep up.

- Use a positive tone and facial expression.

- Avoid body language or facial expressions that may be offensive or misconstrued.

- Periodically check the listener's understanding. Encourage him or her to request clarification when something is not understood.

- Reinforce understanding with visual diagrams and information written in the listener's language.

Courtesy of Srinivas Gosla Reddy, M.B.B.S., B.D.S., M.D.S., Ph.D./ Hyderabad, India.

enhance your interaction with the families. It helps to know the name of your profession in that country's language and to learn some basic words or sentences to use in the assessment (e.g., "How are you?" "Please sit down," "Count from 1 to 20." "Open your mouth." "Stick out your tongue." "Say /æ /and stick out your tongue.").

Interpreters are also very helpful when providing lectures or other forms of education to the local professionals. Although English is the language of medicine and thus many physicians and other health care providers at least understand English, certain considerations must be made when training professionals whose primary language is not English (or the language that you speak).

When giving lectures or seminars to local professionals, it is helpful to have the interpreter translate your slides and handouts to the native language of the participants. In addition, the translator can be helpful in clarifying points and helping with questions during the lecture.

In some cases, the translator is needed to translate throughout the lecture. If that is the case, it is important to give the lecture slowly, pausing frequently for the translator. The use of illustrations and translated slides and handouts is particularly important in this case.

PREPARING FOR INTERNATIONAL TRAVEL

International travel requires some planning, particularly when it is to a developing country with a different language and culture. It is well worth the time to learn about the country and culture before the trip. It is also important to obtain necessary vaccinations and health information. Finally, careful consideration of what to pack can make a big difference in the traveler's comfort during the trip.

Learn about the Culture and Language

Before traveling internationally, whether to teach in-country professionals or to provide direct care, it is important to learn about the culture and language of the host country. As ambassadors of goodwill and humanitarian aid, professionals should make every effort to understand and respect the country's social customs and protocols (Yeow et al., 2002). It is important to know what behaviors are considered polite and which are considered impolite. The role of women in certain societies is important to consider when working with the families. Even if you do not speak the language, it is important to learn how to say "thank you," to memorize certain greetings and phrases, and to know the standard form of addressing children and adults (e.g., señor, señora, etc.).

On a practical note, it may be helpful to learn about the food in the host country, especially if the traveler has allergies or strong aversions to certain types of food. Knowledge about the currency and whether bargaining is expected is helpful when shopping. Tipping customs and standards are also important to know.

Basic knowledge of the language and culture can help the traveler to be more effective as an educator and/or service provider and a good representative of his or her home country. It can also make the trip more interesting and enjoyable.

Documents That You Need

Of course, all individuals must have a passport in order to travel to a foreign country. It is important to note that many countries will not accept a passport that is due to expire in 3 months or less. Some countries also require a visa. This should be determined months before the trip because it can take several months to obtain a visa. It is advisable to keep a copy of the main page of your passport and a copy of your visa in your suitcase. It is also wise to take a copy of your immunization records, written information regarding allergies or special medical issues, and the name and phone number of a contact person in case of emergency. In addition to the copies of travel documents in your suitcase, it is smart to make another set of copies to keep at home.

Protect Your Health

Different parts of the world have different health risks for the traveler. The website for the Centers for Disease Control and Prevention (CDC, 2013) provides specific information, by geographic region, on risks for diseases, insect bites, and food and water contamination. Recommendations for prevention and treatment are also given.

In general, the traveler should determine what vaccinations are recommended for that region of the world and receive them several weeks before the trip. Yellow fever and typhoid vaccinations are commonly recommended. Often the vaccinations are only available through a local health department. If the travel will be in a tropical area, most authorities recommend taking malaria pills before going and using an insect repellent, particularly one containing DEET (N,N-diethyl-meta-toluamide), while there. DEET is especially important for protection against tick bites and mosquito bites, both of which can transmit disease. Clothing to cover arms and legs is also suggested.

Water is often a risk in developing countries. If this is the case, it is best to avoid drinks with ice, as well as salads or raw vegetables (because they are rinsed in water). Your toothbrush should be rinsed with bottled water rather than tap water. It is also wise to avoid swallowing water in the shower.

What to Pack

When packing for international travel, it is good to consider both comfort and culture. Because the days may be very long and may require a lot of walking or standing, comfortable shoes are a must. Many people retain water when traveling, and therefore loose shoes and clothing are preferable.

When selecting clothing, it helps to consider the climate and the probable lack of air conditioning or adequate heating. The cultural norms of dress should also be considered. For example, in Nicaragua, women do not wear

TABLE 23–2 Items to Take for Clinical Use

- Tongue blades
- Dental mirror
- Pen lights and batteries
- Alcohol preps or cloths
- Hand sanitizer
- Box of gloves
- Tissues
- Plastic tubing—pre-cut
- Bending straws
- Cleft palate bottles and nipples
- Therapy tokens
- Rewards (sticker sheets, safety pops, etc.)
- Handouts and diagrams of the velopharyngeal anatomy (in the appropriate language)
- Lavaliere for pen and pen light
- Office supplies: pens, legal pad, paper clips, stapler, etc.
- Scrubs (for observing in surgery)
- Giveaways for parents (pens, hotel-sized toiletries, note cards, etc.)
- Camera
- Fanny pack
- Tote bag
- Small suitcase on rollers

© Cengage Learning 2014

shorts. Therefore, loose-fitting, comfortable, washable, and preferably inexpensive clothes (skirts and dresses for women) should be worn.

For many countries, toilet paper is a luxury and not usually provided in public restrooms, so small packs of tissues should be taken, because they fit well in a fanny pack or pocket.

On surgical mission trips, the clinicians usually need to take everything that will be needed to work with the patients (including pens and paper). A suggested list of items to take for clinical use is found in Table 23–2. A small rolling suitcase can be useful as a portable storage unit for clinical supplies. It is best to take your "supply cabinet" back to the hotel at night because things that are left unattended often disappear.

SUMMARY

There are many organizations that send mission teams to do cleft repair in developing countries. Most organizations realize that educating in-country professionals is the best way to effect long-term change.

Speech-language pathologists can serve on these teams by providing input on which patients are best candidates for surgery. In addition, they can counsel families during the mission. Speech therapy is not realistic on these trips given the limited time available. However, perhaps the best thing that a speech-language pathologist can do is to provide training for in-country professionals who can also train others.

For those who have served on a surgical mission team, most will say that it is a remarkable experience that can change your life. You have the opportunity to work with a group of people who may come from all around the world. All have a strong sense of purpose, dedication, and compassion. They start out as strangers but quickly become friends.

Perhaps the biggest joy, however, is working with children and families who have so little but are so happy and grateful for what they have. By giving our time and efforts to them, we get so much more in return!

FOR REVIEW AND DISCUSSION

1. Why are there still millions of children and adults around the world who are living with an unrepaired cleft?

2. Describe some of the social and educational problems that individuals face in the underdeveloped countries.

3. What are the two primary goals of international not-for-profit organizations that are trying to address the needs of children who are born with clefts or craniofacial conditions? Which goal will make the biggest impact for the future?

4. Describe the role of a speech-language pathologist on a surgical mission team. What are some of the limitations?

5. List the typical clinical and support team members that would be needed on a surgical mission trip. What is the primary role for each professional? What would be the particular challenges for each professional on a surgical mission team?

6. Pretend you are planning to go on your first mission trip. What would you need to do to prepare? What would you take with you?

7. Describe what you would do to screen a large number of patients who speak a language that you do not know.

8. What is the role of the speech-language pathologist during surgery days? What can

you do to maximize the long-term impact of your time and efforts?

9. What are the challenges of obtaining postoperative speech therapy for patients who have a palate repair through one of these surgical missions? What can be done in the future to provide needed postoperative speech pathology services?

REFERENCES

Abenavoli, F. M. (2005). Operation Smile humanitarian missions. *Plastic and Reconstructive Surgery, 115*(1), 356–357.

American Cleft Palate–Craniofacial Association (ACPA). (2009). Parameters for evaluation and treatment of patients with cleft lip/palate or other craniofacial anomalies. American Cleft Palate–Craniofacial Association homepage. Accessed January 20, 2013, from http://www.acpa-cpf.org/uploads/site/Parameters_Rev_2009.pdf.

American Cleft Palate–Craniofacial Association (ACPA). (n.d.[a]). International treatment programs. American Cleft Palate–Craniofacial Association homepage. Accessed January 20, 2013, from http://www.acpa-cpf.org/team_care/position_paper/.

American Cleft Palate–Craniofacial Association (ACPA). (n.d.[b]). Speech samples. American Cleft Palate–Craniofacial Association homepage. Accessed January 20, 2013, from http://www.acpa-cpf.org/education/educational_resources/speech_samples/.

Aziz, S. R., Rhee, S. T., & Redai, I. (2009). Cleft surgery in rural Bangladesh: Reflections and experiences. *Journal of Oral and Maxillofacial Surgery, 67*(8), 1581–1588.

Bermudez, L. E. (2004). Humanitarian missions in the third world. *Plastic and Reconstructive Surgery, 114*(6), 1687–1689; Author reply 1689.

Centers for Disease Control and Prevention (CDC). (2013). *Travelers' health.* Accessed January 20, 2013, from http://wwwnc.cdc.gov/travel.

D'Antonio, L. L., & Landis, P. (1994). *Speech-language pathology services for the individual with cleft lip/palate: A training manual for volunteers to developing nations.* Chapel Hill, NC: American Cleft Palate–Craniofacial Association.

Ducote, C. A. (1998). Speech-language pathology services for individuals with cleft lip/palate in less developed nations: The Operation Smile approach. American Speech-Language-Hearing Association Special Interest Division 5, *Speech Science and Orofacial Disorders, 8*(1), 12–14.

Ducote, C. A. (2005). *Evaluation and treatment of cleft palate speech in developing countries: The Operation Smile approach.* Paper presented at the American Speech and Hearing Association Annual Convention, San Diego, CA.

Ducote, C. A., & Juul, A. M. (1998). *Guidelines for speech-language pathology volunteers on Operation Smile international missions.* New Orleans, LA: Operation Smile Speech Therapy Council.

Fagan, J. J., & Jacobs, M. (2009). Survey of ENT services in Africa: Need for a comprehensive intervention. *Global Health Action, 2.*

Furr, M. C., Larkin, E., Blakeley, R., Albert, T. W., Tsugawa, L., & Weber, S. M. (2011). Extending multidisciplinary management of cleft palate to the developing world. *Journal of Oral and Maxillofacial Surgery, 69*(1), 237–241.

Glazer, C. A., Bailey, P. J., Icaza, I. L., Valladares, S. J., Steere, K. A., Rosenblatt,

E. S., & Byrne, P. J. (2011). Multidisciplinary care of international patients with cleft palate using telemedicine. *Archives of Facial Plastic Surgery, 13*(6), 436–438.

Gupta, K., Bansal, P., Dev, N., & Tyagi, S. K. (2010). Smile Train project: A blessing for population of lower socio-economic status. *Journal of Indian Medical Association, 108*(11), 723–725.

Hartley, S. D., & Wirz, S. L. (2002). Development of a "communication disability model" and its implication on service delivery in low-income countries. *Social Science Medicine, 54*(10), 1543–1557.

Hubli, E. H., & Noordhoff, M. S. (2012, January 5). Smile Train: Changing the World One Smile at a Time. *Annals of Plastic Surgery.*

Kuehn, D. P., & Henne, L. J. (2003). Speech evaluation and treatment of patients with cleft palate. *American Journal of Speech-Language Pathology, 12*, 103–109.

Mossey, P. A., Shaw, W. C., Munger, R. G., Murray, J. C., Murthy, J., & Little, J. (2011). Global oral health inequalities: Challenges in the prevention and management of orofacial clefts and potential solutions. *Advances in Dental Research, 23*(2), 247–258.

Noordhoff, M. S. (2009). Establishing a craniofacial center in a developing country. *Journal of Craniofacial Surgery, 20*(Suppl. 2), 1655–1656.

Operation Smile. (n.d.). Accessed May 31, 2012, from http://www.operationsmile.org.

Prathanee, B., Dechongkit, S., & Manochiopinig, S. (2006). Development of community-based speech therapy model: For children with cleft lip/palate in northeast Thailand. *Journal of the Medical Association of Thailand, 89*(4), 500–508.

RSF-EARTHSPEAK. (2012). RSF-EARTHSPEAK homepage. Accessed May 31, 2012, from http://rsf-earthspeak.org.

Ruiz-Razura, A., Cronin, E. D., & Navarro, C. E. (2000). Creating long-term benefits in cleft lip and palate volunteer missions. *Plastic and Reconstructive Surgery, 105*(1), 195–201.

Saboye, J., ChanchoUe, A. R., Tournier, J. J., & Maurette, I. (2004). Palatovelopharyngoplastie en un temps. Notre experience aux Philippines. *Annales de Chirurgie Plastique et Esthetique, 49*(3), 261–264.

Silver, L. (2000). Creating long-term benefits in cleft lip and palate volunteer missions. *Plastic and Reconstructive Surgery, 106*(2), 516–517.

Smile Train. (n.d.). Accessed January 20, 2013, from http://www.smiletrain.org/.

Thakkar, P., Weatherley-White, R. C., Eiserman, W., Beddoe, M., & Vanderberg, R. (2005). Perceptions, expectations, and reactions to cleft lip and palate surgery in native populations: A pilot study in rural India. *Cleft Palate–Craniofacial Journal, 42*(5), 560–564.

Whitehead, E., Dorfman, V., Tremper, G., Kramer, A., Sigler, A., & Gosman, A. (2012). Telemedicine as a means of effective speech evaluation for patients with cleft palate. *Annals of Plastic Surgery, 68*(4), 415–417.

Winterton, T. (1998). Providing appropriate training and skills in developing countries. *International Journal of Language and Communication Disorders, 33*(Suppl.), 108–113.

Yeow, V. K., Lee, S. T., Lambrecht, T. J., Barnett, J., Gorney, M., Hardjowasito, W., Lemperle, G., et al. (2002). International Task Force on Volunteer Cleft Missions. *Journal of Craniofacial Surgery, 13*(1), 18–25.

APPENDIX A: RESOURCES FOR PARENT INFORMATION AND SUPPORT

Resources for information regarding cleft lip and palate and craniofacial anomalies are available from a variety of sources. The following is a list of some of the national organizations that can be helpful in providing information and resources. This list is not inclusive by any means. In fact, there are many local and state organizations that can provide information and support. Information on other organizations and resources can be found on many of the websites listed.

AboutFace is an organization of individuals and families who have experienced the challenges of facial differences. This organization provides emotional support, information services, and educational programs about living with facial differences. AboutFace focuses on syndromes and conditions, psychosocial issues, public awareness, and integration issues. It provides a variety of resources, including newsletters, videotapes, and publications. There is a national chapter network for local access and networking. For further information:

Phone: (800) 665-FACE [800-665-3223] or (416) 597-2229

Fax: (416) 597-8494

E-mail: info@aboutface.ca

Website: http://www.aboutface.ca

Address: 123 Edward Street, Suite 1003

Toronto, ON, Canada M5G 1E2

The **American Cleft Palate–Craniofacial Association (ACPA)** is a professional organization, founded in 1943, which includes all disciplines involved in the care and treatment of cleft palate and craniofacial anomalies. Members are from the United States and from over 40 countries all over the world. Membership is open to individuals who are qualified to treat or conduct research in the areas of cleft lip, cleft palate, and other craniofacial anomalies. ACPA is dedicated to the study and treatment of all aspects of craniofacial anomalies, including cleft lip and palate. The organization has worked toward establishing standards of care for patients with craniofacial anomalies. Clinical and research information is shared through its quarterly *Cleft Palate–Craniofacial Journal*. Annual professional meetings are held at various locations around the country for the purpose of sharing and exchanging clinical information and the latest research findings. For further information:

Phone: (919) 933-9044
E-mail: info@acpa-cpf.org
Website: http://www.acpa-cpf.org
Address: 1504 East Franklin Street, Suite 102
Chapel Hill, NC 27514-2820

The **Cleft Palate Foundation (CPF)** is a group that is associated with the American Cleft Palate–Craniofacial Association. The CPF has the mission of serving as a resource to families and professionals around the country. Services include a 24-hour toll-free phone number (CLEFTLINE: 1-800-24-CLEFT) that is available to both families and professionals who are seeking information about the evaluation or treatment of individuals with cleft lip, cleft palate, or other craniofacial birth defects. In addition, the CPF provides consumers with booklets on all aspects of cleft lip and palate (available in English and Spanish), craniofacial anomalies, and related syndromes. They provide a bibliography for parents of children with cleft lip/palate and a catalog of informational videocassettes. They can refer families to local and national support groups. Finally, the CPF provides consumers with a list of guidelines for choosing a medical team for cleft palate or craniofacial care, and also provides listings of qualified cleft and craniofacial anomaly teams in the patient's area. For further information:

Phone: (919) 933-9044
Fax: (919) 933-9604
E-mail: info@cleftline.org
Website: http://www.cleftline.org
Address: 1504 East Franklin Street, Suite 102
Chapel Hill, NC 27514-2820

Children's Craniofacial Association offers assistance with doctor referrals and nonmedical assistance. There are annual family retreats and educational programs. The organization has publications about various craniofacial syndromes. For further information:

Phone: (800) 535-3643 or (214) 570-9099
Fax: (214) 570-8811
E-mail: contactCCA@ccakids.com
Website: http://www.childrenscraniofacial.com
Address: 13140 Coit Road, Suite 517
Dallas, TX 75240

FACES: The National Craniofacial Association is a nonprofit organization that serves children and adults with craniofacial disorders by acting as a clearinghouse of information on specific disorders and available resources, providing networking opportunities with other families, publishing a quarterly newsletter, and providing financial assistance to families who cannot afford to travel away from home to a specialized craniofacial medical center. For further information:

Phone: (800) 3FACES3 [800-332-2373]
E-mail: faces@faces-cranio.org
Website: http://www.faces-cranio.org
Address: P.O. Box 11082
            Chattanooga, TN 37401

Let's Face It is an information and support network for people with facial differences, their families, and professionals. Once a year, this organization publishes an extensive manual of organizations and resources for individuals with facial differences. To be placed on their mailing list, just send an e-mail address. For further information:

E-mail: faceit@umich.edu
Website: http://desica.dent.umich.edu/faceit/
Address: University of Michigan
            School of Dentistry/Dentistry Library
            1011 N. University
            Ann Arbor, MI 48109-1078

Parents Helping Parents (PHP) is a parent-directed family resource center serving children with special needs, their families, and the professionals who serve them. This organization provides parent with professional training on how to begin and maintain a parent support network. Publications are available for training and information. For further information:

Phone: (408) 727-5775
Fax: (408) 286-1116
E-mail: info@php.com
Website: http://www.php.com
Address: Parents Helping Parents
            Sobrato Center For Nonprofits–San Jose
            1400 Parkmoor Avenue Suite 100
            San Jose, CA 95126

Smile Train has a free online library and links for articles from around the world on the cause and treatment of clefts. They also have informational booklets for families. For further information:

Phone: (800) 932-9541

E-mail: info@smiletrain.org

Website: http://www.smiletrain.org

Address: 41 Madison Ave., 28th Floor
New York, NY 10010

Appendix B: Cleft Palate Foundation Publications

Reprinted with permission from the Cleft Palate Foundation. Available at http://cleftline.org.

Fact Sheets (Full-Text Online Reports)

- *Answers to Common Questions about Scars* (en español)
- *Bonegrafting the Cleft Maxilla*
- *Choosing a Cleft Palate or Craniofacial Team* (en español)
- *Crouzon Syndrome*
- *Dealing with Your Insurance Company/HMO*
- *Dental Care for a Child with Cleft Lip and Palate* (en español)
- *Financial Assistance* (en español)
- *For the Parents of Newborn Babies with Cleft Lip/Cleft Palate* (en español)
- *Letter to a Teacher*
- *Letter to the Parent of a Child with a Cleft* (en español)
- *Pierre Robin Sequence*
- *Positional Plagiocephaly*
- *Preparing Your Child for Social Situations*
- *Replacing a Missing Tooth*
- *Selected Bibliography for Parents*
- *Special Considerations for Speech and Language Development for the Child Who is Adopted Internationally*
- *Speech Development* (en español)
- *Submucous Clefts*

- *Treacher Collins*
- *Treatment for Adults* (en español)
- *What about Breastfeeding?*
- *Support*

BOOKLET SUMMARIES (SUMMARIES OF DOCUMENTS AVAILABLE FOR ORDERING FROM THE CLEFT PALATE FOUNDATION)

These publications are provided free to families by the Cleft Palate Foundation. To receive a copy of any of the publications below, call the CLEFTLINE: 1-800-24CLEFT or e-mail to admin@cleftline.org.

- *Your Baby's First Year* (en español)
- *Toddlers and Preschoolers* (en español)
- *The School Aged Child* (en español)
- *As You Get Older*
- *Information for Adults*
- *Feeding Your Baby* (en español)
- *Cleft Surgery* (en español)
- *Help with Hearing* (en español)
- *Genetics and You*
- *Treatment Options for Better Speech* (en español)
- *Parameters for Evaluation and Treatment of Patients with Cleft Lip/Palate or Other Craniofacial Anomalies*

GLOSSARY

ablative surgery Surgery that involves removal of a part, such as a portion of the hard palate, due to a malignancy.

acrocentric When the centromere of a chromosome is very close to one end of the chromosome.

active speech characteristics See *compensatory errors*.

acoustic resonance The tendency of an acoustic system to absorb more energy when it is forced or driven at a frequency that matches one of its own natural frequencies of vibration than it does at other frequencies.

acute otitis media Bacterial infection of the middle ear.

adenoid See *adenoids*.

adenoidectomy Surgical procedure to remove the adenoids; done to resolve recurrent infection, improve Eustachian tube function, or eliminate upper airway obstruction.

adenoid facies Facial characteristics due to airway obstruction secondary to adenoid enlargement; characteristics include an open mouth posture, anterior tongue position, the mandible in a forward or downward position, facial elongation, suborbital coloring and puffy eyes, and the appearance of pinched nostrils.

adenoid hypertrophy Excessive enlargement of the adenoid pad.

adenoid pad See *adenoids*.

adenoids A mass of lymphoid tissue that is found on the posterior pharyngeal wall of the nasopharynx on the skull base; also called the *pharyngeal tonsil, adenoid pad,* or *adenoid*.

adenotonsillectomy A surgical procedure where both the tonsil and adenoid tissue are removed; done to resolve recurrent infection, improve Eustachian tube function, or eliminate upper airway obstruction.

adipose Fat tissue.

aerodynamic instrumentation Equipment that can be used to assess airflow and air pressure changes with velopharyngeal opening and closure.

aerodynamics A branch of physics that deals with the mechanical properties of air and other gases in motion, the properties that set them in motion, and the results of that motion.

affricate phonemes Pressure-sensitive consonants that require a buildup of intraoral air pressure and then slow release through a narrow opening; they are produced as a combination of a plosive and fricative and include /ʧ/ and /ʤ/.

ala nasi (pl. alae) Latin for "wing"; the outside curved part of the nostril.

alar base The area where the ala meets the upper lip.

alar rim The outside curved edge of each nostril.

alleles   The alternative forms or variations of a given gene that are found at the same locus on an homologous chromosome.

almost-but-not-quite (ABNQ)   A term used to refer to a small, yet consistent, velopharyngeal gap.

alveolar bone grafting   A surgical procedure of grafting bone, often from the iliac crest (hip), to bridge the gap between the bony segments of the cleft alveolus; this helps to repair the alveolar ridge, serves as the missing nasal floor and piriform (nasal) rim, and provides bone for eruption of teeth.

alveolar ridge   The portion of the maxilla and mandible that form the base and the bony support for the teeth; also called the *alveolus* or simply the *gum ridge*.

alveolus   The socket of the tooth; also known as the *alveolar ridge*.

amino acids   The building blocks of proteins.

amnion   Membrane surrounding the embryo and fetus.

amniotic bands   Strands of tissue from the amnion that have ruptured and float in the amniotic cavity; these strands can attach to limbs, the head, or other body parts, where they act as tourniquets, cutting off blood supply to developing structures, resulting in amputations of limbs and digits, cleft lip, and encephalocele if the cranium is involved.

anodontia   Rare genetic disorder characterized by the congenital absence of all primary or permanent teeth. It is associated with ectodermal dysplasia, which affects the skin.

Angle's classification system   Differentiates normal occlusion and three types of malocclusion.

ankyloglossia   Also known as *tongue-tie;* a condition where the lingual frenulum is short or has an anterior attachment, resulting in restricted movement of the tongue-tip; typically diagnosed if the patient cannot elevate the tongue tip sufficiently to touch the roof of mouth with mouth open, and cannot protrude the tongue-tip past the mandibular gingival ridge or incisors.

ankylosis   Immobility of a moveable part due to restriction.

anotia   Absence of the external auditory canal.

anterior crossbite   A condition where a maxillary tooth or teeth are inside the mandibular arch; may involve any or all of the anterior teeth, such as the central incisors, lateral incisors, or canines; commonly seen in patients with dental or skeletal Class III malocclusion.

anterior nasal spine   The anterior point of the maxilla that corresponds to the base of the columella.

anterior–posterior (AP) view   See *frontal view*.

anticipation   In genetics, the tendency for a disorder to have earlier age of onset or more severe manifestations in successive generations.

antimongoloid slant   Downward slant of the eyes.

apex of the dental arch   The midline point of the dental arch where the left and right halves of the arch join.

apnea   See *sleep apnea*.

apraxia (of speech)   (adj. apraxic) Characterized by difficulty executing volitional oral movements and difficulty in sequencing oral movements for connected speech; can result in an inability to adequately coordinate velopharyngeal movement with the other subsystems of speech (respiration, phonation, and articulation); also called *dyspraxia* or *verbal apraxia.* When it occurs in children and affects speech development, it is called *developmental apraxia* or *childhood apraxia of speech (CAS).*

articulators   The oral structures that move to modify the airstream during speech; these include the lips, jaws (including the teeth), tongue, and velum.

aspiration   Entry of material into the airway; often occurs with swallowing if there is a lack of adequate synchrony of breathing and swallowing.

association   In genetics, when two or more abnormalities appear together frequently but have not yet been classified together as a syndrome.

ataxia   An inability to coordinate muscle activity during voluntary movements, usually due to disorders of the cerebellum or posterior columns of the spinal cord.

atlas   The first cervical vertebrae; articulates with the occipital bone and rotates around the dens of the axis.

atresia   (adj. atretic) Congenital absence or closure of any bodily orifice (opening, passage, or cavity); see *aural atresia.*

atrial septal defect (ASD)   Congenital discontinuity of the tissue that separates the upper chambers of the heart.

atrophy   Shrinkage or degeneration of a structure.

attention deficit-hyperactivity disorder (ADHD)   A cluster of behavioral characteristics involving impaired attention, distractibility, impulsivity, and hyperactivity; there appears to be a genetic basis to this disorder that affects the biochemical function in the brain.

attenuation   The combined absorption and scattering of radiation proton particles by the tissues.

audible nasal emission   Nasal emission through a medium-sized opening; there is some resistance to the flow so that it causes a friction-type sound.

audio   Related to the sense of hearing.

audiologist   A professional who is responsible for testing hearing and middle ear function; the professional who works in conjunction with the otolaryngologist in the monitoring, evaluation, and treatment of hearing loss associated with middle ear disease, structural anomalies, or neurological anomalies that affect hearing recognition and perception.

auditory   Pertaining to the sense of hearing or organs of hearing.

auditory atresia   See *aural atresia.*

auditory cortex   Part of the brain that provides an awareness of sound.

auditory tube   See *Eustachian tube.*

aural   Related to the ear or hearing.

aural atresia   Congenital closure or absence of the auditory canal that usually results in a conductive hearing loss; also called *auditory atresia.*

auricle   The external ear; also called *pinna* or *concha.*

autogenous   Produced by the individual; self-generating.

autosomal recessive   Traits that are manifest only when the trait is present in both copies of a gene.

autosome   (adj. autosomal) Any chromosome that is not a sex chromosome.

backing of phonemes   A compensatory articulation strategy characterized by the production of most phonemes with the back of the tongue, and with the velum or with the posterior pharyngeal wall.

base view X-ray view that allows the examiner to see the entire velopharyngeal sphincter during connected speech, as if looking up through the port; the relative contributions of the velum, the lateral pharyngeal walls, and posterior pharyngeal wall to closure can be determined; also called an *en face view*.

Bell's palsy Facial paralysis due to an infection.

Bernoulli effect The low pressure created behind the fast-moving air column as it passes through the vocal folds. This causes the bottom of the folds to close, followed by the top. The closure of the vocal folds cuts off the air column and releases a pulse of air.

bicuspids Teeth that typically have two cusps.

bifid uvula A congenital split or cleft in the uvula; a stigmata that is frequently associated with a submucous cleft palate.

bilabial competence The ability to achieve bilabial closure at rest and during production of bilabial sounds.

bilabial incompetence The inability to close the lips naturally at rest.

bilabial phonemes Speech sounds that are produced with the lips (e.g., /p/, /b/, /m/, /w/).

biofeedback A technique for making unconscious or autonomic physiological processes perceptible to the senses in order to manipulate them by conscious mental control; techniques are based on the learning principle that a desired response can be learned when it is determined that a specific thought process can produce the desired physiological response.

body section (of a prosthetic device) The anterior or palatal portion of a speech appliance that fits snugly against the contours of the individual's mouth and teeth; the purpose of the body section is to hold the appliance in place against the roof of the mouth or to serve as an obturator to close off a defect in the palate.

bone graft procedure See *alveolar bone graft procedure*.

brachycephaly A short skull.

brachydactyly Abnormally short digits (fingers or toes).

breathiness A vocal quality where the vocal cords are held further apart so that a larger volume of air escapes between them.

Brodie crossbite Occurs when the lingual cusps of all the maxillary posterior teeth are buccal to the mandibular teeth.

buccal (adj.) For the buccinator muscle of the cheeks; pertaining to, in the direction of, or adjacent to the cheek; the part of the dental arch that is posterior to the canine teeth and on the side of the teeth.

buccal crossbite Occurs when one or more maxillary teeth are positioned buccally such that the maxillary lingual cusps reside buccal to the mandibular cusps.

buccal pads Encapsulated fat masses inside the cheek.

buccal sulcus (pl. sulci) The area between the cheeks and teeth.

café au lait macules Pigmented spots the color of "coffee with milk"; characteristic finding of neurofibromatosis 1.

canines Teeth that have one point or cusp; also known as *cuspids*.

cant A slant, as in dental occlusion.

canthus (pl. canthi) The angle or corner of the eye.

capacitance Ability of a transducer to store energy.

caries   Decay in the teeth, resulting in cavities.

carriers   Individuals who have one abnormal copy of a gene and are without detectable abnormalities.

cell cycle   The process of preparing for and undergoing cell division.

central fossa   (pl. fossae) The valley between the buccal cusp and the lingual cusp of a tooth.

central sleep apnea   Suspension of breathing during sleep due to medullary depression, which inhibits respiratory movement.

centromere   The area of constriction of a chromosome that divides the chromosome into two pairs of arms.

cephalogram   See *cephalometric radiograph*.

cephalometric radiograph   A standardized lateral skull film used to measure the jaw relationship and the soft tissue profile of the forehead, nose, lips, and chin; often used in orthodontic and orthognathic surgery planning; often referred to as a *cephalogram*.

cheilorraphy   Cleft lip repair.

childhood apraxia of speech (CAS)   A motor speech disorder, usually of unclear etiology, that affects the child's ability to develop speech; it causes difficulty with the production and sequencing of motor movements for speech; speech is usually characterized by inconsistent errors that increase with utterance length or complexity; also called *developmental apraxia*, *verbal apraxia*, or just *apraxia*.

choana   (pl. choanae) The opening on each side of the posterior part of the vomer that leads from the nasal cavity into the nasopharynx.

choanal atresia   Congenital closure of the choana.

choanal stenosis   A narrowing of the choana.

cholesteatoma   A mass of keratinizing squamous epithelium and cholesterol in the middle ear, usually resulting from chronic otitis media.

chromosome   One of the bodies in the cell nucleus that contains genes; consists of a single linear double strand of DNA with associated proteins that function to organize and compact the DNA in a cell-for-cell division; the 46 chromosomes (23 pairs) contain the complete set of instructions for cell replication and differentiation.

cine study   See *cineradiography*.

cineradiography   Radiography of an organ in motion; an old method for evaluating velopharyngeal function by recording multiple views on motion picture film in order to observe several dimensions; often referred to as a *cine study*.

circular pattern   Pattern of velopharyngeal closure that occurs when all of the velopharyngeal structures contribute equally, and the closure pattern resembles a true sphincter.

circumvallate papilla   A line of prominent taste buds that makes an inverted "V" on the posterior tongue.

Class I occlusion   Normal dental arch relationship, although the teeth may be misaligned; the mesiobuccal (front outside) cusp of the first maxillary molar fits in the buccal (outside) groove of the first mandibular molar.

Class II malocclusion   Abnormal dental arch relationship where the mesiobuccal (front outside) cusp of the first maxillary molar is anterior to the buccal (outside) groove of the first mandibular molar; the maxillary arch is protrusive and too far in front of the mandibular arch.

Class III malocclusion   Abnormal dental arch relationship where the mesiobuccal (front outside) cusp of the first maxillary molar is posterior to the buccal (outside) groove of the first mandibular molar; the maxillary arch is retrusive and too far behind the mandibular arch.

cleft   An abnormal opening or a fissure in an anatomical structure that is normally closed.

cleft lip   A congenital malformation that occurs in utero during the first trimester of pregnancy and involves a fissure of the lip and sometimes alveolus.

cleft muscle of Veau   Refers to abnormal velar muscle insertion due to a cleft palate; the levator veli palatini muscle does not interdigitate in the midline, and both this paired muscle and the palatopharyngeus muscles are inserted abnormally onto the posterior border of the hard palate, rendering them essentially nonfunctional.

cleft palate   A congenital malformation that occurs in utero during the first trimester of pregnancy and involves a fissure in the soft palate and sometimes the hard palate.

cleft palate team (CPT)   A team of professionals that consists of a surgeon, an orthodontist, a speech-language pathologist, and one additional specialist, according to the requirements of the American Cleft Palate–Craniofacial Association; other team members may include an audiologist, dentist, geneticist (dysmorphologist), nurse, oral surgeon (maxillofacial surgeon), and others.

clinodactyly   Deflection or curvature of the digits (fingers or toes).

coarticulation   An abnormal consonant production characterized by one manner of production with simultaneous valving at two places of production.

cochlea   A part of the inner ear that is composed of a bony spiral tube that is shaped as a snail's shell and is responsible for hearing.

coding region   The portions of a gene that determine the amino acid sequence for a polypeptide.

cognition   (adj. cognitive) Refers to the individual's ability to engage in conscious intellectual activities, such as thinking, reasoning, imagining, or learning.

coloboma   A congenital defect, especially of the eye, which often involves a notch of the eyelid margin; usually affects the lower lid.

columella   The "little column" at the lower portion of the nose that separates the nostrils; cartilage and mucosa that are located under the nasal tip and at the lower end of the nasal septum.

compensatory errors   Articulation productions that abnormal in placement due to the individual's response to abnormal structure, such as velopharyngeal insufficiency or dental malocclusion, or abnormal physiology, such as velopharyngeal incompetence; also known as *active speech characteristics*.

complete cleft lip   Involves the entire lip through the nostril sill and the alveolus (or dental arch) all the way to the area of the incisive foramen.

complete crossbite   When the maxilla is very narrow and as a result, the entire maxillary arch is inside the mandibular arch during occlusion.

concha   See *nasal concha*.

conductive hearing loss   A type of hearing loss due to a blockage or problem with sound conduction to the inner ear.

condyle   The rounded articular surface of the bone, such as in the jaw joint.

congenital   A disease or deformity that is present at birth; may be the result of an inherited (genetic or chromosomal) condition or may be caused by something that occurred during the pregnancy (exogenous factors).

congenital palatal insufficiency (CPI)   Velopharyngeal dysfunction with no history of cleft palate, no apparent evidence of submucous cleft, or other known etiology.

conotruncal heart defects   Also known as *outflow tract defects;* these are major abnormalities of the heart's chambers or blood vessels. They include truncus arteriosus, transposition of the great arteries, double outlet of the right ventricle, and tetralogy of Fallot.

consanguinity   Mating between related individuals.

consulting team   A team of professionals whose members provide opinions regarding the total care of the patient; the opinions and recommendations are forwarded to the treating professionals for follow-up.

contiguous gene syndromes   Syndromes caused by deletions large enough to contain several genes, but too small to be seen on routine cytogenetic analysis.

continuous positive airway pressure (CPAP)   An instrument that delivers continuous airway pressure to the nasopharynx by means of a hose and nasal mask; used primarily in the treatment of sleep apnea to prevent pharyngeal collapse; has also been used to provide resistance training to strengthen the velopharyngeal musculature when there is velopharyngeal incompetence.

coronal pattern   A pattern of velopharyngeal closure that is accomplished primarily by the posterior movement of the velum against a broad area of the posterior pharyngeal wall and the possible anterior movement of the posterior pharyngeal wall; there is less contribution of the lateral pharyngeal walls during closure with this pattern.

corpus callosum   Nerve fibers that allow communication between the left and right cerebral hemispheres. Consists mostly of contralateral axon projections. It appears as a wide, flat region just ventral to (below) the cortex.

corticotomy   A partial cut in the bone.

coupling   Sharing of acoustic energy.

craniofacial anomaly   A structural or functional abnormality that affects the cranium or face.

craniofacial team (CFT)   A team of professionals that consists of a craniofacial surgeon, an orthodontist, a mental health professional, and a speech-language pathologist according to the requirements of the American Cleft Palate–Craniofacial Association; other members may include a neurosurgeon, an ophthalmologist, and others.

craniosynostosis   Abnormal development of the cranial skeleton due to premature ossification of one or more cranial sutures, resulting in malformation of the skull with growth; the shape of the skull depends on the sutures that are involved; can cause raised intracranial pressure (ICP) and mental retardation if not treated; can be syndromal, due to genetic factors, or nonsyndromal.

crossbite   A type of dental malocclusion where a maxillary tooth or teeth are inside the mandibular teeth; when the normal overlap of the upper teeth to the lower teeth is reversed, so that the lower teeth overlap the upper teeth buccally; can be anterior or lateral.

cryptorchidism   Undescended testes.

cul-de-sac resonance   Abnormal resonance during speech, which occurs when the transmission of acoustic energy is trapped in a blind pouch in the vocal tract with only one outlet; the speech is perceived as muffled because the sound is contained in a cavity with no direct means of escape.

Cupid's bow   The shape of the top of the upper lip, which includes a rounded configuration with an indentation in the middle.

cusp   The point on a tooth.

cuspids   Teeth that have one point or cusp; also known as *canines*.

cytogenetics   The branch of genetics that is concerned with the structure and function of the chromosomes within the cell; literally means "cell genetics."

cytokinesis   The separation of the cell cytoplasm to form two distinct cells with separate cell membranes.

damping   To slow or stop the vibration or decrease the amplitude of an oscillating system.

deciduous teeth   Primary, or "baby," teeth.

deep bite   When the upper teeth overlap more than 25% of the lower teeth; the lower incisors may be in contact with the alveolar ridge of the palate.

deformation   (syn. deformity) Birth defect that arises as a result of abnormal mechanical or physical forces in the fetal environment on an otherwise normal structure; usually results in the abnormal shape or form of a completely formed organ or structure, such as clubfoot.

deformity   See *deformation*.

dehisce   To pull apart.

dehiscence   A breakdown of a surgical repair or unwanted opening in an area that has been surgically closed.

deletion   In genetics, absence of a piece of a chromosome or genetic material; often results in multiple malformations and developmental handicaps.

denasality   Abnormal resonance due to a lack of vibration of the sound energy in the nasal cavity; total nasal airway obstruction and the resultant effect on resonance.

dental arch   The curved structure in the maxilla and mandible that consists of the alveolar ridge and teeth.

dental elastics   Small rubber bands used to add a dynamic component for pulling teeth or bony segments together.

dental implants   Cylindrical shaped pieces of titanium that can take the place of a missing tooth's root and are able to support crowns and prosthetic devices.

dental occlusion   The manner in which the maxillary teeth and mandibular teeth fit together, or the bite; in normal occlusion the upper arch overlaps the lower arch.

dentition   The teeth taken all together.

dentures   Removable prosthetic teeth that replace an entire dental arch.

deoxyribonucleic acid (DNA)   A nucleic acid made up of building blocks called nucleotides; contained in the nuclei of animal and vegetable cells, it is the component of chromosomes; each DNA molecule contains many genes, which contain hereditary information; DNA consists of two strands that wrap around each other in the shape of a twisted ladder or double helix.

dermatoglyphics   Creases on the hands or changes in the fingerprints that can give clues to early developmental problems.

developmental apraxia   See *childhood apraxia of speech (CAS)*.

diastasis   A separation between two normally joined structures, as in separation of the levator veli palatini muscles when there is a submucous cleft palate.

diastema   A space or opening between the teeth, usually the upper central incisors.

differential pressure   The difference in pressure between the nasal cavity and the oral cavity during speech, as measured simultaneously through aerodynamic instrumentation.

direct instrumental procedures   Instrumental procedures that allow the examiner to visualize the structures of the velopharyngeal valve during speech (and swallowing) and observe abnormalities of velopharyngeal structure or function; includes the use of videofluoroscopy and nasopharyngoscopy.

disruption   A morphologic defect resulting from an extrinsic breakdown or interference with a normal developmental process.

distal   (adj.) Away from the center, midline, or point of origin.

distally   (adv.) See *distal*.

distraction osteogenesis   A method for increasing bone length that involves making a corticotomy in the middle of a bone, then slowly pulling the cut ends apart (distracting) with a mechanical device; new bone is able to regenerate between the cut ends, obviating the need for bone grafts; can be used for maxillary or mandibular advancement.

dolichocephaly   Long, narrow skull seen with prematurity.

dominant inheritance   When only one gene is needed for expression of a trait (e.g., brown eyes); when one allele from one parent is expressed over a contrasting allele from the other parent.

dorsum   The top surface, as on the tongue.

double helix   Coiled ladder of a DNA molecule that consists of two polymers of nucleotides.

duplication   When part of a chromosome is duplicated, often resulting in multiple malformations and developmental handicaps.

dysarthria   A motor speech disorder that affects the oral articulators and is characterized by abnormalities of muscular strength, range of motion, speed, accuracy, and tonicity due to a neurological injury or insult; speech is very slow and characterized by inaccurate movement of the articulators.

dysmorphogenesis   (adj. dysmorphic) The process of abnormal tissue formation, resulting in abnormally formed features.

dysmorphologist   Another term for a geneticist.

dysmorphology   The study of abnormal shape or form.

dysphagia   Abnormality or difficulty in swallowing.

dysphonia   (adj. dysphonic) Refers to voice disorder that results in an alteration in the normal phonatory quality of the voice; characterized by breathiness, hoarseness, low intensity, and glottal fry.

dysplasia   An abnormal organization of cells into tissues and the outcome of the process.

dyspraxia   See *apraxia (of speech)*.

eardrum   See *tympanic membrane*.

ear, nose, and throat (ENT) specialist   See *otolaryngologist*.

ectopic tooth   A normal tooth that erupts in an abnormal position.

ectrodactyly   Deficiency or absence of one or more central digits of the hand or foot. Often called "Lobster-claw syndrome" due to its split hand or foot appearance.

edema   An excessive amount of fluid in cells and tissues, causing swelling.

encephalocele   A congenital gap in the skull with herniation of brain tissue into the nose or palate.

endogenous   A factor from within the organism rather than from the environment, such as the genetic makeup of the organism.

endoscope   A specialized, flexible fiberoptic instrument that consists of an eyepiece at the end of a long tube or scope; used for examination of an internal canal or organ; can be used for evaluation of the velopharyngeal mechanism, pharynx, or larynx; a type of endoscope is a *nasopharyngoscope*.

endoscopy   A procedure that allows the visualization of the interior of a canal or hollow organ by means of a special instrument, usually called an *endoscope*.

en face view   See *base view*.

epibulbar dermoid   A cyst on the eyeball.

epicanthal folds   Folds of tissue that extend from the upper eyelid to the lower part of the orbit at the inner canthus or corner of the eye.

epigenetic disorder   Genetic condition not caused by a change in the DNA.

epiphyseal dysplasia   Underdevelopment or abnormality of the long bones of the extremities.

epitaxis   A nosebleed.

Eustachian tube   The tube that connects the middle ear with the nasopharynx; usually closed at the pharyngeal end at rest, but opens with swallowing and yawning due to the action of the tensor veli palatini muscle; allows ventilation of the middle ear, equalization of air pressure on both sides of the tympanic membrane, and drainage of fluids; also known as the *auditory tube*.

exogenous   A factor that is outside an organism and is not indigenous to that organism, such as drugs or smoke.

exons   Portions of genes that code for amino acids and are separated by introns.

exophthalmos   Protrusion of one or both globes of the eye beyond the socket due to either congenital or pathological factors that provide pressure behind the eye; often associated with craniosynostosis involving the coronal suture.

exorbitism   Excessive protrusion of the globe of the eye from its socket due to shallow orbits.

expressive language   The ability to generate and then transmit a message.

expressivity   The extent to which a gene is apparent in the phenotype.

external auditory canal   A skin-lined canal of the external ear that leads to the eardrum.

external ear   Part of the ear that is comprised of the pinna and the external auditory canal.

fascia   A sheet of fibrous tissue that encloses muscles and muscle groups.

faucial pillars   Bilateral curtain-like structures in the posterior portion of the oral cavity; the anterior faucial pillar is formed as the velum curves downward toward the tongue, and the posterior faucial pillar is just behind the anterior pillar.

faucial tonsils   See *tonsils*.

feeding obturator   A prosthetic appliance that can be used in the first few months of life to assist the infant with cleft palate in feeding; it keeps the tongue from resting inside the cleft and provides a solid surface so that the tongue can achieve compression of the nipple; no longer felt to be needed by most cleft centers.

fiberoptic endoscopic evaluation of swallowing (FEES)   A procedure where a flexible endoscope is used in the evaluation of swallowing disorders; involves the transnasal passage of an endoscope for viewing of the pharyngeal and laryngeal structures to study the integrity of airway protection during swallowing.

fistula   (pl. fistulae or fistulas) An abnormal hole or passage from one between two epithelialized organs that do not normally connect; examples included an oronasal (palatal) fistula or tracheoesophageal fistula.

fixed bridge   Permanently placed prosthetic teeth typically used to replace dental segments.

fluorescent in situ hybridization (FISH)   A procedure used in a cytogenetic laboratory that involves the use of a nucleic acid probe labeled with a fluorescent dye to localize a specified submicroscopic segment of DNA; used to determine deletion of parts of chromosomes, as in the diagnosis of velocardiofacial syndrome.

foramen   (pl. foramina) A normal hole or opening in a bony structure or membranous structure; often serves as a passageway to allow blood vessels and nerves to pass through to the area on the other side.

forme fruste   A partial or arrested form of a cleft lip where the overlying skin is intact, but the underlying muscle, nasal cartilage, and oral sphincter function usually are significantly affected; also called *microform cleft*.

founder effect   When a relatively small number of original ancestors has led to a high frequency of carriers for certain disorders in a population.

fovea palati   (pl. foveae palati) One of the bilateral midline depressions at the junction of the hard and soft palate that are the openings to minor salivary glands.

frenulum   (pl. frenulae) A small frenum; see *frenum* and *lingual frenulum*.

frenum   (pl. frena or frenums) A narrow fold of mucous membrane or web that connects a fixed structure to a movable part and serves to check undue movement; see *frenulum* and *lingual frenulum*.

fricative phonemes   Pressure-sensitive sounds that require a gradual release of air pressure through a small opening; includes /f/, /v/, /s/, /z/, /ʃ/, /ʒ/, /Θ/, /ð/.

frontal view   An X-ray view that allows the examiner to visualize the lateral pharyngeal walls at rest and during speech; the orientation of this view is as if one is looking straight through the nose; also called the *anterior–posterior view* or simply the *AP view*.

fundamental frequency   The lowest frequency of a periodic waveform.

gamete   A sex cell, either an ovum or a sperm cell.

gastrostomy tube (G-tube) feeding   A method of parenteral feeding through the use of a tube that is placed directly into the stomach through an opening that is surgically created.

gene   (adj. genetic) A functional unit of heredity that is submicroscopic, resides at a specific location or locus on a chromosome, and is capable of reproducing itself with each cell division; consists of a sequence of nucleotide bases in a molecule of deoxyribonucleic acid (DNA).

genetics   The science of patterns of heredity.

genioplasty   Horizontal mandibular osteotomy for chin advancement.

genome   Consists of chromosomes and DNA and contains a complete set of instructions for cell replication and differentiation for an organism; see *Human Genome Project*.

genotype   The genetic constitution of an individual.

gingivoperiosteoplasty   A procedure to close the cleft of the alveolus with raised gingival flaps and the underlying periosteum on each edge of the cleft; raw surfaces are advanced and sewn together to allow the bone progenitor cells to lay down bone as the patient grows.

glossopexy   A surgical procedure that involves suturing the tongue tip to the bottom lip to help to keep the airway open in patients with glossoptosis.

glossoptosis   The posterior displacement of the tongue in the pharynx; can cause airway obstruction.

glossus   Related to the tongue.

glottal fricative   A speech sound, /h/, produced by the friction of the airstream as it passes through the glottal opening.

glottal plosive   See *glottal stop*.

glottal stop   A compensatory articulation production characterized by forceful adduction of the vocal folds and the buildup and release of air pressure under the glottis, resulting in a grunt-type sound.

glottis   Space between the vocal cords.

greater segment   Palatal segment on the noncleft side.

hair cells   Sensory cells, as in the organ of hearing, that have hair-like properties.

hard palate   A bony structure that serves as the roof of the mouth and floor of the nasal cavity and separates the oral cavity from the nasal cavity.

harmonics   Component frequencies of a signal that are whole number multiples of the fundamental frequency.

hemangioma   A congenital anomaly in which a proliferation of blood vessels results in a large mass.

hemifacial microsomia   Lack of development of the bones on one side of the face; results in various degrees of both unilateral mandibular hypoplasia and facial weakness.

hemihypertrophy   Where one side of the body grows faster, and therefore is larger, than the other side.

hepatoblastoma   A malignant liver tumor; a risk for individuals with Beckwith-Wiedemann syndrome.

heterogeneity   The mutation of different genes leading to the same phenotype.

heterogeneous   A characteristic where more than one gene can cause the same clinical features.

heterozygous   Having two different copies or alleles of a gene at the same locus on a pair of homologous chromosomes.

holoprosencephaly   Failure of the forebrain to divide into the two hemispheres; often accompanied by a midline deficit in facial development or a midfacial cleft.

homozygotes   Persons with two identical copies of a gene.

homozygous   When genes have two similar alleles.

horizontal plates   Paired plates of the palatine bones located just behind the transverse palatine suture line; forms the posterior portion of the hard palate, ending with the protrusive posterior nasal spine.

Human Genome Project   An international initiative whereby researchers from all over the world are collaborating to compile a comprehensive map of the human genome.

hypernasality   A resonance disorder that occurs when there is abnormal nasal resonance during the production of oral sounds caused by abnormal coupling of the oral and nasal cavities during speech; the perceptual quality of speech is often described as just "nasal," muffled, or characterized by mumbling; it is particularly perceptible on vowels.

hyperplasia   (adj. hyperplastic) Overdevelopment of a structure; an increase in the number of cells in a tissue or organ, not related to tumor formation, whereby that body part is larger than normal.

hypertelorism   Excessive distance between two paired organs, such as the eyes.

hypertrophy   (adj. hypertrophic) Abnormal enlargement of a part of the body due to enlargement of its constituent cells.

hypoglycemia   Low blood sugar.

hyponasality   A type of abnormal resonance that occurs when there is a reduction in nasal resonance during speech due to blockage in the nasopharynx or in the entrance to the nasal cavity; particularly affects the production of the nasal consonants (/m/, /n/, and /ŋ/).

hypopharynx   Part of the pharynx, or throat, that is below the oral cavity and extends from the epiglottis inferiorly to the esophagus.

hypoplasia   (adj. hypoplastic) Underdevelopment or defective formation of a tissue (i.e., bone, muscles, and nerves) or organ, usually due to a decrease in the normal number of cells.

hypospadias   Where the orifice of the penis is proximal to its normal location.

hypotelorism   Narrow-spaced eyes.

hypotonia   (adj. hypotonic) A state of low muscle tonicity and sometimes reduced muscle strength; caused by different diseases and disorders of the brain that affect the motor nerve control or muscle strength.

ideogram   A schematic drawing of the banding pattern of a chromosome.

idiopathic   A condition that appears without apparent cause or etiology.

iliac crest   The superior border of the wing of ilium of the greater pelvis.

imprinting   When some genes function differently, depending on whether they were inherited maternally or paternally.

inaudible nasal emission   Nasal emission due to a relatively large opening; is inaudible because there is very little resistance to the flow and hypernasality masks the sound.

incidence   In epidemiological terms, refers to the number of new cases of a disease or disorder in a given population, such as the number of persons becoming ill with a certain disease.

incisive foramen   A hole in the bone that is located in the alveolar ridge area of the maxillary arch, just behind the central incisors, and forms the tip of the premaxilla.

incisive papilla   The slight elevation of the mucosa at the anterior end of the raphe of the palate.

incisive suture lines   Embryological suture lines in the hard palate that go between the lateral incisors and canines and meet posteriorly at the area of the incisive foramen; the suture lines that separate the premaxilla.

incisors   Teeth that are somewhat shovel shaped; their biting surfaces are thin knifelike edges.

incomplete penetrance   The lack of a recognizable phenotype in an individual who carries a mutation that may cause an autosomal dominant trait or condition.

incus (anvil)   One of the ossicles in the middle ear; articulates with the malleus and the stapes.

indirect instrumental procedures   Provide object data regarding the results of velopharyngeal function, such as airflow, air pressure, or acoustic output, but do not allow visualization of the structures; include the use of aerodynamic instrumentation or the nasometer.

infant oral orthopedics   See *palatal orthopedics*.

inner ear   Part of the ear that consists of the cochlea and semicircular canals.

intelligence   Relates to the ability to learn; a prerequisite for normal language development.

intentional fistula   A nasolabial fistula that is deliberately left in the alveolus (under the lip) at the time of the primary palatoplasty to allow unrestricted facial growth; it is closed with a bone graft at a later time.

interdisciplinary team   A group of professionals from various disciplines who work together to coordinate the care of a patient through collaboration, interaction, communication, and cooperation.

intermaxillary fixation   Wiring the mandible against the maxilla to keep it closed and in place; often done for a period of time after orthognathic surgery.

intermaxillary palatine suture line   See *median palatine suture line*.

interosseous dental implants   Implants that are embedded in the bone so that a speech appliance or denture can be attached and retained.

interphase   The time between cell divisions.

intonation   Refers to the frequent changes in pitch throughout an utterance, as controlled by subtle changes in vocal fold length and mass and pharyngeal cavity size; variation of pitch is used for emphasis, to express feelings, ask a question, and for many other functions.

intraoral air pressure   A buildup of air pressure in the oral cavity that provides the force for the production of oral consonants, particularly plosives, fricatives and affricates.

intravelar veloplasty (IWP)   A surgical reconstruction of the levator veli palatini sling during palatoplasty for correction of a cleft of the velum.

introns   Segments of noncoding DNA that are between the exons, which are the coding portion of all genes.

inversions   When a portion of a chromosome is turned 180 degrees from its usual orientation; may not be associated with any abnormalities in the individual because the total amount of genetic material may be unchanged.

karotype   A gross chromosome analysis that is done by drawing blood, growing the cells in a culture, analyzing the white blood cells, photographing the chromosomes, and then arranging the chromosomes in pairs for display and assessment; a visual profile of an individual's chromosomes

keloid   Excessive scar tissue formed during healing.

labial   (adj.) Relating to the lip; the outer part of the dental arch that touches the lip.

labial tubercle   The prominent projection on the inferior border, or free edge, of the midsection of the upper lip.

labiodental phonemes   Speech sounds that are produced with the bottom lip against the maxillary incisors (i.e., /f/, /v/).

labioversion   When the upper incisors are displaced anteriorly, with overjet greater than 2 mm, causing the maxillary incisors to protrude out toward the lips.

labyrinthitis   Inflammation of the labyrinth, which is sometimes accompanied by vertigo and deafness.

laminar airflow   Airflow that is steady and smooth due to the lack of significant surrounding resistance.

laminography   Use of a radiograph to measure distances and angles between particular landmarks.

language   Refers to the meaning or message that's conveyed back and forth during communication.

laryngeal web   A congenital anomaly that consists of a band of tissue between the vocal folds, usually in the anterior portion of the larynx, that can cause respiratory stridor.

laryngomalacia   Abnormally soft cartilage in the epiglottis and aryepiglottic folds at birth, resulting in loud inspiratory stridor that is particularly pronounced when the infant cries or breathes deeply.

lateral cephalometric X-rays   Still radiographs of the head taken in the sagittal plane.

lateral pharyngeal walls   The side walls of the throat.

lateral view   An X-ray view that shows the velum and posterior pharyngeal wall in a midsagittal plane; the orientation of the lateral view is as if we were able to look through the side of the head to view these structures from the side.

Latham appliance   A two-piece acrylic dental appliance that is used prior to the lip and alveolus repair to close the gap between the greater and lesser maxillary segments from a wide cleft of the primary palate.

Le Fort I osteotomy   A surgical cut in the bone that transversely separates the maxilla just above the base of the nose so that the maxilla and palate can be moved as a single unit.

Le Fort II osteotomy   A surgical cut in the bone that includes both the nasal pyramid and the alveolar arch.

Le Fort III osteotomy   A surgical cut in the bone that includes cheek bones, orbital rims, nasal pyramid, and alveolar arch.

lesser segment   Palatal segment on the cleft side.

levator sling   The levator veli palatini muscles from each side interdigitate and blend together to form a muscle sling.

levator veli palatini   Paired muscle that forms the main muscle mass of the velum, primarily responsible for velar elevation.

lingual   Related to the tongue; also the inner part of the upper and lower dental arch that is in contact with the tongue.

lingual-alveolar phonemes   Speech sounds that are produced with the tongue tip (i.e., /t/, /d/, /n/, /l/).

lingual frenulum   (pl. frenula) A narrow fold of mucous membrane that extends from the floor of the mouth to the midline of the under surface of the tongue; see *frenum* and *frenulum*.

lingual tonsils   A mass of lymphoid tissue located at the base of the tongue and extending to the epiglottis.

lingual tonsil hypertrophy   Abnormal enlargement of the lingual tonsil at the base of the tongue.

linguoversion   When the upper teeth are inside the lower teeth; also known as *anterior crossbite* or *underjet*.

lip adhesion   A simple, straight-line surgical procedure to temporarily repair a cleft lip; this procedure is performed so that subsequent lip pressure draws the segments together, making the final repair more successful.

lip pits   Depressions in the bottom lip that are usually bilateral and are associated with Van der Woude syndrome with cleft palate.

lipodermoids   Fatty tissue.

lobulated tongue   The tongue appears to have multiple lobes, with fissures between each lobe.

lower esophageal sphincter (LES)   Sphincter at the base of the esophagus that relaxes to allow a bolus to enter the stomach.

macro   Large.

macroglossia   Large tongue.

macrostomia   A large mouth opening, often due to failure of fusion between the maxillary and mandibular process of embryonic development of the face.

magnetic resonance imaging (MRI)   A noninvasive method to produce a very clear and detailed view of internal body structures, using a magnetic field and radio waves.

mala   (adj. malar) Relating to the cheek or cheekbone (zygomatic bone).

malar hypoplasia   Lack of cheekbone development.

malformation   Defect in basic embryological plan due to chromosomal or genetic factors.

malleus (hammer)   One of the ossicles in the middle ear; is firmly attached to the tympanic membrane and articulates with the incus.

malocclusion   Abnormal dental or skeletal relationship of the maxillary and mandibular teeth so that the arches do not close together normally during biting.

mandibular hypoplasia   Lack of mandibular development, causing a small, retrusive mandible; see *micrognathia* and *retrognathia*.

manometer   A device that usually consists of a liquid column to measure pressures.

mastoid cavity   A section of the temporal bone that is porous and located just behind the ear.

mastoiditis   Inflammation or infection in any part of the mastoid process.

maxillary hypoplasia   Lack of development of the maxilla, causing midface retrusion or deficiency and concavity of the midface.

maxillary retrusion   Characterized by a small upper jaw (maxilla) relative to the lower jaw (mandible); a common anomaly, especially in individuals with repaired cleft lip and palate secondary to the inherent deficiency in the maxilla due to the cleft and the possible restriction in maxillary growth with the surgical repair; also known as *midface deficiency*.

mean nasalance score   See *nasalance score*.

meatus   An opening, channel or passageway; usually the external opening of a canal; see *nasal meatus*.

meiosis   A special process of cell division that results in gametes (spermatocytes or oocytes) with 23 chromosomes rather than the 46 that are found in somatic cells.

mesial   (adj.) The direction toward the midline, following the curvature of the dental arch.

messenger RNA (mRNA)   Ribunucleic acid (RNA) that has had the introns removed and is transported from the nucleus to the cytoplasm to function as a template for protein synthesis.

metacentric   Chromosomes with a centrally located centromere.

metopic   Related to the forehead or anterior portion of the cranium.

micro   Small.

microcephaly   Small head circumference in comparison to age-matched peers.

microdontia   A condition where some or all of the teeth are unusually small.

microform cleft   See *form fruste*.

microglossia   Small tongue.

micrognathia   A small or hypoplastic mandible; see *mandibular hypoplasia*.

micropenis   Small penis.

microphthalmia   Small eyes.

microstomia   A small mouth opening.

microtia   Hypoplasia or absence of the external ear (pinna or auricle); often accompanied by aural atresia (a blind or absent external auditory meatus).

middle ear   A hollow space within the temporal bone.

middle ear effusion   Collection of fluids within the middle ear space due to the Eustachian tube dysfunction.

middorsum palatal stop   See *palatal-dorsal production*.

midface deficiency   See *maxillary retrusion*.

midface retrusion   Concavity of the midface due to maxillary hypoplasia.

mitosis   The process of separating duplicated chromosomes; the reconstitution of two cell nuclei.

mixed dentition   Presence of both primary and secondary teeth.

mixed resonance   A combination of hypernasality, hyponasality, or cul-de-sac resonance during connected speech.

modified barium swallow (MBS)   See *videofluoroscopic swallowing study (VSS)*.

Moebius syndrome   Involves specific cranial nerve damage with weakness affecting the oral and facial musculature.

molars   Teeth that are designed for grinding; on each side of the maxillary and mandibular arch, there are the first molars (6-year molars), the second molars (12-year molars), and the third molars (wisdom teeth); upper molars have four cusps, two buccal and two palatal (or lingual) cusps, and lower molars have five cusps, three buccal and two lingual cusps.

mongoloid slant   Upward slant of the eyes.

monosomy   Absence of an entire chromosome of a pair of homologous chromosomes.

morphogenesis   The process of embryonic tissue formation.

mosaicism   An anomaly of chromosome division resulting in the presence of cells with two or more different genetic makeups, or a different number of chromosomes, in a single individual.

motor learning   The acquisition of new motor skills in order to be able to execute complex motor movements and motor sequences; is necessary for the individual to perform all complicated motor movements and sequences without conscious thought; the key component of motor learning is feedback.

motor memory   What develops the automaticity of the newly learned motor movement and makes the new learning relatively permanent, although it can degrade with lack of use; the key component of motor learning is practice.

mucoid effusion   A thick, mucus-like fluid in the middle ear.

mucoperiosteum   Tissue that covers the hard palate, consisting of a mucous membrane and periosteum.

mucosa   See *mucous membrane*.

mucous membrane   (adj. mucosal) The lining tissue of the nasal cavity, oral cavity, and pharynx; consists of stratified squamous epithelium and lamina propria; also known as *mucosa*.

mucus   A clear, viscid secretion of the mucous membranes.

multidisciplinary team   A group of professionals from various disciplines who work independently in evaluating and treating patients with complex medical needs; members of this type of team have well-defined roles and cooperate with each other, but there is little communication and interaction among the team members.

multifactorial inheritance   A characteristic in the phenotype that is the result of a combination of many genes at different loci and/or factors from the environment; the combination of genes and other factors all have a small added effect to form the characteristic in the phenotype.

musculus uvulae   A paired muscle that creates a bulge on the posterior nasal surface of the velum during phonation; during contraction, this bulge provides additional bulk and stiffness to the nasal side of the velum and helps to fill in the area between the velum and posterior pharyngeal wall, contributing to a firm velopharyngeal seal.

mutation   A change in the sequence of base pairs in the DNA molecule that is reflected in subsequent divisions of the cell; a change in the chemistry of the gene that is reflected in the subsequent genotype and phenotype; can be as small as a substitution of a single base pair or as large as the deletion of an entire chromosome.

myopia   Nearsightedness.

myringotomy   A surgical puncture of the tympanic membrane so that fluid can be drained or suctioned out of the middle ear.

naris   (pl. nares) Nostril.

nasal airway resistance   Attenuation of the nasal airflow due to any condition that obstructs or restricts the patency of the nasopharynx or nasal cavity.

nasal bridge   The bony structure that is located between the eyes and corresponds to the middle of the nasofrontal suture; also known as *nasion*.

nasal concha   (pl. nasal conchae) A structure that is comparable to a shell in shape, such as the auricle or pinna of the ear or the turbinated bone within the nose; see *turbinates*.

nasal cul-de-sac resonance   Resonance disorder that occurs when sound is partially blocked from exiting the nasal cavity during speech; most noticeable when there is a combination of VPI (which would otherwise cause hypernasality) and also a blockage in the anterior part of the nose.

nasal emission   An inappropriate flow of the airstream through the nose during speech, causing distortion of the speech; usually caused by velopharyngeal dysfunction; also called *nasal escape*.

nasal grimace   A muscle contraction during speech that is typically noted either above the nasal bridge (in the area between the eyes) or around the nares; occurs as an overflow muscle reaction when there is an attempt to achieve velopharyngeal closure; usually accompanied by nasal emission.

nasal meatus   Any of the three passages in the nasal cavity that lie directly under a nasal concha; see *meatus*.

nasal molding   A method of repositioning the nasal septum and ala in the infant prior to cleft lip repair; usually involves an intraoral/nasal appliance combined with taping.

nasal regurgitation   Reflux of fluids into the nasopharynx and nasal cavity during drinking or vomiting.

nasal root   Where the nose begins at the level of the eyes.

nasal rustle   A fricative sound that occurs as air is forced through a small velopharyngeal opening; air stream is released on the nasal side with pressure, resulting in bubbling of nasal secretions; also called *nasal turbulence*.

nasal septum   A wall separating the nasal cavity into two halves; consists of the vomer bone, the perpendicular plate of the ethmoid, and the quadrangular cartilage and is covered with mucous membrane; see *septum*.

nasal sill   The base of the nostril opening.

nasal sniff   An uncommon compensatory articulation production that is produced by a forcible inspiration through the nose; usually substituted for sibilant sounds, particularly the /s/, and typically occurs in the final word position.

nasal snort   A burst of nasal emission that is produced by a forcible emission of air pressure through the nares during consonant production, resulting in a noisy, sneeze-like sound.

nasal turbinates   Bony structures in the nose that are covered with mucosa; the superior and middle turbinates are parts of the ethmoid bone and the inferior turbinate, which is the largest, is its own unique bone; see *nasal concha*.

nasal turbulence   See *nasal rustle*.

nasal twang   Exaggerated nasality as noted in some dialects.

nasal valve   The smallest cross-sectional area or area of constriction in the nasal cavity; typically located approximately 1 cm posterior to the entrance of the nose.

nasal vestibule   The most anterior part of the nasal cavity; it is enclosed by the cartilages of the nose.

nasalance distance   The range between the maximum and minimum nasalance.

nasalance ratio   The minimum nasalance divided by the maximum nasalance.

nasalance score   Represents the relative amount of nasal acoustic energy in the person's speech as determined by the Nasometer; the ratio of nasal acoustic energy over total (oral plus nasal) acoustic energy during speech as determined through the use of the Nasometer; the score represents the mean of the percentage points that are calculated for an entire speech passage; also called *mean nasalance score*.

nasalization of oral consonants   An obligatory distortion due to an open velopharyngeal valve; as a result, oral consonants sound more like their nasal cognates (e.g., m/b, n/d, and ŋ).

nasendoscopy   See *nasopharyngoscopy*.

nasion   See *nasal bridge*.

nasogastric (ng) tube   A tube placed through the nose and down to the stomach and used for feeding.

nasogastric (ng) tube feeding   A method of feeding through the use of a tube that is placed in the nose and goes down to the stomach.

nasogram   A contour display on a computer screen that represents the nasalance results of the spoken passage on the Nasometer.

nasolabial fistula   A fistula in the alveolus (under the lip) that is often deliberately left by the surgeon during the initial repair to allow for maxillary growth. It is later closed by a bone graft; often called an *intentional fistula*.

Nasometer   A computer-based instrument (KayPENTAX, Montvale, N.J.) that measures the relative amount of nasal acoustic energy in a patient's speech.

nasopharyngeal airway tube   A tube that used to improve the airway of infants, such as those with Pierre Robin sequence; the tube is placed in the nose of the infant in such a way that one end sticks out of the nose and the other end extends to below the region of tongue obstruction.

nasopharyngoscope   A type of endoscope that is used for examination of the pharynx, larynx, and velopharyngeal mechanism.

nasopharyngoscopy   A minimally invasive endoscopic procedure that allows visual observation and analysis of the velopharyngeal mechanism or larynx during speech, phonation or swallowing; commonly used in the evaluation of swallowing, upper airway obstruction, and the structure and function of the larynx and vocal cords; also called *nasendoscopy* or *video nasendoscopy*.

nasopharynx   The part of the pharynx, or throat, that lies above the soft palate and just behind the nasal cavity.

necrosis   Abnormal death of cellular tissue due to toxins, infection or trauma.

neurofibromas   Large nerve sheath tumors.

nondisjunction   The failure of one or more chromosomes to separate in cell division.

nonpneumatic activities   As they relate to the velopharyngeal valve: swallowing, gagging, and vomiting.

nosocomial infections   Infections that are acquired while in the hospital.

nucleotides   Building blocks of DNA that consist of a 5-carbon sugar chemically bonded to a phosphate group and a nitrogenous base.

nucleus   A part of a cell that contains genetic material that serves as instructions for cell and tissue functions; it is separated from the rest of the cell by a lipid membrane with specialized proteins.

obligatory distortion   When the articulation placement (the function) of speech is normal, but an abnormality of the structure (i.e., dental malocclusion, velopharyngeal insufficiency, or an oronasal fistula) causes distortion of speech; includes hypernasality, nasal emission, weak consonants, and short utterance length; also known as an *obligatory error* or *passive speech characteristic*.

obligatory error   See *obligatory distortion*.

oblique view   X-ray view that allows the examiner to see the lateral pharyngeal walls and velum during connected speech; used primarily if the base view cannot be obtained due to enlarged adenoids or the inability to hyperextend the neck.

obstructive sleep apnea (OSA)   A period during sleep when the individual is exerting muscular forces to inspire but is unsuccessful in moving air into the lungs due to a blockage in the pharynx; often caused by enlarged tonsils, enlarged adenoids, or pharyngeal hypotonia during sleep.

obturator   A generic term to describe a device that can be used to cover a hole; see *palatal obturator*.

occlusal cant   A sloping, transverse occlusal plane caused by impaired vertical maxillary growth on one side, which is compensated by vertical alveolar growth in the mandible on the same side; common in patients with unilateral cleft lip/palate and those with hemifacial microsomia.

occlusion   The way the maxillary and mandibular teeth fit together when the jaws are closed, as when biting.

occult submucous cleft   A defect in the velum that is under the mucous membrane and not visible on the oral surface; this defect can usually be viewed on the nasal surface of the velum through nasopharyngoscopy.

ocular   Related to the eyes.

oligogenic model   A variation of the multifactorial model of inheritance, where a trait may be determined by the interaction of multiple genes with little environmental influence; a small number of genes may contribute most of the risk.

omphalocele   Where part of the intestines may be outside of the abdomen in the region of the umbilical cord.

oocyte   A female gametocyte involved in reproduction; also an immature ovum, or egg cell.

orifice equation   The formula to calculate the minimal cross-sectional area of the velopharyngeal valve by measuring the differential pressure across the orifice and rate of airflow simultaneously.

ostium   An opening that connects a paranasal sinus to the nose for mucus drainage.

ovum   (pl. ova) Egg cell, a female reproductive cell or gamete.

open bite   Occurs when one or more maxillary teeth fail to occlude with the opposing mandibular teeth; primarily affects the anterior dentition (anterior open bite) and less commonly the posterior dentition (lateral open bite).

ophtha   Related to the eyes.

optic   Related to the eyes.

oral cul-de-sac resonance   Resonance disorder that occurs when sound is partially blocked from exiting the oral cavity during speech; can occur due to microstomia; sounds like mumbling or speaking without opening the mouth normally.

oral frenulae   Oral tissue webs.

oral manometer   An instrument that was used in the past to provide a gross measurement of airflow abilities during blowing or negative pressure during sucking; the patient was required to blow into a catheter or suck the catheter; this is no longer considered valid because information is now available about the physiological differences between blowing or sucking activities and speech.

oral resonance   The result of the sound energy vibrating (resonating) in the oral cavity during speech.

orbicularis oris   The muscle that encircles the mouth and serves to close the lips.

organ of Corti   The part of the inner ear where the mechanical energy introduced into the cochlea is converted into electrical stimulation.

organelles   Internal structures in a cell that perform specific functions such as metabolizing energy, building complex molecules such as proteins, and breaking down waste products).

orifice equation   A formula to calculate the cross-sectional area of the velopharyngeal valve by measuring the differential pressure across the orifice and rate of airflow simultaneously.

orogastric tube feeding   A method of feeding through the use of a tube that is placed in the mouth and goes down to the stomach.

oronasal fistula   See *palatal fistula*.

oropharyngeal isthmus   The opening from the oral cavity to the pharynx; bordered superiorly by the velum, laterally by the faucial pillars, and inferiorly by the base of the tongue.

oropharynx   The part of the pharynx, or throat, that lies below the soft palate at the level of the oral cavity or just posterior to the mouth.

orthodontist   The professional who is responsible for aligning misplaced teeth and correcting discrepancy in jaw size to improve the dental and facial aesthetics and the function of the dentition.

orthognathia   (adj. orthognathic) The study of the causes and the treatment of conditions related to malposition of the bones of the jaw.

orthognathic surgery   Surgery that involves the bones of the upper jaw (the maxilla) and the lower jaw (the mandible).

Orticochea sphincteroplasty   See *sphincter pharyngoplasty*.

osseointegrated implants   Implants that are inserted in the bone; used for retention of bridges and prosthetic devices.

osseointegration   Direct connection between an implant and the bone.

ossicles   (adj. ossicular) Three small bones in the middle ear, the malleus, incus, and stapes, that conduct sound energy from the tympanic membrane to the cochlea.

osteotomy   Surgical cut in a bone so that the bone can be placed in a more functional and appropriate position.

ostium   (pl. ostia) Small opening between a paranasal sinus and the nasal cavity.

otic   Relating to the ear (otitis, otolaryngologist, otorrhea, microtia, etc.).

otitis media   A bacterial infection and inflammation of the middle ear.

otitis media with effusion   An inflammation of the middle ear that is accompanied by a buildup of fluids.

otolaryngologist   The physician who is responsible for monitoring middle ear function and treating middle ear disease, assessing and treating anomalies and disease of the oral cavity, pharynx, nasal cavity, and upper airway and lower airway; also known as the *ear, nose, and throat specialist (ENT)*.

otorrhea   A type of ear disease with discharge.

otoscope   An instrument used to visualize the tympanic membrane.

overbite   The vertical overlap of the upper and lower incisors; can be measured in millimeters but is often reported as a percentage of coverage of the lower incisors by the upper incisors; normal overbite is approximately 2 mm, or about 25%; greater amounts are called either deep overbite or *deep bite*.

overjet   The horizontal relationship between the upper and lower incisors; typically measured in millimeters from the labial surface of the lower incisor to the labial surface of the upper incisor with the teeth in occlusion; a normal amount of overjet is about 2 mm with upper incisors and lower incisors in light contact; excessive overjet is where the maxillary incisors are labioverted or stick out toward the lips.

overlay dentures   Dentures that fit over the existing teeth and usually provide more vertical dimension.

overt submucous cleft   A submucous cleft that can be identified on the nasal surface of the velum based on features such as a zona pellucida (thin zone), bifid or hypoplastic uvula, or apparent diastasis of the levator muscle, which is particularly apparent during phonation.

palatal   (adj.) The inner part of the upper and lower arch that is in proximity to the surface of the hard palate.

palatal-dorsal production   An abnormal articulation production that is often compensatory for anterior oral cavity crowding; produced as a stop consonant that is articulated with the middle of the dorsum against the middle of the hard palate; is usually substituted for the lingual-alveolar sounds (/t/ and /d/), for the velar sounds (/k/ and /g/), and in some cases, for sibilant sounds (/s/, /z/, /ʃ/, /ʒ/, /ʧ/, /ʤ/); also called a *middorsum palatal stop*.

palatal fistula   A hole or opening in the palate that goes all the way through to the nasal cavity; usually the result of failure of the palate to heal after a palatoplasty; also called *oronasal fistula*.

palatal lift   A prosthetic appliance that can be used to raise the velum for speech in cases where the velum is long enough to achieve velopharyngeal closure but does not move well, often due to neurological impairment.

palatal obturator   A prosthetic appliance that can be used to cover an open palatal defect, such as an unrepaired cleft palate or a palatal fistula; this device can be used to improve an infant's ability to achieve compression of the nipple for suction or can be used to close a palatal defect for speech.

palatal orthopedics   A method used to align the alveolar segments in both unilateral and bilateral clefts of the palate prior to surgical correction; also known as *infant oral orthopedics*.

palatal section (of a prosthesis)   The body portion of a prosthetic appliance that fits over the palate.

palatal vault   The rounded dome on the upper part of the oral cavity.

palate   The bony and muscular partition between the oral and nasal cavities.

palatine aponeurosis   A sheet of fibrous tissue located just below the nasal surface of the velum and extending about 1 cm posteriorly from its attachment on the posterior border of the hard palate; consists of periosteum, fibrous connective tissue, and fibers from the tensor veli palatini tendon; provides an anchoring point for the velopharyngeal muscles and adds stiffness to that portion of the velum; also called *velar aponeurosis*.

palatine processes   Paired bones of the maxilla that are just behind the incisive suture lines and form the anterior three quarters of the maxilla.

palatine raphe   The thin white line that can often be seen running longitudinally down the middle of the velum. This is an embryological suture line for the velum.

palatine suture line   Embryological suture line that begins at the incisive foramen and ends at the posterior nasal spine; separates the paired palatine processes of the maxilla and the horizontal plates of the palatine bones; also known as *intermaxillary palatine suture line*.

palatine tonsils   Masses of lymphoid tissue between the anterior and posterior faucial pillars on both sides of the oral cavity; also called simply the *tonsils*.

palatine torus   See *torus palatinus*.

palatoglossus   Paired muscles that act antagonistically to the levator veli palatini to depress the velum or elevate the tongue; these muscles contribute to lowering the velum for the production of nasal speech sounds.

palatomaxillary suture line   See *transverse palatine suture line*.

palatopharyngeus   Paired muscle of the pharynx; the horizontal fibers are thought to be associated with the sphincteric action of the velopharyngeal valve, assisting with velopharyngeal closure by pulling the lateral pharyngeal walls medially to narrow the pharynx.

palatoplasty   Palate repair.

palpebra   (pl. palpebrae, adj. palpebral) Eyelid.

palpebral fissures   Opening between the eyelids.

panendoscope   An older illuminated instrument that included an optical tube that is placed in the mouth and turned upward for visualization of the velopharyngeal sphincter; no longer used.

paranasal sinuses   Four pair of air-filled spaces, including the frontal sinuses (in the forehead area), maxillary sinuses (under the cheeks), ethmoid sinuses (between the eyes), and sphenoid sinuses (deep in the skull).

parathyroid glands   Glands responsible for making parathyroid hormone, which helps regulate calcium levels in the blood.

paresis   (adj. paretic) Weakness of muscle movement; partial or incomplete paralysis or loss of movement.

paring   Skin that is "pared," or sliced off, as in the excess tissue that is trimmed from each side of the prolabium during the initial lip repair.

partial trisomy   Duplication of a piece of a chromosome, rather than the entire chromosome, so that there is a part of a chromosome with the pair.

Passavant's ridge   A shelf-like ridge that projects from the posterior pharyngeal wall into the pharynx during speech; occurs as a result of contraction of specific fibers of the superior pharyngeal constrictor muscles; found in normal speakers and speakers with velopharyngeal dysfunction.

passive speech characteristic   See *obligatory distortion*.

pedigree   Pictorial representation of family members and their line of descent; used by geneticist to analyze inheritance, particularly for certain traits or anomalies.

pedodontist   A term sometimes used for a pediatric dentist.

penetrance   The frequency of the expression of a genotype in a phenotype; if the trait does not appear 100% of the time when the gene is present, then it is said to have reduced penetrance.

periosteum   A thick, fibrous membrane that covers the surface of bone.

peripheral sleep apnea   See *obstructive sleep apnea.*

perpendicular plate of the ethmoid   The bone that projects down to join the vomer and lies between the vomer and the quadrangular cartilage; forms part of the nasal septum.

pharyngeal affricate   A compensatory articulation production that is produced when the tongue is retracted so that the base of the tongue articulates against the pharyngeal wall; is the combination of either a pharyngeal plosive or a glottal stop and a pharyngeal fricative.

pharyngeal cul-de-sac resonance   A resonance disorder that occurs when most of the sound remains in the oropharynx during speech; typically caused by large tonsils that block the exit of the oropharynx and thus the entrance to the oral cavity.

pharyngeal flap   A type of pharyngoplasty designed to be a passive soft tissue obturator of the middle of the velopharyngeal sphincter, to improve or correct velopharyngeal function.

pharyngeal fricative   A compensatory articulation production that is produced when the tongue is retracted so that the base of the tongue approximates, but does not touch, the pharyngeal wall; a friction sound occurs as the air pressure is forced through the narrow opening that is created between the base of the tongue and pharyngeal wall.

pharyngeal plexus   A network of nerves that lies along the posterior wall of the pharynx and consists of the pharyngeal branches of the glossopharyngeal and vagus nerves, which provide motor innervation for the velar muscles that contribute to velopharyngeal closure.

pharyngeal plosive   A compensatory articulation production that is produced with the back of the tongue articulating against the pharyngeal wall; also called *pharyngeal stop.*

pharyngeal stop   See *pharyngeal plosive.*

pharyngeal tonsil   See *adenoid.*

pharyngeal wall augmentation   An implant that is surgically placed or injected in the posterior pharyngeal wall, or a rolled flap on the pharyngeal wall; placed in the area of the velopharyngeal opening to correct velopharyngeal dysfunction.

pharyngoplasty   A surgical procedure of the pharynx that is designed to correct velopharyngeal dysfunction.

pharynx   (adj. pharyngeal) The walls of the throat between the esophagus and nasal cavity.

phenotype   The manifestations of a genotype; range of characteristics associated with a genetic syndrome.

philtral ridges   The raised lines on either side of the philtrum, which are embryological suture lines that are formed as the segments of the upper lip fuse.

philtrum   (adj. philtral) A long dimple or indentation that courses from the columella down to the upper lip and is bordered by the philtral ridges on each side.

phonation   The sound generated by the vocal folds as they vibrate.

phoneme-specific nasal emission (PSNE)   Occurs with the individual has learned to produce pressure-sensitive consonants in the pharynx instead of the oral cavity, despite normal velopharyngeal anatomy and physiology due to mislearning; the airflow is released through the velopharyngeal valve as nasal emission that only occurs on those misarticulated phonemes; usually occurs on sibilant sounds, particularly s/z.

Pierre Robin sequence   A congenital condition that consists of micrognathia, glossoptosis, and cleft palate; there is often upper airway obstruction for several months after birth.

pinna   The delicate cartilaginous framework of the external ear; functions to direct sound energy into the external auditory canal; also known as the *auricle* or *concha*.

piriform (AKA pyriform) aperture   Literally means "pear-shaped opening"; the opening to the nostril or nasal cavity.

pitot tube   A device used to determine airflow velocity.

plagiocephaly   Asymmetric or abnormal skull shape.

pleiotropy   The phenomenon where a single gene can affect multiple unrelated systems.

plosive phonemes   Pressure-sensitive consonants that require a buildup of intraoral pressure prior to a sudden release; include /p/, /b/, /t/, /d/, /k/, /g/.

pneumotachograph   A device that determines the rate of airflow through the use of a flowmeter and a differential pressure transducer; one of the components of aerodynamic instrumentation to measure velopharyngeal orifice area or nasal resistance.

pneumatic activities   As they relate to the velopharyngeal valve: blowing, whistling, sucking, and speech.

polycythemia   An increase in the normal number of red blood cells.

polydactyly   Extra fingers and/or toes.

polymers   Large molecules (macromolecules) composed of repeating structural units.

polymorphism   Variability in genes that contributes to the uniqueness of individuals.

polysomnography   A diagnostic test during which a number of physiologic variables are recorded during an overnight sleep study.

posterior crossbite   Involves any combination of teeth distal (posterior) to the canines where the maxillary teeth are inside the mandibular teeth; usually occurs because the maxilla is too narrow.

posterior nasal fricative   An abnormal articulation production that is produced with the velum somewhat down so that air pressure goes through a velopharyngeal opening, creating a friction sound with audible nasal emission; typically used as a substitution for sibilant sounds, particularly s/z; associated with phoneme-specific nasal emission (PSNE).

posterior nasal spine   A protrusive projection in the middle of the posterior border of the hard palate.

posterior pharyngeal wall   Back wall of the throat.

preauricular tags   Projection of scalp and skin tags from the area of the ear to the cheek.

premaxilla   A triangular-shaped bone that is bordered on either side by the incisive suture lines; this bony segment normally contains the central and lateral maxillary incisors.

premolars   Teeth that typically have two cusps, although they may sometimes have three.

pressure equalizing (PE) tubes   See *ventilation tubes*.

pressure-flow technique   Procedure using aerodynamic instrumentation to evaluate the dynamics of the velopharyngeal mechanism during speech; also used to evaluate nasal respiration and to quantify upper airway obstruction through measurements of nasal airway resistance.

pressure-sensitive phonemes   Speech sounds that require oral air pressure for production; include plosives, fricatives, and affricates.

prevalence   In epidemiological terms, refers to a measure of existing cases of a disorder in a given population.

primary dentition   Stage of dental development where there are 10 teeth in the upper arch, 10 teeth in the lower arch, and usually spacing between all of the primary teeth.

primary palate   The lip and palate anterior to the incisive foramen; includes the lip and alveolus.

prognathia   (adj. prognathic) Protrusive mandible caused by mandibular hyperplasia.

prognathism   A condition where the mandible is bigger than the maxilla.

prolabium   The tissue that normally makes up the central portion of the upper lip between the philtral columns but is isolated when there is a bilateral cleft lip.

proptosis   (adj. proptotic) Protrusion of the eyeball.

prosody   Refers to the stress, intonation, and rhythm of speech.

prosthesis   (adj. prosthetic) A fabricated substitute for a body part that is missing or malformed; also called a *prosthetic device*.

prosthodontist   A dental professional who deals with the restoration of teeth and the development of appliances to replace or improve the appearance of oral and facial structures or to assist with feeding and velopharyngeal closure.

provisionally unique syndromes   Patterns of multiple anomalies in what appears to be an underlying syndrome, although a diagnosis cannot be made because the pattern is not one that has been previously described or reported.

psychologist   The professional who assesses a patient's psychosocial needs and assists the patient and family in dealing with the medical, social, and emotional challenges that occur due to the patient's anomalies.

pterygoid process   A part of the sphenoid bone that contains the medial pterygoid plate, the lateral pterygoid plate, and the pterygoid hamulus, all of which provide attachments for muscles in the velopharyngeal complex.

purines   Nitrogenous bases of nucleotides in a DNA molecule that consists of adenine and guanine.

ptosis   Drooping of the eyelids.

purulent effusion   The fluid in the middle ear that is like pus.

pyrimidines   Nitrogenous bases of nucleotides in a DNA molecule that consist of thymine and cytosine.

quad helix   A palatal expansion device that consists of bands on the most posterior molars, and frequently the primary canines, which are connected by a palatal spring that has two posterior and two anterior loops.

quadrangular cartilage   The cartilage that forms the anterior nasal septum and projects anteriorly to the columella.

radiography   The use of the roentgen rays (X-rays) to image internal body parts.

ramus   The upturned, perpendicular extremity of the mandible on both sides.

raphe   (pronounced *rafay*) A line of union between two bilaterally symmetric structures; the palatine raphe is the midline of the mucosa of the hard palate that runs from the incisive papilla posteriorly over the entire length of the hard palate.

rapid palatal expander   A palatal expansion device that consists of two or four molar bands and a jackscrew connecting them in the middle of the palate; turning the screw creates the necessary force to widen the dental arches.

receptive language   The understanding of a message that is sent.

recessive inheritance   A trait that is expressed only in individuals who are homozygous for the gene involved in that they have inherited the same gene for the trait from both parents (e.g., blue eyes); when the same allele is needed from both parents for expression of a trait.

reduction therapy   A form of speech therapy where a prosthetic device is used to stimulate the movement of the velopharyngeal structures to avoid the need for surgery or reduce the extent of the surgery needed.

replication   The process of making two identical DNA molecules from one, resulting in two double strands, each containing one original and one complementary newly synthesized strand of DNA.

resection   Surgical removal of an organ or piece of a body part.

resonance   (as it relates to voiced speech) The modification of the sound that is generated by the vocal cords through selective enhancement of certain frequencies; this is determined by the size and shape of the cavities of the vocal tract (pharynx, oral cavity, and nasal cavity) and the function of the velopharyngeal valve

retrognathia   (adj. retrognathic) When one or both jaws is located posterior to its normal position; usually used in reference to a retrusive mandible; associated with micrognathia (mandibular hypoplasia).

reverse pull headgear   A device used to advance the maxilla and improve an anterior crossbite.

ribonucleic acid (RNA)   A linear polymer composed of a 5-carbon sugar, similar to DNA; serves to transport genetic information from the nucleus to the cytoplasm of the cell.

ribosomes   Organelles within the cell that function in protein synthesis.

right sided aortic arch   Abnormality where the aortic arch is on the right side rather than the left.

rhinomanometry   Procedure for measuring nasal airway resistance; involves measurement of the pressure encountered by air passing through the nasal cavity.

rhythm   With respect to speech, it refers to the alteration of stressed and unstressed syllables and the relative timing of each.

rolled flap   A flap of tissue is surgically raised from the posterior pharyngeal wall and is rolled up on to itself to form a bulge on the posterior pharyngeal wall; used to fill in a velopharyngeal gap.

rotameter   A device to measure airflow rate; used for the calibration of the pneumotachograph.

rugae   Folds, ridges, or creases in a structure; the transverse ridges in the mucosal covering of the hard palate.

rule of 10s   A guideline for the appropriate time for a cleft lip repair, which says that the infant must be at least 10 weeks of age, 10 pounds, and have a hemoglobin of 10 gm prior to the lip repair.

saccule   A sensory organ within the inner ear that provides a sensation of acceleration.

sagittal pattern   The least common pattern of velopharyngeal closure; the lateral pharyngeal walls move medially to meet in midline to effect closure; the velum may move to close against the lateral pharyngeal walls rather than against the posterior pharyngeal wall.

sagittal plane   The median, longitudinal plane of the body; a plane of view for X-ray procedures.

salpingopharyngeal folds   Folds that originate from the torus tubarius at the opening to the Eustachian tube on both sides of the pharynx and then course downward to the lateral pharyngeal wall; consist of glandular and connective tissue.

salpingopharyngeus   Paired muscle that arises from the inferior border of the torus tubarius and courses vertically along the lateral pharyngeal wall and under the salpingopharyngeal fold; is not felt to have a significant role in achieving velopharyngeal closure given its size and location.

scaphocephaly   Skull that is oblong from front to back; caused by premature closure of the sagittal suture.

sclera   (pl. sclerae) White portion of the eyeball.

secondary palate   Structures that are posterior to the incisive foramen, including the hard palate (excluding the premaxilla) and the velum.

semicircular canals   The loop-shaped tubular parts of the inner ear that provide a sense of spatial orientation; the loops are oriented in three planes at right angles to each other.

sensitivity   The extent to which a test is able to correctly identify positive results; proportion of true positive results as intended to be revealed by a test.

sensorineural hearing loss   A type of hearing loss due to a problem with the creation of nerve impulses within the inner ear or the transmission of the nerve impulses through the brainstem to the auditory cortex.

septum   A thin wall separating two cavities; see *nasal septum*.

sequence   The occurrence of a pattern of multiple anomalies within an individual that arise from a single known or presumed prior anomaly or mechanical factor; where one anomaly leads to the development of the other anomalies, as in Pierre Robin sequence.

serous effusion   Fluid in the middle ear that consists of a very thin, watery liquid.

sex chromosomes   The 23rd pair of chromosomes (X and Y) that function in determining gender.

short utterance length   A leak of airflow through the nose reduces the oral airflow available for connected speech, so more frequent breaths are required for replacement of the airflow; causes utterance length to be shortened

sialorrhea   Drooling.

sibilant phonemes   Speech sounds that are produced by the friction of air pressure as it is emitted anteriorly through the incisors (i.e., /s/, /z/, ʃ/, /ʒ/, /tʃ/, /dʒ/)

Simonart's band   A strand of soft tissue in the area of the cleft lip that is due to partial, yet incomplete, embryonic fusion of the upper lip.

single-tooth crossbite   A crossbite that involves only one upper and one lower tooth.

sinuses   See *paranasal sinuses*.

sleep apnea   Cessation of respiration during sleep due to upper respiratory obstruction or central (neurogenic) causes, or to a combination of both.

soft palate   See *velum*.

somatic cells   All cells in the body with the exception of those for reproduction; body cells as opposed to gamete or sex cells.

sometimes-but-not-always (SBNA)   A term for an individual who demonstrates inconsistent velopharyngeal closure; the individual may be able to achieve total closure with effort but has difficulty maintaining closure consistently and over a prolonged period of time.

somia   Refers to body.

specificity   The extent to which a test correctly identifies true negative results; the proportion of individuals with negative test results for what the test is intended to reveal.

speech aid appliance   See *speech bulb obturator.*

speech bulb obturator   A prosthetic device that can be considered when the velum is too short to close completely against the posterior pharyngeal wall; this device consists of a retaining appliance and a bulb (usually of acrylic) that fills in the pharyngeal space for speech; also known as a *speech aid appliance.*

sphenoid bone   An unpaired bone located at the base of the skull.

sphincter pharyngoplasty   A type of pharyngoplasty to create a dynamic sphincter that encircles the velopharyngeal port; also known as the *Orticochea sphincteroplasty.*

Standard Precautions   Recommended procedures, published by the Centers for Disease Control and Prevention, that are designed to protect the patient, the professional, and all others in a health care environment from the spread of infection.

stapes   One of the ossicles in the middle ear; acts as a piston to create pressure waves within the fluid-filled cochlea.

stenosis   An abnormal narrowing or stricture of a canal (e.g., choanal stenosis, pharyngeal stenosis, or subglottic stenosis).

stertorous   A heavy snoring sound in respiration.

stimulability   The ability to correct an abnormal speech sound production when given minimal cues.

stoma   The surgical opening into the trachea through which the patient can breathe following a tracheostomy.

stomia   Refers to the mouth.

stress   Related to increased muscular effort and subglottic pressure during the production of a syllable; stressed syllables are produced with greater articulatory precision, are longer in duration, and are higher in pitch and intensity than unstressed syllables.

submetacentric   When the centromere of a chromosome is closer to one end than the other.

submucous cleft palate   A congenital defect that affects the underlying structures of the palate, whereas the structures on the oral surface are intact; can involve the muscles of the velum and also those of the bony structure of the hard palate.

suborbital coloring   Darkness under the eyes usually due to lack of sleep; often called "black eyes."

succedaneous teeth   Secondary or permanent teeth.

suckling   An early form of sucking characterized by extension–retraction movements of the tongue.

superior constrictor   Paired muscle of the pharynx; the upper fibers are responsible for the medial displacement of the lateral pharyngeal walls to effectively narrow the velopharyngeal port; also called *superior pharyngeal constrictor.*

superior pharyngeal constrictor   See *superior constrictor.*

supernumerary tooth   An extra tooth; usually erupts in the line of the cleft.

syndactyly   Fusion or webbing of the digits (fingers and/or toes).

syndrome   A pattern of multiple anomalies or malformations that regularly occur together, are pathogenically related, and therefore have a common known or suspected cause; craniofacial syndromes (involving the head and face) cause affected individuals to look alike, even when there is no family relationship (e.g., Down syndrome).

synostosis   Abnormal fusion or premature fusion of the two or more normally separated bones; see *craniosynostosis*.

tailpiece   (of a prosthetic device) The part of a palatal lift or speech bulb appliance that extends posteriorly to either raise the velum or close the nasopharynx behind the velum.

telecanthus   Increased distance between the medial canthi of the eyelids.

temporal bones   Located at the sides and base of the skull.

temporomandibular joint   The joint of the mandible and temporal bone.

tensor veli palatini   Paired muscles that are believed to be responsible for opening the Eustachian tubes to enhance middle ear aeration and drainage.

teratogen   An external chemical or physical agent, such as cigarette smoke, drugs, viruses, or radiation, that can interfere with normal embryological development and result in congenital malformations.

tetralogy of Fallot   Most common congenital heart defect; includes ventricular septal deviation (VSD), dextroposition (right-sided) aortic arch, right ventricular hypertrophy, and pulmonary stenosis; often associated with a syndrome.

thymus   The organ in the chest which is the source of T-lymphocytes.

TONAR   Developed by Fletcher in 1970, this was the first instrument to measure nasal and oral acoustic energy during speech; predecessor to the Nasometer.

tongue-tie   See *ankyloglossia*.

tonsillar hypertrophy   Excessive enlargement of the faucial tonsils.

tonsillectomy   Surgical procedure to remove the tonsils; done to resolve recurrent infection or to eliminate oral cavity obstruction.

tonsils   Lymphoid tissue that is located on either side of the mouth between the anterior and posterior faucial pillars; also referred to as *faucial tonsils*.

torus palatinus   A normal variation, not an abnormality, that consists of a prominent longitudinal ridge, or exostosis, on the oral surface of the hard palate in the area of the median palatine suture line; found most often in Caucasians, particularly those of northern European descent, and reportedly common in the northern Native American and Eskimo populations.

torus tubarius   A ridge in the nasopharyngeal wall, posterior to the opening of the Eustachian tube, caused by the projection of the cartilaginous portion of this tube.

Towne's view   A radiographic view that is sometimes used as an alternative to the base view because it also provides an en face orientation; it allows the examiner to look down into the port.

tracheoesophageal (TE) fistula   Congenital opening between the trachea and the esophagus; causes aspiration during feeding.

tracheostomy   A surgical procedure that involves placement of a tube directly in the trachea; done to relieve upper airway obstruction, which can be life threatening.

transcription   The process of creating a strand of RNA that is complementary to a given strand of DNA.

transdisciplinary team   An interdisciplinary team where members understand the other disciplines and how they relate to the total care of the patient; this understanding of the various disciplines allows them to be able to see the "big picture" in the care of the patient.

transducers   As part of aerodynamic instrumentation, used to convert the detected air pressure or flow into electrical signals for further processing.

translocations   The result of a transfer of genetic material between two or more chromosomes; may not be associated with any abnormalities in the individual because the total amount of genetic material may be unchanged.

transverse palatine suture line   An embryological suture line that separates the paired palatine processes of the maxilla, which form the anterior three-quarters of the maxilla, and the paired horizontal plates of the palatine bones; also known as the *palatomaxillary suture line*.

treating team   Team members who provide a consultation regarding the total care of the patient and also offer treatment.

trigonocephaly   The top of the skull is triangular-shaped with a pointed forehead.

trisomy   A condition where there is an extra chromosome in an homologous pair of chromosomes; for example, trisomy 21 or Down syndrome in humans is a condition where the cell contains 47 rather than 46 chromosomes.

tubercle (of the lip)   The somewhat prominent point at the inferior border of the midsection of the upper lip.

turbinates   See *nasal turbinates*.

turbulent airflow   Airflow that is chaotic due to surrounding obstacles, irregularities, and convolutions.

tympanic membrane   Thin tissue that separates the outer ear from the middle ear; transmits sound energy through the ossicles to the inner ear; also called the *eardrum*.

underbite   The abnormal vertical overlap of the lower incisors over the upper incisors.

underjet   A reversal of the normal incisor position, with the maxillary incisors linguoverted or facing inward toward the tongue; also called *linguoversion* or *anterior crossbite*.

Universal Blood and Body Fluid Precautions (UBBFP)   Guidelines for infection control that were developed by the Centers for Disease Control and Prevention (CDC) in Atlanta.

upper esophageal sphincter (UES)   The upper end of the esophagus that normally is closed but stretches open as the bolus travels through the hypopharynx and into the esophagus.

utricle   A sensory organ within the inner ear that provide a sensation of acceleration.

uvula   A teardrop-shaped structure that is typically long and slender and hangs freely from the back or free edge of the velum; it has no known function.

uvulopalatopharyngoplasty (UPPP)   A surgical procedure for the treatment of the obstructive sleep apnea in adults; involves the excision of the remaining tonsil and resection of the free margin of the soft palate and uvula; the anterior and posterior tonsillar pillars are sewn together to open the oropharyngeal inlet.

Van der Woude syndrome   Includes cleft palate and bilateral lip pits, which are small depressions in the bottom lip; has a 50% recurrence risk for future pregnancies.

variable expressivity   Variability in the clinical presentation (phenotype) of patients with a particular genetic disorder; a gene can result in variations in the phenotype from a very pronounced effect in one individual to a barely noticeable effect in another.

velar affricate   Compensatory production that is produced by a combination of a velar plosive and a velar fricative; see *velar fricative*.

velar aponeurosis   See *palatine aponeurosis*.

velar dimple   The area on the oral side of the velum where it bends during phonation or velopharyngeal closure as a result of the action of the levator veli palatini muscle; can be noted through an intraoral examination.

velar eminence   A bulge on the nasal surface of the velum during phonation, which comes from the musculus uvulae muscles; can be seen through nasopharyngoscopy.

velar fricative   A compensatory articulation production that is produced with the back of the tongue in the same position as for the production of a /j/ (as in "**y**ellow") sound so that a small space is created between the back of the tongue and the velum; a fricative sound is produced as air is forced through that small opening.

velar phonemes   Speech sounds that are produced with the back of the tongue against the velum, including /k/, /g/, and /ŋ/.

velar plosives   Speech sounds that are produced with the back of the tongue against the velum; air pressure is built up behind the tongue and then released suddenly, including /k/ and /g/.

velar stretch   The process where the velum elongates as it elevates to achieve velopharyngeal closure.

veloadenoidal closure   The velum commonly closes against the adenoid during speech in children who have a prominent adenoid pad.

velopharyngeal dysfunction (VPD)   One of the generic terms that is used to describe abnormal velopharyngeal function, regardless of the cause.

velopharyngeal inadequacy (VPI)   One of the generic terms that is used to describe abnormal velopharyngeal function, regardless of the cause.

velopharyngeal incompetence (VPI)   A neuromotor or physiological disorder that results in poor movement of the velopharyngeal structures.

velopharyngeal insufficiency (VPI)   An anatomical or structural defect that precludes adequate velopharyngeal closure by causing the velum to be short relative to the posterior pharyngeal wall.

velopharyngeal mislearning   Inadequate velopharyngeal closure due to faulty learning of appropriate articulation patterns.

velum   The part of the palate that is located in the back of the mouth and consists of muscles that are covered by the same mucous membrane as the hard palate; frequently referred to as the *soft palate*.

ventilation tubes   Small tubes that are surgically inserted in the eardrum to provide an alternate route for air to enter the middle ear for ventilation if the Eustachian tube is nonfunctional; also called *pressure equalizing (PE) tubes*.

ventricular septal defect (VSD)   Congenital discontinuity of the tissue that separates the lower chambers of the heart.

ventricular septum   The tissue that separates the two lower chambers of the heart.

ventral   See *ventrum*.

ventrum   (adj. ventral) The underneath surface of the tongue.

verbal apraxia   See *apraxia (of speech)*.

verbal language   Meaning or message that is conveyed through speech.

vermilion   The red pigmented portion of the upper and lower lips.

video nasendoscopy   See *nasopharyngoscopy*.

videofluoroscopy   An imaging technique used to obtain real-time moving images of internal structures; done through the use of a fluoroscope, which consists of an X-ray source and fluorescent screen; can be used for evaluation of velopharyngeal function or swallowing.

videofluoroscopic speech study   An evaluation of the velopharyngeal mechanism and other oral and pharyngeal structures during speech, using videofluoroscopy.

videofluoroscopic swallowing study   A radiographic procedure that allows an overall view of the oral, pharyngeal, and esophageal phases of swallowing as well as the interactions between the phases; also referred to as a *modified barium swallow (MBS)*.

vocal nodules   Small callus-like masses that typically occur symmetrically on both vocal cords and are due to chronic abuse, misuse, or overuse of the cords.

vomer   A flat bone of trapezoidal shape that is positioned so that it is perpendicular to the palate; the inferior border meets the nasal surface of the maxilla in midline and forms the inferior and posterior portion of the nasal septum.

Waldeyer's ring   A complex of lymphoid tissue, including the adenoids, tonsils, and lingual tonsil, which encircles the pharynx and plays a role in the immune system.

W-arch   A variation of the quad helix palatal expansion device.

weak or omitted consonants   When air is leaked through the velopharyngeal valve, it reduces the amount of airflow that is available in the oral cavity for the production of consonants; causes the consonants to be weak in intensity and pressure or to be omitted.

well-type manometer   Similar to a U-tube water manometer but provides for the direct reading of applied pressures; has a calibrated reservoir filled with water or oil and is used for the calibration of pressure transducers.

white roll   The white border tissue that surrounds the red tissue, or vermilion, of the upper and lower lips.

Wilms tumor   A malignant tumor of the kidney; a risk for individuals with Beckwith-Wiedemann syndrome; a liver tumor called hepatoblastoma X-linked inheritance, an inherited trait from genes located on the X chromosome; the trait is usually more pronounced or is lethal in males because males have only one X chromosome as opposed to females, who have two X chromosomes.

X-linked inheritance   A condition caused by mutations in genes on the X chromosome.

zona pellucida   A bluish area in the middle of the velum that is the result of abnormal insertion of the levator veli palatini muscles, effectively causing the velum to be thin and almost transparent in appearance.

Z-plasty   A plastic surgery technique that is used to lengthen tissue.

zygoma   The bone of the skull that forms the prominence of the cheek and articulates with the frontal, sphenoid, temporal, and maxillary bones. It is also known as the *zygomatic bone* or *malar bone*.

INDEX

Note: Page numbers followed by "f" and "t" indicate figures and tables respectively.